CARE
OF
THE
HIGH-RISK
NEONATE

By

MARSHALL H. KLAUS, M.D.

Professor of Pediatrics,
Case Western Reserve University School of Medicine, and
Director of the Neonatal Nurseries, University Hospitals,
Cleveland, Ohio

And

AVROY A. FANAROFF, M.B. (RAND.), M.R.C.P.E.

Assistant Professor of Pediatrics,
Case Western Reserve University School of Medicine,
Co-Director of the Neonatal Nurseries, University Hospitals,
and Associate Director,
Rainbow Babies' and Children's Hospital,
Cleveland, Ohio

With Critical Comments By

GERARD B. ODELL, M.D.

SAMUEL PROD'HOM, M.D.

LEO STERN, M.D.

W. B. SAUNDERS   *Philadelphia • London • Toronto*

W. B. Saunders Company: West Washington Square
Philadelphia, PA 19105

1 St. Anne's Road
Eastbourne, East Sussex BN21 3UN, England

1 Goldthorne Avenue
Toronto, Ontario M8Z 5T9, Canada

Listed here is the latest translated edition of this book together
with the language of the translation and the publisher.

Spanish (1st Edition) — Editorial Medica Panamericana,
                Buenos Aires, Argentina

Care of the High-Risk Neonate   ISBN 0-7216-5476-2.

Print No.:   18   17   16   15   14   13   12   11   10

This book is dedicated
To our wives, who our efforts tolerated,
Our many teachers, who stimulated,
And the house officers, nurses, and patients, from whom we benefited
While the book was created.

To LOIS, SUSAN, DAVID, ALISA, LAURA, and
SARAH KLAUS; ROSLYN, JONATHAN, and
JODI FANAROFF.

CONTRIBUTORS

RICHARD E. BEHRMAN, M.D.
Professor and Chairman, Department of Pediatrics, College of Physicians and Surgeons, Columbia University, New York, New York

DAVID E. FISHER, M.D.
Assistant Professor of Pediatrics, Abraham Lincoln School of Medicine, University of Illinois, Chicago, Illinois; Director of Neonatology, University of Illinois Hospital, Chicago, Illinois

SAMUEL GROSS, M.A., M.D.
Associate Professor of Pediatrics, Case Western Reserve University School of Medicine, Cleveland, Ohio; Pediatrician, Rainbow Babies' and Children's Hospital, University Hospitals, Cleveland, Ohio

WARREN E. GRUPE, M.D.
Associate Professor of Pediatrics, Case Western Reserve University School of Medicine, Cleveland, Ohio; Director, Pediatric Nephrology, Rainbow Babies' and Children's Hospital, Cleveland, Ohio

SAMUEL J. HORWITZ, M.D.
Assistant Professor of Pediatrics, Case Western Reserve University School of Medicine, Cleveland, Ohio; Associate Clinical Professor of Neurology, Case Western Reserve University School of Medicine, Cleveland, Ohio

JOHN H. KENNELL, M.D.
Professor of Pediatrics, Case Western Reserve University School of Medicine, Cleveland, Ohio

JEROME LIEBMAN, M.D.
Professor of Pediatrics, Case Western Reserve University School of Medicine, Cleveland, Ohio; University Hospitals, Cleveland, Ohio

ANN LLEWELLYN, M.D., M.R.C.P.
Clinical Teacher, Hospital for Sick Children, Toronto, Ontario

DAVID K. MELHORN, M.D.
Assistant Professor of Pediatrics, Case Western Reserve University School of Medicine, Cleveland, Ohio; Pediatrician, Rainbow Babies' and Children's Hospital, University Hospitals, Cleveland, Ohio

GERARD B. ODELL, M.D.
Professor of Pediatrics, Johns Hopkins University School of Medicine, Baltimore, Maryland; Department of Pediatrics, Johns Hopkins Hospital, Baltimore, Maryland

ENRIQUE M. OSTREA, JR., M.D.
Assistant Professor of Pediatrics, Wayne State University, Detroit, Michigan; Department of Pediatrics, Hutzel Hospital, Detroit, Michigan

RONALD L. POLAND, M.D.
Assistant Professor of Pediatrics, Wayne State University, Detroit, Michigan; Department of Pediatrics, Children's Hospital of Michigan, Detroit, Michigan

E. O. R. REYNOLDS, M.D., M.R.C.P.
Consultant Pediatrician, University College Hospital, London, England; Honorary Senior Lecturer in Pediatrics, University College Hospital Medical School, London, England

ARNOLD J. RUDOLPH, M.B.
Professor of Pediatrics and Head of Newborn Section, Baylor College of Medicine, Houston, Texas; Chief of Neonatology, Texas Children's Hospital, Houston, Texas; Director of Nurseries, Jefferson Davis Hospital, Houston, Texas

AVRON Y. SWEET, M.D.
Professor of Pediatrics, Case Western Reserve University School of Medicine, Cleveland, Ohio; Director, Newborn Service, Cleveland Metropolitan General Hospital, Cleveland, Ohio

PAUL SWYER, M.B., M.R.C.P.
Teaching Associate Professor and Director of Neonatal Division, Hospital For Sick Children, Toronto, Ontario

MICHAEL K. WALD, M.D.
Assistant Clinical Professor, Case Western Reserve University School of Medicine, Cleveland, Ohio; Assistant Pediatrician, University Hospitals, Cleveland, Ohio; Attending Pediatrician, Cleveland Metropolitan General Hospital, Cleveland, Ohio

VICTOR WHITMAN, M.D.
Assistant Professor of Pediatrics, Case Western Reserve University School of Medicine, Cleveland, Ohio; University Hospitals, Cleveland, Ohio

FOREWORD

The physiological approach to neonatal care described in this teaching manual is, surprisingly, a very recent development. Care of sick and at-risk newborn infants remained essentially empiric long after advances in scientific medicine had been applied to similar problems in older patients. The curious delay in the development of neonatal and more recently fetal medicine cannot be explained entirely by the very real technical difficulties in making biochemical and physiological observations in very small subjects. Something more intangible stood in the way. There was a generally held fatalistic attitude which had to be overcome before wholehearted exploration could be undertaken, and it was necessary to shift from standardized management according to birth size (a farm-like approach) to focussed attention on the specific problems of each baby. Fatalism was shaken by therapeutic triumphs (especially exchange transfusion), and the importance of an individualized approach was underlined by awesome tragedies caused by routine policies (especially oxygen therapy for premature infants).

A sizable body of evidence has been assembled in the past 10 to 15 years, and perinatal medicine has now acquired a fairly respectable scientific base. Specific treatment of fetus and newborn is now pursued actively; yet, an undercurrent of skepticism continues to haunt the entire enterprise. Has the outlook for intact survival improved? Unfortunately, a firm answer for the skeptics is hard to come by. Analysis of results of new treatments is always difficult without formal trials, and in this field the problem is compounded. There is no practical way to shorten the very long interval between treatment and evaluation of outcome in survivors, and there is no satisfactory way to control the effects of intervening influences. Despite these caveats, favorable reports of long-term outcome of treatments (especially intrauterine transfusion, neonatal resuscitation, and ventilatory support in the respiratory distress syndrome) have been published, and the consistency of these experiences is beginning to lend support to expanded development of perinatal programs.

The immediate problems in sick newborn infants may obscure the fact that the association between poor socioeconomic status and high perinatal risk often overrides all other considerations in determining eventual outcome. Comprehensive measures to improve general health, education, and social circumstances of the disadvantaged must be included in the present concept of perinatal medicine. Students and house officers who are analyzing the complicated derangements of the fetus and newborn cannot afford to ignore the whole patient and his real-life environment.

WILLIAM SILVERMAN

PREFACE

AND HINTS ON HOW TO USE THE BOOK

The principles for the modern care of the newborn were first established in Paris in the 1890s, when Pierre Budin, a French obstetrician, built the first modern nursery for small infants. He laid the foundations for neonatology, as he recognized the relation between incubator temperature and mortality, the importance of controlling infectious disease, and the necessity of keeping the mother of a premature infant near her baby.

The specialty of neonatology was born, flourished briefly, and then lay dormant for many years while physicians devoted their attention to diarrhea and infectious disease. Rigid codes and laws then delayed the adoption in the nursery of many rapid advances occurring in pediatrics.

During the past 15 years, however, neonatology has flowered. This development has been stimulated by many advances in bench biochemistry, by the basic observations of animal and human physiologists in Europe, the United Kingdom, and North America, and by numerous worldwide clinical studies of the normal and sick neonate.

House officers, medical students, nurses, and practicing pediatricians first exposed to the busy neonatal nursery setting must rapidly acquire a whole new set of standards by which to judge the course of their patients. This book was conceived as part of an effort to facilitate this process of adaptation at our hospital. Preliminary versions of some of the chapters have been found helpful in improving our staff's ability to care for high-risk infants, and at the same time many constructive comments have assisted us and been incorporated into this larger volume.

Learning is a personal venture, and we have for this reason deviated from the style of the traditional textbook to employ several techniques which must be appreciated before using this book. The major innovation is the use of questions and case material in each chapter. This was originally suggested by Dr. T. Hale Ham of the Division of Research in Medical Education, Case Western Reserve University. Some readers may be disconcerted by the introduction of material in the questions which has not been mentioned in the text, but this is a device we believe worthy of trial. Reading the text, therefore, will not be complete without going through the questions and cases. It should be emphasized that the questions are not meant to test the reader's comprehension and memory but to illustrate how the information presented in the chapter can be used in patient care, bearing in mind that each individual patient demands a somewhat different body of knowledge and understanding. It is hoped, in other words, that the case problems will act as a kind of "simulator" or "trainer" in preparation for actual patient care.

Neonatology is a rapidly expanding field, and we do not attempt to present comprehensive coverage. Rather, we describe the major principles which must be understood when caring for the sick neonate. Those requiring more specialized information on many syndromes and diseases are referred to such standard texts as Barnett's *Pediatrics,* Cooke's *The Biologic Basis of Pediatric Practice,* the Nelson-Vaughan-McKay *Textbook of Pediatrics,* Schaffer and Avery's *Diseases of the Newborn,* and Warkany's *Congenital Malformations.*

In contrast to other chapters of this book, the authors of the chapters on cardiology and hematology have used case problems as an integral part of the text, as they believe this to be a superior method of education. We have not changed this in any major way, in the hope that the reader might evaluate this for himself.

The sections headed "Unknowns" attempt to show the state of development and knowledge of particular areas of neonatology, and hopefully may stimulate research.

We have purposely attempted to demonstrate that many areas are controversial by asking Doctors Leo Stern, Gerard Odell, and Samuel Prod'hom to comment wherever they found areas of disagreement. Only with time and study will anyone be able to make a final decision in these and other areas.

We are interested in your thoughts and ideas. We hope you will make comments on the enclosed questionnaire and send it to the Division of Research in Medical Education, School of Medicine, Case Western Reserve University.

MARSHALL H. KLAUS
AVROY A. FANAROFF

ACKNOWLEDGMENTS

The field of newborn care has been enriched by investigators from a wide variety of fields whose work has been incorporated into the discipline now known as neonatology. The pioneering work in this country was that of Clement Smith and William Silverman and their many illustrious students.

Fortunately, the authors' past educational experiences have been different, allowing us to present a possibly more comprehensive approach. One of us (M. H. K.) was originally taught and stimulated in pediatrics by Sam Spector, the late Bill Wallace, and Fred Robbins; and in continued interest in the newborn by Kenneth Cross, Julius Comroe, and many exciting years with John Clements.

A. A. F., who trained in South Africa, would like to gratefully acknowledge the guidance, stimulation, encouragement, and training in internal medicine and pediatrics received from many teachers and "chiefs," especially Doctors M. M. Suzman, Seymour Heymann, Sam Javett, Solomon E. Levin, Jacques Theron, Elliot Chesler, and Hessel Utian. Professors H. de V. Heese and Sam Wayburne were especially instrumental, in addition, in nurturing further interest in the problems and welfare of the newly born.

As expected, our thoughts have been influenced by our associates. One of us (M. H. K.) has had the good fortune to work with Bill Tooley, Kurt Weisser, Karl Weaver, Carolyn Piel, Avron Sweet, Phil Sunshine, Irwin Schaeffer, Vernon Thomas, Clifford Barnett, Herb Liederman, Rose Grobstein, and John Kennell; thanks also to Norman Kretchmer, who contributed another view of the newborn. A. A. F. is grateful for the years of association with Arthur Rubenstein, Irving Lissoos, M. Jeffrey Maisels, Mike Plit, Alan Gottlieb, and Rodwin Jackson.

We are also grateful for the continual stimulation of past and present trainees and fellows, with special mention to Belton Meyer, Joseph Dailey, Josephine Chu, Howard Gruber, Roberto Sosa, Chul Cha, and John Kattwinkel. We owe many of our ideas and inspirations to these people.

Special thanks should be given to our Department Chairman, Dr. Leroy Matthews, who has been most thoughtful about arranging time to prepare this work. M. H. K. is especially grateful to Emil Gautier and Samuel Prod'hom for the space given in their unit to work on this book.

We must acknowledge our special gratitude to Dr. T. Hale Ham, who over the past four years has been continually prodding and innovative in his ideas about the book. The Division of Research in Medical Education, which he heads, has been generous in helping to prepare this book. Within that department, Marcia Wile and Treville Leger, supported by the Carnegie Foundation and the National Medical Library, spent countless hours compiling and evaluating the experimental pre-publication of this book. We are also grateful for the long hours and assistance of the medical students, nurses, interns, residents, and practitioners who reviewed the pre-publication effort, shared their insights, and searched out inaccuracies.

We are, of course, especially thankful to Drs. Gerard Odell, Samuel

Prod'hom, and Leo Stern, who gave extra time and energy not only to review the book but also to provide their own critical comments on many of the subjects within the text. These comments have, in most cases, been incorporated into the text itself, so that the reader might appreciate the multiple approaches to the care of the sick neonate. We must also thank Dr. Tom Teree, who reviewed and commented on the book only to see his efforts swept away in the floods which followed Hurricane Agnes.

We would like to pay special tribute to our research associate, Robin White, without whose assistance this book would not have been possible. She has been of inestimable value as an in-house editor, typist, proofreader, and liaison officer. We would also like to acknowledge the expert secretarial assistance and devotion of Beverly Himmelfarb and Ruby Eyke; and the medical illustrations of Betsy Parke.

The authors are grateful to our many colleagues for their contributions or permission to use published and unpublished data. Any error is solely our responsibility.

Our research and the time available to write this book were supported by the generous aid of the Educational Foundation of America and the Grant Foundation, with additional assistance from a grant from the Maternal and Child Health Division of the State of Ohio, and NIH Grant LM00673.

We also thank the W. B. Saunders Company for their patience and continual assistance in producing this book.

M. H. K.
A. A. F.

QUESTIONNAIRE

Please return to:
The Division of Research in Medical Education
Case Western Reserve University, School of Medicine
2119 Abington Road
Cleveland, Ohio 44106

We cordially invite your comments concerning *Care of the High-Risk Neonate* and your suggestions for its next edition. Your response will be part of a post-publication evaluation, supported in part by NIH Grant LM00673 from the National Library of Medicine. The following questions are intended to be evocative rather than exhaustive; your own personal commentary is of primary importance. Please provide us with your comments and return the questionnaire to the above address.

I. What are the strongest features of this book?_____

_____

_____

II. What parts of this book should be revised, and in what way?_____

_____

_____

III. What topics should be added?_____

_____

IV. What topics should be deleted?_____

_____

V. Did you find the case problems useful? Please comment:_____

_____

_____

VI. Did you find the question and answer sections useful? Please comment:_____

_____

_____

Personal Commentary:

QUESTIONNAIRE

Your name (optional)_____Affiliation_____

Please check if you are a faculty member_____

Profession:

PHYSICIAN	**NURSE**	**STUDENT**
____General Practitioner	____Pediatric	____Medical
____House Officer	____Obstetric	____Nursing
____Specialist (specify)	____Other (specify)	____Other (specify)

CONTENTS

CHAPTER 1
RESUSCITATION OF THE NEWBORN INFANT 1
David Fisher and Richard E. Behrman

CHAPTER 2
ANTICIPATION, RECOGNITION, AND TRANSITIONAL CARE OF THE
HIGH-RISK INFANT 23
Arnold J. Rudolph

CHAPTER 3
CLASSIFICATION OF THE LOW-BIRTH-WEIGHT INFANT 36
Avron Y. Sweet

CHAPTER 4
THE PHYSICAL ENVIRONMENT 58
Marshall Klaus and Avroy Fanaroff

CHAPTER 5
FEEDING THE LOW-BIRTH-WEIGHT INFANT 77
Avroy Fanaroff and Marshall Klaus

CHAPTER 6
TRANSPORTATION OF THE HIGH-RISK INFANT 90
Avroy Fanaroff and Marshall Klaus

CHAPTER 7
CARE OF THE MOTHER 98
Marshall Klaus and John Kennell

CHAPTER 8
RESPIRATORY PROBLEMS 119
Marshall Klaus and Avroy Fanaroff

CHAPTER 9
ASSISTED VENTILATION 152
Ann Llewellyn and Paul Swyer

CHAPTER 10
PROBLEMS IN CHEMICAL ADAPTATION 168
Michael K. Wald

CHAPTER 11
NEONATAL HYPERBILIRUBINEMIA 183
Gerard B. Odell, Ronald L. Poland, and Enrique M. Ostrea, Jr.

CHAPTER 12
NEONATAL INFECTIONS 205
Avroy Fanaroff and Marshall Klaus

CHAPTER 13
THE HEART 228
Jerome Liebman and Victor Whitman

CHAPTER 14
THE KIDNEY 256
Warren E. Grupe

CHAPTER 15
HEMATOLOGIC PROBLEMS 270
Samuel Gross and David K. Melhorn

CHAPTER 16
NEUROLOGIC PROBLEMS 287
Samuel J. Horwitz

APPENDICES 301

INDEX 351

CASE PROBLEMS

CHAPTER 1

Case One.   An Asphyxiated Small-for-Dates Infant 17
Case Two.   A Neonatal Emergency in an Infant of a Diabetic Mother 19

CHAPTER 2

Case One.   Transitional Care for Full-Term Infant.................................... 33
Case Two.   Treatment of Infant of Drug-Addicted Mother.................................... 34

CHAPTER 3

Case One.   A Small-for-Dates Infant: Clinical Problems 53
Case Two.   A Small-for-Dates Infant: Respiratory Distress.................................... 54
Case Three.   An Infant of a Diabetic Mother: Clinical Problems.................................... 54

CHAPTER 4

Case One.   An Immature Infant: Early Problems of Temperature Control 73
Case Two.   An Immature Infant: Temperature Control in the First Week of Life 74
Case Three.   A Postmature Infant: Problems of Temperature Control.. 75

CHAPTER 5

Case One.   Hyperalimentation in a Small-for-Dates Infant Following Surgery 86
Case Two.   Feeding a 1200-gm. Immature Infant: The First Four Days................................. 87
Case Three.   Feeding a 1740-gm. Small-for-Dates Infant: The First Week of Life........................ 88
Case Four.   Intravenous Feeding in a Full-Term Neonate Following Surgery............................ 88

CHAPTER 7

Case One.   Discussion with the Parents of an Immature Infant with Respiratory Distress 110
Case Two.   Management of the Parents of an Infant with a Major Malformation 112
Case Three.   A Prenatal Discussion with a Primigravida Diabetic Mother 113
Case Four.   Management of a Mother of a Small Premature.................................... 115
Case Five.   Care of the Family Following the Death of a Neonate 117

CHAPTER 8

Case One.   A Problem in Arterial Blood Sampling in a Sick Infant.. 147
Case Two.   Respiratory Distress in a 2100-gm. Male Infant 149
Case Three.   Respiratory Distress in an 1100-gm. Female Infant 149
Case Four.   Respiratory Distress in a 2000-gm. Male Infant 150

CHAPTER 10
Case One.   A Convulsing Five-Day-Old Infant 179
Case Two: Hypoglycemia in an Infant of a Diabetic Mother 180
Case Three.   Hypoglycemia in a Small-for-Dates Infant... 180

CHAPTER 11
Case One.   A Hemolytic Anemia in a Full-Term Infant... 200
Case Two.   A Modest Elevation of Bilirubin in an Immature Infant of a Diabetic Mother 201
Case Three.   Hyperbilirubinemia in an Immature Infant on a Respirator 203

CHAPTER 12
Case One.   Possible Septicemia in an Immature Infant 223
Case Two.   Fever in an Infant of a Diabetic Mother.. 225
Case Three.   Pathogenic *E. coli* in an Immature Infant with Diarrhea 225
Case Four.   Congenital Infection in a Neonate.. 226

CHAPTER 13
Case One.   Ventricular Septal Defect in an Asymptomatic One-Month-Old Infant...................... 229
Case Two.   Ventricular Septal Defect in the First Days of Life 230
Case Three.   A Large Atrial Septal Defect in a Six-Month-Old Infant 230
Case Four.   A Cyanotic Neonate with a Small Heart and Decreased Pulmonary Vascularity......... 248
Case Five.   A Cyanotic Full-Term Infant with a Quiet Heart and No Respiratory Distress......... 248
Case Six.   A Cyanotic Neonate with a Hyperdynamic Heart.. 249
Case Seven.   A Cyanotic Full-Term Infant in Right Heart Failure................................... 250
Case Eight.   A Cyanotic Three-Week-Old Infant in Heart Failure 250
Case Nine.   Supraventricular Tachycardia and Heart Failure in an Infant................................. 251

CHAPTER 14
Case One.   A Neonate with a Large Left Flank Mass, Appearing Ill 262
Case Two.   Periorbital Edema and Abnormal Urine in a Neonate 264
Case Three.   Pyuria in a Full-Term Neonate 266

CHAPTER 15
Case One.   Blood Loss in a Full-Term Infant 270
Case Two.   Vitamin K Deficiency in a Full-Term Infant.. 273
Case Three.   Low Platelets in a Neonate.. 275
Case Four.   Consumption Coagulopathy in a Full-Term Infant 276
Case Five.   Iron Deficiency Anemia in a Six-Month-Old Infant 278
Case Six.   Vitamin E Deficiency in a Small Premature Infant 281
Case Seven.   A Complicated Case 283

CHAPTER 16
Case One.   Hypotonia and Lethargy in a Full-Term Infant.. 297
Case Two.   Convulsions and "Jitteriness" in a Full-Term Infant 297
Case Three.   Cerebral Dysfunction Following Neonatal Asphyxia.. 299

Chapter 1

RESUSCITATION OF THE NEWBORN INFANT

by
DAVID FISHER, M.D.
and
RICHARD E. BEHRMAN, M.D.

"If the child does not breath immediately upon Delivery, which sometimes it will not, especially it has taken Air in the Womb; wipe its Mouth, and press your Mouth to the Child's, at the same time pinching the Nose with your Thumb and Finger, to prevent the Air escaping; inflate the Lungs; rubbing it before the Fire: by which Method I have saved many."

BENJAMIN PUGH, 1754

Although mouth-to-mouth resuscitation has been known since antiquity and isolated mention of positive pressure ventilation appeared in the literature of the 17th, 18th, and 19th centuries,[21] it was not until the second quarter of the 20th century that a basis for resuscitation of the newborn infant emerged. The use of positive pressure ventilation with an endotracheal tube was described in 1928,[34] as was a positive pressure device with a pressure regulator[48] which, with modifications,[47] is still in use today. With the knowledge available in 1928, one would have expected that an orderly, progressive development of resuscitation techniques would have taken place, but this was not the case.

Until the last decade, methods of resuscitation were based on empirical observations in the human infant without animal experimentation under controlled conditions Since many infants were resuscitated during primary apnea, many methods now discarded seemed to work, including the Blossom positive pressure oxygen-air lock,[13] body rocking,[32, 54] intragastric oxygen, hyperbaric oxygen, analeptic drugs, and electrical stimulation of the phrenic nerve.[20] Studies indicating that some of these methods are of little or no value were only recently reported (body rocking—1962,[6] intragastric oxygen—1963,[43] hyperbaric oxygen—1966[14]). In 1966, it was shown in the monkey[23] that analeptic drugs (lobeline, nikethamide) could be harmful—when given after the last gasp there is a further drop in blood pressure and gasping is not initiated.

This chapter presents an approach to the resuscitation of the asphyxiated human newborn infant. Anticipation is the key to good care; thus, the population of fetuses who are likely to be at risk will be identified and the problem defined. Prenatal detection of fetal distress and the sequential steps necessary to resuscitate the asphyxiated neonate will be discussed. As an adjunct to management, placement of an umbilical vessel catheter may be necessary, and a discussion of techniques and potential complications is included at the end of the chapter.

PATHOPHYSIOLOGY OF ASPHYXIA

An understanding of the pathophysiology of asphyxia is preliminary to considering the approach to resuscitation of an asphyxiated newborn human infant. A significant amount of information is, of necessity, based on animal experiments; however, there is great variability of different species in their response to asphyxia when measured in terms of the time to last gasp or survival time, which are commonly used endpoints.[25] These species differences may be very important factors influencing the course and effect of asphyxia. Furthermore, there are significant differences in degrees of maturation at birth and subsequent rates of development in the diverse species used to study asphyxia, such as the rat, guinea pig, rabbit, cat, sheep, and monkey. Therefore, caution must be exercised when extrapolating such data to the human newborn infant.

The events associated with asphyxia in the human fetus are probably closely analogous to those described for the rhesus monkey. A useful example is the observation of the natural history of total asphyxia at birth in the rhesus monkey fetus delivered by cesarean section, where prior to delivery, catheters were placed in fetal vessels and the head was covered with a saline-filled rubber bag to prevent air breathing during gasping. At delivery, the umbilical cord was immediately tied. (Figure 1–1 illustrates the course of selected physiologic parameters during 10 minutes of total asphyxia and subsequent resuscitation.) Rapid gasps occurred shortly after the onset of asphyxia, accompanied by muscular effort producing thrashing movements of the arms and legs. This ceased after a little more than a minute and usually heralded the onset of *primary apnea* (during which spontaneous respirations can still be induced by appropriate sensory stimuli) which lasted almost a minute. The heart rate dropped considerably but was still approximately 100 beats per minute (normal 180 to 220 beats per minute in an infant monkey). A series of spontaneous deep gasps then followed for four to five minutes, gradually becoming weaker and terminating (*the last gasp*) after approximately eight minutes of total anoxia. *Secondary apnea* (during which spontaneous respirations cannot be induced by sensory stimulus) begins after the last gasp, and death occurs if not reversed within several minutes. The longer the delay in initiating adequate resuscitation measures (artificial ventilation) after the last gasp, the longer the time to the first gasp after resuscitation: for

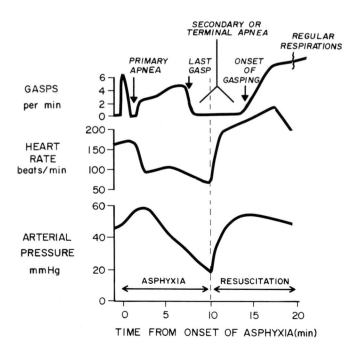

Figure 1–1 Changes in physiologic parameters during asphyxiation and resuscitation of the rhesus monkey fetus at birth. Rhesus monkeys were asphyxiated at birth by tying the umbilical cords while their heads were in saline-filled rubber bags. Resuscitation was by positive-pressure ventilation. (Adapted from Dawes[25] and Adamsons.[3])

every one minute delay, the time to first gasp is increased by about two minutes and the time to onset of rhythmical breathing delayed, on the average, by over four minutes.[3] (See Table 1–4.)

During total asphyxia, dramatic changes occurred in acid-base parameters: pH dropped from 7.3 just prior to asphyxia to 6.8 at 10 minutes; pCO_2 rose from 45 mm. Hg prior to asphyxia to 150 mm. Hg at 10 minutes; and pO_2 fell from 25 mm. Hg. prior to asphyxia to virtually zero at 10 minutes.[25] Concomitantly, the levels of blood lactate, reflecting anaerobic metabolism and accumulation of excess acid, rose rapidly with asphyxia. The concentration of blood lactate fell slowly when positive pressure oxygen ventilation was initiated.

The human fetus and newborn may be less mature and *may* tolerate greater amounts of asphyxia than the rhesus monkey without developing brain damage, and the time to last gasp is probably longer than in the rhesus monkey.[25] The frequency distribution of duration of primary apnea and time to last gasp studied in newborn rabbits shows a reasonably wide range.[14] This variability may also occur in the human infant, with the possibility of a marked prolongation of primary apnea and/or time to last gasp. This means that in the individual newborn patient, the actual time course of asphyxia and the possibility of subsequent manifestations of anoxic brain damage cannot be easily estimated. When an apneic newborn is confronted in the delivery room, it is extremely difficult to determine whether primary or secondary (terminal) apnea is present. The latter must be assumed and resuscitative measures started at once. Retrospectively, on the basis of the infant's response, it may be possible to decide at what degree of apnea resuscitition was started.

CIRCULATORY CHANGES DURING ASPHYXIA

During the course of total asphyxia in the rhesus monkey as seen in Figure 1–1, the blood pressure, after an initial rise, fell steadily. At the same time, the skin became successively blue, blotchy, and then white as the infant responded to the circulatory failure with generalized peripheral vasoconstriction. A recent study[11] of the effects of hypoxia on the rhesus monkey in utero indicated that concomitant with the decrease in cardiac output was a redistribution of the available cardiac output in an attempt to provide oxygenated blood to vital organs—brain, heart, and adrenal glands. This was done at the expense of kidneys, spleen, lungs, and carcass. In this study, mild to moderate asphyxia, as indicated by oxygen uptake and acid-base studies, was induced by a gradual reduction in maternal arterial oxygen tension. Umbilical blood flow decreased by 50 per cent as did fetal oxygen consumption. The oxygenated blood returning to the heart from the ductus venosus contributed a proportionately larger volume to the blood perfusing the brain and heart in control and hypoxic fetuses than did blood from the superior or inferior vena cava. In addition, during hypoxia there was increased shunting of superior vena cava (SVC) blood across the foramen ovale, temporarily maintaining the absolute volume of blood perfusing the heart and brain on a per gram of tissue basis in the face of a falling cardiac output.

Five minutes of total asphyxia in the newborn monkey[33] during the first week of life produced similar alterations in the distribution of cardiac output. With a decrease in cardiac output of 80 per cent the percentage of cardiac output going to the heart, adrenal glands, and midbrain plus brainstem plus cerebellum increased significantly, although not enough to preserve the organ flow per gram of tissue.

The observation of an alteration in the distribution of the circulation during periods of oxygen deprivation is not new. Reflex circulatory adjustments occur in diving seals, with profound bradycardia, decrease in oxygen consumption, decrease in body temperature, and the accumulation of lactic acid in muscle but not in blood.[64] Central blood pressure is usually maintained, and arterial blood contains oxygen while peripheral blood does not. When the seal surfaces, the pre-dive state resumes, and after air breathing starts, the lactic acid is taken away from muscle by the bloodstream and delivered to the liver for metabolism. Similar changes occur during diving in the dolphin[31] and hippopotamus.[30]

It has been postulated that such circulatory adjustments occur in the human infant to protect vital organs from hypoxia occurring at the time of delivery. This is based in part on the observation that the blood lactate level in the newborn increases shortly after the onset of respirations, with higher levels noted in the severely depressed newborn.[41] However, there is a fundamental difference in the stress to the human infant. In the diving mammal, which may remain submerged for 25 minutes, the circulatory changes are not overwhelmed under the conditions of a normal dive; in the asphyxiated primate, however, the circulatory changes are in response to life-threatening pathologic conditions, and the protective effects are quickly overwhelmed after short periods of asphyxia as noted above. Calculations reveal that these circulatory adjustments will account for only a small portion of the increased length of time that the newborn can survive asphyxia.

BIOCHEMICAL CHANGES DURING ASPHYXIA

The most important biochemical event during asphyxia is the conversion from aerobic oxidation of glucose to anaerobic glycolysis in response to hypoxia, with the accumulation of lactate and the development of a metabolic acidosis. Lactate is metabolized by oxidation predominantly in the neonatal liver. There is an increase in lactic acid dehydrogenase (LDH) activity in the liver immediately after birth, which is further increased in response to hypoxia. In addition to the development of severe metabolic acidosis secondary to hypoxia, there is an immediate rapid elevation of pCO_2 during asphyxia. This respiratory acidosis generally occurs first when there is cord compression of the fetus, acute placental insufficiency (placental respiratory acidosis), or obstruction of the airway in a newborn infant. The profound drop in pH is thus a result of a mixed acidosis which is coincident with the hypoxia.

Free fatty acids (FFA) and glycerol, both products of neutral fat hydrolysis, increase in blood in response to hypoxia. It has been postulated that a decrease in transfer of glucose across the placenta secondary to hypoxia may mobilize FFA by release of epinephrine and norepinephrine.[70]

Hepatic glycogen is mobilized immediately after birth to provide a continuing source of glucose to the brain when the maternal blood glucose supply is terminated. At the time of delivery, maternal blood glucose is usually elevated secondary to sympathetic stimulation, and the neonate has a parallel elevation, although the levels are lower than in maternal blood. The mobilization of hepatic glycogen during hypoxia makes it extremely unusual to find hypoglycemia in the infant being resuscitated because of asphyxia, and administration of a hypertonic glucose solution under such circumstances is probably of little value. Although a beneficial effect (prolongation of last gasp) from the infusion of alkali and glucose has been reported in the rhesus monkey asphyxiated at birth, the glucose levels were not low even in the control group, and the effect may be related to improvement in the circulating vascular volume. Recent data[45] in fetal and newborn lambs suggest that the *hypertonicity* of the infused solution (glucose, saline, or sodium bicarbonate), regardless of the effect of pH, may be responsible for increasing pulmonary blood flow and cardiac output.

Animal studies indicate that initially ATP levels are maintained at the expense of phosphocreatine. As the level of high-energy phosphate falls, cell processes begin to fail, including resynthesis of acetylcholine and the "sodium pump," which results in cell losses of potassium and amino acids.[61] The cell accumulates carbon dioxide, inorganic phosphate, ammonia, and γ-aminobutyric acid (GABA), which is a neuroinhibitory substance.[61] These changes take considerably longer to occur in the newborn infant with immature nervous tissue than in the adult animal.

Recent studies[22, 28, 40, 57] suggest that brain tissue can utilize glycerol[69] and ketone bodies (β-hydroxybutyrate, acetoacetate) as metabolic substrate; however, the oxygen requirements are high and it is unlikely that this pathway is utilized under conditions of hypoxia and glycogen depletion.

ABILITY OF THE NEWBORN TO SURVIVE ASPHYXIA

There are several factors which enable the newborn infant to tolerate asphyxia better than the adult. The lower metabolic rate of particular tissues is probably most important. The relatively immature brain of the newborn animal has a resting metabolic rate which is only a fraction of that observed in the adult. The state of activity of a given tissue, as well as the temperature, is also significant. For example, the metabolic requirements of the myocardium are probably initially increased during asphyxia. Environmental temperatures outside the neutral thermal range may also increase metabolic requirements.

Another major factor is the availability of substrate for anaerobic degradation. The substrate may be locally stored, as with myocardial glycogen, or mobilized via the circulation to supply the brain with carbohydrate from liver glycogen. Although glucose represents the main metabolic fuel for brain tissue, glycerol, free fatty acids, and ketone bodies may also provide metabolic fuel to a limited extent.

An intact circulation is of major importance in the ability to survive asphyxia, and it was shown as early as 1812 by Le Gallois (cited by Dawes[25]) that rabbits asphyxiated by immersion in water or opening of the thorax gasped significantly longer than those from which the heart was removed. An intact circulation is also able to redistribute lactate and hydrogen ion to tissues still being perfused (that may have a lower hydrogen ion production), and thus provide a means of buffering cerebral cells during asphyxia.[125] It is an adjunct to this that sodium bicarbonate, administered during asphyxia, may exert a beneficial effect if CO_2 gas is being removed.

In summary, as shown in the rat brain,[44] immature brain tissue with a low rate of energy metabolism can possibly increase the rate of anaerobic glycolysis and use the available energy more efficiently, so that proteosynthesis continues and biochemical ultra structure is maintained within recoverable limits in response to hypoxia. Unfortunately, severe sustained hypoxia will overcome these protective mechanisms, and brain damage or death of the newborn animal or human will occur.

PRENATAL DETECTION AND MONITORING

Recent advances in medical instrumentation have made it practical to monitor the human fetus during labor. The major effort must be directed toward identifying the pregnant woman who has an increased likelihood of delivering an infant who is at increased risk from asphyxia or other causes—the so-called high-risk pregnancy. Women who fall into this group (see Table 1–1) should ideally be referred to a facility equipped to provide appropriate observation, diagnosis, and treatment during pregnancy, labor, delivery, and the immediate neonatal period. This is one of the effective ways to reduce perinatal mortality. Although many pregnancies identified as high-risk by one or more of the criteria noted will prove to be uneventful, at least those requiring special management can be identified. Monitoring or intensive observation can be divided into: (1) evaluation of the function of the feto-placental unit during pregnancy, (2) estimation of duration of gestation, and (3) acute monitoring of the fetus during labor and delivery.

FUNCTION OF THE FETO-PLACENTAL UNIT

Serial determinations of urinary estriol excretion over 24 hours is useful in evaluating the feto-placental unit, since the major precursor of estriol, dehydroepiandrosterone, is made in the fetal adrenal gland and not the placenta, while the synthesis of estriol from dehydroepiandrosterone occurs in the placenta.[60] Serial measurements are necessary because of the daily variation in levels and difficulty in collecting accurate 24-hour urine specimens.[37]

The large variation in estriol levels and the difficulty in interpreting these by themselves have led a number of investigators to utilize the estriol/creatinine ratio as a more exact parameter. To a large extent, this might obviate the difficulties encountered in measurement of estriol levels alone in the urine.

L. STERN

Included in the group of high-risk pregnancies where this study is of frequent value are those complicated by diabetes mellitus, hypertension, preeclampsia, prolonged pregnancy ($\geq$42 weeks), and previous unexplained fetal loss.[38] Falling values indicate that the fetus is not in good health, either because of fetal asphyxia or because of an inadequately functioning placenta, and death in utero is very likely without obstetric intervention. Surgical intervention to deliver the fetus requires that the gestation is far enough advanced ($>$32 weeks) that the newborn infant will be at less risk from premature delivery than from remaining in utero. Continuously very low levels are seen in a mother carrying an anencephalic infant, in isolated adrenal cortical hypoplasia, in fetal death, and in a mother who has received high doses of corticosteroids. In a mother carrying an infant with severe erythroblastosis, the maternal urinary estriol does not fall until fetal death. However, the level of amniotic fluid estriol (a glucosiduronate conjugate, most likely produced in the fetal liver and excreted in the fetal

TABLE 1-1 CRITERIA FOR IDENTIFICATION OF HIGH-RISK PREGNANCY*

THE PATIENT	MEDICAL HISTORY	PREVIOUS PREGNANCY HISTORY	PREGNANCY-RELATED MEDICAL CONDITIONS (PAST OR PRESENT)
Teenage (<16 at conception)	Hypertension	Grand multiparity	Toxemia
Elderly (>40 at conception)	Renal disease	Previous surgical delivery	Bleeding after 12 weeks' gestation
	Diabetes	Previous prolonged labor	Multiple pregnancy (present)
Underweight or overweight (2 S. D.	Cancer	(>24 hours)	Abnormal presentation or
from mean when compared	Thyroid disease	Previous fetal loss	position of fetus (present)
to standard chart appropriate	Cardiovascular	Previous live premature	Hydramnios
for race and/or ethnic group)	disease	infant	General anesthesia during
Low socioeconomic status	Rh sensitization	Previous infant death in	pregnancy
	Tuberculosis	first week of life	Administration of certain drugs
	Lupus erythematosus	Previous "damaged" infant	to mother (propylthiouracil)
	Mental retardation	(birth trauma, cerebral	Anemia (Hb <8 gm per 100 ml.)
	Alcoholic or narcotic	palsy, mental retardation,	Indifference to health needs
	addict	etc.)	(multiple missed appointments,
	Major psychoses		failure to follow recommenda-
	Neurologic disease		tions)
	Severe anemia (sickle-cell,		
	thalassemia)		

S. D. = Standard Deviation.
*Adapted from Gold.[36]

urine) correlates with fetal status, values below 100 μg per liter being associated with an unhealthy fetus.[38]

ESTIMATION OF GESTATIONAL AGE

If the fetus threatened by asphyxia is being monitored as a potential candidate for early delivery, then an estimate of the duration of pregnancy must be made as accurately as possible in order to avoid delivering a small premature infant at less than 32 weeks' gestation. Although pregnancy can usually be dated reliably from the onset of the last menstrual period, errors up to a month are not rare. Several methods now available to help assess intrauterine growth depend on the evaluation of amniotic fluid or the use of ultrasound.

Amniotic fluid studies include spectrophotometric analysis, determination of the creatinine level, and cytology. The cytologic study evaluates the percentage of fetal sebaceous gland cells (which have cytoplasm stained orange with Nile blue) compared to fetal squamous cells (which stain pale blue). The percentage of sebaceous gland cells increases with advancing gestation to about 20 per cent at term.[4] Similarly, creatinine values, probably reflecting maturation of the fetal kidneys, increase with progression of gestation. A combination of these two tests may be reliable in distinguishing between pregnancies less than 35 and greater than 36 weeks' gestation.[12] High ratios of amniotic fluid lecithin to sphingomyelin are also indicative of fetal (pulmonary) maturity, and are most valuable in estimating the level of lung maturation. It appears to be most helpful in determining when delivery of an infant will not result in respiratory distress syndrome. The estimation of saturated lecithin has been remarkably simplified with a new technique devised by Clements et al.[17] The test (the "shake test") requires about 20 minutes. (It is most important that the procedure be followed *exactly*.)

Ultrasound determination of the fetal biparietal diameter is done by controlled beaming of high-frequency, low-energy sound waves at the fetus. The echo signals reflected back from tissue interfaces can provide a two-dimensional picture of the fetal head at its widest diameter. Serial determinations of biparietal diameter can provide a rate of growth that is useful in predicting gestational age[15] with the accuracy of perhaps plus or minus two weeks. On the other hand, since the range of normal values for a given gestational age progressively increases during the third trimester of pregnancy, a single determination of biparietal diameter may give an estimation of gestational age in error by as much as six weeks.[15, 50] A recent study[16] suggests that measurement of the fetal lumbar spine on a roentgenogram of the mother can provide an estimation of gestational age plus or minus two weeks, with 90 per cent accuracy in a fetus with a cephalic presentation.

MONITORING THE FETUS DURING LABOR

Selected high-risk pregnancies should be closely monitored during labor. Forty-seven of 83 *term* intrapartum fetal deaths recently reported[51] occurred in mothers who had at least one of the criteria for high risk based on the individual pregnancy history alone. Careful monitoring with appropriate operative intervention might salvage a significant number of these infants.

The contribution that intrapartum death makes to the stillbirth rate and thus to overall perinatal mortality should not be underestimated. In most series, unexplained peripartum asphyxia (so called) accounts for approximately one-third or greater of all stillbirths. A very high proportion of these are in turn intrapartum deaths in which the fetus was apparently alive and in good condition at the start of labor, but in which fetal death subsequently occurred before labor was completed. It is in this group that monitoring during labor has been shown to be not only efficacious but also highly effective in reducing fetal losses.

L. STERN

Counting the fetal heart rate (FHR) between contractions using a stethoscope is an inadequate method of determining early evidence of fetal distress, since significant rate changes occur early during a contraction and persist for a short time after the contraction is over (Figure 1–2). This is the period when a fetal heart is least audible with a stethoscope. By continuously monitoring intrauterine pressure and FHR, using continuous ultrasound (Doptone) or, when the fetal scalp is accessible, a scalp clip attached to recording electrodes, significant abnormalities can be detected at a time when operative intervention has a greater chance of producing a live, neurologically intact newborn infant.

Transient tachycardia with heart rates

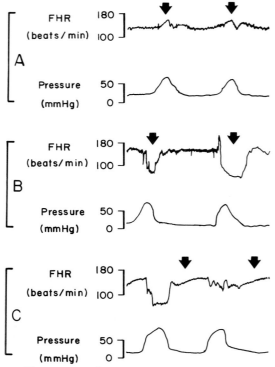

Figure 1–2 Changes in fetal heart rate during uterine contractions as reflection of fetal distress. The arrows indicate transient tachycardia (*A*), variable deceleration (*B*), and variable deceleration with slow recovery after uterine relaxation (*C*). FHR = fetal heart rate. Pressure is uterine pressure. See text for explanation.

over 160 beats per minute (Figure 1–2*A*) may be an isolated early finding. It is frequently followed by a "variable deceleration," (Figure 1–2*B* and *C*) or "late deceleration" (Figure 1–3) pattern of fetal heart rate associated with uterine contractions. Any of these patterns is compatible with fetal distress.

Amnioscopy with direct inspection and assessment of the amniotic fluid for meconium staining, etc., has been considered by some to be an adjunct to scalp sampling as well as a method of selection as to who should be sampled and who possibly anticipated. The procedure is open to

some debate as to its usefulness because of the relatively subjective nature of the examination; nevertheless, in capable hands and in the absence of external monitoring techniques, it has afforded a useful guide as to which fetus is at risk.

L. STERN

Sampling blood from the fetal scalp during labor is another method used for monitoring the fetus of selected high-risk pregnancies or when fetal distress is suspected. The procedure can be done when membranes are ruptured, the cervix is dilated several centimeters, and the fetal vertex is close to or below the ischial spines.[67] A fetal scalp puncture (only a few millimeters deep) is made under direct visualization, and a sample is collected in a heparinized polyethylene tube. The values for acid-base parameters on fetal scalp blood correspond to those obtained from the umbilical cord at cesarean section.[62,67] The most reliable parameter reflecting the presence of fetal hypoxia and acidosis has been pH.[8] There is a high correlation with fetal distress when the fetal scalp pH is below 7.15 in the presence of normal maternal blood pH. However, a significant number of infants with low pH are born vigorous and with essentially normal acid-base status.[67] Improved reliability is obtained by monitoring fetal heart rate as well as fetal scalp blood where facilities are available to do both. Continuous fetal heart rate monitoring is the preferred method in general, as it is easier to use and is a more reliable index of fetal distress. Complications associated with fetal scalp blood monitoring include excessive fetal blood loss, newborn infections, and unnecessary obstetrical intervention in labor.

TREATMENT OF FETAL DISTRESS (ASPHYXIA) IN UTERO

Administration of a high concentration of oxygen to the mother of a distressed fetus

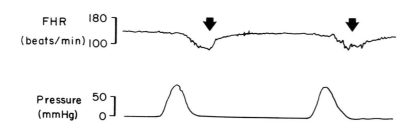

Figure 1–3 Changes in fetal heart rate during uterine relaxation as reflection of fetal distress. The arrows indicate late deceleration pattern with slow recovery after uterine relaxation. FHR = fetal heart rate. Pressure is uterine pressure. See text for explanation.

is one of the few methods of treating fetal asphyxia. Experiments in the rhesus monkey suggest that umbilical blood flow is not adversely affected, and that there is an increased amount of oxygen transferred to some hypoxic fetuses.[10]

Repositioning the mother in labor occasionally may relieve fetal asphyxia caused by mechanical compression of the umbilical cord.[66] Maternal hypotension, secondary to compression of the inferior vena cava, may produce fetal asphyxia by decreasing uterine blood flow and oxygenation. This may be relieved by rotating the mother from a supine to a lateral position.

Preliminary observations in the rhesus monkey[68] and in humans[39] suggest that sodium bicarbonate instilled into the amniotic sac may be able to correct to a degree the metabolic acidosis related to fetal hypoxia. If further study is confirmatory, then such treatment may provide a reasonable temporizing measure while preparing for operative intervention.

When a decision is made to intervene operatively for a fetus in distress, the pediatrician should be immediately alerted so that there is adequate preparation for prompt resuscitation of the newborn infant if necessary.

Editors' Comment: We have found the indications listed in Table 1–2 useful for alerting our pediatric staff.

RESUSCITATION TECHNIQUES

Many early methods depended on uncomfortable stimuli to initiate the onset of respirations, including gentle, intermittent traction on the tongue, spanking the feet or buttocks, dilation of the anal sphincter, and alternately immersing the infant in hot and cold water.[59] There is little experimental basis for these methods and they should be avoided, as injury may be produced and they waste time which can be used more effectively.

Hypothermia has been recommended for resuscitation[55] of the asphyxiated human newborn based on findings in the guinea pig, rabbit, piglet, kitten, and puppy, which were cooled to 15°C. Presumably, at such a low temperature, homeostatic mechanisms are not functioning and metabolic activity is greatly reduced.[52, 55] A significant benefit

TABLE 1–2   OBSTETRICAL INDICATIONS FOR ALERTING
THE HIGH-RISK NURSERY*

The obstetric nursing staff should notify the high-risk nursery when any of the following are noted:

FACTORS SUGGESTING FETAL DISTRESS
Meconium staining with vertex presentation
Persistent fetal heart rate >160 per minute
Persistent fetal heart rate <120 per minute
Irregular fetal heart rate

MATERNAL PROBLEMS
Toxemia
Intrauterine growth retardation
Diabetes
Erythroblastosis
Abruptio placentae, placenta previa
Dystocia
Elderly primigravida
Prematurity
Gestation > 42 weeks
Maternal fever
Premature rupture of membranes > 24 hours
Vaginal bleeding other than "show"
Multiple gestation
Abnormal presentation

*Adapted from Merenstein and Blackmon.[53]

from cooling was not noted in the rhesus monkey asphyxiated at birth.[24] An adequate controlled study in the human is not available. Until this debatable issue is settled, *we strongly recommend that the asphyxiated newborn be placed in a neutral thermal environment for resuscitation.*

Considerable misunderstanding exists regarding the difference between cooling and true, deep hypothermia. The latter is usually carried out in an operating room with controlled artificial ventilation as a patient is being prepared for cardiovascular surgery, and ultimately results in a lower metabolic rate from slowing of all metabolic processes. By contrast, so-called little bit of cooling results in no such advantage, since it merely raises oxygen consumption and increases the metabolic rate. A distinction must be made between these two forms of the application of a cold environment.

The need to keep an infant warm during the resuscitation procedure needs to be re-emphasized. Not only is attention to the thermal environment frequently forgotten in the rush and bustle of apparently heroic procedures such as intubation, mouth-to mouth respiration, and intracardiac adrenalin but also the administration of cold oxygen which has not been prewarmed may only further compound the cooling engendered, since it has been clearly shown that regardless of the environmental temperature, a cold stimulus administered either to the trigeminal area or the forehead itself can result in significant elevations of oxygen consumption. These cold stimuli, in addition to causing an obligatory increase in metabolic rate, will also result in vasoconstriction, further potentiating any acidosis and subsequent poor perfusion of the tissues with tissue hypoxia. In addition, there is an increase in free fatty acids in the cold, with subsequent inverse depression of glucose. Finally, the free fatty acid increase may also subsequently result in an earlier predisposition to kernicterus at lower levels of bilirubin, since the fatty acids compete with bilirubin for the albumin molecule.

L. STERN

Mouth-to-mouth resuscitation has been used as a last-resort resuscitative measure for many years and has been supplanted by positive-pressure ventilation by one of several different methods: a pressure-controlled ventilator connected to a tight-fitting face mask or endotracheal tube; a ventilation bag similarly connected; or mouth-to-endotracheal-tube ventilation.

Current resuscitation methods based on the previous discussion of asphyxia are directed toward providing oxygen and removing carbon dioxide by positive-pressure ventilation, maintaining the circulation by external cardiac massage (described in neonatal resuscitation in 1962[56]), and providing alkali for buffering the excess acid produced during anaerobic metabolism. If blood loss has occurred, transfusion or infusion of a plasma expander may be required.

This is one of the major pediatric emergencies. There is no substitute for adequate training and periodic review of the techniques required to resuscitate a newborn infant. When a potential problem is anticipated at the time of delivery, based on the identification of a high-risk pregnancy or evidence of fetal distress (asphyxia) during labor, the physician on call for the delivery room should be alerted. He can then arrive early enough to set out the necessary equipment and see that it is functioning properly. Another major advantage of arriving before the delivery is that useful information may be obtained from the obstetrician concerning the pregnancy and labor which may make it possible to anticipate the kind of problems that may be present at birth. (If the pediatrician arrives after the delivery, he is obviously at a disadvantage with respect to organizing equipment and obtaining the relevant history. In addition, it may be difficult to accurately assess the time sequence of events following delivery of the infant.)

The brightness of the laryngoscope blade should be checked, as well as the patency of the endotracheal tubes with obturators (Figure 1–4). The resuscitation bag should be checked for proper function, and appropriate adapters should be available to connect the bag to the endotracheal tube. The oxygen flowmeter and suction equipment should be checked for proper function. The necessary syringes, needles, umbilical vessel catheters, and drugs ($NaHCO_3$, 10 per cent dextrose in water, epinephrine 1:10,000) should all be available. If a resuscitation unit is available, this usually provides a heat source to keep the infant warm. Otherwise, a radiant heater should be on hand.

The first critical decision that must be made is to evaluate the severity of depression of the newborn infant, which dictates the course of immediate management. The most practical emergency guideline can be based on the Apgar scoring chart (Table 1–3). An infant with an Apgar score of 0 to 2 is considered asphyxiated until proven otherwise. The assistance of another skilled person should be requested immediately to assist in this infant's resuscitation. Very brief (15-second) suctioning should be done initially

TABLE 1–3   APGAR SCORE*

SIGN	SCORE		
	0	1	2
Heart rate	Absent	Below 100	Over 100
Respiratory effort	Absent	Weak, irregular	Good, crying
Muscle tone	Flaccid	Some flexion of extremities	Well flexed
Reflex irritability (Catheter in nose)	No response	Grimace	Cough or sneeze
Color	Blue, pale	Body pink Extremities blue	Completely pink

*Adapted from data of Apgar.[5]

to clear the airway, preferably under direct laryngoscopic visualization. It is most important that prolonged suctioning be avoided because it wastes time and there is evidence that it may produce reflex bradycardia.[18]

An endotracheal tube should be inserted (Figures 1–5 and 1–6) and there should be adequate ventilation with oxygen by positive pressure established by mouth-to-tube or bag-to-tube inflation of the lungs. In either case, ventilation should be at the rate of approximately 50 times per minute, and the inspiratory phase should be slightly less than half the time of a ventilation cycle so that adequate passive emptying of the lungs can occur before the next inflation. Approximately 20 to 25 centimeters of water pressure is needed to inflate the lungs of a normal newborn infant, but pressure twice as high may be necessary initially. The adequacy of ventilation can be determined best by observing the chest wall excursion and/or listening to the chest with a stethoscope. If mouth-to-tube ventilation is initiated, the puffs of air-oxygen should be expelled only with pressure from the mouth. If the expiratory lung volume of the adult is used, too much pressure may be generated and the procedure may be complicated by the development of a pneumomediastinum and/or pneumothorax. Bag-to-tube or bag-to-mask ventilation is probably preferable, as it is easier to monitor the infant's respiratory excursions and to help direct the resuscitation effort. If the initial heart rate is over 100 beats per minute, primary apnea is more likely and a brief (15 to 20-second) attempt to resuscitate, using a tight-fitting face mask and positive pressure oxygen by bag, can be made. If there is no immediate re-

sponse, indicated by an increase in heart rate, endotracheal intubation should be performed.

The infant with primary apnea or gasping at the time resuscitation is started will usually respond promptly to suction or the administration of oxygen by face mask with

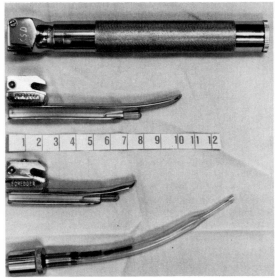

Figure 1–4 Equipment for intubation of the newborn. Note in particular the difference in length between the size 1 (term infant) and size 0 (premature infant) blades. The size 0 blade will not be long enough for adequate visualization of the larynx in the near-term infant. Note the short distal segment of the Cole endotracheal tube (preferred) which passes between the vocal cords and the wider portion, and which prevents the tube from being advanced too far and reduces the length of high resistance to air flow with ventilation.

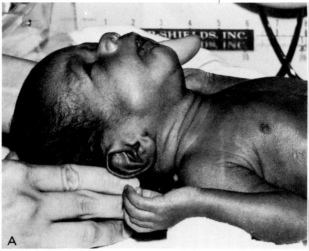
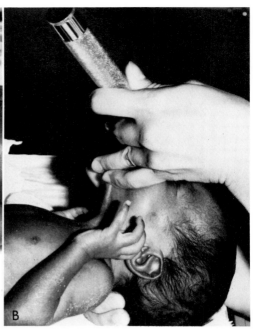

Figure 1-5 Note the positioning of the head for intubation with chin up and shoulders slightly elevated. The laryngoscope is held in the left hand and the fourth and fifth fingers can help control the position of the head. When held properly, the blade should be easy to control and soft tissue injury avoided.

an increase in heart rate, spontaneous increased gasping, improved color, and some spontaneous movement.

If after clearing of the airway the infant does not improve with positive-pressure ventilation through an endotracheal tube, he has reached the stage of secondary apnea and can be presumed to be severely acidotic. At this point, the administration of $NaHCO_3$ (3 mEq. per Kg.) via an umbilical vein catheter is indicated. The $NaHCO_3$ should be diluted with equal volumes of H_2O and given over a period of 20 to 30 seconds.

If after several minutes of resuscitative effort, including adequate ventilation and administration of bicarbonate, the Apgar score is 1 to 2 with a falling heart rate or a heart rate below 50 beats per minute, 1 to 2 ml. of 1:10,000 epinephrine should be given (if the heart beat is detectable, the epinephrine can be given via the umbilical catheter; if not detectable, it should be given by direct cardiac puncture) and external cardiac massage started in an attempt to maintain perfusion of critical organs (heart muscle and brain) with oxygenated blood. External cardiac massage may be needed immediately after establishing ventilation and administration of alkali if the heart rate is still severely depressed. Closed chest cardiac massage should be done at a rate of 120 compressions per minute with a lung inflation every two to three seconds. The infant should be resting on a firm surface for external cardiac massage to be effective. Use of the fingertips of the index and middle fingers over the middle third of the sternum provides adequate force to depress the sternum the desired one-half to three-quarters of an inch.[56]

The infant with an Apgar score of 3 to 6 when first seen has probably had mild to moderate asphyxia. If apnea is present it is usually primary, and gasping respiratory efforts can be anticipated. In such situations, brief suctioning of the airway followed by oxygen ventilation by positive-pressure mask and bag often will result in rapid improvement. In the rare infant who becomes worse over several minutes and the Apgar score drops into the range of the severely asphyxiated infant (Apgar 0 to 2), subsequent management should proceed as for severe asphyxia.

The infant with an Apgar score above 7 will rarely need any resuscitation unless the Apgar score drops suddenly several minutes after birth. If this occurs, then management is as described above. It is important to avoid prolonged vigorous nasopharyngeal suctioning of these infants, as it may cause reflex bradycardia and apnea.

The physician should be familiar with both the premature (size 0) and infant

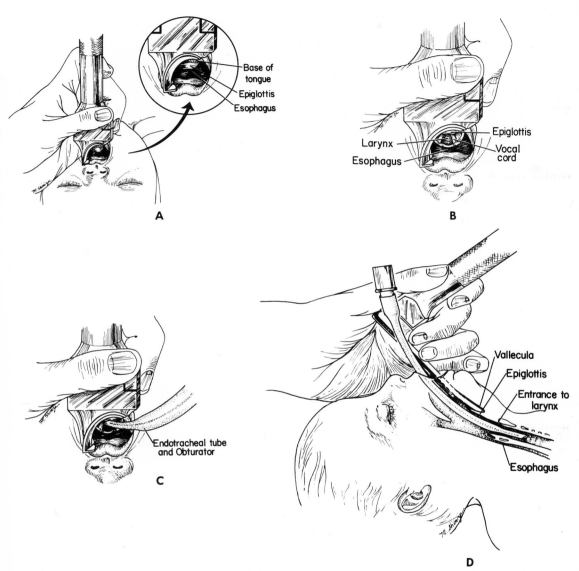

Figure 1-6 Technique of endotracheal intubation. The Miller blade should be inserted near the midline and moved to the left side of the mouth, gently deflecting the tongue. As it is advanced, the base of the tongue and epiglottis are visualized. The blade should be advanced in the same plane of movement into the vallecula (see *D*); as the blade is gently raised, the epiglottis swings anteriorly, revealing the opening of the larynx. If secretions or meconium are noted, gentle suctioning should be done before insertion of the endotracheal tube. On certain occasions when the epiglottis is not adequately raised, the blade tip may be placed posterior to the epiglottis, which can then be gently raised to expose the vocal cords. The endotracheal tube is advanced from the right corner of the mouth and inserted while maintaining direct visualization. The laryngoscope blade is then carefully withdrawn while the position of the tube is maintained by the right hand on the infant's face. Note the tip of the blade in the vallecula.

(size 1) Miller laryngoscope blades. The infant size is more flexible, in that the length is adequate for all newborns even if somewhat cumbersome. On the other hand, the premature blade is not long enough to permit adequate visualization of the larynx in the newborn weighing over 2500 gm.

The endotracheal tube should be the largest one which fits the trachea easily. A Cole tube size 14, 16 or 18 F should be used in a term newborn infant. A smaller size (10 or 12 F) may be necessary in the very small infant. Under no circumstances should a size 8 F tube be used, as a suction catheter cannot be passed and the airway flow resistance is extremely high. A relatively stiff obturator should be available in the endotracheal tube.

Editors' Comment: We prefer the use of clear tubes, and have not found it necessary to use obturators.

This is of particular value in the very small infant, where the angle of access to the trachea is more acute than in the larger infant. Sometimes a helpful procedure to aid visualization of the larynx is gentle, downward, external pressure over the trachea.

Infrequently, an infant may be depressed secondary to narcotic sedation of the mother, and improvement may occur after administration of a narcotic antagonist, nalorphine (0.2 mg. given by umbilical vein). However, an airway should be established first and adequate ventilation initiated before considering this diagnosis. Similarly, hypovolemic shock, when diagnosed, may require treatment with blood or a plasma expander after clearing the airway and establishing good ventilation. (See Figure 8–8 and Table 8–4 for normal blood pressure values and the predictive value of blood pressure.)

After successful resuscitation of the newborn infant, a feeding tube should be passed into the stomach and any secretions and/or air removed by gentle suction.

BRAIN DAMAGE FOLLOWING ASPHYXIA AND RESUSCITATION

It is hoped that by appropriate intervention with adequate resuscitative measures, the severely asphyxiated infant can be saved and brain damage prevented or minimized. Brain injury occurs when prolonged hypoxia overwhelms the compensatory mechanisms previously described. The damage may be severe and manifested early in the form of a seizure disorder, cerebral palsy, or profound developmental retardation. Damage also may be reflected by very subtle neurologic findings in early childhood or as a learning disorder at school age.

Behavioral abnormalities have been described in experimental animals following various periods of asphyxiation and resuscitation.[9, 58] Similarly, characteristic pathologic changes in the brain have been described in the nonhuman primate,[58] and in the human fetus and newborn.[19, 52]

The Apgar scoring system has shown a significant relationship between one-minute and five-minute scores and neonatal mortality and morbidity.[27] The initial assessment (one-minute score) identifies the neonatal infant needing immediate attention (Apgar score 0 to 6) and helps estimate the degree of asphyxia likely to be present. The five-minute Apgar score is more closely correlated with neonatal mortality and morbidity. Based on the information presented above, it might be anticipated that infants with prolonged hypoxia resulting in a stage of secondary apnea will be more depressed and take longer to resuscitate, most probably resulting in a low Apgar score at five minutes of age. Of those infants with a five-minute score of 0 or 1, 44 per cent did not survive the second day of life, and 49 per cent did not survive the neonatal period (to 28 days).[27] Follow-up of infants with a 0 to 3 five minute Apgar score compared to a 7 to 10 score indicated that, at one year of age, neurologic abnormality appeared in over three times as many infants with a 0 to 3 score.[28] If the data is rearranged, either on a weight basis or by individual Apgar scores, the higher the score, the lower the associated mortality and long-term morbidity.

The assessment of lactic acid levels between zero and four hours of age has been shown to be a valuable objective index of asphyxia. There is a statistically significant correlation between lactic acid level and cumulative Apgar score, with the two following exceptions: (1) low Apgar scores and low lactic acid levels (found in infants depressed from anesthesia of the mother), and (2) high lactic acid levels with good Apgar scores (found in small-for-dates infants suffering from subacute and chronic fetal distress).

S. PROD'HOM

It can be concluded that every effort should be made to identify potential obstetric pathologic conditions, manage the pregnancy as optimally as possible, and be prepared to skillfully resuscitate an asphyxiated newborn when necessary. The goal is to present each mother with a healthy newborn infant who has maximal potential for growth and development.

UMBILICAL VESSEL CATHETERIZATION

A central catheter inserted into the inferior vena cava via the umbilical vein or into the aorta via an umbilical artery may be required in the management of the sick neonatal infant for intermittent sampling of blood to monitor acid-base status and for infusion of parenteral fluids. Use of central catheters requires careful consideration of the risks involved and a decision as to whether the need for the catheter outweighs the risk of the catheterization procedure and the subsequent presence of an indwelling catheter.

Radiopaque catheters should be used and the position of the placed catheter should be verified by X-ray, preferably including a lateral view as well as anteroposterior.[7] Catheters should be removed or repositioned if they are in a dangerous location. An umbilical vein catheter can be located in a branch of the portal vein, and under such circumstances infusion of a hypertonic solution, such as a sodium bicarbonate and hypertonic glucose solution, has been responsible for areas of liver necrosis without perforation of the vein wall.[49, 63, 65] Portal vein thrombosis has also occurred with and without infection. In addition, at least 17 cases of spontaneous perforation of the colon following exchange transfusion via an umbilical vein catheter have been reported. X-ray verification of catheter tip location was not done in any of these cases; most likely the catheter tip was in the portal vein and the cause of perforation was local necrosis of bowel wall following hemorrhagic infarction secondary to retrograde microemboli or obstructive hemodynamic changes.[35]

Editors' Comment: We use mainly umbilical artery catheterization, limiting the umbilical vein to emergency situations.

Umbilical artery catheters must also be precisely located. A major objective is to avoid the area of the origins of the renal arteries, as a catheter may occlude a renal artery and catheters in the area may produce thrombosis. Both situations result in renal infarction.

Other major complications of catheter-ization include thrombosis of the vessel around the catheter and subsequent release of microemboli on the venous or arterial side of the circulation. It has been postulated that the catheter tip can traumatize the vessel wall with release of tissue thromboplastin and exposure of platelets to collagen with subsequent aggregation and activation of the intrinsic coagulation pathway.[49] Alternatively, the presence of the catheter may acitvate the Hageman factor (XII) and trigger off the intrinsic coagulation pathway.[49]

Editors' Comment: Hemorrhage, either as a result of loose connections or careless use of the stopcocks, or at the time of removal of the catheter, is a major complication of arterial catheters, and great care must be taken to prevent this. It has been our practice not to inject a heparin-containing solution for at least four hours prior to removal of the catheter.

In general, umbilical vein catheterization is technically easier. However, since a major indication for catheterization is to monitor the acid-base status of the small premature infant in cardiorespiratory distress, the umbilical artery catheter is usually preferred. In addition, there may be an advantage to infusing fluids and drugs through an arterial catheter, since the solution enters a fast-flowing stream of blood, and greater dilution in a capillary network will occur before the infusate reaches the heart.[46] In addition, systemic blood pressure can be monitored continuously through the catheter when the necessary equipment is available.

We do not use an umbilical vein catheter anymore at all, except for exchange transfusions.

S. PROD'HOM

The umbilical vessel catheter should be removed as soon as possible and a peripheral I.V. substituted, if necessary.

In the undistressed newborn infant requiring parenteral fluids, *under no circumstances should an umbilical vessel catheter be used when a peripheral I.V. could be started* via a scalp vein or extremity vein.

Technique of Catheterization

In the small premature infant, the entire procedure should be done in the incubator or under a radiant heater to avoid chilling the infant. In the delivery room, a radiant heater and/or heating blanket should be used.

When not precluded by the emergency (i.e., acute asphyxia), the following protocol should be followed. The operator carefully scrubs hands and arms to the elbows and puts on sterile gloves. A 3.5 (infants <1500 gm.) or 5 French catheter with rounded tip, which has a radiopaque line and end hole (Argyle Umbilical Artery Catheter), is attached to a syringe by a three-way stopcock and the system filled with heparinized isotonic saline (prepared by adding 250 units of heparin to a 250-ml. bottle of sterile isotonic saline). (Appendix 8 lists the equipment found on the catheterization tray.) Before proceeding, the length of the catheter to be inserted should be marked according to the location desired (Figure 1–7). After carefully preparing the umbilical stump and surrounding abdominal wall with an antiseptic solution, sterile towels are placed around the stump and a "circumcision drape" placed with the hole over the stump. The cord stump is then grasped at the base with a gauze sponge and the stump of cord is cut to within about one and one-half centimeters of the abdominal wall with a scissors or surgical knife blade. The exposed vessels are identified—a thin-walled oval vein and two smaller, thick-walled round arteries with tightly constricted lumens.

The lumen of the vessel to be used is gently dilated with a curved eye dressing

forcep or small obturator. The catheter is then inserted and gently advanced. Obstruction at the level of the abdominal wall may be relieved by gentle traction on the umbilical cord stump accompanied by steady but gentle pressure for about 30 seconds. If an umbilical vein catheterization is performed, the next site of obstruction is the portal system (the catheter meets resistance several centimeters before the distance marked on the catheter is reached). The catheter should be withdrawn several centimeters, gently rotated, and reinserted in an attempt to get the tip through the ductus venosus into the inferior vena cava. Occasionally, it will not be possible to get the catheter into the inferior vena cava for anatomical reasons, and vigorous attempts to advance the catheter are to be avoided. If an umbilical artery catheterization is performed, obstruction may occur at the level of the bladder. It may be overcome by gentle, steady pressure for 30 seconds. If not successful, 0.1 to 0.2 ml. of 2 per cent lidocaine (*without epinephrine*) can be injected via the catheter (remove the catheter first to add lidocaine to the tip of the catheter) to relieve the vasospasm. If unsuccessful, the other artery should be used. If the leg on the side of catheterization blanches, the catheter should be removed immediately and the other umbilical artery used.

An umbilical vessel catheter should be tied in place with a silk suture around vessel and catheter and sutured to the umbilical stump or taped to the abdominal wall. *Disastrous hemorrhage can occur if the catheter is inadvertently pulled out or the stopcocks are disconnected by the activity of the infant.* The position of the catheter must be identified by X-ray immediately after insertion.

If the X-ray after umbilical vessel catheterization indicates that the catheter has been inserted too far, it may be gently withdrawn an estimated amount for appropriate placement. If the catheter is not in far enough, it must be completely withdrawn and a new sterile one inserted after appropriately preparing the area again with antiseptic solutions, and so forth.

When no longer needed, the catheter should be removed using sterile technique and the vessel tied off with a silk suture (3-0 or 4-0).

The policy in our department is not to use the umbilical vein for either sampling or infusions unless a peripheral vein is simply unobtainable or urgency demands immediate access to a venous site. While we would agree with the risks of umbilical artery

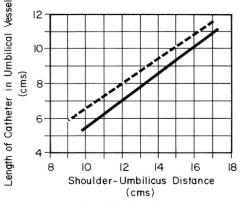

Figure 1–7 Determination of length of catheter to be inserted for appropriate arterial or venous placement. The length of the catheter read from the diagram is to the umbilical ring; the length of the umbilical cord stump present must be added. The shoulder-umbilicus distance is the perpendicular distance between parallel lines at the level of the umbilicus and through the distal ends of the clavicles. (Adapted from data of Dunn.[29])

sampling, the incidence of complications is proportional also to the experience of the operator, and units in which the most inexperienced house offier is responsible for the procedure will, of necessity, carry a much higher incidence of such occurrences. Reports of these complications, therefore, have only a limited value. All of them can be imagined without having to have them described. The use of multiple peripheral arterial punctures (i.e., radial, temporal, and brachial) in the hands of skilled personnel has proved useful, particularly where long-term sampling is not required and several early determinations may suffice. In the final analysis, this procedure, like any other, may be weighed for its risk/benefit ratio (i.e., is the information to be obtained of such value that it will exceed the risk of complications from the procedure itself?).

L. STERN

PRACTICAL HINTS

1. *All* newborn infants have some degree of respiratory acidosis and hypoxia at birth.

2. The asphyxiated newborn infant has more profound hypoxia and respiratory acidosis. An additional metabolic acidosis may be found if asphyxia has been present for a short time. These infants may also be hypothermic and require warming.

3. The resuscitation of the asphyxiated newborn must include both ventilatory (pCO_2, pO_2, and mechanical effect of inflation of the lung) and metabolic (bicarbonate) correction. In some infants, metabolic resuscitation should be started *as promptly* as ventilatory resuscitation.

4. Acidosis cannot be diagnosed clinically and must be suspected in any infant with a history of asphyxia.

5. Newborn infants may have cardiorespiratory problems because of asphyxia, maternal drugs (anesthesia, reserpine, etc.), intrathoracic disease (pneumothorax, diaphragmatic hernia, or paralysis, etc.), anemia, hypotension, hypoglycemia, etc. The reason should be sought.

6. Stimulating drugs (caffeine, etc.) do not have a place in the treatment of asphyxia; however, antidotes should be considered (e.g., nalline for overdose of morphine).

7. Umbilical arterial catheters are not without morbidity and should be used only when deemed clinically necessary.

CASE PROBLEMS

The clinical relevance of this information can best be understood by the following case ex- amples and the questions they raise. The answer to each question follows immediately after the question, but we encourage the reader to think out his own answers before reading the answer.

Case One

E. A., an 1800-gm. male infant, was delivered after a 38-week gestation. The fetal heart rate varied widely (40 to 110 beats per minute) 30 minutes prior to delivery. The amniotic fluid was heavily meconium-stained. At the age of one minute, the infant was noted to be limp, cyanotic, with a pulse rate of 84 per minute, making no spontaneous effort to breathe, and unresponsive to stimuli. The rectal temperature was 38°C. The one-minute Apgar score was 2. At the age of two minutes, the pulse was 40 per minute, with no respirations.

How would you now proceed to establish respiration?

With a birth weight of 1800 gm. at 38 weeks, this infant is small-for-gestational-age. (The antenatal diagnosis might have been made by lag in fundal growth and a fall in maternal estrogen output.) Under these circumstances, prolonged labor, difficult delivery, or excessive sedation must be avoided, as the small-for-dates infants are particularly prone to perinatal asphyxia. As there was fetal distress, evidenced both by a fall in fetal heart rate and the passage of meconium prior to delivery, the problem should have been anticipated and a person skilled in resuscitation of the newborn present at the delivery. Fetal scalp sampling might also have indicated this problem. Low Apgar scores are correlated with metabolic acidosis, which requires early correction. This, together with the fall in pulse rate from 84 to 40 beats per minute and apnea, is urgent indication for resuscitation as follows:

(a) Clear the upper airway by a short period of gentle suction with direct vision of pharynx and larynx. (b) Establish adequate ventilation with oxygen by positive pressure, either with mask and bag, or preferably with endotracheal tube. If there is no immediate response to mask and bag ventilation, then an endotracheal tube should be passed and positive-pressure ventilation carried out in this manner. (c) With the heart rate only 40 beats per minute, after ventilating the lungs a few times, closed chest cardiac massage should be commenced. (d) An umbilical venous catheter should be inserted and 3 to 4 mEq. per Kg. of sodium bicarbonate, diluted with equal parts of sterile water, should be administered over a one-minute period. (e) Heat loss should be minimized during resuscitation by keeping the infant warm and dry. Attempt to maintain the skin temperature between 36 and 36.5° C.

Once respiration has been established and the circulation restored, the infant can be further assessed. The small-for-gestational-age infant is likely to develop hypoglycemia, and the blood sugar should be monitored. Blood gases, an X-ray of the chest, and a hematocrit are necessary in the further management of this infant.

What is the significance of the 38° C temperature?

An elevated temperature, 38° C within the first two minutes of life, further indicates uteroplacental insufficiency during the latter stages of labor. Under normal circumstances the placenta acts as a heat exchanger, and if there is any interference in placental blood flow, the infant is unable to dissipate the heat he produces; hence, there will be a rise in body temperature. As there is frequently marked vasoconstriction and poor peripheral circulation associated with severe asphyxia, these infants lose heat at a slightly slower rate after delivery. (The elevated temperature does not mean infection.) This is usually not observed because rectal temperatures are rarely taken so quickly after birth. It should be emphasized that asphyxiated infants have a lower body temperature at one hour when compared with normal infants (see page 59 and Figure 4–1).

Should this infant receive antibiotics?

Although he required resuscitation and an umbilical venous catheter, there is no evidence that he is infected. The risks of infection following these procedures are admittedly slightly increased, but unless he aspirated meconium and has evidence of an aspiration pneumonia, antibiotic therapy is probably not indicated.

Was this infant in primary or secondary apnea?

In attempting to determine whether the infant was in primary or secondary apnea, the history of whether the infant cried or breathed before becoming apneic is obviously impor-

tant. If either of these took place, it is primary apnea. In this case, there is no indication of this having taken place, and it is the events during the recovery which will aid in arriving at the diagnosis. If the color is restored before the onset of breathing, then the infant is usually in secondary apnea. On the other hand, if gasping commences quickly before the onset of the improvement in color, then the infant is in primary apnea. A number of infants in primary apnea will commence gasping while preparation is being made to start the resuscitation with the initial handling, suction, or oxygen blowing over their faces. In primary apnea, the heart rate and blood pressure are maintained, and there is some muscle tone present. Although the vast majority of infants that require resuscitation will be in primary apnea, this infant was probably in secondary apnea.

What are the effects of analeptic drugs during secondary apnea?

There are absolutely no indications for the use of analeptic drugs during secondary apnea. They will have no effect in restoring normal ventilation and circulation. Once secondary apnea has occurred, it is only by assisted ventilation, re-establishment of the circulation, and/or resuscitation with bicarbonate that normal circulation and respiration can be established. Actually, analeptic drugs *may* increase the length of apnea and cause a further drop in blood pressure.

What is the relationship between the duration of asphyxia and the re-establishment of spontaneous respiration?

The duration of asphyxia prior to artificial ventilation appears to influence the re-establishment of gasping and spontaneous ventilation. For each minute after the last gasp that ventilation is delayed, there is a further delay of two minutes before gasping begins again, and four minutes before rhythmic breathing is established. Thus, the longer artificial ventilation is delayed during secondary apnea, the longer it will take to resuscitate the infant. (See Table 1–4.)

What factors prolong the interval until the last gasp?

Although there are a number of factors prolonging the interval until the last gasp, including the maintenance of pH, hypother-

TABLE 1-4 EFFECT OF DELAYING RESUSCITATION IN NEWBORN MONKEYS*

DURATION OF ASPHYXIA (MINUTES)	MINUTES OF ASSISTED VENTILATION BEFORE:	
	Gasping	Breathing
10.0	2.3	9.7
12.5	9.4	20.5
15.0	13.6	30.0

*Adapted from James.[42]

mia, and the administration of analgesic or anesthetic agents, only the maintenance of pH will protect against permanent cerebral damage. Cooling alone does not reinitiate gasping in secondary apnea, nor does it produce in the experimental animal a significant difference in time to the last gasp unless the cooling is initiated prior to the asphyxia.

What are the beneficial effects of alkali infusion?

The beneficial effects of correcting pH in addition to protecting against cerebral damage include: (a) increased myocardial responsiveness to sympathetic amines, (b) a fall in pulmonary vascular resistance with increased pulmonary blood flow, (c) correction, by the administration of bicarbonate, of the shift in the oxygen dissociation curve to the right with acidosis.

What are some of the sequelae that may be anticipated after asphyxia?

(a) Lungs—respiratory distress syndrome. (b) Heart—cardiomegaly and heart failure. (c) Kidney—anuria, hematuria, proteinuria. (d) Brain—cerebral edema; seizures; cerebral hemorrhage; tremulousness; irritability; intraventricular hemorrhage, particularly in premature infants, often 48 hours after a severe asphyxial episode. (e) The onset of disseminated intravascular coagulation. (f) Following severe asphyxia with any cellular damage there will be a rise in serum potassium. The serum sodium may be influenced by the renal status as well as the amount of sodium administered in the form of bicarbonate. The blood sugar rises during a period of asphyxia. (g) Traumatic purpura—the distribution will depend on the type of delivery; thus, there may be extensive purpura, bruising of legs after breech delivery, or facial purpura if the umbilical cord was tight around the neck. (h) Edema.

What prognostic significance does the onset of convulsions at the age of 12 hours have in an asphyxiated infant?

The etiology of the convulsions must be known in order to make a meaningful answer. A number of infants will have seizures following a severe asphyxial episode as a result of the ensuing cerebral edema. Provided that at the time of discharge from the hospital there are no neurologic deficits detectable, the prognosis for normal development neurologically is surprisingly excellent, irrespective of the symptomatology in the early neonatal period.

Case Two

A repeat cesarean section was performed on a well-controlled Caucasian diabetic at 38 weeks' gestation. The male infant, B. W., weighed 3900 gm. and at one minute was found to be hypotonic, making gasping respirations. His pulse rate was 120 per minute, and he was slightly cyanotic. The one-minute Apgar score was 5. There was some improvement when the airways were cleared and oxygen was administered. The heart rate remained 100 per minute and the respiratory rate at five minutes was 40 per minute. He remained slightly hypotonic and had a slightly pale color. At age 15 minutes, respirations were noted to be 60 per minute. He had gasping movements with the use of accessory muscles of respiration and his mouth opened with each respiration. The rectal temperature was 35° C. He had good air entry, with no cyanosis.

What investigations should be carried out immediately?

Factors predisposing to asphyxia in this case are diabetes and cesarean section. There is no information as to the type of anesthesia used for the cesarean section, which may also be a contributing factor. The Apgar is in the 4 to 7 range, so this infant is in no immediate danger. Significantly, his color is poor and he is using the accessory muscle of respiration with an open mouth, which indicates air hunger. The poor color may reflect poor peripheral circulation, or may be genuine pallor due to the anemia. Air hunger may be due to airway obstruction, but there is good air entry and no cyanosis at 15 minutes, so this is unlikely; it may be a result of lack of oxygen-carrying capacity. The urgent investigations required, therefore, include: (a) hematocrit, (b) blood pressure, and (c) blood gases, including pH, pO_2, pCO_2, and bicarbonate. A blood sugar is not necessarily indicated at this stage, as it is extremely unlikely that hypoglycemia is the cause of the above symptomatology. However, determination of the blood sugar by Dextrostix will be a useful base line in the further management of this infant. Chest X-ray is also required. In this infant, a diagnosis of anemia and hypotension was established. The hematocrit was 32 per cent and the blood pressure 30 mm. (Note: The blood pressure may be falsely high with acidosis. When this is corrected, vasodilation occurs and the pressure can fall precipitously. See pages 126 and 127.)

The anemia was partially corrected by the administration of whole blood, 10 to 15 ml. per Kg. at 30 minutes. While waiting for the blood to be collected, the circulation was supported with an infusion of normal saline (10 ml. per Kg.).

It is not uncommon for anemia to occur following cesarean section. Blood loss from the infant may occur if the placenta is incised. In addition, the infant does not get the full placental transfusion, because the normal gravitational effect is lost and the cord is often clamped before the first breath, before the transfusion from placenta to baby. Other features to be searched for in a full-term anemic infant include concealed hemorrhage, such as ruptured viscus (e.g., liver and/or spleen). If the etiology *cannot* be established, the mother should be studied for evidence of fetal-maternal bleeding.

Is gastric aspiration essential immediately after delivery by cesarean section?

Although it has been established that the gastric contents are greater following ce-

sarean section than vaginal delivery, it is not essential immediately to aspirate the stomach. It is important that the procedure be delayed until normal ventilation has been established; otherwise, apnea, bradycardia, and even cardiac arrest may be induced when an attempt is made to aspirate the stomach.

What methods should be used to maintain temperature during resuscitation?

The most important source of heat loss in the immediate neonatal period is evaporative. The infant should be dried and a source of heat thereafter should be available, either in the form of a radiant warmer or by placing the infant in a blower-warmed incubator as soon as possible. (Note how quickly this infant dropped his temperature after delivery.) If oxygen is required, it should be warmed and humidified.

At one hour, the infant appeared in no distress; however, *at three hours,* he was found to be retracting, grunting, tachypneic, and cyanotic, with poor air entry on auscultation, and a hyperinflated chest.

What investigations would you now perform?

At three hours, a new problem is now evident. There is definite evidence of respiratory distress, and the etiology of this requires urgent elucidation. In view of the fact that the chest is hyper-inflated, it is more than likely that this infant has either an aspiration syndrome or an aspiration syndrome complicated by pneumothorax. There are no predisposing features of pneumonia. This infant requires an urgent chest X-ray, a repeat hematocrit, a blood sugar, and blood gases in order to direct further management. (X-ray revealed a mild aspiration with right-sided pneumothorax.)

REFERENCES

1. Adamsons, K., Jr.: Brain damage in the fetus and newborn from hypoxia or asphyxia. *In* James, L., Myers, R., and Gaull, G., Eds.: *Report of 57th Ross Conference on Pediatric Research.* Columbus, Ross Laboratories, 1967, p. 75.
2. Adamsons, K., Jr., Behrman, R., Dawes, G., et al: The treatment of acidosis with alkali and glucose during asphyxia in foetal rhesus monkeys. J Physiol *169*:679, 1963.
3. Adamsons, K., Jr., Behrman, R., Dawes, G., et al: Resuscitation by positive pressure ventilation and tris-hydroxy-methylaminomethane of rhesus

monkeys asphyxiated at birth. J Pediat 65:807, 1964.

4. Andrews, B.: Amniotic fluid studies to determine fetal maturity. Pediat Clin N Amer 17:49, 1970.

5. Apgar, V.: A proposal for a new method of evaluation of the newborn infant. Anesth Analg 32:260, 1953.

6. Avery, M., and O'Doherty, N.: Effects of body-tilting on the resting end-expiratory position of newborn infants. Pediatrics 29:255, 1962.

7. Baker, D., Berdon, W., and James, L.: Proper localization of umbilical arterial and venous catheters by lateral roentgenograms. Pediatrics 43:34, 1969.

8. Beard, R., Morris, E., and Clayton, S.: pH of foetal capillary blood as an indicator of the condition of the fetus. J Obstet Gynaec Brit Comm 74:812, 1967.

9. Becker, R.: Learning ability after asphyxiation at birth, especially as it concerns the guinea pig. In Windle, W., Hinman, E., and Bailey, P., Eds.: Neurological and Psychological Deficits of Asphyxia Neonatorum. Springfield, Charles C Thomas, 1958, p. 44.

10. Behrman, R., Peterson, E., and deLannoy, C.: The supply of O_2 to the primate fetus with two different O_2 tensions and anesthetics. Resp Physiol 6:271, 1969.

11. Behrman, R., Lees, M., Peterson, E., et al: Distribution of the circulation in the normal and asphyxiated fetal primate. Amer J Obstet Gynec 108:956, 1970.

12. Bentrem, G., Perkins, P., and Waxman, B.: Newer methods of evaluating fetal maturity. Amer J Obstet Gynec 106:917, 1970.

13. Bloxsom, A.: Resuscitation of the newborn infant. J Pediat 37:311, 1950.

14. Campbell, A., Cross, K., Dawes, G., et al: A comparison of air and O_2, in a hyperbaric chamber or by positive pressure ventilation, in the resuscitation of newborn rabbits. J Pediat 68:153, 1966.

15. Campbell, S. and Newman, G.: Growth of the fetal biparietal diameter during normal pregnancy. J Obstet Gynaec Brit Comm 78:513, 1971.

16. Chang, L., Woesner, M., Nakamato, M., et al: Device to estimate fetal age. Obstet Gynec 38:154, 1971.

17. Clements, J., Platzker, A., Tierney, D., et al: Assessment of the risk of the respiratory distress syndrome by a rapid test for surfactant in amniotic fluid. New Eng J Med 286:1077, 1972.

18. Cordero, L., Jr. and Hon, E.: Neonatal bradycardia following nasopharyngeal stimulation. J Pediat 78:441, 1971.

19. Corner, G., and Anderson, G.: Asphyxia of the human fetus in relation to brain damage. In Windle, W., Hinman, E., and Bailey, P., Eds.: Neurological and Psychological Deficits of Asphyxia Neonatorum. Springfield, Charles C Thomas, 1958, p. 173.

20. Cross, K., and Roberts, P.: Asphyxia neonatorum treated by electrical stimulation of the phrenic nerve. Brit Med J 1:1043, 1951.

21. Daily, W., and Northway, W., Jr.: Perspectives in mechanical ventilation of the newborn. Advances Pediat 18:253, 1971.

22. Daniel, P., Love, E., Moorehouse, S., et al: Factors influencing utilization of ketone-bodies by brain in normal rats and rats with ketoacidosis. Lancet 11:637, 1971.

23. Daniel, S., Dawes, G., James, L., et al: Analeptics and the resuscitation of asphyxiated monkeys. Brit Med J 2:562, 1966.

24. Daniel, S., Dawes, G., James, L., et al: Hypothermia and the resuscitation of asphyxiated monkeys. J Pediat 68:45, 1966.

25. Dawes, G.: Foetal and Neonatal Physiology. Chicago, Year Book Medical Publishers, 1968.

26. Dawes, G., Hibbard, E., and Windle, W.: The effect of alkali and glucose infusion on permanent brain damage in rhesus monkeys asphyxiated at birth. J Pediat 65:801, 1964.

27. Drage, J., and Berendes, H.: Apgar scores and outcome of the newborn. Pediat Clin N Amer 13:635, 1966.

28. Drahota, Z., Hahn, P., Mourek, J., et al: The effect of aceto-acetate on oxygen consumption of brain slices from infant and adult rats. Physiol Bohemoslov 14:134, 1965.

29. Dunn, P.: Localization of the umbilical catheter by post-mortem measurement. Arch Dis Child 41:69. 1966.

30. Elsner, R.: Diving bradycardia in the unrestrained hippopotamus. Nature 212:408, 1966.

31. Elsner, R., Kenney, D., and Burgess, K.: Diving bradycardia in the trained dolphin. Nature 212: 407, 1966.

32. Eve, F.: Artificial circulation produced by rocking. Brit Med J 2:295, 1947.

33. Fisher, D., Paton, J., Mangurten, H., et al: The effect of phenobarbital on asphyxia of the newborn monkey. Pediat Res 5:415, 1971.

34. Flagg, P.: Treatment of asphyxia in the newborn. JAMA 91:788, 1928.

35. Friedman, A., Abellera, R., Lidksy, I., et al: Perforation of the colon after exchange transfusion in the newborn. New Eng J Med 282:796, 1970.

36. Gold, E.: Identification of the high-risk fetus. Clin Obstet Gynec 11:1069, 1968.

37. Greene, J., Jr., and Beargie, R.: The use of urinary estriol excretion studies in the assessment of the high-risk pregnancy. Pediat Clin N Amer 17: 43, 1970.

38. Greene, J., Jr., and Tweeddale, D.: Endocrine indices of fetal environment. Clin Obstet Gynec 11: 1106, 1968.

39. Hamilton, L., and Behrman, R.: Intra-amniotic infusion of bicarbonate in the treatment of human fetal acidosis. Amer J Obstet Gynec 112:834, 1972.

40. Hawkins, R., Williamson, D., and Krebs, H.: Ketone-body utilization by adult and suckling rat brain in vivo. Biochem J 122:13, 1971.

41. James, L.: In Biochemical aspects of asphyxia at birth. Ross Conf Pediat Res 31:66, 1959.

42. James, L.: Onset of breathing and resuscitation. J Pediat 65:807, 1964.

43. James, L., Apgar, V., Burnard, E., et al: Intragastric oxygen and resuscitation of the newborn. Acta Paed Scand 52:245, 1963.

44. Jilek, L., Travnickova, E., and Trojan, S.: Characteristic metabolic and functional responses to oxygen deficiency in the central nervous system. In Stave, U., Ed.: Physiology of the Perinatal Period. New York, Appleton-Century-Crofts, 1970.

45. Johnson, G., Kirschbaum, T., Brinkman, C., III, et al:

Effects of acid base and hypertonicity on fetal and neonatal cardiovascular hemodynamics. Amer J Physiol *220*:1798, 1971.

46. Kitterman, J., Phibbs, R., and Tooley, W.: Catheterization of umbilical vessels in newborn infants. Pediat Clin N Amer *17*:895, 1970.

47. Kreiselman, J.: An improved apparatus for treating asphyxia of the newborn infant. Amer J Obstet Gynec *39*:888, 1940.

48. Kreiselman, J., Kane, H., and Swope, R.: A new apparatus for resuscitation of asphyxiated newborn babies. Amer J Obstet Gynec *15*:552, 1928.

49. Larroche, J.: Umbilical catheterization: its complications. Biol Neonat *16*:101, 1970.

50. Lee, B., Major, F., and Weingold, A.: Ultrasonic determination of fetal maturity at repeat cesarian section. Obstet Gynec *38*:294, 1971.

51. Lilien, A.: Term intrapartum fetal death. Amer J Obstet Gynec *107*:595, 1970.

52. Lindberg, R.: *In* Brain damage in the fetus and newborn from hypoxia or asphyxia. James, L., Myers, R., and Gaull, G., Eds.: *Report of the 57th Ross Conference on Pediatric Research.* Columbus, Ross Laboratories, 1967, p. 12.

53. Merenstein, G., and Blackmon, L.: *Care of the High Risk Newborn.* San Francisco, Children's Hospital, 1971.

54. Millen, R., Rowson, A., and Mayberger, H.: Prevention of neonatal asphyxia with the use of a rocking respirator. Amer J Obstet Gynec *70*:1087, 1955.

55. Miller, J.: New approaches to preventing brain damage during asphyxia. Amer J Obstet Gynec *110*:1125, 1971.

56. Moya, F., James, L., Burnard, E., et al: Cardiac massage in the newborn infant through the intact chest. Amer J Obstet Gynec *84*:798, 1962.

57. Owen, O., Morgan, A., Kemp, H., et al: Brain metabolism during fasting. J Clin Invest *46*:1589, 1967.

58. Ranck, J., Jr., and Windle, W.: Brain damage in the monkey, Macaca mulatta, by asphyxia neonatorum. Exp Neurol *1*:130, 1959.

59. Resuscitation of newborn infants. Obstet Gynec *8*:336, 1956.

60. Reynolds, J.: Assessment of fetal health by analysis of maternal steroids. J Pediat *76*:464, 1970.

61. Richter, D.: *In* Brain damage in the fetus and newborn from hypoxia or asphyxia. James, L., Meyers, R., and Gaull, G., Eds.: *Report of the 57th Ross Conference on Pediatric Research.* Columbus, Ross Laboratories, 1967, p. 56.

62. Saling, E.: A new method of safe-guarding the life of the foetus before and during labor. J Internat Fed Gynec Obstet *3*:100, 1965.

63. Sarrut, S., Alain, J., et Alison, F.: Les complications précoces de la perfusion par la veine ombilicale chez le prématuré. Arch Franc Pediat *26*:651, 1969.

64. Scholander, P.: The master switch of life. Sci Amer *209*:92, 1963.

65. Scott, J.: Iatrogenic lesions in babies following umbilical vein catheterization. Arch Dis Child *40*:426, 1965.

66. Seeds, A.: Adverse effects on the fetus of acute events in labor. Pediat Clin N Amer *17*:811, 1971.

67. Seeds, A., and Behrman, R.: Acid-base monitoring of the fetus during labor with blood obtained from the scalp. J Pediat *74*:804, 1969.

68. Seeds, A., Bissonnette, J., Lim, H., et al: Changes in rhesus monkey fetal and maternal acid-base measurements following amniotic fluid bicarbonate or tris infusion. Amer J Obstet Gynec *107*:232, 1970.

69. Sloviter, H., Shimkin, P., and Suhara, K.: Glycerol as a substrate for brain metabolism. Nature *210*:1334, 1966.

70. Stave, U., and Wolf, H.: Metabolic effects in hypoxia neonatorum. *In* Stave, U., Ed.: *Physiology of the Perinatal Period.* New York, Appleton-Century-Crofts, 1970.

Chapter 2

ANTICIPATION, RECOGNITION, AND TRANSITIONAL CARE OF THE HIGH-RISK INFANT

by
ARNOLD J. RUDOLPH, M.B.

"Everything ought to be done to ensure that an infant be born at term, well-developed, and in a healthy condition. But in spite of every care, infants are born prematurely...."

PIERRE BUDIN, *The Nursling*

Appraisal of the newborn infant, just as in older children, requires a knowledge of the history of the infant. It must be remembered that he *does* have a past history, for he is not really "new" but only newly born. One cannot stress sufficiently the importance of this past history (that is, the maternal history, prior to conception and throughout the pregnancy; the course of labor and delivery; and any signs of fetal distress), because the infant will, on examination, reflect the sum total of his genetic and environmental past and the minor or major insults to which he has been subjected.

Normal development of the fetus is threatened by a myriad of factors, both singly and in combination. Maternal complications (obstetrical factors) play a threatening role, but of greater importance are the environmental factors (unfavorable social conditions, nutritional deficits, etc.). An interaction between many of these factors occurs and adversely affects the perinatal mortality rate and the quality of survivors. Such factors have resulted in the identification of high-risk pregnancies and high-risk infants.

A high-risk pregnancy is one in which the fetus has a significantly increased chance of death, either before or after birth, or later disability. Some fetuses may be damaged early, others late; many infants will be born prematurely or they may be unusually small for their gestational age. A few will be too large or will have remained in utero too long. Each situation has its special hazards. The high-risk infant is thus one, regardless of gestational age or birth weight, whose extrauterine existence is compromised by a number of factors (prenatal, natal, or postnatal), and who is in need of special medical care.

ANTICIPATION AND RECOGNITION OF HIGH-RISK FACTORS

The list of medical and obstetrical problems of pregnancy, labor, and delivery known to affect the infant, and problems in the infant per se making him high risk, is lengthy (Appendix 4).

A patient may make her first prenatal visit soon after she misses a period. It is becoming increasingly apparent, however, that by the time pregnancy has been confirmed, the fetus has already passed the most critical period in its development. If anything is to be done to influence the events in the pre- or peri-conceptional period, probably the most dangerous time in any individual's lifetime, it must be done before rather than after the woman thinks she is pregnant. Under these circumstances, it becomes advisable to have patients see their doctor before they expect to start a pregnancy.

PRECONCEPTIONAL VISIT

The physician has an excellent opportunity in a pre-conceptional visit for discussion and counseling the aspiring mother. The mother has certain intrinsic attributes, such as her age, stature, nutritional status, immunologic make-up (Rh and ABO factors), and past obstetric performance. These tend to be unchangeable and may to some extent be influenced by the extrinsic features of her socioeconomic level. The interaction of all of these factors has a definite influence on the course of pregnancy, labor, and delivery. In general, a healthy woman will have the lowest risk of pregnancy problems and adverse outcomes.

Past illnesses can be discussed and the physician can become aware of unfavorable factors in the family history, such as diabetes or congenital abnormalities. Occasionally, abnormalities which might or might not influence the course of a pregnancy will make further investigation desirable. It is usually better to carry out such investigations before rather than after conception has taken place. The physician can check on immunizations in the mother and previous illnesses, such as rubella, syphilis, etc.

The prospective mother should be given advice about the importance of an adequate diet and the effects of smoking (pregnant women who smoke give birth to smaller babies). Nutritional state and general health are greatly influenced by the level of indigency, educational background (ignorance of a balanced diet), and ethnic eating habits. There are no conclusive reports on the effect of chronic malnutrition in the mother as a single factor on the fetus, but it is known that malnutrition in the fetus does have an effect on tissue replication and growth, especially brain tissue.

The fetal and neonatal hazards of maternal medication should be discussed. All drugs may be teratogenic and there seems to be no satisfactory way of determining which ones are safe; therefore, obstetricians have retreated into a position approaching therapeutic nihilism. Such a policy may indeed be a wise one, since in several reported studies the average woman takes between 4 and 10 different drugs during pregnancy, with the consequence that now the fetus is potentially at greater risk from well-intentioned medicaments than from the vicissitudes of pregnancy and delivery.

The noxious effects of therapeutic drugs taken during pregnancy range from fetal death to various types of malformations involving different organ systems with varying degrees of severity (Appendix 7). Many of these drugs may influence profoundly the developmental processes in the fetus and newborn.

The newborn infant's response to drugs may not only be a quantitative difference but also a profound qualitative difference. These differences are even more striking when one considers the developing embryo. During the first weeks of embryonic development, characterized by a period of rapid cell division and differentiation of organ systems, drugs such as thalidomide, aminopterin, and others may result in complete disruption of the embryo or a nonlethal aberration producing a congenital defect. These agents may be relatively benign in their effects on the older fetus.

Other factors to be considered in the effects of maternal medication on the fetus and newborn are the distribution, metabolism, and excretion of the drug. Permeability of the blood-brain barrier to pharmacologic agents is generally greater in the neonate than in the adult. For example, the neonate has an increased sensitivity to morphine, which readily traverses the immature blood-brain barrier of the neonate and attains concentrations three to four times greater than those in adults given comparable doses. Barbiturates penetrate the unmyelinated white matter of the neonatal brain more rapidly than they penetrate the gray matter and produce much longer sleeping times in neonatal than in adult animals given equal doses per unit of body weight.

At birth, there is significant limitation of the activity of drug-metabolizing enzymes (located primarily in the liver) which convert drugs into products which are generally less active or toxic than the parent compounds. Studies have also shown impaired capacity in infants for conjugation of chloramphenicol, acetylation of sulfonamides, and other effects. Excretion regulates the actual removal of an unchanged drug and its metabolites from the body, mainly in urine and feces. As the glomerular filtration rate of the immature newborn is 30 to 40 per cent of that in the adult, drugs and their metabolites are removed more slowly and can achieve higher tissue levels. This limited excretory function has significant clinical implications. In newborns less than 48 hours of age, tetracycline, streptomycin, kanamycin, chloramphenicol, ampicillin, penicillin, methicillin, colistin and cephaloridine have extremely long plasma half-lives and may readily accumulate to reach toxic levels if dosage regimens are not altered. The limited excretory function can also serve as a positive therapeutic function. For example, small doses of penicillin G, the least toxic of the penicillins, can be given every 12 hours to the newborn and will still provide drug levels which are effective in combating infection.

The pre-pregnancy visit provides an opportunity to inquire into the patient's drug usage, regular or sporadic, and to advise discontinuing all but the essential drugs. While much has been written about the teratogenic effects of many drugs, until recently little attention has been paid to fetal hazards from environmental pollution with certain nonessential trace elements, such as mercury and lead. Minamata Bay disease is an example of mercury contamination in which pregnant women give birth to infants with congenital neurologic problems.

PRENATAL CARE

During the course of prenatal examination, the first warning signs of fetal danger invariably occur. Complications of pregnancy known to be associated with fetal risk can be identified in prenatal visits. During pregnancy, the mother may suffer from acute medical illnesses (infections, toxemia, drug addiction) and obstetric problems (acute bleeding, premature labor) that may affect the fetus.

Infections known to influence the fetus and newborn are rubella (German measles), syphilis, gonorrhea, toxoplasmosis, cytomega-lovirus disease, genital herpes, and others (see page 211).

The chronically ill mother presents other problems. Chronic kidney disease, for example, is associated with vascular insufficiency and hence inadequate uterine arterial blood flow, and the mother may give birth to an infant with an intrauterine growth retardation. The mother with congenital heart disease may present similar problems. Maternal diabetes, subjecting the fetus to an abnormal metabolic environment, also creates problems for the fetus.

Fetal factors require consideration. These include the undesirable effects of multiple births, including twin-to-twin (feto-fetal) transfusion syndrome and discrepancy in size of twins; abnormalities in presentation; and cord anomalies.

Recently, lack of prenatal care has been shown to be the single most important factor predisposing to serious illness in low-birth-weight infants during the first nine months of life. Hence, lack of prenatal care would appear to continue to affect the infant following labor and delivery.

It has been shown that intensive inpatient prenatal care applied to high-risk cases pays good dividends. Efficiently organized prenatal care remains the mainstay of successful reproduction. During the last decade, it has been supplemented by a more direct approach, in selected cases, to what has come to be known as the "feto-maternal unit," by which is meant the placenta, the amniotic fluid, and the fetus. The emphasis in medical care of the newborn has been on instituting aggressive action at the birth of the infant. The events preceding the delivery are equally important. In fact, the product delivered — the infant — is probably more influenced by factors present during its in utero development than by those during delivery. For example, a malnourished mother or one with hypertension during pregnancy can give rise to a small-for-dates infant; the mother exposed to teratogens or infectious agents may give birth to an infant with abnormalities; and the uncontrolled diabetic mother may have a stillborn infant. The course of neonatal events rests in great measure on antepartum factors, and, in some instances no amount of effort or expertise in neonatal management can alter these undesirable outcomes. The pediatrician, no matter how proficient, can make only limited progress in further reducing perinatal loss unless presented with a healthier infant.

The emphasis of obstetric teaching, practice, and research has thus increasingly been directed toward securing the fetal welfare by increased antenatal care and the application of intrauterine diagnosis in selected cases.

APPROACHES TO FETAL ASSESSMENT

The mainstay of intrauterine diagnosis is the study of the feto-maternal unit, and there is now a rapidly growing battery of investigations under review or in active clinical use (Appendix 2).

Recognition of the importance of the placenta in relation to fetal functions made a study of placental function a priority. In the early 1950s, it was shown that reduced excretion of pregnanediol in the maternal urine was associated with defective placental function and increased incidence of fetal hypoxia (distress). At the present time, estriol, another metabolite of placental and fetal origin, is more commonly assayed; it has proved useful as a means of detecting placental dysfunction once the fetal risk factor is originally identified during prenatal care. Serial levels are principally indicative of fetal well-being. Sudden drops or disappearance of urinary estriol previously present in serial samples is an ominous sign for the fetus. Recent reports suggest that enzyme assays can give information about placental damage and dysfunction in much the same way that enzyme studies are used to indicate damage to cardiac or hepatic tissue.

The amniotic fluid which is obtained by amniocentesis during pregnancy has been increasingly studied during the last decade. It was originally examined for bilirubin in suspected cases of Rh hemolytic disease, as a guide to the severity of the hemolytic process. Amniotic fluid can be obtained as early as the 12th to 14th week of gestation and reflects extensive metabolic processes, primarily of the fetus but also of the placenta and mother. It is now also examined for many other substances of fetal origin, including creatinine, urea, meconium, and cells from the fetal skin. As the fetus matures, increasing amounts of urea and creatinine are excreted from its kidneys, and increasing numbers of squamous cells are shed from its skin. Estimation of these substances and cells provides information about the maturity of the fetus.

Rising concentrations of creatinine during gestation can be correlated with fetal gestational age. Creatinine concentrations less than 1.8 mg. per 100 ml. occur prior to the 36th week and greater than 1.8 mg. per 100 ml. after the 36th week of gestation. The reason for this increase has been explained variously as being due to maturing kidney function or decreasing amniotic fluid volume, or that it reflects the increasing muscle mass.

Good correlation with pulmonary maturity is seen in the sudden increase at 35 to 36 weeks' gestation of the lecithin to sphingomyelin ratio in the amniotic fluid. This increased ratio indicates pulmonary maturity, as the saturated lecithins and related phospholipids arise principally from the fetal lung.

Fetal cells found in the amniotic fluid can be examined directly for Barr bodies for sex determination. They may be cultured for chromosomes, and more refined studies can be carried out for the identification of genetic and metabolic errors in the unborn fetus. If fetal cells in amniotic fluid are stained with Nile blue sulfate (viable cells stain orange), gestational age can be determined. Prior to 34 weeks' gestation, the number of orange-stained cells in amniotic fluid is less than one per cent; between 34 and 38 weeks, one to 10 per cent; between 38 and 40 weeks, 10 to 50 per cent; beyond 40 weeks, over 50 per cent. Biopsies of fetal skin stained with Nile blue sulfate suggest histologically that orange-stained cells in amniotic fluid originate from fetal sebaceous glands. Their presence in large numbers reflects the functional maturity of these glands.

In later pregnancy, the fluid can be visually inspected by amnioscopy. With this technique the fluid is visualized through intact membranes and, if meconium is seen, fetal distress is diagnosed and action taken to deliver the infant. Amnioscopy can also be used to obtain fetal scalp blood samples during labor, and the prevailing pH level gives a direct indication of the status of the fetus. A pH of 7.2 or less strongly suggests fetal distress.

In recent years, a variety of electronic techniques have been developed to assess the fetal heart rate during labor. These include electrocardiography, phonocardiography, and the application of the Doppler principle to record fetal heart action. The latter method is now being used most extensively. By using simultaneous recording of the fetal heart rate and uterine contraction waves, it is possible to see how the fetal heart behaves during and after uterine contractions; significant abnormalities have now been identified and assessed against other investigations. It is currently considered that simultaneous fetal heart and uterine contraction records can best provide early information about impending distress in labor. Currently, in many centers, labor in high-risk cases is being continuously monitored in intensive care units set aside especially for this purpose.

During the last decade, examination of the fetus itself has been greatly enhanced by ultrasonic scanning, which is used to measure the diameters of the fetal skull (biparietal diameter). This enables obstetricians to estimate the fetal maturity at the time of the examination or, in serial observations, to assess the rate of fetal growth. The objective examination of maturity and fetal growth provided by this technique is proving accurate, and therefore of the greatest value in clinical management, as fetal size can be estimated in utero with virtually no danger to the fetus. Ultrasonography has also been of value in localization of the placenta, diagnosis of multiple pregnancy, and the diagnosis of fetal abnormalities.

The dangers of radiation dictate that examination by X-ray to determine fetal size should be discouraged. The classic approach is to X-ray the fetus for ossification centers in distal femoral and proximal tibial epiphyses. The radiologic presence of the distal femoral epiphysis generally occurs at 36 weeks' gestation and that of the proximal tibial epiphysis at 38 weeks' gestation. However, the gestational age of the fetus can be predicted accurately only to within a range of plus or minus seven weeks, and infants with intrauterine growth retardation may have absent or markedly smaller epiphyses than normal.

A recent approach to diagnosis of gestational age is with the intra-amniotic injection of radiopaque iodized lipid (ethyliodophenylundecylate). This compound dissolves in vernix and thus outlines the fetal skin on X-ray prior to 38 weeks' gestation; from 38 to 40 weeks' gestation, limbs and abdomen are patchily outlined; after 40 weeks, only the back and head are visible. This procedure is based on the natural history of the vernix, which covers the fetus from about the 20th to 38th week; beyond the 38th week, the vernix begins to disappear and by term it usually is absent.

TRANSITION

Birth is an obligatory exchange of environments, and with the dynamic changes occurring during this transition, the signs of disease are frequently difficult to differentiate from the rapidly changing signs that accompany these physiologic adjustments. Every infant, whether sick or well, mature or immature, must pass through a process of transition if he is to survive and adapt successfully to extrauterine life.

Transition to extrauterine life is a complex process. It encompasses, first, *changes in function* of organ systems (onset of respiration, changeover of fetal to neonatal circulation with change in cardiovascular hemodynamics, alterations of hepatic and renal functions, and clearance of meconium from the bowel). Secondly, there is a *reorganization of metabolic processes* to achieve a new steady state or postnatal homeostasis. These processes include enzyme induction, increase in blood oxygen saturation, decrease in postnatal acidosis, and a recovery of neural tissues following the intense input of stimuli from labor and delivery.

Only after *changes in function and reorganization* are progressing satisfactorily will the infant be able to proceed with his primary task — that of growth and development. For most infants, transition is so smooth as to appear superficially uneventful; for some, transition is delayed or complicated, and for a small percentage of infants, transition is never achieved.

The marked individual differences in clinical behavior may be related to a wide range of prenatal and natal influences which do not cease to function at the infant's birth but remain to modify the complex adaptation from intrauterine to extrauterine life (Figure 2–1). Adequate evaluation of the infant's condition must take into consideration all factors which determine the success of neonatal adjustments. These include:

1. *The state of maturity at the time of birth* — length of gestation is a factor of vital importance, since it determines the state of maturation (anatomic and physiologic) reached by the fetus in preparation for the exigencies of birth.

2. *The inherent vitality* — how perfect the infant is at birth as the result of his past history.

   a. Congenital anomalies

   b. Results of adverse conditions of

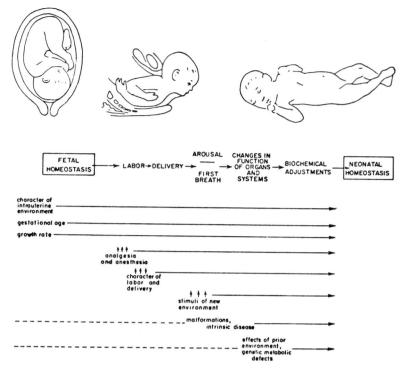

Figure 2–1 The course of events ensuing between fetal homeostasis and neonatal homeostasis. Factors influencing the sequence are shown in the lower portion of the diagram.[13]

fetal environment due to maternal infections, medications, metabolic disorders, and/or dietary deficiencies.

3. *The degree to which pathologic processes interfere with the normal course of events.*

    a. Those which are the direct result of the birth process include: pure trauma—fractured clavicle, etc., intracranial hemorrhage; anoxia from various causes—drugs, anesthesia, placenta previa, abruptio placentae

    b. Those due to pathologic variations of certain physiologic peculiarities of the newborn—tetany, jaundice, hypoglycemia, hemorrhagic disease of the newborn, breast enlargement, infants of diabetic mothers

    c. Those due to postnatal hazards—e.g., infections.

In many cases, two or all three of these factors are involved—for example, the premature infant who acquires infection postnatally, or the premature infant whose inherent vitality has been adversely affected by maternal health factors.

REACTION OF THE INFANT TO DELIVERY

As labor progresses, the biochemical milieu undergoes progressive change and sensory input to the fetus increases (e.g., amniotomy, oxytocic stimulation of labor, forceps application, fundal pressure, varying methods of delivery, and various agents administered to the mother, such as drugs, anesthetics, glucose, and hyperventilation).

The stimuli of labor are reinforced by the avalanche of new stimuli encountered immediately upon emergence of the infant from an intrauterine existence (dark, warm, and watery, where there was minimal sensory stimulation, and respiration and nutrition were performed by the maternal organism) into a new environment in which the medium is air, temperatures are unstable, sensory stimuli are increased and constant, and the physiologic functions of respiration and nutrition must be performed by him. The sum of the stimuli causes a massive sympathetic reaction.

These changes are reflected in the changes in fetal and neonatal heart rate at the time of delivery. In vigorous high-Apgar-score term infants at the end of labor, the fetal heart rate fluctuates around a base-line rate with a rapid return to this base line after either tachy-cardia or bradycardia. These wide swings mirror the intensity of the input reaching the fetus at the end of labor and the rapidity of his response to these stimuli. Following delivery there is an abrupt increase in heart rate. For a short time, oscillations occur around a higher base line, then the rate begins to fall irregularly.

In infants with a suboptimal response to delivery and low one-minute Apgar scores, the heart rates may remain at an extremely low or extremely high level and do not return promptly to base-line heart rate levels after the wide oscillations. The inability to return to base-line rate constitutes an autonomic imbalance.

On delivery, if the infant is vigorous and reactive to the experience of being born, a characteristic series of changes in vital signs and clinical appearance takes place. These include a first period of reactivity, a relatively unresponsive interval, and a second period of reactivity (Figure 2–2).

In the first 15 to 30 minutes of life (first period of reactivity), the infant exhibits changes which are at first predominantly sympathetic, including tachycardia (mean peak heart rate of 180 beats per minute occurs at three minutes of age), with some lability of the heart rate and irregular respirations (peak 60 to 90 minutes), transient rales, grunting, flaring of the alae nasi and retraction of the chest, a falling body temperature, increased tonus, and alerting exploratory behavior.* Brief periods of apnea and sternal retraction are not unusual during this period. The parasympathetic system is also active, as bowel sounds become evident during the first 15 minutes and oral mucus may be visible. This massive reaction dissipates rapidly, and after the first period of reactivity (usually between 10 and 60 minutes of age), heart and respiratory rates decline while the diffuse, apparently purposeless motor activity reaches a peak and then diminishes. With return of tonus to normal and diminished responsiveness, color should be excellent. A fast respiration rate without dyspnea should not be alarming at this time. An increase in the anteroposterior diameter (barrelling) of the chest may be noted accompanying the periods of shallow, rapid respiration. The chest, however, is not fixed in this position; the barrelling disappears promptly with any change in respiratory pattern if the infant is handled or begins to cry spontaneously. It recurs with resumption of

_____

*Characteristic reactions and responses with alerting exploratory behavior include nasal flaring or "sniffing" unrelated to respiratory activity; movements of the head from side to side; spontaneous startles and Moro reflexes; sucking, chewing, pursing, swallowing, grimacing, smacking, etc.; tremors of the extremities and mandible; opening and closing of the eyelids; short, rapid, jerky movements of the eyeball; outcries and sudden onset and cessation of crying.

Figure 2–2 A summary of the physical findings in normal transition (the first 10 hours of extrauterine life in a representative high-Apgar-score infant delivered under spinal anesthesia without premedication).[12]

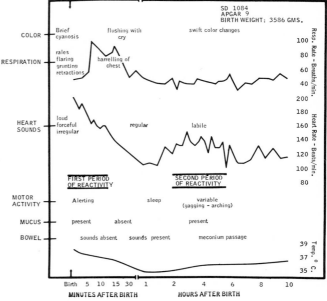

rapid, shallow, synchronous breathing. The abdomen should be rounded and bowel sounds audible.

Peristaltic waves beginning in the left upper quadrant of the abdomen and moving from left to right (gastric peristalsis) may occasionally be visible during periods of quiet activity or sleep. Small amounts of watery mucus may be visible at the lips. General responsiveness declines and the infant sleeps. Heart rate at this time (average 120 to 140 beats per minute) is relatively unresponsive. After sleep, the infant enters a second period of reactivity (between two and six hours of age). Responsiveness returns and may become exaggerated. This is not unlike the reactivity of a patient following anesthesia. The infant again exhibits tachycardia, brief periods of rapid respiration, and abrupt changes in tonus, color, and bowel sounds. Oral mucus may again become prominent, and gagging and vomiting are not unusual; the infant becomes more responsive to exogenous and endogenous stimuli, and heart rate becomes labile. The bowel is cleared of meconium. In some infants, the secondary reactivity period results in waves of heightened autonomic activity. Wide swings in heart rate (bradycardia to tachycardia) occur, along with the passage of meconium stools, the handling of mucus, vasomotor instability, and irregular respiration with apneic pauses. The second period of reactivity may be brief or last over a period of several hours. As it diminishes, the infant appears to be relatively stable and ready for feeding.

The sequence of clinical behavior just described appears to occur generally after birth, regardless of gestational age or route of delivery. The time sequence of changes is altered, however, in infants who are immature or who have demonstrated difficulty in establishing respiration promptly on delivery (low-Apgar-score infants). The length of time these two periods last is also affected by the length and difficulty of labor, the amount of stress to the fetus during labor, maternal medication and/or anesthesia, and other factors. All the events occurring during labor and delivery need to be carefully monitored and recorded, since they may profoundly influence the immediate as well as the long-term outcome of the newborn.

COMPLICATED TRANSITION (APPENDIX 3)

Complicated transition or neonatal morbidity occurs when the process of transition is disturbed by the addition of one or more adverse factors. These additional factors influence transition and alter its pattern. Although patterns of postnatal events are altered, these events still occur, since every infant must pass through the transition process before he is truly an extrauterine independent being.

At this point, a few comments should be made regarding the occurrence of convulsions in the neonatal period. Seizures, unless terminal, seldom occur during severe depression but are noted more frequently following a general improvement in the infant's condition (improved responsiveness, spontaneous activity, and improved color). Stereotyped repetitive movements may precede definite convulsions. Factors which render the brain irritable and lower seizure threshold are pH change from acidosis to relative alkalinity, falling blood sugar, falling ionized calcium and magnesium levels, the re-entry of oxygen to previously hypoxic neural tissues, and the presence of cerebral edema.

In addition to the general pattern outlined in Appendix 7, certain medications administered to the mother may have specific effects. Infants whose mothers have received Rauwolfia compounds prior to delivery may show combinations of the following: hypertonus, bradycardia, nasal stuffiness with intermittent dyspnea, vasodilation, tremors, and low body temperature. These effects would not be expected to lower one-minute Apgar scores, since they become evident some hours after delivery. The duration seldom exceeds two to five days.

Phenothiazines, given as premedication, may be associated with transient hypotonus during the first hours, unresponsiveness, decreased spontaneous activity, and marked vasomotor instability. After chronic high dosage late in pregnancy, the infant may show altered clinical behavior of two types: the changes described above, beginning after delivery and lasting from hours to several days; and agitation, tremors, hand posturing, and hypertonus, a phase of variable duration from weeks to months.

PHYSICAL EXAMINATION OF THE NEWBORN

Serial evaluation of the infant is more valuable than a single examination at any particular age. *Optimum evaluation would include a delivery room examination, a natal day examination, and a more detailed examination after the infant is 24 hours old.* With such serial evaluation, it is possible to determine the infant's progress in his transition and to detect problems which are interfering with transition. The detailed examination after 24 hours of age provides a good base line for judging the infant's future growth and development. Details of the physical examination of the infant have been well described in textbooks.

DELIVERY ROOM EXAMINATION

The Apgar score, which consists of an evaluation of five factors (heart rate, respiratory effort, muscle tone, responsiveness, and color) at one minute after delivery gives an immediate appraisal of the infant's condition. This "instant physical" assesses the cardiopulmonary and neurologic function. The results are reproducible and significantly related to neonatal mortality. Perhaps the greatest value of the score lies in the clarity of the picture of the infant's clinical condition which the number representing the total and component score conveys to those accustomed to its use.

A second scoring at five minutes after delivery gives added information concerning the infant's recovery and progress. Statistically, mortality and the clinical course of survivors have been related to both one- and five-minute Apgar scores.

In addition to the Apgar score, the infant is checked for cyanosis or pallor (anemia), congenital anomalies, state of maturity and evidence of neonatal disease. The infant with respiratory distress may be evaluated by the Silverman-Andersen retraction score.

Following this immediate appraisal or "instant physical" in the delivery room, there has been a supervisory limbo of the infant's first hours when he is "nobody's baby" until seen by the pediatrician. Thus, the early detection of problems not apparent in the delivery room frequently falls to nursery attendants. Our concern at Jefferson Davis Hospital, Houston, over this limbo period instigated the concept of the transitional care nursery.

NATAL DAY EXAMINATION

Ideally, the examination of a newborn should be gentle, rapid, and sufficiently thorough to obtain the desired information. Since much of the examination is based on observation, the first portion may be performed while the infant is still in the incubator.

POSTNATAL DAY EXAMINATION

Examination of the infant performed after he is 24 hours old would be of great value as a base line for following the infant's growth and development in future years. After he is 24 hours old, the infant has largely recovered from the intense sensory experiences accompanying labor and delivery; thus, a complete examination at this time is advantageous. During the first hours post delivery, excessive handling of the infant, particularly the premature, may be followed by clinical deterioration. The infant is still under the influence of maternal anesthesia and analgesia, and body temperature may be low. Re-examination after the infant is 24 hours old may reveal new findings, since many neonatal problems may not be evident during the first day. These include cephalhematoma, bleeding into tissues, fat necrosis, jaundice, apneic episodes, seizures, intestinal obstruction, genitourinary disorders, and other conditions.

RECOMMENDATIONS FOR CARE OF THE NEWBORN

1. Newborn infants should be regarded as recovering patients (few surgical procedures stress the patient more than the birth process) and kept under close surveillance during the first few hours after birth.

2. Assign a specific person (physician or nurse) to each delivery. This person is responsible for obtaining a pertinent history of pregnancy, labor, and delivery.

3. On delivery, place the infant in a prewarmed incubator or infant warmer. Apgar score is checked at one and five minutes (if low, until a good score is reached) and appropriate care is given.

4. Transfer infant to transitional care (recovery) nursery where trained personnel are more aware of the changes during the transitional state. They will observe the infant frequently and intensively until he has achieved a smooth transition. A vital signs sheet, preferably begun in the delivery room, is continued in the nursery (Appendix 1). In this manner, departures from the orderly progress of transition may be noted at their

early appearance. Neonatal intensive care nurseries are used in some areas for transitional care.

Editors' Comment: We have one slight disagreement. See p. 102.

5. All infants should remain in the transitional care nursery for at least six to eight hours or until stabilized. Infants who prove to be normal, as evidenced by a smooth transition, or infants with transient difficulties should be transferred to regular nurseries. If transition is complicated, appropriate measures should be taken in the management of the infant.

6. The equipment necessary for proper functioning of the transitional care nursery does not differ from that necessary in the intensive care area. The following equipment is recommended:

    a. Resuscitation equipment—respirators, etc.

    b. Environmental control equipment—radiant warmers, oxygen hoods, etc.

    c. Physiologic monitoring devices—apnea and cardiac monitors, etc.

    d. Electrocardiograph

    e. Portable X-ray

    f. Laboratory facilities—for monitoring of blood gases, glucose, calcium, hematocrit, etc.

If the infant requires continued monitoring, it is recommended that he be transferred to the intensive care area. The length of stay of the infant in the transitional care nursery should be determined by the physician.

In conclusion, the course of the *individual* infant during the natal day is *unpredictable* and *variable*. Optimal care of the neonatal patient should be prospective and anticipatory.

QUESTIONS

True or False

Lack of prenatal care is the single most important factor predisposing to serious illness in low-birth-weight infants during the first nine months of life.

Serious illnesses requiring re-hospitalization of low-birth-weight infants following discharge from the nursery were related to four specific sociomedical factors, of which failure of the mother to receive prenatal care was the most important.[16] Therefore, the statement is true.

Chronic malnutrition in the mother has deleterious effects on the infant.

There are no conclusive reports on the effect of chronic malnutrition in the mother as a single factor on the fetus, but it is known that malnutrition in the fetus does have an effect on tissue replication and growth, especially brain tissue. Infants of mothers who are narcotic or alcohol addicts eat poorly and deliver small-for-gestational-age infants. Therefore, the statement is true.

Match the following clinical findings in the neonate with the most likely maternal medication:

    A. Paralytic ileus   1. Thiazides

    B. Neonatal goiter   2. Reserpine

    C. Congenital   3. Aminopterin
       malformations

    D. Nasal stuffiness   4. Potassium iodide
       with intermittent
       dyspnea

    E. Thrombocytopenia   5. Hexamethonium

    A-5, B-4, C-3, D-2, E-1.

Withdrawal symptoms are seen in neonates delivered to narcotic addicts, but not in infants of chronic alcoholic mothers

In recent years, there have been several reports of a withdrawal syndrome in infants of alcoholic mothers. The clinical picture is much like that of delirium tremens seen in the adult. The infants often become hypoglycemic, also. Therefore, the statement is false.

Barbiturates produce more depression in the neonate than in older children.

Barbiturates penetrate the unmyelinated white matter of the neonatal brain more rapidly than they penetrate the gray matter, and therefore produce much longer sleeping times in neonatal than in adult animals, given equal doses per unit of body weight. Therefore, the statement is true.

The limited excretory function of the neonatal kidney serves as a positive therapeutic function.

Because of the limited excretory function of the neonatal kidney, small doses of penicillin can be given every 12 hours to the newborn and still provide effective blood levels. The renal function should also be taken into consideration when prescribing other antibiotics (e.g., chloramphenicol, methicillin, ampicillin, etc.), as they have long half-lives and may accumulate to toxic levels if dosage regimens are not altered. Therefore, the statement is true.

Match the following findings in the infant with the most likely maternal infection:

A. Meningoencephalo-myocarditis
B. Anencephaly
C. Granulomatosis infantiseptica
D. "Celery stick" appearance of long bones

1. Listeriosis
2. Rubella
3. Coxsackie virus
4. Influenza

A-3, B-4, C-1, D-2.

A sudden decrease in amniotic fluid lecithin/sphingomyelin ratio at 36 weeks' gestation indicates fetal distress.

The lecithin/sphingomyelin ratio *increases* suddenly at 35 to 36 weeks' gestation. This is evidence of fetal (especially pulmonary) maturity. It does *not* indicate fetal distress. Therefore, the statement is false.

High levels of urinary estriol indicate fetal well-being.

A sudden fall in urinary estriol, especially if being followed serially, is an ominous sign for the fetus. Therefore, the statement is true.

The absence of a distal femoral epiphysis on a fetogram accurately predicts a gestational age of less than 36 weeks.

The gestational age of the fetus can be predicted accurately only within a range of plus or minus seven weeks by looking for the distal femoral epiphysis. Infants with intrauterine growth retardation may have absent or smaller epiphyses than normal. Therefore, the statement is false.

Barrelling (increased AP diameter) of the chest is frequently seen in normal infants.

During normal transition in the unresponsive period between the first and second periods of reactivity, increase in the anteroposterior diameter of the chest may be noted accompanying the periods of shallow rapid respiration. The chest is not fixed in this position, since, if the infant cries or is handled, the barrelling disappears promptly only to return with resumption of rapid, shallow breathing. The same pattern may be seen in infants affected by maternal medication. Therefore, the statement is true.

Gastric peristalsis (peristalsis from left to right) is always indicative of bowel obstruction.

Gastric peristalsis is often noted during the transition period, especially in the relatively unresponsive interval between the first and second periods of reactivity. Therefore, the statement is false.

A scaphoid abdomen is diagnostic of an esophageal atresia or diaphragmatic hernia.

Although the diagnosis of esophageal atresia without a fistula or diaphragmatic hernia should always be considered, a scaphoid abdomen is noted frequently during transition in infants with low Apgar scores or infants depressed by maternal medication. Therefore, the statement is false.

Seizures (unless terminal) seldom occur in the severely depressed neonate.

In the majority of infants with convulsions, it has been noted that when they are severely depressed they seldom convulse. As their condition improves with increased responsiveness, spontaneous activity, and improved color, the brain becomes more irritable and the seizure threshold is lowered. Similarly, transplacental sedation will raise the seizure threshold. Therefore, the statement is true.

The clinical behavior during transition of the small-for-dates infant follows the course of that of an immature infant of comparable weight.

The more mature infant of low birth weight reacts like a larger infant of comparable gestational age. Small-for-dates infants have neurologic hyperexcitability and a lowered threshold for seizure activity. Therefore, the statement is false.

CASE PROBLEMS

Case One

B. A. is a 21-year-old gravida 2 para 1 mother admitted in labor with no history of prenatal care. Her blood pressure was 150/100, and she had 3+ proteinuria. She was treated with magnesium sulfate and thiazides. Two hours later she delivered a 3000-gm. male infant under caudal analgesia with mepivacaine. The infant was flaccid at birth, with an Apgar score of 3 at one minute, but resuscitation was initiated successfully.

Describe the possible effects of the maternal medication.

Mepivacaine when used for caudal analgesia has caused intoxication and death of the fetus if accidentally injected into the fetal scalp. Magnesium sulfate administered to the mother in large doses may cause severe neonatal depression. Thiazides have been reported to cause thrombocytopenia.

Describe the pattern of transition expected in this infant.

Transition would be complicated and the infant would manifest a combination of the changes seen during transition in low-Apgar-score infants and those depressed by maternal medications (Appendices 3 and 7).

What complications could be expected during recovery?

During recovery, the infant may possibly require ventilatory assistance and parenteral fluids, as respiration and sucking and swallowing responses are often poor. The infant will require close observation for onset of hypoglycemia, apneic attacks, and seizures.

Case Two

G. S. is a 20-year-old gravida 2 para 1 mother with an uncomplicated pregnancy who delivered a 2700-gm. male infant under spinal anesthesia. The infant had an Apgar score of 8 at one minute, and the initial physical examination of the infant was described as normal. At eight hours of age, the infant began to cry constantly, became extremely hyperactive, tremulous, and had vasomotor instability. Apart from the above findings, physical examination was again unremarkable. The hematocrit was 54, blood glucose was 100 mg. per 100 ml., and calcium was 9 mg. per 100 ml.

What would be the first approach in establishing a diagnosis?

Obtain a detailed history from the mother, especially in regard to medications. Of prime concern in this infant is a "withdrawal syndrome." One will repeatedly find that a personal interview of the mother is critical in delineating problems in a neonate. The infant

was normal at birth and had no metabolic problems. The mother was an addict.

Is the fact that transition was apparently normal surprising?

Transition may be normal, as the infant has adapted to his abnormal intrauterine environment, and it is only when withdrawal effects occur that he becomes symptomatic. Withdrawal effects occurring during the course of transition will alter the pattern, but if they occur after transition is achieved, the clinical behavior during transition can be normal.

Having established a diagnosis, how would you manage the infant?

Management of these infants consists in giving specific therapy and supportive care. Withdrawal effects may be relieved by the administration of paregoric, starting with one to two drops per Kg. every four to six hours. If necessary, this dose may be increased once symptoms are under control. Paregoric is gradually withdrawn by reducing the dose about 10 per cent daily. It may be necessary to continue therapy for several weeks. Chlorpromazine and diazepam have been used with good results. Swaddling of the infant is of great value and will decrease the amount of medication required. These infants may require supportive therapy for diarrhea, vomiting, and dehydration.

REFERENCES

1. Adamsons, K., Jr., and Joelsson, I.: The effects of pharmacologic agents upon the fetus and newborn. Amer J Obstet Gynec 96:437, 1966.
2. Anderson, J.: High-risk groups—Definitions and identifications. New Eng J Med 273:308, 1965.
3. Babson, S., and Benson, R.: Management of High-Risk Pregnancy and Intensive Care of the Neonate. St. Louis, C. V. Mosby Co., 1971.
4. Baker, J.: The effects of drugs on the fetus. Pharmacol Rev 12:37, 1960.
5. Barrett-Connor, E.: Infections and pregnancy: a review. Southern Med J 62:2715, 1969.
6. Brosens, I., and Gordon, H.: The estimation of maturity by cytological examination of the liquor amnii. J Obstet Gynaec Brit Comm 73:88, 1968.
7. Brosens, I., Gordon, H., and Baert, H.: Prediction of fetal maturity with combined cytological and radiological methods. J Obstet Gynaec Brit Comm 76:20, 1969.
8. Cohlan, S.: Fetal and neonatal hazards from drugs administered during pregnancy. New York J Med 64:493, 1964.
9. Desmond, M., and Rudolph, A.: Progressive eval-

uation of the newborn. Postgrad Med *37*:207, 1965.

10. Desmond, M., and Rudolph, A.: The clinical evaluation of the low-birthweight infant with regard to head trauma. *In* Angle, C., and Bering, E. Jr., Eds.: Physical Trauma as an Etiologic Agent in Mental Retardation, *Proceedings of a Conference on the Etiology of Mental Retardation, October 13–16, 1968, Omaha, Nebraska,* p. 241.

11. Desmond, M., Rudolph, A., and Phitaksphraiwan, P.: The transitional care nursery. Pediat Clin N Amer *13*:651, 1966.

12. Desmond, M., Franklin, R., Blattner, R., et al: The relation of maternal disease to fetal and neonatal morbidity and mortality. Pediat Clin N Amer *8*:421, 1961.

13. Desmond, M., Franklin, R., Vallbona, C., et al: The clinical behavior of the newly born. I. The term baby. J Pediat *62*:307, 1965.

14. Donald, I.: Sonar as a method of studying prenatal development. J Pediat *75*:326, 1969.

15. Fulginiti, V.: Bacterial infections in the newborn infant. J Pediat *76*:646, 1970.

16. Glass, L., Kolka, N., and Evans, H.: Factors influencing predispostion to serious illness in low birthweight infants. Pediatrics *48*:368, 1971.

17. Gluck, L., Kulovich, M., Borer, R., et al: Diagnosis of the respiratory distress syndrome by amniocentesis. Amer J Obstet Gynec *109*:440, 1971.

18. Gold, E.: Identification of the high risk fetus. Clin Obstet Gynec *11*:1069, 1968.

19. Gold, E.: Interconceptional nutrition. J Amer Diet Assn *55*:27, 1969.

20. Greene, J. Jr., and Beargie, R.: The use of urinary estriol excretion studies in the assessment of the high risk pregnancy. Pediat Clin N Amer *17*:43, 1970.

21. Hendricks, C.: Delivery patterns and reproductive efficiency among groups of differing socio-economic status and ethnic origins. Amer J Obstet Gynec *97*:608, 1967.

22. Moya, F., and Thorndike, V.: Passage of drugs across the placenta. Amer J Obstet Gynec *84*:1778, 1962.

23. Nadler, H.: Prenatal detection of genetic defects. J Pediat *74*:132, 1970.

24. Nadler, H., and Gerbie, A.: Present status of amniocentesis in intrauterine diagnosis of genetic defects. Obstet Gynec *38*:789, 1971.

25. Nora, J., Nora, A., Sommerville, R., et al: Maternal exposure to potential teratogens. JAMA *202*:1065, 1967.

26. Overall, J. Jr., and Glasgow, L.: Virus infections of the fetus and newborn infant. J Pediat *77*:315, 1970.

27. Palmisano, P., and Polhill, B.: Fetal pharmacology. Pediat Clin N Amer *19*:3, 1972.

Chapter 3

CLASSIFICATION OF THE LOW-BIRTH-WEIGHT INFANT

by
AVRON Y. SWEET, M.D.

"...there are tiny, puny infants with great vitality. Their movements are untiring and their crying lusty, for their organs are quite capable of performing their allotted functions. These infants will live, for although their weight is inferior...their sojourn in the womb was longer."

PIERRE BUDIN, *The Nursling*

In the past, newborn infants weighing 2500 gm. or less were arbitrarily identified as *premature,* while those weighing more were designated *full term.* When it became widely accepted that all neonates of 2500 gm. or less at birth were not prematurely born (<37 weeks' gestation), the designation *low birth weight* was applied to them instead. Accordingly, *low birth weight* now refers to all infants whose weight at birth is 2500 gm. or below, irrespective of the cause and without regard to the duration of gestation.

The concept that small neonates did not constitute a homogeneous group, and that babies of low birth weight were often truly undernourished full-term infants, did not gain wide acceptance and attention until after the meticulous studies of Gruenwald[27] demonstrated fetal malnutrition, or chronic fetal distress as he termed it. The idea of intrauterine growth retardation had been proposed earlier,[67] but Gruenwald's work and the wide support of his concepts did much to curtail the use of birth weight alone as a measure of maturity of newborn infants. The importance of birth weight was not diminished, but the necessity for relating it to the duration of gestation was established. This is important clinically because growth-retarded infants differ from their gestational-age or birth-weight peers in immediate clinical problems, physical growth, mental and neurologic outlook, incidence of congenital abnormalities, and several physiologic parameters.

Almost simultaneously, Lubchenco[38] presented standards of intrauterine growth of Caucasian infants in which birth weight was related to gestational age. The graphic display of the relationship provides a useful and simple method for determining the appropriateness of weight with respect to gestational age in a given infant. The reliability of weight measurement and determination of gestational age are critical. Unfortunately, the accuracy of the determination of the duration of gestation from obstetrical information is sometimes difficult whether based on menstrual history or obstetrical milestones such as quickening, appearance of fetal heart sounds, fundal height, etc. A reliable assessment of gestational age was not attainable until a method was devised which was based on the infant himself.

We are indebted to a lineage of French

36

physicians whose studies resulted in techniques which provide a means of assessment of gestational age based on neurologic evaluation of the newborn.[5, 33, 49, 50, 60] Of equal importance has been the establishment of the relationship of gestational age to a variety of external physical characteristics of the neonate.[21, 22, 64] Although the techniques have faults, it is possible to assess each neonate with reasonable accuracy. By these means, newborn infants can now be categorized as *appropriate (in weight) for gestational age (AGA), small for gestational age (SGA)*, also referred to as *small-for-dates*, and *large for gestational age* (LGA). At the same time, they may be identified as *preterm* (<37 weeks' gestation), *term* (37 to 42 weeks' gestation) or *post-term*, also referred to as *postmature* (>42 weeks' gestation). (See Figure 3–1).

Based on this classification, the clinician can now anticipate clinical problems peculiar to the category to which the patient belongs. Furthermore, he is better able to prognosticate with respect to growth and development, and to seek out inapparent congenital abnormalities intelligently.

This chapter presents procedures for classifying young neonates, the physical differences between immature infants and small-for-gestational-age infants, and the clinical significance of these differences. (Antenatal evaluation of fetal maturity is considered in Chapter 2.)

BASIC CONSIDERATIONS

An understanding of the dimensional changes that occur in small-for-gestational-age infants or appropriately sized infants has resulted from the application of new techniques which permit the determination of cell number and cell size. These techniques are based on the assumption that the proteins of any organ are contained within the cells, and that the amount of DNA within the diploid nucleus of all cells of a given species is constant (k). Accordingly, the measurement of the DNA and total protein content of an organ permits the estimation of cell size (protein/DNA) and number (DNA/k). These techniques have been used in valuable studies of animals with and without growth retardation and in studies of normal and malnourished human infants.

During early fetal life, virtually all growth is due to increases in cell number. Increases in cell size become more dominant during the

Figure 3–1 The birth weights of liveborn singleton Caucasian infants at gestational ages from 24 to 42 weeks. (Adapted from Battaglia and Lubchenco.[8])

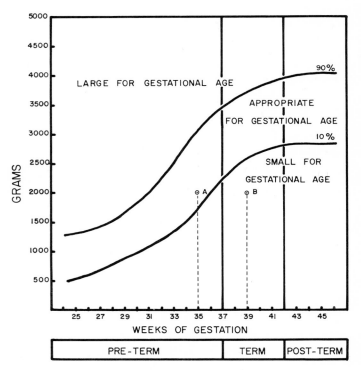

latter part of gestation. It is not clear how long the increase in cell number continues nor what variations occur in different organs.

Interference with the growth of the fetus during the period of increase in cell number results in organs containing fewer cells, but cells of normal size. If the insult occurs during the period of growth characterized by increase in cell size, then the cells will be normal in number but small in size. For example, with an intrauterine insult throughout the periods of increase both in cell number and size, cells will be few in number and small in size. The classic example of this is the infant with the rubella syndrome.

Studies of the human brain have shown that brain cell number continues to increase after delivery. However, there is some disagreement as to when cell number no longer increases, and estimates vary between 8 and 15 months beyond 40 weeks' gestation. Thus, malnutrition at any time up to 15 months should be regarded as a potential hazard to brain development.

Total brain DNA content is directly and linearly related to head circumference if no abnormal accumulation of intracranial fluid is present. Postmortem studies of marasmic infants have shown brain weight and protein to be reduced proportionate to head circumference. These findings strongly support the use of changes in head circumference as a measure of postnatal brain growth.

Retardation of brain development in small-for-dates infants, the failure to catch up postnatally, and the enhancement of the problem by postnatal malnutrition suggest that a permanent impairment in function will occur. Supporting this are the observations that South African children malnourished during infancy were later found to have smaller body and head sizes and lower intelligence quotients than controls.[59]

Furthermore, in New South Wales, nearly 15 per cent of 1300 mentally retarded patients with intelligence quotients below 50 had been small-for-gestational-age at birth.[11]

All studies of undergrown infants, however, do not reveal significant mental retardation.[6] Drillien[18] found that small-for-dates infants born into high socioeconomic group families did as well as or better than their peers at the age of 10 to 12 years, while small-for-dates infants of lower socioeconomic groups functioned below their matched peers. She found intellectual function to be low if congenital anomalies were present.

The brain is not the sole organ affected by intrauterine growth retardation. Brain and skeletal growth, together with the heart and lung, appear to be the least affected, while the adrenals, liver, spleen, and thymus are severly reduced in size.[41]

Bone growth has also been found to be impaired with intrauterine growth retardation. Fibular length is sometimes diminished, and there is a delay in the time of appearance of the distal femoral and proximal tibial epiphyses. (X-rays are thus of little value in establishing gestational age.)

Careful study of weight gain in the immediate neonatal period indicates that some small-for-dates infants between 1500 and 2500 gm. birth weight tend to exceed the grid for expected growth of "premature" infants,[16] and that they do not exhibit appreciable weight loss in the first days of life, which is so characteristic of AGA preterm infants.[3] Postnatal catch-up growth is variable and unpredictable. Some growth-retarded infants eventually catch up to their gestational-age peers, and some do not. This again suggests a lack of homogeneity in the small-for-dates group. It is of interest that Wilson et al,[69] in their small sample, found that those infants who failed to catch up had serious congenital anomalies. Other studies have shown that small-for-dates infants remain small, but they make no mention of abnormalities.[20, 45]

When infants of low birth weight are properly classified, it is usually discovered that about one-third are small-for-gestational age, while two-thirds are appropriate-for-gestational age and preterm (gestational age < 37 weeks).

ETIOLOGY

The *causes* for the early delivery of most of the infants who are appropriately sized remain obscure; however, small-for-gestational-age infants may be associated with: (1) intrauterine malnutrition, (2) infection, (3) congenital anomalies or genetic factors, and (4) miscellaneous factors.

Malnutrition

Although it has been demonstrated that nutritional inadequacy causes intrauterine growth retardation in a variety of laboratory animals, there is no comparable evidence in the human. This difference may well be explained by the comparatively slow growth of the human fetus relative to the size of its mother. A nutritional problem of even short duration might prove catastrophic to the fast-growing rat; however, the rate of growth of the human fetus is not nearly so demanding, thereby requiring a protracted and severe nutritional insult to produce an effect (Figure 3–2). Furthermore, the evidence which indicates that nutritional factors play a role in human fetal growth offers no clue as to whether the problem derives from inadequate calories or specific deficiencies such as certain fats, proteins, vitamins, etc.

Nutritional inadequacy was the accepted cause of prematurity when the term referred to all infants weighing 2500 gm. or less at birth. It is evident that many such infants were the products of women from areas of urban poverty. Naeye et al[44] found that women considered to be poor (as determined by weekly income and family size) more often delivered stillborn or liveborn infants who died within 48 hours of age and were smaller than comparable infants of more affluent mothers. Having removed from consideration infants with other known causes of growth retardation, they assumed that intrauterine growth was retarded because of poor maternal nutrition.

In an attempt to evaluate the effects of maternal nutritional deprivation upon the fetus, Smith[57, 58] reviewed hospital records in Rotterdam before, during, and after the "hunger winter" in northern Holland toward the end of World War II. During 1944 and 1945, there was a paucity of food to the point of near (sometimes actual) starvation. Women who were pregnant during this period delivered infants who tended to be only 200 gm. or so below expected weight at birth when compared to mean birth weights of infants born before and after the episode. It appears that no significant undergrowth of infants in utero occurred during the hunger winter if food supplies were restored before the last weeks of pregnancy. If, however, the last weeks of pregnancy occurred during the time of severe food shortage, the infants were somewhat underweight. A similar trend was noted in Japan.[29]

Winick's studies favoring nutritional inadequacy as a cause of growth retardation in man impressively demonstrate poor placental growth in nutritionally deprived pregnant women.[59, 70] Less direct studies suggest impaired brain growth in the intrauterine-growth-retarded infants of poorly nourished mothers.

The occurrence of monochorionic twins with grossly disparate size in association with vascular communications in the placenta may produce a type of malnutrition in the small

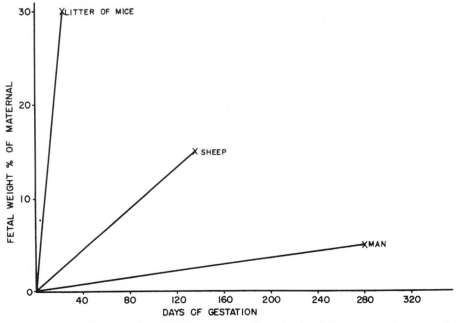

Figure 3–2 Products of conception of three mammalian species in per cent of maternal weight.[58]

twin. This is referred to as the twin trans-fusion syndrome or the parabiosis syndrome. Aside from differences in weight, length, and head size, there is comparable discrepancy in the size of all organs. The smaller (donor) infant is anemic, while the large recipient infant is polycythemic. Naeye[40] found the anemic member is always on the arterial side of the placental shunt, while the plethoric recipient is on the venous side. Often the smaller twin is dead, and may present as a fetus papyraceous. The smaller of the pair is small-for-dates. Peculiarly, hypoglycemia is not prominent in the smaller of these twins, whereas in the usual circumstances in which there is discordance, the smaller tends to be hypoglycemic. Hyperbilirubinemia, probably as a consequence of polycythemia, is common in the recipient twin, who also is prone to develop cardiac failure because of hyper-volemia. Hyaline membrane disease is not un-common, and may be found in either twin. In the common occurrence of discordance, the infants are of rather good size (1500 gm. or more), whereas with the parabiosis syn-drome, the infants tend to be very small and usually immature. In Shanklin's group of seven such twins, both members of five sets were 815 gm. or less, one pair weighed 1270 and 1125 gm. respectively, and one pair weighed 2960 and 2100 gm.[53]

Infection

Certain intrauterine infections are known to cause diminished fetal growth. Newborn infants with overt cytomegalic inclusion dis-ease may be small-for-gestational-age. On the other hand, the disease may occur without clinical signs in small infants of young pri-miparous mothers. Whether these represent small-for-dates infants is not clear.

Similarly, congenital rubella is associ-ated with infants who are undergrown, partic-ularly if they demonstrate the "expanded" rubella syndrome. In a study of 58 infants with congenital rubella who were born in New York City during the 1964 outbreak, 60 per cent fell below the 10th percentile for weight and 90 per cent fell below the 50th per-centile.[13] While some other viruses are capable of causing malformations and runting in animals, only rubella and cytomegalo-viruses are clearly known at present to cause a disparity in weight and gestational age in man.

Although congenital syphilis has been

identified as a cause of prematurity, Naeye[42] found no evidence of intrauterine growth re-tardation by examination of body weight, organ size, or cell number in organs of infected infants as compared to controls.

There is some question as to the effect of intrauterine toxoplasmosis on fetal growth. It does result in infants of low birth weight, but these infants were not classified as to whether they were small- or appropriate-for-gestational-age.

Bacterial infections are known to occur in utero, but they are not associated with the problem of growth retardation. In the main, these infections occur just prior to or during labor (possibly causing premature labor), so that insufficient time can elapse to cause growth difficulties.

Genetic or Inherited Factors

With the separation of the true premature (< 37 weeks) from the small-for-dates infant, it became apparent that congenital mal-formations occur most frequently in under-grown infants. Van den Berg and Yerushalmy[66] reviewed the records of 469 liveborn infants weighing between 1501 and 2500 gm. and found that SGA infants with the longest gestation had the highest incidence (18 per cent) of *severe* malformations.

Drillien[17, 18] also found the frequency of congenital malformations to increase as small-ness-for-gestational-age increases. The more severe the intrauterine growth retardation, the more likely is the chance for malformation. Usher[61] found congenital malformations to oc-cur 10 to 20 times more frequently in SGA infants than in AGA infants. (Congenital heart disease occurred in six per cent of the SGA infants.)

Inadequate sex chromosome, as exempli-fied by the female Turner's syndrome (45/XO), is associated with fetal growth retardation. Reisman[48] suggests that material on the short arm of the X chromosome is important for intrauterine as well as postnatal growth, and that a homologous locus is present on the Y chromosome. Individuals with excessive numbers of X or Y chromosomes, such as 47/XXY (Klinefelter's syndrome). XO/XX mosaicism, etc., do not exhibit growth re-tardation at birth. Infants with the various autosomal trisomies are well known to be SGA. Those with trisomy-21 have been found to weigh 10 to 15 per cent less than normal at birth; half weigh less than 2700 gm.[56] Similarly, infants with trisomies 16-18 and 13-15 are undergrown.[68]

Inherited disorders without chromosomal abnormalities often occur in infants who are small-for-dates. This is obvious in such situations as diastrophic dwarfs, achondroplastic dwarfs and the like, but it is also true of disorders in which mass is diminished for reasons other than diminutive or missing anatomic parts, such as arms or legs.

A woman who has produced a small-for-dates infant is likely to do so in subsequent pregnancies. There are families in which infants are SGA without associated abnormalities except for mental retardation. A family has been reported by Warkany et al[67] in which four generations contained several members who were below the expected weight at birth, and virtually all went on to be of normal size.

Most infants with anomalies tend to have problems that are immediately evident by physical examination at birth, or manifest themselves in the first few days of life. Because urinary tract abnormalities may be silent, it is often questioned whether excretory urograms and other diagnostic studies are necessary to demonstrate abnormalities in SGA infants who appear to be normal otherwise. We do not study these patients unless there are physical findings suggestive of abnormalities, such as enlargement of one or both kidneys, ear abnormalities, or the presence of a single palmar crease together with a single umbilical artery. Significantly, the majority of congenital anomalies in SGA infants are not associated with demonstrable chromosomal peculiarities, nor is there a specific pattern of abnormalities identified with SGA neonates.

Although the presence of congenital anomalies is commonly associated with intrauterine growth retardation, there are certain notorious exceptions. Infants with transposition of the great vessels are large-for-gestational-age. Infants of diabetic mothers are very commonly large-for-dates even though anomalies are present.

Other Factors

A wide variety of miscellaneous circumstances are associated with aberrations of intrauterine growth.

As a rule, products of multiple births are small-for-dates. This is usually apparent only if birth occurs after 35 weeks of gestation,[36] presumably because the placenta becomes inadequate to meet the needs of more than one fetus.

Mothers who smoke cigarettes during pregnancy produce infants who are small-for-dates.[1] Moderate smokers have double the incidence in nonsmokers, while that of heavy smokers is threefold. The cause of this is not known, but it is assumed to be a result of the vascular effects of smoking.

The relationship between smoking and intrauterine growth retardation exists not only statistically on the basis of experience with human infants. Indeed, in the British Perinatal Mortality Survey Report, it appears as the single most obvious statistical correlate between a maternal factor and the occurrence of the underweight-for-gestational-age product of the pregnancy. In addition, however, animal experiments have suggested that it is not merely the smoke, but in fact a constituent of the tobacco which is responsible for this growth retardation, since rabbits exposed to tobacco smoke had fetuses grossly underweight, whereas those in which the smoke was produced from other substances (lettuce) did not show such growth retardation.

L. STERN

At high altitudes, the infant tends to be small in weight for the duration of the pregnancy, although linear growth is unaffected.[36] The reason for this phenomenon is not known.

Finally, certain noxious agents have a damaging effect upon the fetus. X-irradiation causes microcephaly and intrauterine growth retardation. Aminopterin and other antimetabolites given to the mother result in growth impairment, malformations of the brain and cranial vault, as well as other anomalies, depending on when the drug is taken.

Infants born to drug addicts are often small-for-gestational-age.

It appears to be specifically infants born to heroin-addicted mothers who are small-for-gestational-age, whereas the so-called soft drug addicted parents do not have any such apparent relationship. Heroin, however, may have some positive advantages to the fetus, although the heroin withdrawal syndrome (methadone itself also produces a similar syndrome) may be violent and, if unrecognized and uncontrolled, can often terminate fatally for the baby. There is evidence accumulating which suggests that heroin may be an important enzyme inducer and that infants born to heroin-addicted mothers show a greater maturation of pulmonary function (with a lower incidence of the respiratory distress syndrome); there is also the possibility that there may be enhanced induction of glucuronyl transferase (with subsequent less hyperbilirubinemia).

L. STERN

From the standpoint of discernible pathology, gross anatomic lesions of the placenta play a very minor role in fetal growth impairment, while minute lesions may be of importance. In any event, identifiable placental pathology is surprisingly not a major etiologic factor[9, 10, 27, 53] associated with low-birth-weight infants.

Toxemia and Hypertension

In the past, it was widely believed that toxemia causes prematurity. It can now be stated that hypertensive mothers who may or may not have toxemia deliver a higher than expected percentage of preterm and small-for-dates infants or both. The actual basis for this association is not clear; however, it is well known that, with toxemia, placental infarcts are numerous and widespread. Possibly the placenta is involved in the general vascular changes associated with these conditions, so the perfusion of the placenta is not adequate to meet the needs of the rapidly growing fetus during the latter part of gestation.

CLINICAL PRINCIPLES

ASSESSMENT OF GESTATIONAL AGE

The assessment of a neonate as small-for-gestational-age, appropriate-for-gestational-age, or large-for-gestational-age is of immediate clinical value to the physician. As observed in Table 3–3, the clinical course, outcome, and problems are quite different for each group of infants. Hypoglycemia and congenital malformations, as well as pulmonary aspiration, are far more common in infants who are SGA, while hyaline membrane disease, hyperbilirubinemia, etc., are more common in the preterm, immature AGA infants. The need for *precision* in the estimation of gestational age cannot be overemphasized, and is illustrated in Figure 3–1. Note that if there is an incorrect estimation of gestational age by four weeks, an AGA infant weighing 2 Kg. at 35 weeks who is incorrectly assessed as having a gestational age of 39 weeks will be labeled as a small-for-gestational-age term infant.

Therefore, there must be accuracy in estimating the gestational age of infants. Although the mother's dates are useful, they are sometimes confusing because of irregular menstrual periods, bleeding in the first trimester, and the irregular or abnormal growth of the fetus.

In the past 15 years, several methods using the physical characteristics of infants have been developed which avoid this dependency on maternal information. Three methods which are most commonly used to determine gestational age are:

1. The use of external physical characteristics.
2. The neurological evaluation.
3. Scoring systems combining the external physical characteristics and the neurologic evaluation.

External Physical Characteristics of Newborn Infants According to Gestational Age. Certain external physical characteristics of newborn infants have developmental patterns which progress in an orderly fashion during gestation. From these, scoring systems have been established by which each physical characteristic is weighed (scored) increasingly as it changes with gestation. (For an example, see Figure 3–3.) By means of a chart, the total score is equated with the duration of pregnancy. These are described in conjunction with the neurologic examination (see below). This method is described in Table 3–1 (as adapted by Dubowitz et al[19]).

Assessment of Gestational Age by Neurologic Examination. Contrary to the assessment of gestational age by physical criteria, which can be performed immediately after birth, neurologic evaluation requires the infant to be in a quiet, rested state. Accordingly, examination is possible during the latter part of the first day of life in some infants, but for many it cannot be done until the second or third day. In addition, "depressed," asphyxiated, neurologically-damaged, or otherwise sick infants are difficult to assess. It is unfortunate that the neurologic assessment as a means of judging gestational age is not always practical at the time it is needed most.

Judgment of gestational age according to posture, passive range of motion of certain parts, active tone, righting reactions, and a variety of reflexes has been beautifully described by Amiel-Tison.[5] This method is depicted in Figure 3–4 and described in Table 3–2 (as adapted by Dubowitz et al[19]). For reference to the original method, see Appendix 14.

Scoring System for Assessing Gestational Age from Physical and Neurologic Findings. Dubowitz and colleagues[19] devised a scoring system combining neurologic findings similar to those of Amiel-Tison[5] and physical characteristics described by Farr et al.[22] Tables 3–1 and 3–2 and Figures 3–4 and 3–5 describe

(*Text continued on page 46.*)

TABLE 3–1 SCORING SYSTEM OF EXTERNAL PHYSICAL CHARACTERISTICS*

EXTERNAL SIGN	SCORE**				
	0	1	2	3	4
Edema	Obvious edema of hands and feet; pitting over tibia	No obvious edema of hands and feet; pitting over tibia	No edema		
Skin texture	Very thin, gelatinous	Thin and smooth	Smooth; medium thickness. Rash or superficial peeling	Slight thickening. Superficial cracking and peeling, especially of hands and feet	Thick and parchment-like; superficial or deep cracking
Skin color	Dark red	Uniformly pink	Pale pink; variable over body	Pale; only pink over ears, lips, palms, or soles	
Skin opacity (trunk)	Numerous veins and venules clearly seen, especially over abdomen	Veins and tributaries seen	A few large vessels clearly seen over abdomen	A few large vessels seen indistinctly over abdomen	No blood vessels seen
Lanugo (over back)	No lanugo	Abundant; long and thick over whole back	Hair thinning especially over lower back	Small amount of lanugo and bald areas	At least $1/2$ of back devoid of lanugo
Plantar creases (Figure 3–3)	No skin creases	Faint red marks over anterior half of sole	Definite red marks over > anterior $1/2$; indentations over < anterior $1/3$	Indentations over > anterior $1/3$	Definite deep indentations over > anterior $1/3$
Nipple formation	Nipple barely visible; no areola	Nipple well defined; areola smooth and flat, diameter < 0.75 cm.	Areola stippled, edge not raised, diameter < 0.75 cm.	Areola stippled, edge raised, diameter > 0.75 cm.	
Breast size	No breast tissue palpable	Breast tissue on one or both sides, < 0.5 cm. diameter	Breast tissue both sides; one or both 0.5 to 1.0 cm.	Breast tissue both sides; one or both > 1 cm.	
Ear form	Pinna flat and shapeless, little or no incurving of edge	Incurving of part of edge of pinna	Partial incurving whole of upper pinna	Well-defined incurving whole of upper pinna	
Ear firmness	Pinna soft, easily folded, no recoil	Pinna soft, easily folded, slow recoil	Cartilage to edge of pinna, but soft in places, ready recoil	Pinna firm, cartilage to edge; instant recoil	
Genitals: Male	Neither testis in scrotum	At least one testis high in scrotum	At least one testis right down		
Genitals: Female (with hips $1/2$ abducted)	Labia majora widely separated, labia minora protruding	Labia majora almost cover labia minora	Labia majora completely cover labia minora		

*Adapted by Dubowitz et al[19] from Farr et al.[22]
**If score differs on two sides, take the mean.

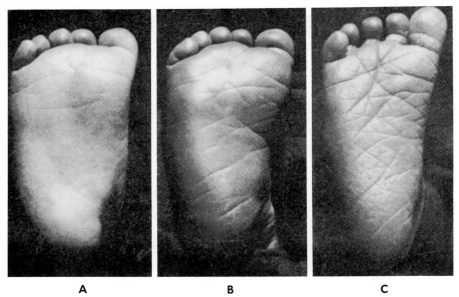

| | A | B | C |

Figure 3–3 Plantar aspect of the foot in infants of varying gestational ages.[64] *A*. Thirty-six weeks' gestation. Note the transverse creases on the anterior third only. *B*. Thirty-eight weeks' gestation. Note transverse creases extend to heel. *C*. Forty weeks' gestation. Note transverse crease over entirety of the sole, and additional wrinkling.

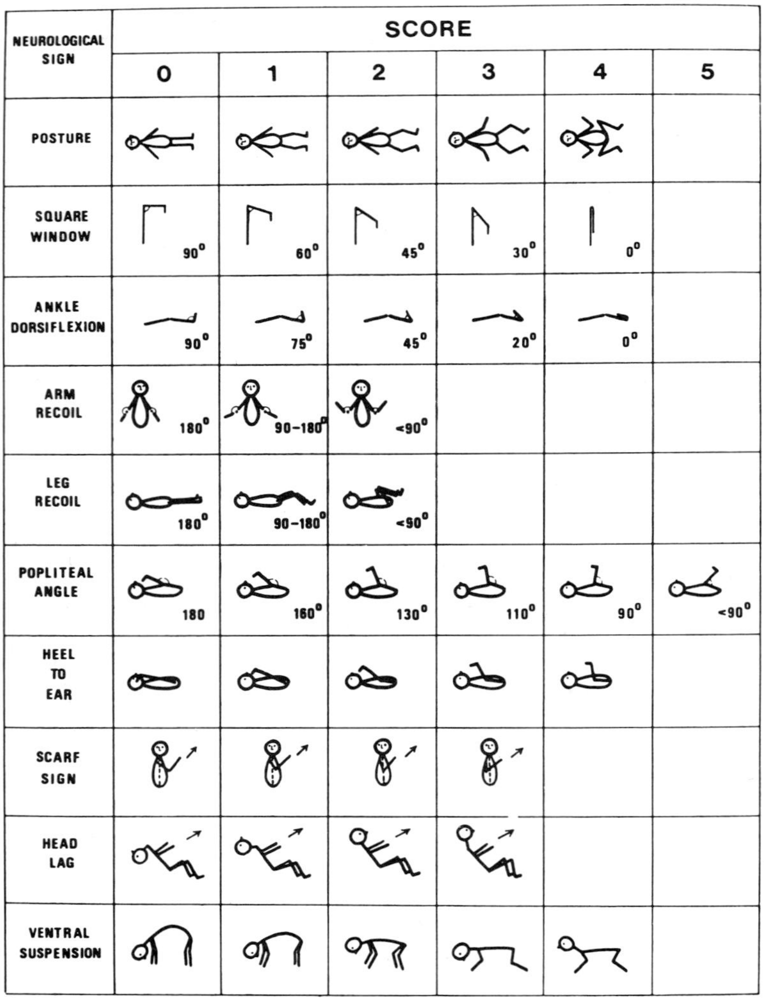

NEUROLOGICAL SIGN	SCORE					
	0	**1**	**2**	**3**	**4**	**5**
POSTURE						
SQUARE WINDOW	90°	60°	45°	30°	0°	
ANKLE DORSIFLEXION	90°	75°	45°	20°	0°	
ARM RECOIL	180°	90–180°	<90°			
LEG RECOIL	180°	90–180°	<90°			
POPLITEAL ANGLE	180	160°	130°	110°	90°	<90°
HEEL TO EAR						
SCARF SIGN						
HEAD LAG						
VENTRAL SUSPENSION						

Figure 3–4 The scoring of neurologic findings according to Dubowitz et al[19] from Amiel-Tison.[5] (To be used in conjunction with Table 3–2.)

TABLE 3-2 TECHNIQUES OF NEUROLOGIC ASSESSMENT*

POSTURE
With the infant supine and quiet, score as follows:

arms and legs extended,	= 0
slight or moderate flexion of hips and knees	= 1
moderate to strong flexion of hips and knees	= 2
legs flexed and abducted, arms slightly flexed	= 3
full flexion of arms and legs	= 4

SQUARE WINDOW
Flex the hand at the wrist. Exert pressure sufficient to get as much flexion as possible. The angle between the hypothenar emenence and the anterior aspect of the fore- arm is measured and scored according to Figure 3–4. Do not rotate the wrist.

ANKLE DORSIFLECTION
Flex the foot at the ankle with sufficient pressure to get maximum change. The angle between the dorsum of the foot and the anterior aspect of the leg is measured and scored as in Figure 3–4.

ARM RECOIL
With the infant supine, fully flex the forearm for five seconds, then fully extend by pulling the hands and release. Score the reaction according to:

remain extended or random movements	= 0
incomplete or partial flexion	= 1
brisk return to full flexion	= 2

LEG RECOIL
With the infant supine, the hips and knees are fully flexed for five seconds, then extended by traction on the feet and released. Score the reaction according to:

no response or slight flexion	= 0
partial flexion	= 1
full flexion (less than 90° at knees and hips)	= 2

POPLITEAL ANGLE
With the infant supine and the pelvis flat on the examining surface, the leg is flexed on the thigh and the thigh fully flexed with the use of one hand. With the other hand the leg is then extended and the angle attained scored as in Figure 3–4.

HEEL TO EAR MANEUVER
With the infant supine, hold the infant's foot with one hand and move it as near to the head as possible without forcing it. Keep the pelvis flat on the examining surface. Score as in Figure 3–4.

SCARF SIGN
With the infant supine, take the infant's hand and draw it across the neck and as far across the opposite shoulder as possible. Assistance to the elbow is permissible by lifting it across the body. Score according to the location of the elbow:

elbow reaches the opposite anterior axillary line	= 0
elbow between opposite anterior axillary line and midline of thorax	= 1
elbow at midline of thorax	= 2
elbow does not reach mid- line of thorax	= 3

HEAD LAG
With the infant supine, grasp each forearm just proximal to the wrist and pull gently so as to bring the infant to a sitting position. Score according to the relationship of the head to the trunk during the maneuver:

no evidence of head support	= 0
some evidence of head support	= 1
maintains head in the same anteroposterior plane as the body	= 2
tends to hold the head forward	= 3

VENTRAL SUSPENSION
With the infant prone and the chest resting on the examiner's palm, lift the infant off the examining surface and score according to the posture shown in Figure 3–4.

---

*According to Dubowitz et al[19] from Amiel-Tison.[5] To be used in conjunction with Figure 3–4.

and depict the procedures for the neurologic evaluation. The changes in external physical characteristics are weighed according to their appearance as pregnancy progresses. Tables 3–1 and 3–2 describe these findings and provide an appropriate score.

The score obtained from the assessment of each of the 10 neurologic signs (Figure 3–4) are summed and added to the scores of each of the 11 external signs (Table 3–1). The total score is located on the horizontal axis of Figure 3–5, and a perpendicular line is drawn to the diagonal. At the point of intersection, a horizontal line is drawn to the vertical axis, which indicates the gestational age in weeks. This method is accurate to within two weeks.

Dr. Ballard of Cincinnati has produced an abbreviated version of the system of Dubowitz et al (Figure 3–6), in which certain neurologic criteria are retained which do not require the infant to be alert and vigorous. This appears to be the simplest and most practical technique presently available; however, the precision of the total score is currently being evaluated.

I believe that every infant should be evaluated physically and neurologically as soon as possible after birth. It is important to adhere closely to the directions of *the original author* and to use the same method in following the neurologic development. Only by repetition can one obtain proficiency, reliability, and reproducibility. Under the best circumstances, physical and neurologic examination is only accurate to within plus or minus two weeks, so history and all other factors must be taken into consideration when determining gestational age.

The weight, length, and head circumference of all newborn infants should be compared to a set of normal standards. In this way, a number of SGA and LGA infants who would not otherwise be recognized will be identified.

Estimation of Gestational Age by Head Circumference. Occasionally there are circumstances which do not permit assessing gestational age from physical characteristics, and the infant is too ill to allow an accurate neurologic evaluation. Because the brain is one of the least affected structures during intrauterine growth retardation secondary to malnutrition, head circumference has been used to estimate gestational age.[37] The head circumference is measured and the value is located on the 50th percentile of Figure 3–7.

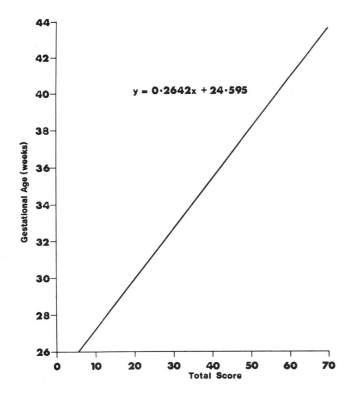

$$y = 0.2642x + 24.595$$

Figure 3–5 Graph for ascertaining gestational age from the total score of physical and neurologic development according to Dubowitz et al.[19]

Neuromuscular Maturity

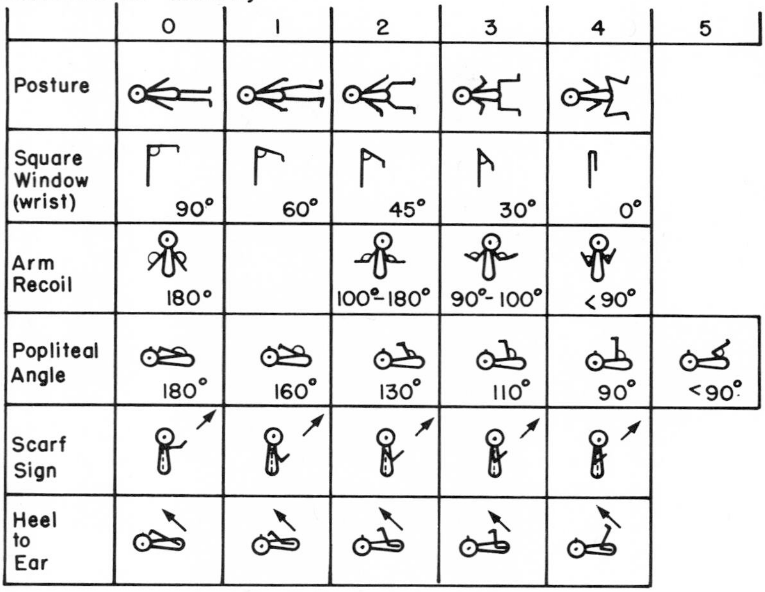

	0	1	2	3	4	5
Posture						
Square Window (wrist)	90°	60°	45°	30°	0°	
Arm Recoil	180°		100°–180°	90°–100°	<90°	
Popliteal Angle	180°	160°	130°	110°	90°	<90°
Scarf Sign						
Heel to Ear						

Apgars _____ 1 min _____ 5 min

Age at Exam _____ hrs

Race _____ Sex _____

B.D. _____

LMP _____

EDC _____

Gest. age by Dates _____ wks

Gest. age by Exam _____ wks

B.W. _____ gm. _____ %ile

Length _____ cm. _____ %ile

Head Circum. _____ cm. ____ %ile

Clin. Dist. None _____ Mild _____

                Mod. _____ Severe _____

PHYSICAL MATURITY

Skin	gelatinous red, transparent	smooth pink, visible veins	superficial peeling &/or rash few veins	cracking pale area rare veins	parchment deep cracking no vessels	leathery cracked wrinkled
Lanugo	none	abundant	thinning	bald areas	mostly bald	
Plantar Creases	no crease	faint red marks	anterior transverse crease only	creases ant. 2/3	creases cover entire sole	
Breast	barely percept.	flat areola no bud	stippled areola 1–2 mm bud	raised areola 3–4 mm bud	full areola 5–10 mm bud	
Ear	pinna flat, stays folded	sl. curved pinna; soft with slow recoil	well-curv. pinna; soft but ready recoil	formed & firm with instant recoil	thick cartilage ear stiff	
Genitals ♂	scrotum empty no rugae		testes descending, few rugae	testes down good rugae	testes pendulous deep rugae	
Genitals ♀	prominent clitoris & labia minora		majora & minora equally prominent	majora large minora small	clitoris & minora completely covered	

MATURITY RATING

Score	Wks
5	26
10	28
15	30
20	32
25	34
30	36
35	38
40	40
45	42
50	44

Figure 3–6 Assessment of gestational age. University of Cincinnati. (With thanks to Dr. J. Ballard.)

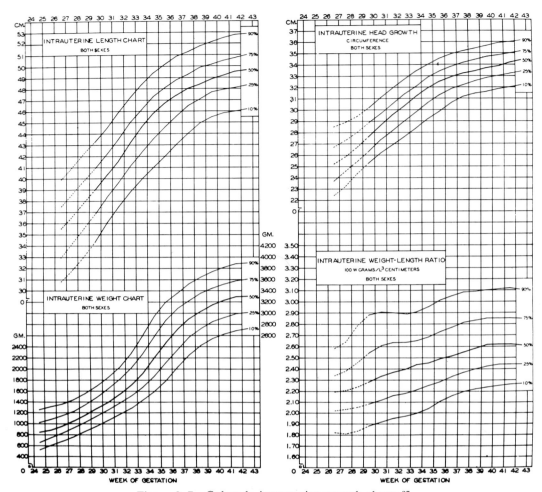

Figure 3–7 Colorado intrauterine growth charts.[37]

The gestational age is then read off the horizontal axis. Obviously, this may be grossly inaccurate if primary CNS disease, such as hydrocephalus or microcephaly, is present.

Intrauterine Growth Curves. It should be apparent that impaired growth may vary in duration and cause, and that small-for-dates infants are not a homogeneous group. Without a comparison to expected norms, proper classification of infants cannot be made. The most commonly used normal values are those compiled by Lubchenco et al,[38] which have been used to construct smoothed curves as shown in Figure 3–1. As with all such data, they are compiled from records which are deemed to contain reliable obstetrical data and exclude infants with obvious problems which are known to cause abnormal birth weight–gestational duration relationships, such as

hydrocephaly, anencephaly, and maternal diabetes. The data of Lubchenco and her colleagues are from singleton Caucasian infants born at high altitude (Denver, Colorado). Figure 3–7 shows similar data of singleton Caucasian infants born at sea level.[63] Curves constructed from values of gestational ages and birth weights of singleton Negro infants of indigent families[26] are shown in Appendix 13. Similar data concerning monochorionic and dichorionic twins[43] have also been used in constructing curves (Appendices 11, 12).

The curves alluded to above are constructed from values of birth weights attained by infants born at specific weeks of gestation (by history). The lowest 10 per cent of values in each week of gestation represents the 10th percentile, etc. An infant whose birth weight is on or below the 10th percentile curve is considered to be small-for-gestational-age, while a large-for gestational-age infant has a birth weight on or above the 90th percentile curve.

Since the curves considered to represent normal intrauterine growth for any particular segment of the population are constructed from values obtained from a large number of pregnancies exclusive of those with vague or obviously erroneous histories and malformed products, inapparent errors tend to be few, and therefore fail to skew the data because of the overwhelming volume of correct information.

APPEARANCE AT BIRTH— SMALL-FOR-GESTATIONAL-AGE INFANTS

The majority of small-for-dates infants are born at or near term, and of those who weigh less than 2500 gm. at birth, about one-third are full term.[12, 28]

They appear thin and wasted. The skin is loose, often dry, and frequently scaling. Meconium staining of the skin, nails, and umbilical cord is common. There is little subcutaneous tissue. The face is not full nor do the trunk and extremities seem to have as much musculature as expected. While weight is low, quite often length is not affected and head size may be normal. Hair on the head tends to be sparse. These babies are usually alert, active, and seem hungry, although not necessarily from the first minutes of life. These infants often do not urinate in the first hours of life and may go for 24 hours or more without voiding if fluids are not provided early. The cord dries more rapidly than that of normal infants.

The spectrum of small-for-dates infants includes those who are proportionately small without wasting, meconium staining, etc. These neonates seem to have been undergrown for a long time and appear old for their size. It is in this group that anomalies tend to occur. Aside from the evident problems of the rubella syndrome and the various trisomies, congenital heart disease and genitourinary and alimentary tract abnormalities are encountered. The presence of a unilateral or bilateral single palmar crease, single umbilical artery, and peculiarities of the ears may serve as additional clues that hidden problems exist.

The clinical problems encountered by the SGA infant are different from those seen in the AGA, preterm infant, and some of these are tabulated in Table 3–3 and considered below.

CLINICAL PROBLEMS

Neonatal *asphyxia* tends to be more common and accentuated in small-for-dates infants. This is especially true in markedly undernourished patients. These infants sometimes require immediate metabolic and ventilatory resuscitation with close attention to temperature control. The problem of poor growth in utero may be recognized by measurement of fundal height, babies' head circumference by ultrasound, and urinary estriols. Persons skilled in resuscitation should be present at the delivery of infants who have recognized intrauterine growth retardation.

In contrast to the AGA, preterm infant, whose prime *pulmonary problem* is hyaline membrane disease, SGA infants are prone to aspiration of amniotic fluid, often containing meconium, and hence aspiration pneumonia, which may be complicated by pneumothorax. In addition, pulmonary hemorrhage occurs frequently.

Hypoglycemia. This condition occurs most frequently during the neonatal period among infants of diabetic mothers, small-for-dates infants (including the smaller of discordant twins), and stressed small, preterm infants. Neonatal symptomatic hypoglycemia (blood glucose concentration <20 mg. per 100 ml.) is more common in males and predominantly small-for-gestational-age infants.[15] It is seen most frequently (50 per cent) among the SGA infants who are markedly wasted with weights below the third percentile for gestational age.[61] Hypoglycemia is most likely to occur during the first 12 hours of life, but may appear as late as 48 hours. Blood sugars should be carefully monitored in SGA infants and an early feeding regimen commenced. (For the management of symptomatic hypoglycemia, see Chapter 10.)

Thermal Regulation. Because of differing body composition and basal metabolic rates,[52, 55] the usual tables for the neutral thermal environment which are based on weight do not apply for SGA infants. Incubator settings should be determined by closely monitoring the infant's temperature, attempting to maintain abdominal skin temperature, between 36.0 and 36.5° C.

Polycythemia. A central hematocrit

TABLE 3–3 A COMPARISON OF PROBLEMS IN
SMALL-FOR-GESTATIONAL-AGE AND IMMATURE INFANTS

	SMALL-FOR-GESTATIONAL-AGE	IMMATURE
Gestation	28–44 weeks	<37 weeks
Birth weight of siblings	Low	Normal
Pulmonary	Aspiration syndrome Pneumothorax Pulmonary hemorrhage	Hyaline membrane disease
Infection (congenital)	++	+
Hyperbilirubinemia	+	++++
Hypoglycemia	+++	+
Congenital malformation	+++	±
Intracranial hemorrhage	++	+
Apnea	+	+++
Blood	Polycythemia	Normal
Feeding	Large gastric capacity	Small capacity
Future retarded growth	++	0

> 60 per cent has been described by several authors[14, 31, 32] in small-for-dates infants. In addition, infants with intrauterine growth retardation have been found to have increased red blood cell volume,[62] elevated erythropoietin levels,[23, 24] and reduced 2,3-diphosphoglycerate in the erythrocyte.[25]

The cause of the polycythemia in SGA infants is unknown. Hypoxemia below that usually found in utero has been suggested.[27] Maternal-fetal transfusion has also been considered but the demonstration of higher than expected percentage of fetal hemoglobin in the blood of small-for-dates infants tends to discount this.

The polycythemic infant is usually asymptomatic, but some manifest one or more clinical abnormalities. Symptoms may be related to increased viscosity, which rises precipitously as hematocrit values reach 70 per cent. These include tachypnea, intercostal retraction, grunting, nasal flaring, tachycardia with or without cardiac failure, pleural effusion, scrotal edema, priapism, and convulsions. Hyperbilirubinemia is not uncommon.

Treatment of symptomatic infants consists of bloodletting with or without fluid replacement. A small decrease in hematocrit results in a large decrease in blood viscosity with improvement in symptoms. It has been our practice to provide a volume of plasma equal to the quantity of blood removed. Although one might attempt to calculate how much blood to remove and how much plasma to give to attain some arbitrary hematocrit value, it is simplest to use the calculations as a rough guide and use serial hematocrit determinations as a means of deciding when to stop. The usual hematocrit value aimed for is 50 to 60 per cent.

PRACTICAL HINTS

1. A small-for-dates infant usually requires his major care during the first three or four days of life. If at all possible, the diagnosis of growth retardation should be anticipated and delivery should take place at a center with a special high-risk nursery. The expected risk

of neonatal mortality or morbidity based on perinatal data should be ascertained prior to delivery from tables constructed for this purpose. (Appendices 5, 6, 10).

2. Every neonate requires an immediate assessment for early recognition of any problem. The first step in this process is to classify the baby as mature, immature, or postmature, and small-for-gestational-age, appropriate-for-gestational-age, or large-for-gestational-age.

3. The gestational age as calculated from an adequate maternal history of menstrual periods should not be downgraded. Estimates calculated in this fashion should be seriously considered when caring for a neonate.

4. It is so important for assessment of gestational age to be done for each infant that a scoring sheet should be part of every newborn infant's record.

5. Infants of the same weight but varying gestational ages may have different obstetrical complications and problems in the neonatal period, and as a result, a different prognosis.

6. Neonatal asphyxia tends to be more common and accentuated in small-for-dates infants. The problem of poor growth in utero may be recognized by measurement of fundal height, babies' head circumference by ultrasound, and urinary estriols. Persons skilled in resuscitation should be present at the delivery of infants who have recognized intrauterine growth retardation.

7. The incidence of major congenital anomalies is higher in the growth-retarded infant than in AGA, preterm infants. Greater care must be exercised to search for congenital malformations in undergrown infants.

8. The growth-retarded infant with a placenta of normal weight for gestational age has a high risk of having a major congenital anomaly, and should be followed closely for the detection of hidden genitourinary or cardiovascular anomalies.

9. Neonatal symptomatic hypoglycemia is commonly found (15 per cent) in infants who are small-for-gestational-age. Blood sugar should be closely monitored in these infants (see Chapter 10).

10. Polycythemia is a common finding in the small-for-dates infant. Although usually asymptomatic, he may occasionally present with tachypnea, intercostal retractions, grunting, nasal flaring, tachycardia with or without failure, pleural effusions, scrotal edema, and possibly convulsions, all of which can sometimes be relieved by reducing the hematocrit. Central hematocrit should be checked and appropriate therapy instituted (see Chapter 15).

11. The infant with intrauterine growth retardation secondary to malnutrition tends to have a greater brain weight and smaller thymus, adrenal, liver, and spleen weights than does the AGA, preterm infant of the same body weight. If head size is also reduced, search for congenital infection (e.g., CID, rubella).

12. The neonatal mortality rate is higher for the AGA, preterm infant than for the growth-retarded baby of the same weight (see Appendix 10).

QUESTIONS

True or False

The brain is the most severely stunted organ in infants with intrauterine growth retardation secondary to malnutrition.

The brain is usually the least affected organ. Therefore, the statement is false.

The intrauterine twin transfusion (parabiosis) syndrome results in twins of unequal size, and the larger will usually be polycythemic. Neither twin is prone to hypoglycemia.

In other instances of twin discordance the smaller twin is usually hypoglycemic. The above statement, however, is true.

Transposition of the great vessels is associated with large-for-dates infants.

Infants with transposition of the great vessels are usually large-for-gestational-age. Therefore, the statement is true. The explanation for this is unknown. (Infants of diabetic mothers are also commonly large-for-gestational-age when the mother's blood glucose is not tightly controlled during late pregnancy. However, it has been recently observed that if the mother's blood glucose is closely controlled — below 120 mg. per 100 ml. — the infants are not large.)

Significant retardation of brain growth during intrauterine life can be compensated for by good nutrition following birth.

Retardation of brain growth signifies that severe intrauterine malnutrition occurs during a period in which brain cells are increasing in number. Therefore, normal nutrition following birth will probably not compensate for the retarded head growth. The statement is false.

Although an infant has suffered intrauterine growth retardation secondary to malnutrition, there is no increased risk of developing problems during labor.

Small-for-dates infants usually have low levels of liver and cardiac glycogen and are not prepared for the rigors of labor. Although mild-to-moderate degrees of asphyxia are noted in every infant at birth, it appears to be accentuated in small-for-dates babies. Therefore the statement is false.

Twin pregnancies are unlikely to yield small-for-dates infants if delivery occurs at 30 to 34 weeks' gestation.

There is usually a relative reduction in weight only if the infants are delivered after 35 weeks' gestation. The statement is therefore true.

Neurologic assessment of gestational age of every neonate while still in the delivery room might well afford an opportunity to more accurately identify high-risk infants.

Neurologic assessment is not highly reliable in the first hour of life. The statement is therefore false. The state of wakefulness, hunger, irritability, or effects of maternal sedation may all affect the neurologic examination. When discordance is found between gestational and neurologic age, repeat the examination—further studies are required.

Small-for-dates infants have a higher mortality rate than preterm infants who are appropriate in weight for gestational age.

Immature infants have a higher mortality. North,[46] for example, found the mortality of AGA preterm babies to be seven per cent with three per cent in weight-matched SGA infants. Therefore the statement is false.

In small-for-dates infants, the chance of malformation is unrelated to the degree of undergrowth.

The greater the degree of growth retardation, the greater the chance of malformation. Therefore the statement is false.

Small-for-dates infants have low fat stores, but a normal amount of brown fat.

Brown fat is also reduced with malnutrition. Therefore, these infants have a decreased ability to control their body temperature in a cool environment. The statement is false.

By and large, brown and white fat are not interconvertible in the normal newborn infant. Studies among gypsy children in Hungary and subsequently experimentally in rabbits have demonstrated that infants (and experimental animals) who die of starvation or undernutrition have their white fat stores depleted but their brown fat stores intact. Conversely, wellnourished infants dying in the cold, and experimental rabbits who have been well nourished but subjected to cold stress, show depletion of brown fat but have their white fat intact.

L. STERN

Carbohydrate stores of small-for-dates infants are low, and their oxygen consumption per unit weight is higher than AGA preterm infants.

Based on their body weight, infants who are small-for-gestational-age have a high oxygen consumption. Therefore the statement is true. (When compared to controls of the same weight, the growth-retarded infants appeared to have an increased oxygen consumption; however, if the infants were assigned the body weights expected for their gestational ages, no differences in oxygen consumption were noted.[55])

Small-for-dates infants have an alert appearance not found in other newborns.

Small-for-dates infants do appear alert. Therefore the statement is true.

The ratio of fetal to adult hemoglobin synthesis is greater in small-for-dates infants than in normally grown infants.

Usually, as pregnancy progresses in the normal infant, there is a decrease in the proportion of fetal to adult hemoglobin. This is not true in the small-for-dates infant, and supports Gruenwald's hypothesis that intrauterine hypoxemia is an important cause of growth retardation,[27] since, in vitro, a decrease in oxygen tension or glucose in the environment results in an increase of fetal hemoglobin synthesis as compared with adult hemoglobin synthesis.[7] Therefore the statement is true.

Large parents tend to have large babies.

Infants of large parents do tend to be large at birth, and they contribute significantly to the category of large-for-gestational-age neonates.[20] The statement is therefore true.

Gross placental lesions are frequently found in association with growth-retarded infants.

Gruenwald[27] found that it was unusual for intrauterine growth retardation to be associated with small placentas, and conspicuous gross lesions were relatively rare. While minute lesions may be of importance, in only a small number of instances do gross lesions of the placenta provide an explanation for the inappropriate growth. Identifiable placental pathologic conditions are not a major etiologic factor. Therefore the statement is false.

It is important to differentiate between low-birth-weight infants who are small-for-gestational-age and those who are appropriate-for-gestational-age. Check the following statements, marking which are correct:
  A. *Estimation of bone development by X-ray is a precise measure of gestational age.*
  B. *Maturity of organs correlates better with birth weight than with gestational age.*
  C. *With intrauterine malnutrition, birth weight and length will show greater reduction than head circumference.*
  D. *Hyperbilirubinemia is a major problem in small-for-gestational-age infants.*

A. Although organ maturation parallels gestational age, delay in the appearance of ossification centers makes radiologic investigation unreliable for estimating gestational age. Therefore the statement is false.

B. Organ maturity correlates best with gestational age. The statement is therefore false.

C. In late intrauterine malnutrition, there is a decrease only in weight. The statement is therefore true.

D. Liver function in SGA infants is similar to that of term infants; thus, hyperbilirubinemia is not a major problem in the absence of blood-group incompatibility or polycythemia. Therefore the statement is false.

Around eight per cent of all infants with birth weights greater than 2500 gm. have gestational ages less than 37 weeks, and masquerade as full-term infants.

This statement is true, and these infants should definitely be identified. Often their poor sucking reflex, limpness, and poor temperature control incorrectly suggest to the parents and physician that they are ill. They are subject to the diseases of immaturity (hyaline membrane disease, hyperbilirubinemia, etc.) and must be observed closely in the early hours and days after birth.

CASE PROBLEMS

Case One

A 1600-gm. infant presents no problems in the delivery room, is 42 cm. in length, has a head circumference of 32 cm., and no evidence of physical abnormality. Assessment of gestational age from menstrual history and neurologic examination indicates he was born at 38 weeks' gestation.

The most likely complication in the next 12 hours is: (check one)
  A. *Hypoglycemia.*
  B. *Hypocalcemia.*
  C. *Septicemia.*
  D. *Apneic episodes.*

This patient is small-for-dates, and therefore hypoglycemia (blood glucose concentration less than 20 mg. per 100 ml.) is the most likely complication of those listed to appear in the first 12 hours of life. Therefore the answer is A. Neither hypocalcemia nor septicemia is a particular problem of small-for-dates infants. Apneic episodes are generally observed in very immature infants.

It is likely he will: (check any which are appropriate)
  A. *Lose little if any weight in the first 24 hours of life.*
  B. *Not reach birth weight for 5 to 10 days after an initial fall in weight.*
  C. *Gain more slowly than an AGA infant of the same birth weight.*
  D. *Gain more rapidly than an AGA infant of the same birth weight.*

It is likely he will lose little if any weight

in the first 24 hours, and will gain more rapidly than an AGA infant of the same birth weight. This is true for the first few weeks of life; thereafter, the rate of gain will decrease and he will probably be smaller than his preterm weight peer. The answers are A and D.

He has a greater chance than an AGA infant of the same weight of having: (check any which are appropriate)
   A. Syphilis.
   B. A serum bilirubin greater than 12 mg. per 100 ml.
   C. A congenital anomaly.
   D. Mental retardation evident later in life.

He has a greater chance than an AGA infant of the same weight of having a congenital anomaly and/or mental retardation later in life. Syphilis is not a cause of intrauterine growth retardation, and hyperbilirubinemia is less frequent in small-for-dates infants than in AGA infants of equal weight. Therefore the answers are C and D.

Case Two

A 1600-gm. infant is delivered of a pre-eclamptic primipara. The infant is cyanotic, poorly responsive to stimuli, and ventilates poorly. She is meconium-stained and by examination deemed to be of 37 weeks' gestation. Resuscitation is successful, but grunting respiration, flaring of the alae nasi, intercostal retractions, hyperinflation of the chest, and dusky skin color in room air are present.

The most likely cause of the problem is: (check one)
   A. Hyaline membrane disease.
   B. Massive aspiration.
   C. Hypoglycemia.
   D. Intraventricular hemorrhage.

In a small-for-dates infant, this clinical picture is usually due to massive aspiration. Hyaline membrane disease may occur in an infant of 37 weeks' gestation, but it is not the most likely cause of these symptoms. Therefore the answer is B.

The most likely complications are: (check any which are appropriate)
   A. Pneumonitis.
   B. Pneumothorax.
   C. Hemorrhagic disease of the newborn.
   D. Seizures.
   E. Apneic episodes.
   F. Jaundice.

The most likely complications are pneumonitis due to meconium aspirated with the amniotic fluid, and pneumothorax. (Pneumothorax is a common occurrence in infants with meconium aspiration.) Therefore the answers are A and B.

In our view, the pneumothorax which occurs with meconium aspiration is often more dangerous than that which follows hyaline membrane disease in that it much more often results in tension pneumothorax with sudden shifts and the danger of death from kinking of the great vessels. The explanation of this may lie in the difference in lung compliance in the two diseases, since, in infants with the respiratory distress syndrome, the stiffness of the lung may in part minimize the shift imposed by an extrapulmonary collection of air.

L. STERN

It is necessary immediately to: (check any which are appropriate)
   A. Obtain an X-ray of the chest.
   B. Obtain an X-ray of the skull.
   C. Perform a lumbar puncture.
   D. Give oxygen.
   E. Give glucose.

Every cyanotic, poorly responsive infant requires oxygen. An X-ray of the chest is necessary to verify the lung disease, evaluate its extent, and note the presence or absence of complications. X-ray studies of the skull and examination of cerebrospinal fluid are inappropriate to the problem. Although there is nothing to be gained by the immediate administration of glucose, it is important to make frequent assessment of the blood glucose concentration. Therefore the answers are A and D.

Case Three

S. A. is the 2350-gm. product of the 31-week gestation of a 20-year-old primigravida diabetic on 58 units NPH insulin per day. The mother has been well controlled during pregnancy, and had a normal labor and delivery. One-minute Apgar = 8; five-minute Apgar = 10. Length is 41 cm. and head circumference is 27 cm. The infant began grunting and retracting, and was transferred to the intensive-care nursery. An X-ray of the chest was obtained.

This infant of a diabetic mother (IDM) is:
(choose one)
  A. SGA and preterm.
  B. LGA and preterm.
  C. AGA and preterm.
  D. SGA and term.

A. Although infants of diabetic mothers may be SGA and preterm, you have not carefully read the data.

B. This infant, as are the majority of infants of diabetic mothers, is large-for-gestational-age. He is also preterm (31 weeks' gestation).

C. This infant is preterm, but large for 31 weeks' gestation.

D. Incorrect. This infant is neither SGA nor term.

The respiratory distress in this infant is most likely due to: (check any which are appropriate)
  A. Pneumothorax.
  B. Aspiration pneumonia.
  C. Intrapulmonary hemorrhage.
  D. Hyaline membrane disease.

Pneumothorax, aspiration pneumonia, and intrapulmonary hemorrhage occur more commonly in SGA infants. Therefore the answer is D. This is a preterm infant, and hyaline membrane disease is more likely. An X-ray is essential to determine the nature of the problem.

The following metabolic derangement may be anticipated: (check any which are appropriate)
  A. Hypocalcemia.
  B. Hypoglycemia.
  C. Acidosis.
  D. Hyperbilirubinemia.
  E. All of the above.

A. Hypocalcemia occurs commonly in IDM. Therefore the statement is correct.

B. This statement is correct. The quantitative blood sugar was 11 mg. per 100 ml. The infant responded to I.V. glucose.

C. With RDS, the combination of respiratory and metabolic acidosis is to be expected. Therefore the statement is correct.

D. Hyperbilirubinemia is to be anticipated, particularly in this immature infant with respiratory distress and hypoglycemia. Therefore the statement is correct.

E. These infants present complex management problems in the early neonatal period. All the above statements are correct.

Neurologic evaluation of the infant at age 21 days revealed features appropriate for an infant of 34 weeks' gestation. Is this normal?

The gestational age is now 34 weeks (31 weeks at delivery plus three weeks postnatal age). Neurologic maturation is dependent on gestational age, so the parents should be advised accordingly. Therefore the answer is yes. Preterm infants are often erroneously labeled as slow or retarded because no allowance is made for this.

The following factors adversely influence the outcome of the fetus in diabetic mothers: (check any which are appropriate)
  A. Previous history of stillbirth.
  B. Hypoglycemia.
  C. Keto-acidosis.
  D. The dose of insulin the mother requires.
  E. The duration of her disease.
  F. Development of hydramnios.

A. Diabetic mothers with a history of a previous normal pregnancy have fewer problems than those with a history of stillbirth or previous neonatal death. Therefore the statement is true.

B. Maternal hypoglycemia does not have an adverse effect on the fetus. The statement is therefore false.

C. Keto-acidosis during pregnancy may be disastrous for the fetus and result in the infant's demise. Therefore the statement is true.

D. There is no good correlation between the dose of insulin the mother requires and the perinatal course. Therefore the statement is false.

E. The longer the mother has been diabetic and the greater the vascular involvement, the worse the outlook for the infant. The statement is therefore true.

F. False.

While we would agree that the advent of polyhydramnios, which is rather common in infants of diabetic mothers, may not afford an index as to the severity of the degree to which the diabetic mother's infant will be affected, the polyhydramnios on occasion may reflect serious congenital malformations, particularly those associated with high obstruction in the gastrointestinal tract. The answer to this question is, therefore, perhaps not quite so "false" as the author indicates, since congenital malformations may be more common in infants of diabetic mothers than among infants born to mothers not so affected.

L. STERN

REFERENCES

1. Abernathy, J., Greenberg, B., Wells, H., et al: Smoking as an independent variable in a multiple regression analysis upon birth weight and gestation. Amer J Public Health 56:626, 1966.
2. Aherne, W., and Hull, D.: Brown adipose tissue and heat production in the newborn infant. J Path Bact 91:223, 1966.
3. Ahlfors, C., and Brown, E.: Personal communication.
4. Allen, D., and Jandl, J.: Factors influencing relative rates of synthesis of adult and fetal hemoglobin in vitro. J Clin Invest 39:1107, 1960.
5. Amiel-Tison, C.: Neurological evaluation of the maturity of newborn infants. Arch Dis Child 43:89, 1968.
6. Babson, S., and Kangas, J.: Preschool intelligence of undersized term infants. Amer J Dis Child 117:553, 1969.
7. Bard, H., Makowski, E. L., Meschia, G., et al: The relative rates of synthesis of hemoglobins A and F in immature red cells of newborn infants. Pediatrics 45:766, 1970.
8. Battaglia, F., and Lubchenco, L.: A practical classification of newborn infants by weight and gestational age. J Pediat 71:159, 1967.
9. Beltran-Paz, C., and Driscoll, S.: cited in Benirschke, K., and Driscoll, S., Eds.: *The Pathology of the Human Placenta.* New York, Springer-Verlag New York, Inc., 1967.
10. Benirschke, K., and Driscoll, S.: *The Pathology of the Human Placenta.* New York, Springer-Verlag New York, Inc., 1967.
11. Collins, E., and Turner, G.: The importance of the "small-for-dates" baby to the problem of mental retardation. Med J Aust 2:313, 1971.
12. Colman, H., and Rienzo, J.: The small term baby. Obstet Gynec 19:87, 1962.
13. Cooper, L., Green, R., Krugman, S., et al: Neonatal thrombocytopenic purpura and other manifestations of rubella contracted in utero. Amer J Dis Child 110:416, 1965.
14. Cornblath, M., and Schwartz, R.: *Disorders of Carbohydrate Metabolism in Infancy.* Philadelphia, W. B. Saunders Company, 1966.
15. Cornblath, M., Wybregt, S. H., Baens, G. S., et al: Symptomatic neonatal hypoglycemia. Studies of carbohydrate metabolism in the newborn infant. VIII. Pediatrics 33:388, 1964.
16. Dancis, J., O'Connell, J., and Holt, L., Jr.: A grid for recording the weight of premature infants. J Pediat 33:570, 1948.
17. Drillien, C.: Intellectual sequelae of "fetal malnutrition." *In* Waisman, H., and Kerr, G., Eds.: *Fetal Growth and Development.* New York, McGraw-Hill Book Co., 1970.
18. Drillien, C.: The small-for-dates infant: Etiology and prognosis. Pediat Clin N Amer 17:9, 1970.
19. Dubowitz, L., Dubowitz, V., and Goldberg, C.: Clinical assessment of gestational age in the newborn infant. J Pediat 77:1, 1970.
20. Engleson, G., Rooth, G., and Tormblom, M.: A follow-up study of dysmature infants. Arch Dis Child 38:62, 1963.
21. Farr, V., Kerridge, D., and Mitchell, R.: The value of some external characteristics in the assessment of gestational age at birth. Develop Med Child Neurol 8:657, 1966.
22. Farr, V., Mitchell, R., Neligan, G., et al: The definition of some external characteristics used in the assessment of gestational age of the newborn infant. Develop Med Child Neurol 8:507, 1966.
23. Finne, P.: Erythropoietin levels in cord blood as an indicator of intrauterine hypoxia. Acta Paediat Scand 55:478, 1966.
24. Finne, P.: Erythropoietin production in fetal hypoxia and in anemic uremic patients. Ann NY Acad Sci 149:497, 1968.
25. Fiori, R., and Scanlon, J.: Erythrocyte levels of 2,3-diphosphoglycerate in the syndrome of fetal malnutrition. Amer J Obstet Gynec 111:681, 1971.
26. Freeman, M., Graves, W., and Thompson, R.: Indigent Negro and Caucasian birth weight–gestational age tables. Pediatrics 46:9, 1970.
27. Gruenwald, P.: Chronic fetal distress and placental insufficiency. Biol Neonat 5:215, 1963.
28. Gruenwald, P.: Infants of low birth weight among 5,000 deliveries. Pediatrics 34:157, 1964.
29. Gruenwald, P., Funakawa, H., Mitani, S., et al: Influence of environmental factors in foetal growth in man. Lancet 1:1026, 1967.
30. Halvorsen, S., and Finne, P.: Erythropoietin production in the human fetus and newborn. Ann NY Acad Sci 149:576, 1968.
31. Haworth, J., Dilling, L., and Younoszai, M.: Relation of blood glucose to hematocrit, birth weight, and other body measurements in normal and growth-retarded newborn infants. Lancet 2:901, 1967.
32. Humbert, J., Abelson, H., Hathaway, W., et al: Polycythemia in small for gestational age infants. J Pediat 75:812, 1969.
33. Koenigsberger, M.: Judgment of fetal age. I. Neurologic evaluation. Pediat Clin N Amer 13:823, 1966.
34. Lochridge, S., Pas, R., and Cassady, G.: Reticulocyte counts in intrauterine growth retardation. Pediatrics 47:919, 1971.
35. Lubchenco, L.: Assessment of gestational age and development at birth. Pediat Clin N Amer 17:125, 1970.
36. Lubchenco, L., Hansman, C., and Bäckström, L.: Factors influencing fetal growth. *In* Jonxis, J., Visser, H., and Troelstra, J., Eds.: *Nutricia Symposium: Aspects of Praematurity and Dysmaturity.* Springfield, Charles C Thomas, 1968.
37. Lubchenco, L., Hansman, C., and Boyd, E.: Intrauterine growth in length and head circumference as estimated from live births at gestational ages from 26 to 42 weeks. Pediatrics 37:403, 1966.
38. Lubchenco, L., Hansman, C., Dressler, M., et al: Intrauterine growth as estimated from liveborn birth weight data at 24 to 42 weeks of gestation. Pediatrics 32:793, 1963.
39. Mehrizi, A., and Drash, A.: Birth weight of infants with cyanotic and acyanotic congenital malformations of the heart. J Pediat 59:715, 1961.
40. Naeye, R.: Human intrauterine parabiotic syndrome and its complications. New Eng J Med 268:804, 1963.
41. Naeye, R.: Abnormalities in infants of mothers with toxemia of pregnancy. Amer J Obstet Gynec 95:276, 1966.
42. Naeye, R.: Fetal growth with congenital syphilis: A quantitative study. Amer J Clin Path 55:228, 1971.
43. Naeye, R., Benirschke, K., Hagstrom, J., et al: Intra-

uterine growth of twins as estimated from live-born birth-weight data. Pediatrics *37*:409, 1966.

44. Naeye, R., Diener, W., Dellinger, W., et al: Urban poverty: Effects on prenatal nutrition. Science *166*:1026, 1969.

45. Neligan, G.: The clinical effects of being "light for dates." Proc Roy Soc Med *60*:881, 1967.

46. North, F., Jr.: Small-for-dates neonates. I. Maternal, gestational, and neonatal characteristics. Pediatrics *38*:1013, 1966.

47. Ounsted, M.: Foetal growth. *In* Gairdner, D., and Hull, D., Eds.: *Recent Advances in Paediatrics.* London, Churchill Ltd., 1971. 4th Edition.

48. Reisman, L.: Chromosome abnormalities and intra-uterine growth retardation. Pediat Clin N Amer *17*:101, 1970.

49. Saint-Anne Dargassies, S.: La maturation neuro-logique du prématuré. Etudes Néonatales *4*:71, 1955.

50. Saint-Anne Dargassies, S.: The full term newborn; neurological assessment. Biol Neonat *4*:174, 1962.

51. Schlesinger, E., and Allaway, N.: The combined effect of birth weight and length of gestation on neonatal mortality among single premature infants. Pediatrics *15*:698, 1955.

52. Scopes, J., and Ahmed, I.: Minimal rates of oxygen consumption in sick and premature newborn infants. Arch Dis Child *41*:407, 1966.

53. Shanklin, D.: The influence of placental lesions on the newborn infant. Pediat Clin N Amer *17*:25, 1970.

54. Shelley, H.: Carbohydrate reserves in the newborn infant. Brit Med J *1*:273, 1964.

55. Sinclair, J., and Silverman, W.: Intrauterine growth in active tissue mass of the human fetus, with particular reference to the undergrown baby. Pediatrics *38*:48, 1966.

56. Smith, A., and McKeown, T.: Prenatal growth of mongoloid defectives. Arch Dis Child *30*:257, 1955.

57. Smith, C.: Effects of maternal undernutrition upon the newborn infants in Holland (1944–1945). J Pediat *30*:229, 1947.

58. Smith, C.: Prenatal and neonatal nutrition. Pediatrics *30*:145, 1962.

59. Stoch, M., and Smythe, P.: Does undernutrition during infancy inhibit brain growth and subsequent intellectual development? Arch Dis Child *38*:546, 1963.

60. Thomas, A., and Saint-Anne Dargassies, S.: *In Etudes Neurologiques sur le Nouveau-né et le Jeune Nourisson.* Paris, Masson et Cie, 1952.

61. Usher, R.: Clinical and therapeutic aspects of fetal malnutrition. Pediat Clin N Amer *17*:169, 1970.

62. Usher, R., and Lind, J.: Blood volume of the newborn premature infant. Acta Paediat Scand *54*:419, 1965.

63. Usher, R., and McLean, F.: Intrauterine growth of liveborn Caucasian infants at sea level: Standards obtained in 7 dimensions of infants born between 25 and 44 weeks of gestation. J Pediat *74*:901, 1969.

64. Usher, R., McLean, F., and Scott, K.: Judgment of fetal age. II. Clinical significance of gestational age and an objective method for its assessment. Pediat Clin N Amer *13*:835, 1966.

65. van den Berg, B., and Yerushalmy, J.: The relationship of the rate of intrauterine growth of infants of low birth weight to mortality, morbidity, and congenital anomalies. J Pediat *69*:531, 1966.

66. van den Berg, B., and Yerushalmy, J.: The statistical approach to fetal growth. *In* Waisman, H., and Kerr, G. R., Eds.: *Fetal Growth and Development.* New York, McGraw-Hill Book Co., 1970.

67. Warkany, J., Monroe, B., and Sutherland, B.: Intra-uterine growth retardation. Amer J Dis Child *102*:249, 1961.

68. Warkany, J., Passarge, E., and Smith, L.: Congenital malformations in autosomal trisomy syndromes. Amer J Dis Child *112*:502, 1966.

69. Wilson, M., Meyers, H., and Peters, A.: Postnatal bone growth of infants with fetal growth retardation. Pediatrics *40*:213, 1967.

70. Winick, M.: Cellular growth of the human placenta. III. Intrauterine growth failure. J Pediat *71*:390, 1967.

71. Winick, M.: Changes in nucleic acid and protein content of the human brain during growth. Pediat Res *2*:352, 1968.

72. Winick, M.: Cellular growth in intrauterine malnutrition. Pediat Clin N Amer *17*:69, 1970.

Chapter 4

THE PHYSICAL ENVIRONMENT

by

MARSHALL KLAUS, M.D.

and

AVROY FANAROFF, M.B. (Rand.),
M.R.C.P.E.

"The foetus was no larger than the palm of his hand, but the father. . . put his son in an oven, suitably arranged . . . making him take on the necessary increase of growth, by the uniformity of the external heat, measured accurately in the degrees of a thermometer."

LAWRENCE STERNE, *Tristram Shandy*

The low-birth-weight infant is particularly dependent on the physician to provide the ideal "external milieu" in order to ensure optimal neurologic and physical development, not mere survival. In as much as the ideal amount of light, sound, cutaneous stimulation, humidity, and temperature at different ages are at present unknown, this is not a simple task.

Animal studies, however, reveal that apparently minor changes in the environment may result in profound temporary or permanent developmental alterations in the organism. These studies suggest that the complete physical environment of the immature infant must be thoroughly explored. Extreme caution is necessary before introducing any major alterations in present care procedures.

With this in mind, the multiple aspects of the physical environment — most especially the thermal environment — will be considered in this chapter.

THE THERMAL ENVIRONMENT

HISTORY

An understanding of the thermal requirements of the high-risk infant was slow to develop. Pierre Budin,[9] historically the first neonatologist, had perhaps the earliest insight into the clinical importance of the thermal environment. In 1907, in his book *The Nursling,* he emphasized the need for temperature control. He observed that if the infant's temperature remained between 32.5 and 33.5° C (90.5 and 92.3° F), only 10 per cent of the infants survived; however, if the infant's body temperature was maintained in the normal range (between 36 and 37° C, 96.8 and 98.6° F), 77 per cent survived. He recommended an air temperature of 30° C (86° F) for the small (1 Kg.), fully clothed infant. Sadly, his observations were neither fully understood nor appreciated in the first fifty years of this century.

Blackfan and Yaglou,[6] working between 1926 and 1933 with a group of infants fully clothed and weighing between 1360 and 2270 gm., observed that high relative humidity and an air temperature of about 25° C (77° F) were required to maintain equilibrium of body temperature. When comparable groups of infants were placed in a slightly higher thermal environment with a lower relative humidity, they noted wider fluctuations in temperature, an increase in the incidence of diarrhea, a decrease in weight gain, and an increased mortality.

Although their observations became the basis of care (and gospel), several significant but unstudied changes were made in the infants' environment during the next 29 years. Not only the humidity but also the particulate water was increased to such an extent that infants in incubators were often not visible. In the late 1940's, to improve observation, the infant was undressed and left nude without increasing the incubator temperature. In retrospect, the clinical value of the two variables, temperature and humidity, were confused during these years.

The relative importance of incubator temperature and relative humidity was finally resolved by Silverman in three sequential analyses, the design of which has become a model for further studies of the neonate.[34,35,36] In his first study, he compared high and low humidity in two groups of infants. Infants in the high humidity group had a lower mortality but higher rectal temperatures. In the second study, to end the confusion caused by two variables, he controlled the humidity and examined the effect of varying environmental temperature. He noted a striking difference in survival rates (Table 4–1). With only a 4° F increase in incubator temperature (29.9 to 33.6° C, 85 to 89° F) he observed a 15 per cent increase in survival at the higher temperature (68.1 per cent vs. 83.5 per cent), with the biggest difference appearing in the smallest infants.

In a further study, controlling environmental temperatures but varying humidity demonstrated no difference in survival.

About the same time, Cross,[12] working in England, observed a drop in oxygen consumption in normal full-term infants when they were placed in a low-oxygen environment (15 per cent) and suggested that this might explain the unusual ability of newborn mammals to survive prolonged periods of asphyxia. As a defense against asphyxia, oxygen consumption would be reduced. However, the infants breathing 15 per cent oxygen had lower body temperatures.

June Hill,[26] working in Cross' laboratory with kittens and guinea pigs, in part clarified the exciting studies of Cross and explained the profound effects of environmental temperature on survival observed by Silverman. She found that in 20 per cent oxygen, oxygen consumption and rectal temperatures varied with the environmental temperature (Figure 4–1). She noted *a set of thermal conditions at which heat production (measured as oxygen consumption) is minimal yet core temperature is within the normal range (neutral thermal environment).* When the animals were cooled while breathing 20 per cent oxygen, their oxygen consumption markedly increased and body temperature was maintained. However, when they were given 12 per cent oxygen and cooled, oxygen consumption did not increase and the animals' body temperatures dropped. This, as well as the work of Bruck[7] and others, has emphasized that the human

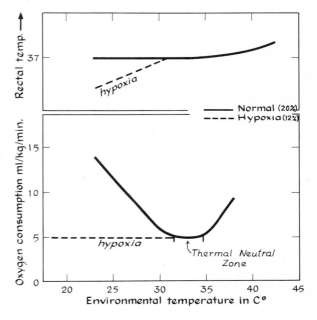

Figure 4–1 Effect of environmental temperature on oxygen consumption, breathing 20 per cent or a hypoxic mixture.

TABLE 4-1 SURVIVAL RATE BY BIRTH-WEIGHT GROUPS[37]

BIRTH WEIGHT	NUMBER OF INFANTS	SURVIVAL RATE*	
		"Normothermic" Incubator 89° *Per Cent*	"Hypothermic" Incubator 85° *Per Cent*
1501 + gm.	84	92.9	78.6
1001–1500 gm.	70	85.7	77.1
<1001 gm.	28	50	14.3
	Overall	83.5	68.1

*In each birth-weight category, survival was greater among infants in normothermic incubators.

infant is a homeotherm and not a poikilotherm, as is a turtle. When the infant is cooled and not hypoxic, he attempts to maintain body temperature by increasing the consumption of calories and oxygen to produce additional heat. Homeotherms possess mechanisms which enable them to maintain body temperature at a constant level with more or less accuracy despite changes in the environmental temperature. In contrast, the turtle drops his body temperature if placed in a cool environment.

The increased survival rate in the warmer environment observed by Budin and Silverman resulted from the decreased oxygen consumption and carbon dioxide production as environmental conditions approximated the neutral thermal environment. (An immature infant with a minimal ability to transfer oxygen and excrete carbon dioxide across his lungs has the least chance of becoming hypoxic or developing a respiratory acidosis—increased $PaCO_2$—if maintained in an environment which minimizes oxygen consumption or metabolic rate.)

These observations became the stimulus for an intense study of temperature control which has continued to the present. The physiologic and clinical highlights of these investigations will be summarized in the next section.

PHYSIOLOGIC CONSIDERATIONS

Heat Production

The heat production within the body is a side-product of metabolic processes and must equal the heat that flows from the surface of the infant's body over a given period of time if the mean body temperature is to remain constant. A characteristic of the home-othermic infant is the ability to produce extra heat in a cool environment. In the adult, additional heat production can come from: (1) voluntary muscle activity, (2) involuntary tonic or rhythmic muscle activity (at high intensities it is characterized by a visible tremor known as "shivering"), and (3) non-shivering thermogenesis. The latter is a cold-induced increase in oxygen consumption and heat production, which is not blocked by curare—a drug which prevents muscle movements and shivering. In the adult, shivering is quantitatively the most significant involuntary mechanism of regulating heat production, while in the infant, nonshivering thermogenesis is probably most important. From animal studies it can be inferred that in the human infant, the thermogenic effector organ—brown fat—contributes the largest percentage of nonshivering thermogenesis.

More abundant in the newborn than in the adult, brown fat accounts for about two to six per cent of total body weight in the human infant. Sheets of brown fat may be found at the base of the neck, between the scapulae, in the mediastinum, and surrounding the kidneys and adrenals. Brown fat differs both morphologically and metabolically from the more abundant white fat. The cells are rich in mitochondria and contain numerous fat vacuoles (as compared with the single vacuoles in white fat). There is also an abundant blood and sympathetic nerve supply. Its metabolism is stimulated by noradrenalin released through sympathetic innervation resulting in triglyceride hydrolysis. In hibernators, the brown adipose tissue has a brown appearance which gave it its name. Its contribution to extra heat production in the infant animal varies with the species.

There exists considerable misunderstanding as to the origin of the term "brown fat." For a long time it was supposed that the brown appearance derived from the high concentration of catecholamines found therein, with the excess dopamine granules giving the color to it. Indeed, however, it is the rich blood supply of the tissue which gives it its brown appearance. The blood supply is in turn a reflection of the high metabolic activity of the tissue, and therefore the name, though essentially a misnomer, has remained in common usage.

L. STERN

The evidence that brown fat plays a role in the responses of the newborn infant includes: (1) the increase in oxygen consumption (60 per cent) without an appreciable increase in physical activity following an I.V. administration of noradrenalin; (2) the rise in the renal noradrenalin excretion simultaneously with the increase in oxygen uptake in cold-exposed newborn infants while adrenalin secretion is small; and (3) the discovery by Silverman[37] that during cold exposure in humans the nape of the neck is warmer than any other skin, corresponds with the fact that in the rabbit exposed to cold, local heat production occurs in the large mass of brown adipose tissue in the interscapular region. Furthermore, Dawkins[14] showed, in cooled infants, a rise in plasma glycerol with only a slight rise in free fatty acids (FFA), suggesting that part of the FFA are immediately oxidized at the site of liberation, the brown fat. These results strongly suggest that brown adipose tissue is a major source of additional heat when the human newborn is exposed to cold.

The early rise in plasma glycerol following cold exposure is always followed by a considerable rise in free fatty acids as the cold exposure is prolonged. It has been estimated that approximately 10 per cent of the free fatty acids produced from the breakdown of neutral fat are oxidized directly in the tissue, and a further 20 per cent released into the plasma, where they do serve as an adequate reflection of the cold exposure. The remaining 70 per cent are recombined with triglycerides to again form neutral fat. At first glance, the reaction may appear to be, therefore, quite inefficient. However, it has been shown that this apparently purposeless recyclization is indeed a highly exothermic reaction; it is presumably this which forms the major source of heat production in the brown adipose tissue.

L. STERN

Heat Loss

Heat transfer or loss within the body to the environment can be divided into two portions: (1) from within the body to the surface (internal gradient), and (2) from the body surface to the environment (external gradient). The physiologic control mechanisms of the infant may alter the internal gradient (i.e., vasomotor) to change skin bloodflow. The external gradient is of a purely physical nature. Both the large surface-to-volume ratio of the infant (especially those below 2 Kg.) in relation to the adult and the thin layer of subcutaneous fat increase the heat transfer in the internal gradient—less insulation.

The heat transfer from the surface of the body to the environment involves four components: loss by (1) radiation, (2) conduction, (3) convection, and (4) the evaporation of water. This heat transfer is complex and the contribution of each component depends on the temperature of the surroundings (air and walls), air speed, and water vapor pressure. Of special clinical importance to the pediatrician is the increase in convective losses as air speed increases, and the considerable increase in radiant loss from the infant's skin to the cold walls of incubators. This is of major significance when the infant is nude and the incubator has only a single plastic wall. In this situation, the room temperature will have a major effect on the temperature of the inside wall of the incubator.

It should be stressed that radiant heat loss is independent of the surrounding air temperature; consequently, the temperature inside the incubator will not help very much in stemming loss to the cold, outside wall. The converse of this phenomenon occurs with radiant heat gain, whereby an incubator placed in the bright sunlight will result in a rise in the temperature of the infant—an elevation which is often mistaken for sepsis, and which results in needless investigative procedures and often therapy for the infant.

L. STERN

The effect of environmental temperature on heat production (oxygen consumption) is considered in Figure 4–2. As the environmental temperature is decreased below Point A (critical temperature), oxygen consumption increases. Body temperature, however, is maintained if heat production is adequate.

However, if cooling is severe and body temperature drops below Point B, with cold paralysis of the temperature regulation center, oxygen consumption also drops—two to three times for every 10° fall in body temperature. This is known as the "Q-10 Effect."

From Figure 4–2 it can be seen that oxygen consumption is minimal in two areas

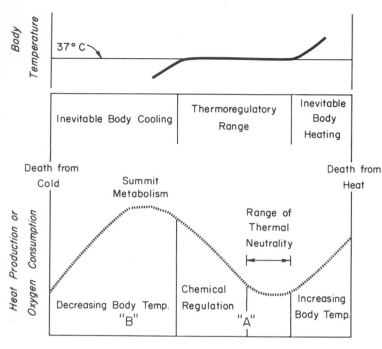

Figure 4–2 Effect of environmental temperature on oxygen consumption and body temperature. (Adapted from Merenstein and Blackmon.[29])

—the neutral thermal environment and severe hypothermia. The cardiac surgeon sometimes works in the latter (temperatures below Point B); the neonatologist attempts to maintain the infant in a warm environment (the neutral thermal environment, or the so-called zone of thermal comfort). It is most important clinically to note that the infant may not be in a neutral thermal environment and yet the rectal temperature may be in the normal range. As emphasized by Hey,[21] ". . . body temperature alone fails to indicate whether a baby is subjected to thermal stress: it can only alert us to situations in which the thermal stress has been so severe that the baby's normal thermoregulatory mechanisms have been at least partially overpowered." When the infant is in an environment above the neutral thermal zone, hyperthermia rapidly occurs. Hyperthermia develops more rapidly in the neonate than in the adult. The infant has a lower capacity for heat storage because of the higher temperature of the body shell and the larger surface-to-volume ratio. Thus, the thermoregulatory system of the homeothermic infant adjusts and balances heat production, skin blood flow, sweating, and respiration in such a way that the body temperature remains constant within a control range of environmental temperatures. The control range refers to the range of environmental temperatures at which body temperature can be kept constant by means of regulation. The control range of the infant is more limited than that of the adult because of less insulation. For the nude human adult, the lower limit of the control range is 0° C (32° F), while in the full-term infant it is 20 to 23° C (68 to 73.4° F). It is necessary to note here that the insufficient stability of body temperature in the small premature does not indicate an immaturity of temperature regulation, for the system is intact. As pointed out by Bruck,[8] the insufficient stability "seems to be due to the discrepancy between efficiency of the effector systems and body size." The newborn infant has a well-developed temperature regulation but a narrower control range than the adult.

In Utero

While in utero, the heat produced by the infant is dissipated through the placenta to the mother (Figure 4–3). Normally, the core temperature of the infant is higher than that of the mother. This system works well for the infant except during periods when the mother has an increasing body temperature. During these febrile periods, the infant's

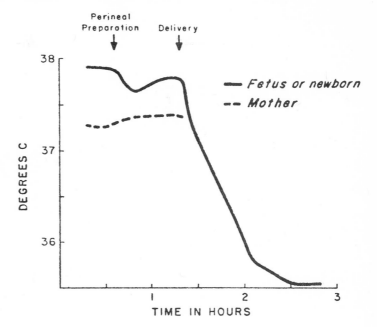

Figure 4–3 Colonic temperatures of mother and fetus during labor, and that of the newborn after delivery.[2]

After Birth

At birth, the infant's core temperature drops rapidly, owing mainly to evaporation from its moist body. The infant's small amount of subcutaneous tissue and large surface area-to-mass ratio compared to the adult, together with the cold air and walls of the delivery room, also result in large radiant and convective heat losses. Thus, under normal delivery room conditions, deep body temperature of human newborns can fall 2 to 3° C unless special precautions are taken.

Although moderate to severe cooling may result in metabolic acidosis, a lower arterial oxygen level, and hypoglycemia in the newborn infant, very slight cooling of the infant may be beneficial in its adaptation to extrauterine life. Cooling of the skin receptors may play a significant role in initiating respiration while possibly stimulating the onset of thyroid function. The vasoconstriction and peripheral resistance observed with cooling also alter systemic vascular resistance, thereby reducing the right to left shunting of blood through the ductus arteriosus.

Despite the possible advantages of slight cooling, the neonatologist has chosen to warm the infant following delivery to prevent metabolic acidosis and possibly dangerous reflex responses to cooling. Many devices are now available which allow the newborn infant to

temperature will be raised even higher than the mother's temperature.[1]

be in a warm environment while still in the delivery room, although the mother and obstetrician are cool.

PRACTICAL APPLICATIONS

Nutrition and Temperature

As a result of the relationship between metabolic rate and body temperature, both fluid and nutritional requirements for growth are intimately linked with temperature regulation. This is especially important in the small premature infant maintained in a cool environment. His caloric intake is limited by the small capacity of his stomach. Fewer calories would be required for maintenance of body temperature if he were in a warmer environment; thus, in the neutral thermal environment, caloric intake can be more effectively utilized.

The insensible loss of water parallels the metabolic rate, with 25 per cent of total heat produced being dissipated in this manner. Thus, an elevated metabolic rate results in elevated fluid losses and hence, increased fluid requirements.

The neutral thermal temperature allows for smaller feedings and reduced caloric requirements for growth.

Glass, Silverman and Sinclair[18] were able to quantitate the effect of temperature control on growth, comparing twelve matched healthy small infants aged one week and between 1 and 2 Kg. in weight. These infants were divided into a "warm" group (abdominal skin temperature maintained at 36.5° C (97.7° F) and a "standard" group (abdominal skin temperature maintained at 35° C (95° F). Both groups received 120 calories per Kg. per day. They showed a significantly more rapid increase in body weight and length in the warm group; however, their cold resistance (ability to prevent a fall in deep body temperature in a cool environment) was diminished. Identical growth rates could be obtained by increasing caloric input in the standard group.

It is therefore difficult to decide if the premature infant, after the early neonatal period (two weeks), should be maintained in the neutral thermal environment for optimal growth or be prepared for the rigors of a cold apartment.

Heating Equipment

Maintenance of an infant in the neutral thermal environment minimizes heat production, oxygen consumption, and nutritional requirements for growth. Unfortunately, equipment (usually incubators) presently available are not easily adjusted to maintain an infant in the neutral thermal environment.

In the United States, the most commonly used heating device for the nude infant is an incubator with a single plastic wall.[17] The infant is heated by convection. Because the temperature of the plastic walls cannot be controlled, the radiant heat loss of the infant to the wall of the incubator is variable. Figure 4-4 indicates how the incubator wall temperature drops with cooler room temperatures—a major disadvantage when nursing a sick infant. If the nursery is cool (23.8 to 15.6° C, 75 to 60° F) or if the incubator is placed near a cool window or wall, it will be difficult—usually impossible—to locate and maintain the neutral thermal environment. The infant will lose heat to the cold incubator wall and will needlessly increase oxygen and caloric consumption in his efforts to stay warm. The magnitude of this loss can be predicted if room temperature is known. Hey and Katz[21] found that operative temperature (true environmental temperature, taking into account radiation and convection) fell one degree below incubator temperature for every seven degrees that incubator air exceeded room temperature (Figure 4-5). Unless the incubator, room air, and radiant surfaces have

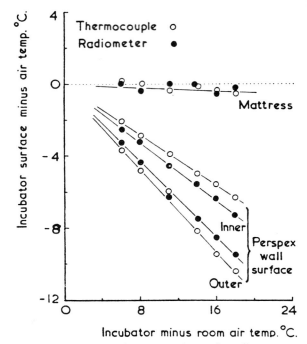

Figure 4-4 Thermocouple and radiometer estimates of the relation between incubator air and mean surface temperatures in a natural convection incubator.[24]

similar temperatures, innumerable thermal conditions can exist.

Different types of adaptations will prevent radiant heat loss and allow a precise and controlled thermal environment.

One method is to warm the nude infant with warm air and heated incubator walls, using either a layer of warm water or electrically conductive plastic paneling.[24]

These expensive procedures have been obviated by Hey, who has developed a small clear plastic heat shield to be used within the traditional single-walled incubator (Figure 4-6). The warm incubator air heats the plastic wall of the shield to the same temperature as the air within the incubator. The infant radiates only to the warm inner plastic wall, as radiant waves from the infant (2 to 9 microns) will not penetrate the plastic wall.

Radiant heat panels[4] placed above the infant without a complete enclosure have been used. Again they have the disadvantage that changing room temperature makes the location and maintenance of the neutral thermal environment almost impossible. It

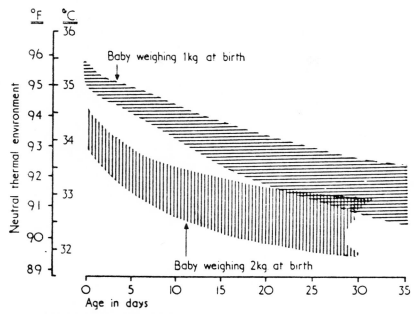

Figure 4–5 The range of temperature to provide neutral environmental conditions for a baby lying naked on a warm mattress in draught-free surroundings of moderate humidity (50 per cent saturation) when mean radiant temperature is the same as air temperature. The hatched area shows the average neutral temperature range for a healthy baby weighing 1 Kg. (▤) or 2 Kg. (▥) at birth. "Optimum" temperature probably approximates to the lower limit of the neutral range as defined here. Approximately 1° C should be added to these operative temperatures in order to derive the appropriate neutral air temperature for a single-walled incubator when room temperature is less than 27° C (80° F), and rather more if room temperature is very much less than this.[21]

is, however, useful for short-term warming in the delivery room and for procedures.

An alternative approach which has been revived and studied in detail by Hey and O'Connell[25] is to care for the infant dressed (cot-nursed) rather than naked. As shown in Table 4–2, the resistance to heat loss is increased by 1.25 units when the infant is dressed in a shirt, diaper, and gown, but only an aditional resistance of 0.61 units is added when a flannellette sheet and two layers of cotton blanket are added. The many advantages of cot nursing are appreciated by inspecting Figure 4–7, which illustrates the range of environmental temperatures over which an infant should be expected to main-

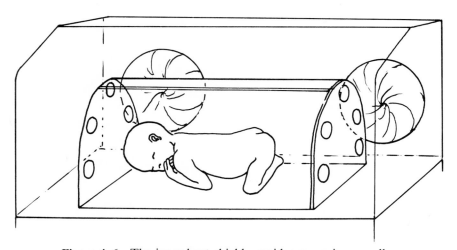

Figure 4–6 The inner heat shield provides warm inner walls.

TABLE 4–2   RESISTANCE TO HEAT LOSS IN CLO UNITS FOR A BABY WEIGHING
2.5 KG. LYING ON A FOAM MATTRESS IN A COOL DRAUGHT-FREE ENVIRONMENT[25]

	NAKED	CLOTHED	COT-NURSED
Effect of body tissue	0.29	0.29	0.29
Effect of still air	0.78	0.78	0.78
Effect of clothing	—	1.25	1.25
Effect of bedding	—	—	0.61
Total resistance	1.07	2.32	2.93

tain his rectal temperature between 36.5 and 37° C (97.7 and 98.6° F) for a period of time, and the required levels of heat production. For neutral thermal conditions in the nude infant, an operative temperature of 32.5° C (90.5° F) is required, while only 25° C (77° F) is necessary when cot nursed. As emphasized by Hey, the major additional advantage is the larger latitude of safe environmental temperatures when infants are cot nursed. If the incubator temperature drops 2° C, the naked infant must increase heat production by 35 per cent to prevent a fall in deep body temperature, while a 2° C increase would result in the infant becoming febrile. Similar changes in room temperature would have a negligible effect on the cot-nursed infant. Hey calculated that for the same effects in the cot-nursed infant, the room temperature must fall to 19° C (66.2° F) or rise to 31° C (87.8° F). Lightly dressed infants of around 1 Kg. will drop the lower end of their neutral thermal environment to slightly above 31° C (88° F) and minimize the effects of fluctuation in environmental temperature. Cot nursing may be clinically useful when continuous observation is not required.

A completely different approach to caring for an infant in the neutral thermal environment is to servo the heating device (whether it is a heat panel or incubator) to the infant's abdominal skin temperature. If the infant's skin temperature drops, the warming device increases its heat output. The temperature of the skin at which the incubator is servoed is critical. Silverman's studies showed that maintaining the abdominal skin temperature at 36.5° C (97.7° F) minimizes oxygen consumption; at an abdominal skin temperature of 37.2° C (98.9° F), oxygen consumption increases six per cent; and at an abdominal skin temperature of 35.9° C (96.6° F), oxygen consumption increases 10 per cent.[10, 33]

Two disadvantages of servo-controlled equipment are the increased expense and the required re-orientation of both nurses and physicians when evaluating the infant's condition — both the infant and the incubator temperature must be compared together, lest the infant's true condition be masked. When an infant who is servo-controlled starts to become febrile, the incubator temperature drops, but there is no change in body temperature. In the other direction, when an infant who is being servo-controlled dies, his body temperature will be maintained because the incubator temperature will rise.

The use of a servo-controlled incubator may deprive the physician of one of the earlier indices of sepsis in a newborn — that is, the inability of the infant to maintain his own temperature. This sign, which is often also seen in intracranial hemorrhage or other CNS injury, may be extremely valuable in alerting the attending personnel to an impending and potentially reversible disaster.

L. STERN

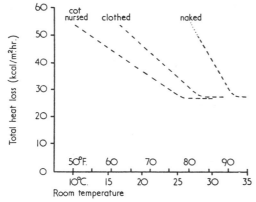

Figure 4–7 The relation between heat loss and room temperature in a typical baby weighing ween 2 and 3 Kg. when more than two days old. Clothes and bedding increase the resistance to heat loss and decrease the temperature necessary to provide thermoneutral conditions.[25]

If and when the thermal conditions can be described and controlled, the neutral thermal environment for any nude infant can easily be located by using the studies of Scopes.[32] Bruck determined the neutral thermal environments for infants of different ages and weights. Generally, the thinner, smaller and younger the infant, the higher the environmental temperature required to achieve the neutral thermal environment[20, 22] (Figure 4–8).

Table 4–3 is a general guide for roughly locating the neutral temperature if the temperature of the walls of the incubator is warm and within a degree of the incubator air temperature. When estimating neutral temperatures in single-walled incubators, add 1° C to all the temperatures in the table for every seven degrees that incubator air temperatures exceed room temperature (see Figure 4–5).

DISORDERS OF TEMPERATURE REGULATION

Hypothermia

Hypothermia should be anticipated in low-birth-weight infants, and the routine use of low-reading thermometers (from 33.8° C, 85° F) is advocated in their care, as temperatures below 34.4° C (94° F) are frequently not immediately detected with the routine clinical thermometers. Hypothermia is seen particularly following resuscitation of asphyxiated premature infants. It may be an early sign of sepsis or evidence of intracranial pathology such as meningitis or cerebral hemorrhage.

Neonatal Cold Injury

Neonatal cold injury following extreme hypothermia occurs under both warm and cool climatic conditions, particularly with domiciliary maternity services. Low-birth-weight infants are almost exclusively affected, except for full-term infants with problems such as intracerebral hemorrhage and major congenital malformations.

Clinical Features. A slight drop in temperature may produce profound metabolic change;[3] however, a significant drop must occur before clinical features are evident.

The infants will feed poorly, are lethargic, and feel cold to the touch. Mann[28] describes an "aura" of coldness about the body and skin over the trunk; the periphery feels intensely cold and "corpse-like." Core temperatures will be depressed, often below 32.2° C (90° F).

The most striking feature is the bright red color of the infant. This red color (which may lead the physician astray, as the infant "looks so well") is due to the failure of dissociation of oxyhemoglobin at low temperatures. Central cyanosis or pallor may be present.

Respiration is slow, very shallow, irregular, and often associated with an expiratory grunt. Bradycardia occurs proportionate to the degree of temperature drop.

Activity is lessened. Shivering is rarely observed. The central nervous depression is constant, and reflexes and responses are diminished or absent. Painful stimuli (e.g., injections) produce minimal reaction and the cry is feeble. Abdominal distension and vomiting are common.

Edema of the extremities and face is common, and sclerema is seen, especially on the cheeks. (Sclerema is hardening of the skin, associated with reddening and edema. It is observed particularly with cold injury, infection, and near the time of death.)

Metabolic derangements include: metabolic acidosis, hypoglycemia, hyperkalemia, elevated blood urea, and oliguria.[17]

A problem encountered is massive intrapulmonary hemorrhage in association with a generalized bleeding diathesis (a common finding at autopsy).

Treatment. The infant should be warmed slowly, with the ambient air temperature set approximately 1.5° C warmer than abdominal skin temperature. (The basis for this is depicted in Figure 4–9,[1] showing oxygen consumption to be minimal when the temperature gradient between body surface and environment is <1.5° C, although the rectal temperature may be subnormal.) Skin temperature should be recorded every 15 minutes.

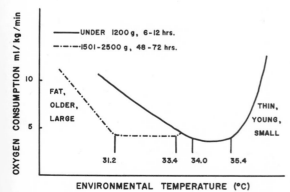

Figure 4–8 The neutral thermal environment for two different sizes of infants.

TABLE 4–3   NEUTRAL THERMAL ENVIRONMENTAL TEMPERATURES*

AGE AND WEIGHT	STARTING TEMPERATURE (°C)	RANGE OF TEMPERATURE (°C)
0–6 Hours		
Under 1200 gm.	35.0	34.0–35.4
1200–1500 gm.	34.1	33.9–34.4
1501–2500 gm.	33.4	32.8–33.8
Over 2500 (and >36 weeks)	32.9	32.0–33.8
6–12 Hours		
Under 1200 gm.	35.0	34.0–35.4
1200–1500 gm.	34.0	33.5–34.4
1501–2500 gm.	33.1	32.2–33.8
Over 2500 (and >36 weeks)	32.8	31.4–33.8
12–24 Hours		
Under 1200 gm.	34.0	34.0–35.4
1200–1500 gm.	33.8	33.3–34.3
1501–2500 gm.	32.8	31.8–33.8
Over 2500 (and >36 weeks)	32.4	31.0–33.7
24–36 Hours		
Under 1200 gm.	34.0	34.0–35.0
1200–1500 gm.	33.6	33.1–34.2
1501–2500 gm.	32.6	31.6–33.6
Over 2500 (and >36 weeks)	32.1	30.7–33.5
36–48 Hours		
Under 1200 gm.	34.0	34.0–35.0
1200–1500 gm.	33.5	33.0–34.1
1501–2500 gm.	32.5	31.4–33.5
Over 2500 (and >36 weeks)	31.9	30.5–33.3
48–72 Hours		
Under 1200 gm.	34.0	34.0–35.0
1200–1500 gm.	33.5	33.0–34.0
1501–2500 gm.	32.3	31.2–33.4
Over 2500 (and >36 weeks)	31.7	30.1–33.2
72–96 Hours		
Under 1200 gm.	34.0	34.0–35.0
1200–1500 gm.	33.5	33.0–34.0
1501–2500 gm.	32.2	31.1–33.2
Over 2500 (and >36 weeks)	31.3	29.8–32.8
4–12 Days		
Under 1500 gm.	33.5	33.0–34.0
1501–2500 gm.	32.1	31.0–33.2
Over 2500 (and >36 weeks)		
4–5 days	31.0	29.5–32.6
5–6 days	30.9	29.4–32.3
6–8 days	30.6	29.0–32.2
8–10 days	30.3	29.0–31.8
10–12 days	30.1	29.0–31.4
12–14 Days		
Under 1500 gm.	33.5	32.6–34.0
1501–2500 gm.	32.1	31.0–33.2
Over 2500 (and >36 weeks)	29.8	29.0–30.8
2–3 Weeks		
Under 1500 gm.	33.1	32.2–34.0
1501–2500 gm.	31.7	30.5–33.0
3–4 Weeks		
Under 1500 gm.	32.6	31.6–33.6
1501–2500 gm.	31.4	30.0–32.7
4–5 Weeks		
Under 1500 gm.	32.0	31.2–33.0
1501–2500 gm.	30.9	29.5–32.2
5–6 Weeks		
Under 1500 gm.	31.4	30.6–32.3
1501–2500 gm.	30.4	29.0–31.8

*Adapted from Scopes and Ahmed.[32] For his table, Scopes had the walls of the incubator 1° to 2° warmer than the ambient air temperatures.

Generally speaking, the smaller infants in each weight group will require a temperature in the higher portion of the temperature range. Within each time range, the younger the infant, the higher the temperature required.

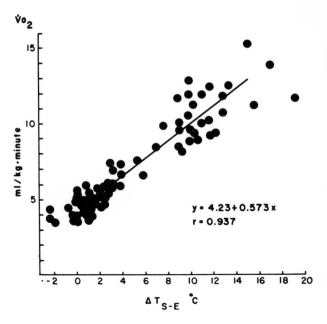

Figure 4–9 Oxygen consumption and temperature gradient between body surface (skin of abdominal wall) and environment (ΔT_{S-E}) of mature human newborns with varying deep body temperatures. Difference between the temperatures of ambient air and surfaces surrounding the newborn is less than 2° C.[3]

Oxygen is administered, blood sugar monitored closely, and the metabolic acidosis corrected with sodium bicarbonate as required.

Feed only by intravenous infusion or gavage of dextrose solution until the temperature is 35° C (95° F). Hypothermic infants should not be permitted to feed by nipple.

Antibiotics are only administered when infection is suspected or documented.

Hyperthermia

Elevation of the deep body temperature may be due to an excessive environmental temperature, infection, dehydration, or alterations of the central mechanisms of heat control associated with cerebral birth trauma or drugs.

The question of systemic infection is invariably raised in infants with elevated deep body temperatures. Due consideration should also be taken of the environmental conditions that alter heat control. It is not uncommon to find an elevated core temperature following the increased heat input with the commencement of the use of bilirubin reduction lights. On rare occasions, if an incubator is placed in the sunlight, the short wavelength radiant emission goes through the plastic wall and can overheat the infant, since long wavelength reradiation through the plastic wall is prevented (the "Greenhouse effect," Figure 4–10).

Asphyxia

Research continues while arguments rage on the relationship between temperature and birth asphyxia. For many years it was believed that any asphyxiated infant should be maintained at lower temperatures with a hope of diminishing permanent cerebral sequelae and increasing survival. Some experimental studies in animals cooled before asphyxia begins support this view.

With newborn infants, prolonged resuscitative attempts often are carried out on a damp towel, with precipitous drops in body temperature. Clinically relevant experimental studies in which cooling was begun at the end or during the asphyxia show that a cool environment offers no advantage to the infant — in fact, a disadvantage, the time to the last gasp being reduced.[1]

Temperature responses following delivery are sometimes a guide to the state of the infant during delivery.[11] If the infant was severely asphyxiated or hypoxic, temperature control is reflexively turned off and body temperature is often not maintained immediately after delivery.

Resuscitative procedures should be performed with due attention to heat control:

1. Evaporative losses may effectively be reduced by immediately drying the infant.

2. Conductive losses can be eliminated by laying the infant on a dry, warm towel or cloth.

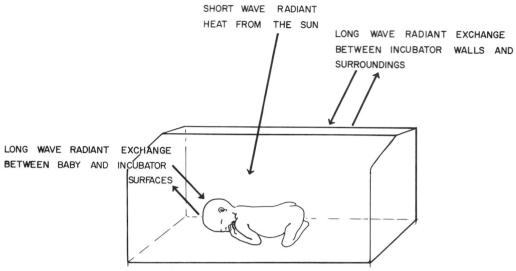

SHORT WAVE RADIANT HEAT FROM THE SUN

LONG WAVE RADIANT EXCHANGE BETWEEN INCUBATOR WALLS AND SURROUNDINGS

LONG WAVE RADIANT EXCHANGE BETWEEN BABY AND INCUBATOR SURFACES

Figure 4–10   "The greenhouse effect." (Adapted from Hey and Mount.[24])

3. Radiant source of heat in the form of a radiant warmer will provide a heat-giving environment. These are ideal for resuscitation, as the infant can be maintained nude and is readily accessible. Abdominal skin temperature should be monitored.

4. Convection is to be controlled—no drafts in the room—and the oxygen is to be warmed.

Apnea

Despite the beneficial effects of maintaining a warm environment, a possible disadvantage is its effect on respiratory control.

1. Immersing a normal infant in a bath equal to the maternal temperature stops respiration. Rapid warming is also associated with apneic episodes.

2. Observations in a group of low-birth-weight infants[13] having apneic attacks reveal that lowering the servo-controlling temperature less than 1° C significantly reduced the number of episodes.

We suggest therefore that a premature infant having apneic attacks should be maintained closer to the low range of neutral thermal environment.

THE SENSORY ENVIRONMENT

LIGHT, SOUND, TOUCH

Although historically more attention has been directed toward the thermal and bacteri-

ologic aspects of the environment, studies in animals and a small number of recent observations in human infants suggest that sensory stimuli may play a major role in neurologic and physical maturation and may be especially crucial in furthering the organization of many higher order processes.

Hasselmeyer[19, 39] reported that simply fondling the premature infant for five minutes out of every hour for two weeks altered bowel motility, crying, activity, and possibly growth. In another study, Freedman, Boverman and Freedman[16] found that rocking one identical twin increased its growth rate above that of the unrocked twin. Siqueland and Lipsitt[38] found that when one experimental group of premature infants was rocked by nurses, given increased visual stimuli, sung to, and in general provided with increased sensory stimulation characteristic of warm mothers during their early weeks of life, they were different from the controls in a learning situation four months later. The stimulated infants at four months of age were better learners and more able to control their own environmental visual inputs.

Phototherapy for hyperbilirubinemia and increasing illumination in the nursery have focused attention on the light requirements of the newborn. It should be remembered that light has a profound effect on biologic rhythm.

As we begin a major consideration of the effects of sensory stimuli, the most difficult criterion in every study will be: Is it beneficial or harmful to the infant? The stimulation must be appropriate to his state of development and to his individual requirements, as there is danger in overstimulation of the immature organism. Animal as well as human studies indicate that the kinds of stimulation which most mothers and sensitive nurses offer naturally, as responses to the infant's behavior, could be the basis for enlarging these infants' experiences and furthering their development in the early crucial period. A recent suggestion is to permit the premature or newborn to decide on the amount of sensory stimulation. An example is the rate of sucking determining the intensity of light or the volume of a sound.

Here again we must measure the effects of sound, light, etc., not only on the immediate weight gain or activity but also on the later and long-term effects, such as age of sexual maturation, school performance, and length of survival.

The final environment, the ideal "external milieu," comprised of thermal and sensory considerations, must optimize both immediate and ultimate neurologic and physical development.

QUESTIONS

True or False

Provided that the rectal temperature is maintained between 36.5 and 37° C (97.7 and 98.6° F), the infant can be considered to be in the "neutral thermal environment."

A single measurement of temperature is of little value in defining the neutral thermal environment. The infant may have an elevated metabolic rate and be "working" to maintain normal body temperature. Therefore the statement is false.

Neutral thermal environment takes into account ambient air temperature, air flow, relative humidity, and temperature of surrounding objects.

The neutral thermal environment is that set of thermal conditions associated with minimal metabolic rate in a resting subject; thus, potential heat loss by conduction, convection, radiation, and evaporation must be considered. Therefore the statement is true.

Swaddling the infant should not influence the temperature settings of the incubator in order to achieve neutral thermal environment.

The use of the Scopes tables for achieving neutral thermal environment refers to a set of specific conditions; namely, that the incubator wall temperatures are a degree higher than the air temperature, and that the infants are nude. All the processes of heat exchange are altered and reduced by clothing the baby. The ambient air temperature inside the clothing is warmer than ambient incubator air and humidity is higher, too. Therefore the statement is false.

Overheating the infant produces no noticeable clinical effects and can only be detected by monitoring deep body temperature.

Overheating will of course be documented by monitoring deep body temperature. However, the infant will be noted to be flushed and panting. He will hyperventilate and initially show irritability. Sweating may occur but is reduced in immature infants. With prolonged hyperthermia, stupor, coma, and convulsions may occur and brain damage may be irreversible. The statement is false.

The stimulus for an increased metabolic rate begins immediately after onset of cold stimulus even before the deep body temperature has fallen.

Bruck has shown that it is not necessary for body temperature to fall before there is an increase in metabolic rate. Therefore the statement is true. Even mild cold stress (e.g., blowing cold air on the face) may result in significant increase in oxygen consumption. This occurs when unwarmed oxygen is blowing over the infant's face.

The lower end of the range of the neutral thermal environment is referred to as the "critical temperature." It varies with size, age, and clinical condition. Premature, appropriate-for-gestational-age infants have higher critical temperatures than term infants.

The above data are of value in using the charts of Scopes and Ahmed, and Hey and Katz, in order to place and maintain the infants in the neutral thermal environment. The statement is true.

Maintaining an infant with RDS at the neutral thermal environment plays an insignificant part in overall management.

Many infants with respiratory distress syndrome have a limited capacity to transfer oxygen, and the maintenance of the neutral thermal environment is most important in their care. Therefore the statement is false.

The rate of growth in body weight and length can be influenced by environmental temperature.

Infants kept at a warmer environment showed significantly greater increase in body weight and length over those maintained in a cooler environment, when both groups had the same caloric intake. Infants in a cooler environment require more calories to regulate body temperature and thus have fewer available for growth. Therefore the statement is true.

When an infant who is being monitored in a servo incubator develops a fever, this is reflected by a rise in incubator temperature.

As the infant's temperature rises, the abdominal skin temperature which is controlling the infant will also rise, resulting in a fall in incubator temperature. Thus, a drop in incubator temperature reflects a rise in the temperature of the infant and vice versa. Therefore the statement is false.

Heat loss from the lungs may be diminished by maintaining the infants in supersaturated warm air.

Heat loss from the airways of the lung due to evaporation of H_2O as inspired air is warmed and saturated with water vapor can be diminished by increasing environmental humidity. Therefore the statement is true.

What is "dehydration fever?"

Dehydration fever occurs usually in fully breast-fed infants aged 48 to 72 hours. The infants are febrile but appear well, with temperatures up to 103° F (39.4° C). They may manifest features of dehydration with poor tissue turgor and often show weight losses in excess of 10 per cent of birth weight. Urine volume diminishes and hematocrit and serum proteins are elevated. It occurs from diminished fluid intake in breast-fed infants. The infants are alert, and the fever subsides with administration of fluids, either orally or by I.V.

The newborn infant who has not been asphyxiated exhibits poikilothermic behavior when subjected to cold stress.

The newborn infant exhibits homeothermic behavior—that is, an elevation in metabolic rate (or oxygen consumption) when subjected to cold stress. Therefore the statement is false. In the face of severe hypoxemia, metabolic rate is not increased with cooling.

The greatest source of heat loss in the immature infant is from the lungs.

Radiant heat loss is loss to immediate surrounding cooler solid objects, (e.g., wall of incubator) and accounts for the majority of heat lost in the immature infant. Therefore the statement is false.

Radiant heat losses are similar in adults and immature infants, as they are both homeotherms.

Radiant heat loss is of less significance in adults because they are clothed, and has no bearing on the question of homeothermy. A homeotherm is an animal which attempts to maintain a constant body temperature despite alterations in environment, e.g., increases metabolic rate in a cool environment. Therefore the statement is false.

The environmental temperature has a profound effect on mortality and morbidity.

Survival rates for immature infants during the first five days of life are much improved by maintaining infants in a neutral thermal environment. Therefore the statement is true. It is important to note that the "thermal environment" for the premature infant varies with size and age. (Consult Table 4–3 for the actual temperatures.)

Shivering and increased muscular activity play significant roles in maintaining body temperature in a cool environment in newborns.

At present there is no doubt that the newborn infant is able to employ nonshivering thermogenesis for cold defense. However, no successful attempts have been made to estimate the relative contributions of nonshivering thermogenesis and shivering to the total cold-induced oxygen consumption. Therefore the statement is false.

The newborn infant loses equal amounts of heat per unit of body mass compared with the adult.

While at birth the infant's body mass is about five per cent of the adult, the surface area is nearly 15 per cent. There is also less subcutaneous tissue, resulting in a higher thermal conductance and thus a higher skin temperature at lower ambient temperatures. Bruck has estimated that because of the above, the heat loss of the newborn infant per unit of body mass is about four times that of the adult. Therefore the statement is false.

Full-term infants who have been cold-stressed at birth may have a normal pH and low HCO_3.

A compensated metabolic acidosis possibly secondary to lactic acid production is sometimes observed. Therefore the statement is true.

Lowering of the body temperature is beneficial in resuscitating asphyxiated newborns.

There is insufficient evidence to indicate that lowering of the body temperature of depressed or asphyxiated newborns is of value in changing mortality or morbidity. Therefore the statement is false.

The duration of quiet sleep is markedly reduced when small nude infants are exposed to an environmental temperature of only 1 to 2° C below the lower limit of the presumed range of thermal neutrality.

It has been suggested by some investigators that the temperature range in which the least amount of oxygen is consumed is also the temperature range of thermal comfort for the neonate. Therefore the statement is true.

Swaddled, full-term babies may not cry or otherwise call attention to the fact that they are under severe cold stress.

This statement is true, and is particularly important since the upper limit of heat production is reached for cot-nursed, full-term infants when the room temperature falls to about 10° C (50° F). In some situations at night, bedrooms get colder and the infants become hypothermic.

CASE PROBLEMS

Case One

L. A. is a 1480-gm. (3 lbs. 4 oz.) male infant delivered vaginally at 32 weeks in an outlying hospital following an uneventful pregnancy and the spontaneous onset of premature labor. Apgar at one minute = 8, and at five minutes = 9.

The onset of grunting was noted at age 1 hour, and the infant was first seen at age 2 hours, following transfer to an incubator with 70 per cent oxygen, at which time he was grunting 100 per cent of the time with minimal retractions and peripheral cyanosis.

Length was 42 cm., head circumference 28.5 cm., rectal temperature was below 34° C (93.2° F), pulse 144 per minute, and respirations 64 per minute. Mean arterial blood pressure was 40 mm. Hg.

Other than the respiratory problem, the physical examination was unremarkable and the neurologic features confirmed a gestational age of 32 weeks.

Investigation revealed the following:

A. Hematocrit 52

B. Arterial blood gases: pH = 7.22, pO_2 = 102 mm. Hg, pCO_2 = 35.0 mm. Hg, HCO_3 = 14.1 mEq.

C. Dextrostix 90 mg. per 100 ml.

Tabulate from the information given the problems that require your immediate attention.

a. Hypothermia—temperature below 34.4° C (94° F).

b. Metabolic acidosis—pH = 7.22

c. Grunting and retracting—the etiology of this will have to be elucidated.

How would you proceed to warm this infant?

The infant should be warmed gradually. Environmental temperature and abdominal skin temperature should not differ by greater than 1.5° C. Rapid warming may be complicated both by apneic attacks and an increase in metabolic rate aggravating, for example, the respiratory problems of the infant. Once the infant is in a heat-gaining environment, metabolic rate falls to minimal levels. There is no urgency to increase body temperature rapidly.

Assuming a rectal temperature of 33° C (91.4° F) and an abdominal skin temperature of 32.5° C (90.5° F), what would your incubator and oxygen hood temperature settings be in a double-walled box?

After consulting the Scopes tables, you should set the incubator at 34.0° C (93.2° F) with the hood at the same temperature.

Two hours after admission, the status of the patient is as follows:

rectal temperature 35.2° C (95.4° F)
skin temperature 35.4° C (95.7° F)
pulse 156 per minute
respiration 64 per minute
environmental oxygen 60 per cent

arterial blood gases: pH = 7.321, pO₂ = 66 mm. Hg, pCO₂ = 57 mm. Hg, HCO₃ = 28.9 mEq. per liter
incubator temperature 34.5° C (94.1° F)
hood temperature 34.3° C (93.7° F)
grunting less than 50 per cent of the time
moderately active

Should the temperature settings be altered now?

Temperature settings are appropriate and the infant is progressing well. Acidosis has been corrected by administration of sodium bicarbonate and the infant's temperature is increasing significantly. There appears to be no worsening of RDS.

Should oral feedings be commenced now?

There are three reasons why this infant should not be fed orally at this stage: (1) respiratory distress, (2) weight less than 1500 gm., (3) hypothermia. Oral feeding should not be carried out for the first 48 to 72 hours in distressed infants under 1500 gm., as mortality is significantly reduced by I.V. feeding. Regardless of weight, no infant with a temperature below 34.4° C (94° F) probably should be allowed to nipple.

Case Two

Baby D. O. was an 1160-gm. product of a 31-week gestation. No problems were encountered in the immediate neonatal period, and the pregnancy had been uncomplicated. Delivery was under caudal anesthesia by forceps. Apgar at one minute = 6. On the second day of life, the rectal temperature was noted to be 36.8° C (98.2° F). The incubator temperature at this time was 34.1° C (93.4° F).

Is this infant in the neutral thermal environment?

It is impossible to say — more data are required.

What additional data would you require to define the neutral thermal environment?

To define the neutral thermal environment, you also require the temperature of the mattress with regard to conductive heat loss, the air flow in the incubator, the relative humidity, and the temperature of the inner walls of the incubator to determine the radiant heat losses which can occur to the surrounding walls of the incubator. A continuous recording of the abdominal skin temperature would permit a rough idea of whether or not the infant is in the neutral thermal zone. If a servo incubator is controlled to maintain an abdominal skin temperature of 36.5° C (97.7° F), oxygen consumption has been found to be minimal. In this case, the abdominal skin temperature was 34.9° C (94.8° F), the side wall of the incubator was 32.5° C (90.5° F), and the relative humidity was 80 per cent. We can assume the temperature of the mattress to be the same as the incubator air temperature.

With this available data, would you say that the infant is in the neutral thermal environment?

No, the infant is not in the neutral thermal environment. Our indications of this are that the abdominal skin temperature is only 34.9° C (94.8° F), even with the incubator air at 34.1° C (93.4° F). If you refer back to the table of Scopes and Ahmed, the appropriate temperature for this infant to be in the neutral thermal environment is an environmental temperature of 34 to 35° C (93.2 to 95° F), providing that the walls are 1° C higher than the air. Note that the side wall temperature is only 32.5° C (86.5° F). He is losing heat by radiation.

How could you diminish radiant heat loss in this infant?

Radiant heat losses may be diminished by using a radiant warmer or by placing a plastic heat shield inside the single-walled incubator.

On the fourth day of life, the rectal temperature was 37° C (98.6° F), the abdominal skin temperature was 36.8° C (98.2° F), incubator air was 34° C (93.2° F), and the side wall (using radiant heat shield) was 34° C (93.2° F). The infant was having recurrent apneic attacks responding to stimulation. What measures may be taken to reduce the number of apneic attacks after checking the calcium, sugar, etc.?

In some babies, lowering of the environmental temperature diminishes the number of apneic spells. It might be useful to try to servo this infant at an abdominal skin temperature of 35.9° C (96.6° F) in an attempt to reduce the number of attacks.

Would this alteration in temperature affect the nutritional requirements of this infant?

Yes. With the abdominal skin temperature at 35.9° C (96.6° F), both the oxygen and caloric requirements will be slightly increased.

Case Three

Baby H. is a girl delivered after a 42-week pregnancy, weighing 1600 gm. No problems were noted in the immediate neonatal period. The neurologic examination was appropriate for an infant with a 42-week gestation, with the exception that there was diminished neck flexor tone. Head circumference was 33 cm. This infant was unable to increase her metabolic rate with cold stress.

How can the optimal thermal environment be found?

This is a difficult question to answer because no tables are available for this age and weight. The problem may best be managed by servoing the incubator and maintaining the abdominal skin temperature at 36.5° C (97.7° F).

REFERENCES

1. Adamsons, K., Jr.: The role of thermal factors in fetal and neonatal life. Pediat Clin N Amer *13*: 599, 1966.
2. Adamsons, K., Jr., and Towell, M.: Thermal homeostasis in the fetus and newborn. Anesthesiology *26*:531, 1965.
3. Adamsons, K., Jr., Gandy, G., and James, L.: The influence of thermal factors upon oxygen consumption of the newborn human infant. J Pediat *66*:495, 1965.
4. Agate, F., and Silverman, W.: The control of body temperature in the small newborn infant by low-energy infra-red radiation. Pediatrics *31*:725, 1963.
5. Benzinger, T.: Clinical temperature — the new physiologic basis. JAMA *209*:1200, 1969.
6. Blackfan, K., and Yaglou, C.: The premature infant: a study of the effects of atmospheric conditions on growth and development. Amer J Dis Child *46*:1175, 1933.
7. Bruck, K.: Temperature regulation in the newborn infant. Biol Neonat *3*:65, 1961.
8. Bruck, K.: Heat production and temperature regulation. *In* Stave, U., Ed.: *Physiology of the Perinatal Period.* New York, Appleton-Century-Crofts, 1970.
9. Budin, P.: *The Nursling.* London, Caxton Publishing Co., 1907.
10. Buetow, K., and Klein, S.: Effect of maintenance of "normal" skin temperature on survival of infants of low birth weight. Pediatrics *34*:163, 1964.
11. Burnard, E., and Cross, K.: Rectal temperature in the newborn after birth asphyxia. Brit Med J *2*:1197, 1958.
12. Cross, K., Tizard, J., and Trythall, D.: The gaseous metabolism of the newborn infant breathing 15% oxygen. Acta Paediat *47*:217, 1958.
13. Dailey, W., Klaus, M., and Meyer, H.: Apnea in premature infants: monitoring, incidence, heart rate changes, and effect of environmental temperature. Pediatrics *43*:510, 1969.
14. Dawkins, M., and Hull, D.: Brown adipose tissue and the response of newborn rabbits to cold. J Physiol *172*:216, 1964.
15. Day, R.: Respiratory metabolism in infancy and childhood. Amer J Dis Child *65*:376, 1943.
16. Freedman, D., Boverman, H., and Freedman, N.: Effects of kinesthetic stimulation on weight gain and on smiling in premature infants. Paper presented at the Meeting of the American Orthopsychiatry Association, San Francisco, April 1966.
17. Gandy, G., Adamsons, K., Jr., and Cunningham, N.: Thermal environmental and acid-base homeostasis in human infants during the first few hours of life. J Clin Invest *43*:751, 1964.
18. Glass, L., Silverman, W., and Sinclair, J.: Effects of the thermal environment on cold resistance and growth of small infants after the first week of life. Pediatrics *41*:1033, 1968.
19. Hasselmeyer, E.: The premature neonate's response to handling. Amer Nurs Assoc *11*:15, 1964.
20. Hey, E.: The relation between environmental temperature and oxygen consumption in the newborn baby. J Physiol *200*:589, 1969.
21. Hey, E., and Katz, G.: The optimum thermal environment for naked babies. Arch Dis Child *45*:328, 1970.
22. Hey, E., and Maurice, N.: Effect of humidity on production and loss of heat in the newborn baby. Arch Dis Child *43*:166, 1968.
23. Hey, E., and Mount, L.: Temperature control in incubators. Lancet *2*:202, 1966.
24. Hey, E., and Mount, L.: Heat losses from babies in incubators. Arch Dis Child *42*:75, 1967.
25. Hey, E., and O'Connell, B.: Oxygen consumption and heat balance in the cot-nursed baby. Arch Dis Child *45*:335, 1970.
26. Hill, J.: The oxygen consumption of newborn and adult mammals: Its dependence on the oxygen tension in the inspired air and on environmental temperature. J Physiol *149*:346, 1959.
27. Hill, J., and Rahimtulla, K.: Heat balance and the metabolic rate of newborn babies in relation to environmental temperature; and the effect of age and of weight on basal metabolic rate. J Physiol *180*:239, 1965.
28. Mann, T., and Elliott, R.: Neonatal cold injury due to accidental exposure to cold. Lancet *1*:229, 1957.

29. Merenstein, G., and Blackmon, L.: *Care of the High-Risk Newborn*. San Francisco, Children's Hospital, 1971.

30. Mestayan, J., Jarai, I., Bata, G., et al: The significance of facial skin temperature in the chemical heat regulation of premature infants. Biol Neonat 7:243, 1964.

31. Scarr-Salapatek, S., and Williams, M.: A stimulation program for low-birth-weight infants. Amer J Public Health 62:662, 1972.

32. Scopes, J., and Ahmed, I.: Range of critical temperatures in sick and premature newborn babies. Arch Dis Child 41:417, 1966.

33. Silverman, W., and Agate, F.: Variation in cold resistance among small newborn animals. Biol Neonat 6:113, 1964.

34. Silverman, W., and Blanc, W.: The effect of humidity on survival of newly born premature infants. Pediatrics 20:477, 1957.

35. Silverman, W., Agate, F., and Fertig, J.: A sequential trial of the nonthermal effect of atmospheric humidity on survival of newborn infants of low birth weight. Pediatrics 31:719, 1963.

36. Silverman, W., Fertig, J., and Berger, A.: The influence of the thermal environment upon the survival of newly born premature infants. Pediatrics 22:876, 1958.

37. Silverman, W., Zamelis, A., Sinclair, J., et al: Warm nape of the newborn. Pediatrics 33:984, 1964.

38. Siqueland, E., and Lipsitt, L.: Learning ability and its enhancement. *In* Henkes, J., and Schain, R., Eds.: *Learning Disorders in Children*. Report of the 61st Ross Conference on Pediatric Research, Columbus, Ross Laboratories, 1971, pp. 52–55.

39. Solkoff, N., Yaffe, S., Weintraub, D., et al: Effects of handling on the subsequent development of premature infants. J Dev Psych 1:765, 1969.

40. Stephenson, J., Du, J., and Oliver, T.: The effect of cooling on blood gas tensions in newborn infants. J Pediat 76:848, 1970.

Chapter 5

FEEDING THE
LOW-BIRTH-WEIGHT INFANT

by

AVROY FANAROFF, M.B. (Rand.),

M.R.C.P.E.

and

MARSHALL KLAUS, M.D.

We have the baby weighed today
The nursing time is set,
At last we find we are so wise
We can begin to standardize
No baby now need fret;
In spite of this the baby grows
But why it does God only knows.

JOHN RUHRÄH, (1872–1935)

The feeding of a small infant presents a major challenge to the physician responsible for the care of low-birth-weight infants, since specific feeding practices alter mortality,[9] and probably morbidity. Dietary mixtures for the low-birth-weight infant are a highly controversial subject, and as noted by Barness:[5] "It is likely that no area in the care of the newborn infant is less critically or more controversially approached than his feeding. What, When, How, and How Often to Feed are questions surrounded by emotions, beliefs, fads, and even commercialism, all of which tend to obscure the basic goals of infant feeding."

Whereas the full-term healthy neonate will tolerate periods of prolonged starvation together with wide variation in both quantity and composition of formula, the low-birth-weight infant is much more vulnerable.[1, 7, 8, 27–29, 34, 45] The food intake must satisfy the requirements for growth as well as replacing the mineral losses in the urine, feces, and sweat, and nitrogen losses due to tissue breakdown. In planning the feeding schedule, careful consideration must be taken not only of the weight but also of the gestational age of the infant, because the gastro-intestinal capacities, metabolic rates, and requirements of fuel and water will differ with differing gestational ages (see Chapter 3).

Guidelines for feeding the low-birth-weight infant will be presented in this chapter, but it will not include a schema for feeding the healthy full-term neonate.

PHYSIOLOGIC CONSIDERATIONS

The objective of feeding is to meet the metabolic requirements of a number of developing organ systems. A major obstacle has been to find a yardstick. What represents optimum nutrition and how should it be evaluated? At present, the adequacy of growth is judged according to increments of weight, length, and head circumference as plotted on growth charts.[3] (See Figure 5–1 and Appendices 15 and 16.) Because the optimum positions on the charts are unknown, an attempt is made to maintain growth within or above the percentiles at birth.[4] But the evaluation of nutrition should include not only short-term effects on growth but also ultimate intelligence, and length and quality of survival.[8, 16]

Name _____   History No. _____

Birth Weight _____Gms   Length _____Cm.   Head Circ. _____Cm

                                                         Chest Circ. _____Cm

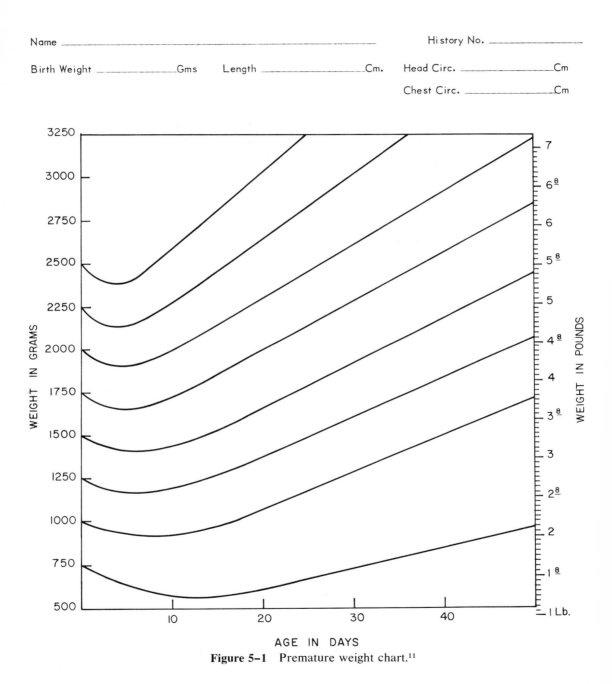

Figure 5–1   Premature weight chart.[11]

The exact quantity and combination of substances required by all the developing organ systems are unknown for the full-term infant.[12, 19, 28] For the immature or under-nourished infant, the problem is even more complex.

NUTRITIONAL REQUIREMENTS

The caloric, water, electrolyte, mineral, and vitamin requirements of the low-birth-weight infant are dependent upon body stores, absorption, rate of utilization and expenditure, and excretion of the substances. The metabolic rate and body composition of infants with a similar weight but a dissimilar gestational age are different; hence, their requirements will also differ.

Water

The water content of the human infant decreases progressively from 85 per cent of body weight at 28 weeks' gestation to 70 per cent at full term. Low-birth-weight infants are particularly vulnerable to excess fluid losses in the early neonatal period because of increased water content in the skin, a thinner epidermis, and increased skin permeability. The actual clinical requirements of water are highly variable and dependent on the state of the infant. Very small and immature infants kept in a single-walled incubator, feeding frequently, with increased activity, and cardiac or respiratory disease, may require large amounts of water.[17] The requirements are greater in addition if there are excessive losses via the gastrointestinal tract, insensibly by skin or lungs, or if a large electrolyte load is given.

Large fluid losses are most easily recognized clinically by close observation of body weight. Losses in excess of 10 per cent of birth weight in the first three to four postnatal days are excessive. There may be, in addition, an associated rise in hematocrit or serum sodium and also frequent apneic episodes. The ability of the immature kidney to conserve water is limited.

The fluid volume required to administer the necessary 120 calories per Kg. per day will depend on the caloric density (number of calories per ml.) of the formula. Assuming a caloric density of 24 calories per 30 ml., which may be achieved by the third to fourth day of life, the daily fluid requirement will be 150 ml. per Kg. per day. Infants receiving 140 to 160 ml. water per Kg. per day are usually in positive water balance. However, some infants may require from 180 to 200 ml. per Kg. per day.

The ability of the low-birth-weight infant to take in this quantity of fluid is influenced by the capacity of the stomach. Particularly in infants with birth weights below 1250 gm., it is easy inadvertently to exceed this, which will result in abdominal distention and vomiting, frequently complicated by aspiration. This is probably a major factor in the increased mortality of early oral feeding of low-birth-weight infants.[42]

As with many other techniques in a nursery, the efficacy of oral feeding is dependent upon the skill and experience of the nurses involved. A blanket statement, therefore, regarding its desirability or lack thereof is not warranted, as the success or danger of the procedure is probably more dependent upon who is doing it than upon the procedure itself.

L. STERN

Calories

The caloric requirements are related to the cell mass and number. Thus, infants with the same weight may require different caloric intakes to achieve the same weight gain. In most instances, 120 calories per Kg. per day will provide maintenance for the normal infant and allow sufficient calories for growth.[24, 36] Some infants, particularly those small-for-gestational-age who have a higher metabolic rate, require more calories.[36]

The distribution of the caloric expenditure is outlined in Table 5–1. It will be noted that in the low-birth-weight infant, a significant portion of the calories are not absorbed.

For each gram of weight gain, between two and three calories must be stored, of which 60 to 80 per cent is water, 13 per cent protein, and the rest fat.[24] In order to maintain

TABLE 5–1 PARTITION OF DAILY CALORIC EXPENDITURE IN A TYPICAL GROWING PREMATURE INFANT[36]

ITEM	CAL. PER KG. PER 24 HOURS
Resting caloric expenditure	50
Intermittent activity	15
Occasional cold stress	10
Specific dynamic action	8
Fecal loss of calories	12
Growth allowance	25
Total	120

the rate of intrauterine growth, the low-birth-weight infant needs to store 20 to 40 calories per Kg. per day.

Considerable awe appears to be inspired by the determination for the infant to maintain the rate of intrauterine growth, even though he is no longer in the intrauterine state. The evidence that this is beneficial, mandatory, or necessary, is not apparent; indeed, efforts to do so have often resulted in serious disturbances from excessive and overzealous nutritional attempts. It remains to be proved that maintenance of an intrauterine growth rate in the extrauterine situation is beneficial and/or that the failure to grow at this rate is in fact detrimental to the developing organism.

L. STERN

Most immature infants sleep approximately 60 per cent of the time and are in a state of quiet wakefulness for a further 25 per cent, during which metabolic rate will be low. Fifteen per cent of the time they are feeding and crying. If the metabolic rate is increased, so too are the caloric requirements necessary for growth. This is observed when the environmental temperature is outside the neutral thermal range,[20] with increased muscular activity, persistent respiratory problems, increased cardiac output, or infection.

We aim to achieve the recommended intake of calories as quickly as possible; however, in practice this usually takes at least a week to ten days.

Protein[13, 21, 38]

While it is agreed that the protein requirement in infancy is greater than that for the adult, the optimal protein intake has not been established. We presently use a protein intake of 4 to 5 gm. per Kg. per day where protein accounts for about 10 per cent of the caloric intake. A normal newborn will grow provided he receives at least 2 gm. of protein per Kg. per day; however, edema and low plasma protein levels are sometimes noted at this level.

Infants with large protein intakes (>7 gm. per Kg. per day) gain more rapidly and retain more nitrogen. This is associated with earlier maturation of the kidney (urine concentrating capacity and acidification is improved). However, part of this extra weight gain may be increased fluid retention associated with a higher ash content and the relative inability of the premature infant to excrete the large solute loads. Infants fed high-protein diets have protein casts in the urine, more often become febrile, have increased lethargy, feed poorly, and possibly have more apnea. Late metabolic acidosis of prematurity is also seen in infants receiving large protein intakes. The effects of the high protein intake on brain maturation are unknown. Studies are underway evaluating the long-term effects of different protein intakes in the neonatal period and the results are eagerly awaited.[22] Using the "humanized" commercial formulas which contain less than 2 gm. protein per 100 ml., most infants will receive about 4 gm. per Kg. per day if the recommended fluid and caloric requirements discussed above are met.

Vitamins and Minerals

The low-birth-weight infant, in addition to daily requirements, needs to replenish stores, as perinatal storage of many substances normally occurs during the last trimester of pregnancy. The daily nutritional and vitamin requirements are outlined in Table 5-2.

TABLE 5-2 DAILY NUTRITIONAL AND VITAMIN REQUIREMENTS FOR LOW-BIRTH-WEIGHT INFANTS

NUTRIENTS, TOTAL	PER KILOGRAM	VITAMINS, TOTAL PER DAY	
Calories	110–140	A	1500–2500 I.U.
Water	130–200 ml.	Thiamine	0.4 mg.
Protein	4–6 g.	Riboflavin	0.5 mg.
Carbohydrate	10–15 g.	Pyridoxine	0.25 mg.
Fat	5–7 g.	B_{12}	1.0 μg.
Sodium	0.5–2 mEq.	C	30–50 mg.
Chloride	0.5–2 mEq.	D	400 I.U.
Potassium	0.5–2 mEq.	E	5–100 I.U.
Calcium	4–6 mEq.	Niacin	6.0 mg.
Phosphorus	2–4 mEq.	Panthenol	– –
Magnesium	0.5–1 mEq.	Folic acid	0.35 mg.
		K	1.5 mg.
Iron	6 mg. per day		

Because of rapid growth, the vitamin requirements of low-birth-weight infants may exceed intake, and supplementation is necessary. Most commercial formulae have vitamin supplements. However, in order to ingest the minimal daily requirements, the infant must drink a quart of formula per day. This is obviously impossible in the smaller infant, whose vitamin intake must be supplemented commencing on the 5th to 10th days of life.

Apart from vitamins D and E, most vitamin deficiencies are relatively rare in the absence of malabsorption syndromes. Rickets may be seen in rapidly growing low-birth-weight infants not receiving vitamin supplements.[32] Vitamin E absorption, requirements, and deficiency are considered in detail in Chapter 15.

GROWTH IN THE PERINATAL PERIOD

In nongenerating organs, such as the brain, liver, and kidney, three periods of cellular growth have been defined. The first period is characterized by an increase in cell number or hyperplasia. This is followed by a period during which the cells increase in both number and size. The third period consists mainly of an increase in cell size.[44]

From studies of cell size and number, one may determine the state of the organ, and if it is small, whether this is a result of a reduction in cell size, cell number, or a combination of both. Undernutrition during the period of hyperplasia will decrease the rate of cell division and may lead to permanent decrease in the number of cells in the organ. Undernutrition during the phase of increase in cell size will result in a temporary decrease in cell size which is reversible once normal feeding or nutrition is reinstated. This is noted clinically among slightly small-for-gestational-age infants secondary to placental insufficiency. They gain weight once normal nutrition is re-established.

FUNCTIONAL CAPACITY — GASTROINTESTINAL TRACT

Sucking and Swallowing[25, 26]

Sucking and swallowing are established prenatally but are not fully developed until after birth. The patterns of suck and esophageal and gastric motor function differ in the immediate neonatal period and the period thereafter. In the full-term, the esophageal response to deglutition is uncoordinated during the first day.

Normally, sucking precedes swallowing, which in turn inhibits respiration. At the time of swallowing, the nasal passages are open and the epiglottis closed, so that air enters the stomach. Thereafter, the epiglottis opens and air goes into the trachea. The inhibition of respiration during swallowing safeguards against aspiration. Coordination of this mechanism develops at approximately 32 to 34 weeks' gestation. Before this time, the premature infant displays discoordinate activity, and aspiration is possible.

When presented with a stimulus, infants first "mouth" the nipple before making sucking attempts. Sucking varies with nipple flow and the type of food. Slower sucking is seen with glucose water than with formula. The "mature suck swallow pattern" consists of prolonged sucking bursts with multiple swallows occurring simultaneously with sucking. *In immature infants, the suck pattern* is characterized by short sucking bursts which are preceded or followed by swallows. Simultaneous contractions are seen throughout the esophagus but peristalsis is only evident with prolonged sucking bursts. This "immature suck pattern" persists for some time in the small premature infant and may represent a developmental protective mechanism which prevents overloading of an esophagus not yet ready to transmit a large bolus.

In the majority of term and premature infants, the inferior esophageal sphincter mechanism which is located at or above the effective diaphragmatic hiatus has poor tone. Barrie[6] demonstrated that all infants, even those fed through a nasogastric tube, regurgitated milk into the lower half of the esophagus and also showed altered or abnormal patterns of breathing associated with feeding. He noted an increase in respiratory rate and attributed this to mechanical interference with diaphragmatic movement. In contrast, Russell and Feather,[35] studying the effects of feeding on respiratory mechanics in healthy newborn infants, demonstrated no adverse effects of small feeds on the work of breathing, compliance, respiratory rate, and minute volume.

In immature infants, periodic breathing with apnea often occurs within 15 minutes following feeding.[10] Radiologically, large amounts of air are found in both the stomach and the esophagus. (For a further discussion of apnea, see pp. 144 and 145.)

Gastric Activity in Emptying

At birth, the stomach contains swallowed liquor amnii to which is added respiratory mucus, blood, and occasionally meconium. The gastric muscle coats are thin, motility is diminished, and emptying time is prolonged. The anatomical capacity is probably small and regurgitation is common. Gastric activity and emptying is dependent on the type of meal ingested and its volume. The higher the concentration of the glucose solution, the slower the gastric emptying. However, despite the slow emptying of 10 per cent glucose, this solution may be preferable to five per cent glucose when oral glucose is used for intermittent feeding, because more glucose is delivered to the small intestine per unit time.[30]

In our experience, the use of glucose and water solutions as a form of nutrition has not been very rewarding. Even 10 per cent glucose (admittedly twice as strong as five per cent) does not basically provide very many calories, and efforts to increase this much beyond 15 per cent glucose generally result in diarrhea. More calories can be obtained by the use of an equivalent volume of milk, and this form of oral nutrition is, in our view, always preferable to glucose and water solutions.

L. STERN

Emptying is also retarded with more fat and larger protein particles. Isosmotic food passes through more readily than extremely hypo- or hypertonic foods.

PRINCIPLES

1. A new formula should not be used until it has been proved by adequate studies.[28] Experimental feeding practices should be limited to centers where critical analysis is available. When evaluating the results of any feeding study, one must distinguish the truly premature infants from those small-for-gestational-age, and must also match birth weights, gestational ages, and sex. In comparing the results, one should study weight gain, increase in length, changes in head circumference, morbidity, and mortality, and such difficult parameters to evaluate as school performance and length of life.

2. The institution of early feeding will shorten the period required to regain birth weight. It should be noted that even with the present techniques of extrauterine nutrition, infants with birth weights less than 1500 gm. usually weigh only approximately 2.5 Kg. at what for them would be a gestational age of 40 weeks, compared with the mean birth weight of 3 to $3\frac{1}{2}$ Kg. if existence continued to term in utero.

3. While the protein, CHO, fat, fluid, and electrolyte requirements necessary for increase in size are known, *bigger is not necessarily better.* (In animals, length of survival can be altered by changing the quantity of early feeding. Overfeeding predisposes to obesity — early overfeeding causes more rapid maturation but the animals also die at a younger age.) Early malnutrition may result in permanent dwarfing, diminished intelligence, and increased susceptibility to disease.

4. The term fetus receives large quantities of iron and other minerals during the last two months of gestation. Deficiency disease must be prevented by adequate supplementation of minerals and vitamins. The preterm infants are delivered before receiving these stores, which need to be repleted as well as daily maintenance requirements provided.

5. Extrauterine adaptation should be normal *before the first feed.* The infant should be warm, breathing normally, and have good color, tone, and cry.[2] The technique of feeding will be determined by both birth weight and gestational age. The gag reflex is *not* complete until eight months' gestation. Before this time, infants should be gavage fed, supplemented by I.V. (see Practical Considerations). Note that the presence of normal sucking does not guarantee a completely adequate gag reflex. If the infant has a moderate-to-severe pulmonary problem, do not feed him orally.

6. The gastric capacity of the small infant is limited; thus, he may require small amounts of formula at frequent intervals. *Spitting should not be tolerated* in small infants where danger of pulmonary aspiration is great. If spitting is noted, reduce the volume of formula per feed.

7. Because of the increased fluid content, the stomach of infants born by cesarean section and infants of diabetic mothers may be aspirated before the first feed.

8. Early feeding of low-birth-weight infants is associated with a higher blood sugar, lower bilirubin, less dehydration, and a more rapid return to birth weight.[7, 27, 29, 34, 37, 45] Nonetheless, the immature infants do not achieve normal birth weight at the expected gestation time. Late feeding of calories and fluid may reduce the chance for normal development.

In infants less than 1500 gm., maintain I.V. administration from three hours of age until oral intake is around 110 ml. per Kg. In the smaller infants, this may be for a long period of time.

9. Small-for-gestational-age infants are prone to hypoglycemia and cannot tolerate prolonged fasting.

10. Low-birth-weight infants during the period of rapid "catch-up" growth may require increased vitamin intake to prevent deficiency diseases such as rickets.[32]

PRACTICAL CONSIDERATIONS

1. The commencement of feedings should be determined by the tone, color, and respiratory patterns of the immature infant and should be individualized. There should be no fixed feeding orders written for low-birth-weight infants. If the infant has respiratory distress or is hypothermic, oral feedings should be withheld and fluids and calories given by intravenous route.

2. *The first feed.* Early feeding (I.V. and/or oral) of newborn infants—premature and full term—results in a reduction in the degree of hyperbilirubinemia, less hypoglycemia and dehydration, and a significantly higher survival rate (only in infants <1500 gm.). Infants less than 1500 gm. should probably receive all their fluids and calories intravenously for the first 24 to 48 hours. A most important controlled study revealed a steep reduction in mortality for infants weighing less than 1500 gm. who received parenteral fluids early (six hours) when compared to those given nasogastric fluids early, or to those who were starved.

Surprisingly to most pediatricians, Olson[33] found that five per cent glucose water instilled into the respiratory tree in rabbits caused changes similar to milk. Sterile water, which causes no pulmonary reaction, would theoretically thus be the choice for the first feed. However, when an infant aspirates, the lung is invaded not only by the feed but also by the other gastric contents including HCl, which will cause a severe chemical pneumonia. We still use the traditional five per cent glucose water for the first feed (four to six hours of age), exercising caution in selecting infants who have had normal extrauterine adaptation, using careful technique, and avoiding large volumes.

The finding by Olson (see above) that five per cent glucose and water appears to be as harmful to the lung in the newborn rabbit as milk casts serious doubt on the rationale which has made five per cent or 10 per cent glucose and water the first drink of the newborn infant. Since there appears to be no evidence to support it, there would seem to be little value in maintaining this so-called traditional initial feeding, and our own view therefore is to go immediately to a milk formula as the baby's first drink.

L. STERN

3. A significant study evaluating the effect of a feeding gastrostomy on the survival of infants with birth weights between 750 and 1250 gm. showed that the mortality with gastrostomy was higher than with routine feedings.[39] Gastrostomy should be reserved only for infants requiring surgical correction of anatomical malformations, e.g., tracheo-esophageal fistula.

4. Infants over 34 weeks' gestation or those between 32 and 34 weeks who show an ability to both suck and swallow may be fed by nipple. Those who do not have an adequate gag reflex (<32 weeks) should be gavage fed.

Procedure for Gavage Feeding. Use No. 5 or 8 French polyethylene feeding tube.

a. With the baby's head turned to the side, measure the length from xiphoid to tip of ear lobe plus ear to nose, and mark tube.

b. Pass the catheter through the nose or mouth to this mark.

c. Check that the catheter is in the stomach by first placing the proximal end of the catheter under water to determine that air is not returned with each respiration and then inject a small amount of air and listen over the stomach for bubbling. Aspirate the contents of the stomach and test the reaction.

d. If the gastric content is thick and/or contains blood and mucus, a small stomach washout with sterile water (5 to 10 ml.) may be given.

e. Feedings are to be introduced by gravity and are not to be injected with syringe under pressure.

f. When removing the tube, pinch it closed as it is withdrawn to avoid dripping fluid into the pharynx.

5. In order to accommodate the relatively large fluid load and because of the diminished gastric capacity, we use frequent small feeds, feeding infants <1250 gm. as often as hourly. The feeds are increased progressively as per feeding schedule, making sure that a given amount is tolerated before increasing the amount. Oral feeding is supplemented initially by I.V. fluid.

TABLE 5-3 COMPOSITION OF FORMULA COMMONLY USED IN NURSERY (per 100 ml.)

	HUMAN MILK	COW'S MILK*	ENFAMIL	ENFAMIL 24	SIMILAC	SIMILAC 24	SIMILAC PM 60/40	SMA	NUTRAMAGEN
Protein (gm.)	1.25	3.3	1.5	1.8	1.8	2.2	1.6	1.5	2.2
Fat (gm.)	3.5	3.7	3.7	4.5	3.6	4.3	3.5	3.5	2.6
Carbohydrate (gm.)	7.0	4.8	7.0	8.3	7.0	8.4	7.5	7.0	8.5
Ash (gm.)	0.2	0.7	0.34	0.41	0.4	0.5	0.2	0.25	0.6
Calories (no.)	67.0	66.0	67.0	81.0	68.0	81.0	67.0	67.0	67.0

*Cow's milk included for comparison.

Composition of Formula. The composition of some of the formulas used in our nursery is outlined in Table 5–3. We use formula closely resembling breast milk (humanized milk) for feeding low-birth-weight infants. Despite what you may hear to the contrary from well-meaning salesmen, these products resemble each other very closely and changes from one brand to another will be tolerated by most infants. Obviously, breast milk can be used, and may have advantages to the neonate other than nutrition alone. A special formula, of which there are many available, may be required for infants with special dietary problems, e.g., galactosemia, milk intolerance, etc.

A SUGGESTED FEEDING SCHEDULE

The first feeding is 5 to 10 per cent glucose in water or sterile water. If the glucose is tolerated, formula is commenced. Formula feeding should be 20 cal. per 30 ml. for the first 48 to 72 hours and then increased to 24 cal. per 30 ml. For infants with a poor gag reflex (gestational age 32 to 34 weeks), it is *most* important that the chosen volume will not result in *any* vomiting or spitting.

Supplement daily oral intake with I.V. infusion so that total fluid intake is between 120 and 150 ml. per Kg. per day. To achieve minimum weight loss in some infants, 150 to 200 ml. per Kg. per day may be required.

Maintain I.V. infusion of 10 per cent glucose, commencing at age three to six hours at a rate of 80 to 100 ml. per Kg. per day. After 24 hours, add maintenance sodium chloride and potassium. Check urine every eight hours and if glycosuria develops, reduce concentration of I.V. to 7.5 per cent or five per cent glucose. When oral feedings have reached 100 to 120 ml. per Kg. per day, discontinue I.V.

The use of intravenous fluids, particularly in small infants, is clearly beneficial under these situations. Little attention, however, is usually paid to the question of calcium in these solutions; this, coupled with an already easy tendency to hypocalcemia, may result in an augmented iatrogenic hypocalcemia from the use of calcium-free fluids. In our experience, this is frequently associated with apneic spells which can be abolished when the cause is recognized and calcium is administered, either orally or added to the intravenous fluids. It is our policy to monitor calcium along with the other electrolytes, and to provide for its addition to either the intravenous or oral portions of the feeding as indicated.

L. STERN

For Infants Weighing 1250 Gm. or Less at Birth (after 24 to 48 hours of I.V. feeding)

First feeding—1 ml. five per cent glucose in water. If this is tolerated, give a second such feeding after one hour.

If the first two feedings are tolerated, the infant is scheduled to be fed every hour. Five per cent glucose in water is increased 1 ml. every hour until 3-ml. volumes have been given twice and tolerated.

Start formula, 3 ml. every hour, which may be slowly increased in volume by 1 ml. until maximum of 6 ml. is given every hour. Then the quantity remains the same at least until 144 hours (six days) of age. If the infant is less than 1100 gm., stop at 5 to 6 ml. (120 to 144 ml. per Kg. per day; 100 to 120 cal. per Kg. per day) and continue this amount for 6 to 10 days. This is usually only achieved at between 7 and 14 days of age. Aspiration is a major problem in this group. Small infants may require hourly feedings for a long period of time.

Aspirate the stomach before giving feed and measure the residue. Replace the aspirate plus the amount needed to achieve the desired volume. If residue is equal to the desired volume, no formula is added.

When an infant is gaining and tolerating hourly feeding well, increase up to 8 ml. per hour then move to a two-hourly schedule as follows: first hour—9 ml., second hour—7 ml., third hour—10 ml., fourth hour—6 ml., and so on, thus gradually changing to a larger volume.

If a feeding is not tolerated, return to the next lower volume given, offer it times six and start increasing volume again.

For Infants Weighing 1250 to 1500 Gm. at Birth

First feeding—3 ml. of 5 to 10 per cent glucose in water. If this is tolerated, give 5 ml. glucose in water after two to three hours.

Thereafter formula is fed every two to three hours, starting with a volume of 5 ml. and increasing it 1 ml. every other feeding until the infant is getting 10- to 14-ml. volumes. Then the amount stays the same for 72 hours.

If a feeding is not tolerated, go back one step.

For Infants Weighing 1501 to 2000 Gm. at Birth

First feeding—5 ml. of 5 to 10 per cent glucose in water. If this is tolerated, give 8 ml. five per cent glucose in water after two to three hours.

Formula feedings may then be given every two to three hours, starting with 8 ml. and increasing 1 ml. every other feeding until 14-ml. volumes are taken.

Thereafter, increments of 2 to 4 ml. may be made daily until calculated requirements are met.

If a feeding is not tolerated, go back one step.

For Infants Weighing 2001 Gm. or More at Birth

First feeding—15 ml. of five per cent glucose in water. If tolerated, repeat 15 ml. five per cent glucose in water.

The third feeding is given three hours after the second, and is formula. If the third feeding is tolerated, regular three-hour feedings are given, starting with 15 ml. and increasing 5 ml. every other feeding until 30-ml. feedings are given.

If a feeding is not tolerated, go back one step. N.B. In small-for-gestational-age infants, 10 to 15 per cent glucose orally may be utilized from soon after birth. (These infants usually feed well and will tolerate larger volumes than the immature infants.) Blood sugar must be carefully monitored (every two hours for 12 hours) and an I.V. instituted if hypoglycemia develops and is not immediately controlled by oral feeding.

A new method has been evolved by Professor Visser in Rotterdam,[40] who continually infuses formula using a burette attached to the nasogastric feeding tube. The oral intake is supplemented by intravenous fluid for at least a week in the smaller infants. With this technique, larger volumes can be fed, resulting in a more rapid weight gain.

PRACTICAL HINTS

1. DO NOT starve infants for too long.
2. DO NOT nipple too early. All infants <32 weeks will require gavage feeding.
3. DO NOT increase the quantity too rapidly.
4. DO NOT nipple feed infants with respiratory rates above 60 per minute and those who are hypothermic. Do not feed those infants receiving assisted ventilation with mask and bag.
5. DO NOT feed infants delivered with maternal hydramnios or who have excess

mucus until a tube has been passed into the stomach.

6. Weigh small infants (less than 1500 gm.) twice daily during the first two weeks. Loss of weight is variable in rate and degree but can be measured accurately and is a useful clinical index of fluid requirements.

7. Keep accurate records of fluid and caloric intake. The basis for the infant not gaining weight can then be readily established.

8. Consult nurses before increasing volume or changing method of feeding.

9. Encourage the mother to come and feed her infant after he has taken easily from the nipple. Never ask the mother to do anything at which she will not succeed.

10. Beware of any new preparation—the use of new formulas has resulted in vitamin B, folic acid, and protein deficiency as well as hypernatremia.

11. Poor sucking after a period of normal feeding should be regarded as a danger signal and may be the first indication of serious infection.

12. Large-for-gestational-age, preterm infants often are lethargic and feed poorly. They may be erroneously diagnosed as being infected or cerebrally damaged.

UNKNOWNS

1. Ideal timing and composition of the first and subsequent feeds are unknown. What are the effects associated with a higher protein intake (and its attendant elevated blood amino acids such as phenylalanine, tryosine, etc.) on the subsequent neurologic development of low-birth-weight infants? Is the myelin composition different in artificially fed infants as compared to breast-fed infants?[14] (Galactose is necessary for the synthesis of sphingolipids, a principal lipid in myelin—there is less galactose in artificial formulas than in breast milk.)

2. Do the differences in tissue composition resulting from the use of artificial formula as opposed to breast milk result in disease in adult life? For example, do present feeding practices and particularly overfeeding in early life relate to "those burdens of adult life—obesity, atherosclerosis, and hypertension . . . ?"[15]

3. What is the ideal thermal environment in which to raise and nourish the newborn infant? What are the proper criteria for assessing adequacy of nutrition? Should we only use increasing length, weight, and head circumference?

4. The sensory needs of the infant at feeding time are unknown. Feeding represents a pleasurable experience and his major contact with his environment. Factors related to his handling and technique of feeding may subsequently influence development. It is of interest that non-caloric input, such as rocking the baby between feeds, favorably influences amount of weight gain.

5. Undernutrition due to uteroplacental dysfunction cannot be remedied by special oral feedings administered to the mother. It is not unreasonable that in the near future we will be able to influence the growth of undergrown fetuses in utero, and since 30 to 40 per cent of infants weighing less than 2.5 Kg. at birth are small-for-gestational-age, this will involve a large number of infants. How can we give additional nutrition to the fetus in utero?

CASE QUESTIONS

Case One (Compiled by M. Wald, M.D.)

J. K. is a 1250-gm. white female born to a 38-year-old woman at approximately 34 weeks' gestation. She exhibited no evidence of respiratory distress. Physical and X-ray examination following transfer at two days of age revealed evidence of small bowel obstruction, malnutrition, and a gestational age of about 34 weeks. Surgery revealed jejunal atresia and a malrotation requiring a jejunostomy. A long recovery course is anticipated.

If hyperalimentation is started, how should the orders read? Please consider and calculate all of the infant's needs.

With poor endogenous protein and energy stores, high metabolic requirements, major surgery, and a short bowel, this infant is likely to die without nutritional support. The technical arrangements for total intravenous support should be made at time of surgery. Calculate the hyperalimentation solution as follows:

a. Meet *protein* needs first. 3.5 to 4.0 gm. per Kg. as protein hydrolyzate. Aminosol (Abbott) is usually used because of its low electrolyte content. This infant's protein needs will be met by 100 ml. of five per cent Aminosol—five per cent dextrose solution, which also provides 40 calories.

b. Consider *caloric* needs next. This infant is dysmature and for good growth should receive a total of 120 to 140 calories per Kg. Many babies will tolerate this caloric load as glucose, but some may better tolerate a glucose-fructose mixture. Alcohol has also been suggested as an energy source. This infant's caloric needs will be met by 62 ml. 50 per cent glucose in water, providing an additional 124 calories.

c. *Water* needs must be considered next. Although maintenance water requirements are 80 to 100 ml. on intravenous therapy, infants receiving a full protein allowance need considerably more: 150 to 170 ml. per Kg. The total volume per day for this baby should be 200 ml.

d. Additional requirements:

Sodium 3 to 4 mEq. per Kg.	3 per cent NaCl 6 ml.
Potassium 3 mEq. per Kg.	Monobasic K phosphate 2M 2 ml. (Provided by NaCl.)
Chloride 3 to 4 mEq. per Kg.	10 per cent Ca gluconate 2.5 ml. (Provided as K phosphate.)
Calcium 0.5 mM. per Kg*	50 per cent Mg SO_4 0.15 ml.
Phosphorus 3 mM. per Kg.*	
Magnesium 0.5 mM. per Kg*	

Vitamins: A, D, E, C, B_1, B_2, B_6, pantothenate, niacin. As M.V.1. (U.S. Vitamin and Pharmaceutical Corp.) 1 ml.

Trace minerals, iron, or other nutrients may be added, if available, or plasma and blood transfusions can be given biweekly.

e. Orders to pharmacy: Basic solution for J.K.**

5% Aminosol 5% Dextrose	100 ml.
50% D/W	62 ml.
3% NaCl	6 ml.
2M KH_2PO_4	2 ml.
10% Calcium gluconate	2.5 ml.
50% $MgSO_4$	0.15 ml.
Multivitamin infusion	1 ml.
Distilled water	26 ml.
Total:	200 ml.

The solution for parenteral nutrition should only be prepared in the pharmacy under a laminar flow hood, not on the ward.

*We know nothing about the actual intravenous requirements of these substances.

**See Appendix 17 for sample order sheet.

Administration. See Filler[18] and Wilmore and Dudrick[43] for catheter technique and equipment. Attention to utmost detail is mandatory. The full-strength solution at maximum rate will not be tolerated until three to four days after surgery. Start with two-thirds dilution with additional distilled water at two-thirds of maximum rate,

Basic solution	100 ml.
Distilled water	50 ml.

Infuse at 5.5 ml. per hour = 133 ml. per 24 hours. Increase both *rate* and *concentration* gradually thereafter.

Precautions. Monitor daily: blood glucose, sodium, potassium, CO_2 content and pH, BUN, serum osmolarity, urine volume, specific gravity, urine glucose, urine osmolarity, weight, clinical state of hydration, and serum proteins.

Twice a week: hematocrit and ammonia level.

Continued search for infection.

The danger of infection under conditions of intravenous hyperalimentation should not be underestimated. There is an extremely high incidence of infection, particularly with Candida, and especially in situations in which high glucose-containing formulas are used. This infection appears to be only minimally affected by the use of small millipore filters, and increasing reports have appeared of serious systemic candidiasis with meningitis, osteomyelitis, septic arthritis, and ensuing death. For the moment, it is our view that unless specifically indicated because of surgical procedures which may limit the absorptive surface of the GI tract, intravenous hyperalimentation is not currently to be routinely recommended.

L. STERN

Case Two

L. M. is a 1200-gm., normal male born at 30 weeks' gestation who appeared in no distress during the first hours of life. By history and physical and neurologic examination, he appears appropriately sized for gestational age.

How and what should this infant be fed for the first four days of life? Please write your orders.

Intravenous maintenance should be begun by three to four hours of age, using a peripheral vein ideally, unless an umbilical catheter is otherwise justified. The solution should contain 10 per cent glucose.

At 24 hours of age, a solution of 10 per cent glucose with 20 mEq. per liter sodium chloride plus 20 mEq. per liter potassium chloride is substituted. The rate should be 4 ml. per hour (100 ml. per Kg. per day).

Oral feeding by nasogastric tube should begin at 36 to 48 hours of age with 2 ml. of water and be repeated in one hour. Formula (20 calories per 30 ml.) may then be fed, 3 ml. per hour, aspirating for gastric residue before each feeding (be sure to replace aspirate).

Increase by 1 ml. per feeding after 24 hours, then cautiously in 1 ml. steps every other feeding. At four days of age, intake will *probably* be 4 to 5 ml. per hour (80 to 100 ml. per Kg. per 24 hours) by nasogastric tube if all goes well. At this point, intravenous fluids may be tapered.

Water needs vary, and may be higher than these allowances in very small infants. If proper amounts of water are being provided:

a. Weight loss should not exceed 8 to 10 per cent of birth weight at four days.

b. Urine osmolarity should not exceed that of plasma.

c. Plasma osmolarity and serum sodium values should remain normal. Failure to achieve these goals calls for an increase in the intravenous water allowance.

Case Three

A 1740-gm. female was born at 40 weeks' gestation to a primigravida who had no problems during pregnancy, labor, or delivery. A physical examination, including a neurologic examination for gestational age, agreed with the mother's dates. There were no physical abnormalities nor any suggestion of intrauterine infection.

What are this infant's nutritional requirements? How and what should this infant be fed during the first week of life?

Assuming this infant's low birth weight stems from intrauterine malnutrition, her caloric requirements will be high (120 to 150 calories per Kg. per day) for growth. She is at risk of hypoglycemia. Fortunately, she may feed well from a very early age. Feedings should be started at two to six hours of age and offered on a three-hour schedule. If she takes them well, there may be no further problem. If she does not, intravenous caloric supplements with 10 per cent glucose and maintenance electrolytes should be given. Dextrostix monitoring at two-hour intervals is sufficient guard against hypoglycemia as long as the baby remains well.

Case Four

N. D. is a 3340-gm., normal male born at 40 weeks' gestation following a difficult labor. The infant was covered with meconium at birth and had moderate respiratory distress. X-ray revealed aspiration syndrome and duodenal atresia. It was anticipated that there would be at least a 10-day period before oral feedings would be instituted.

How should this infant's caloric, fluid, and electrolyte requirements be met?

This infant, unlike the baby in Case One, has better caloric stores. Provided he is able to begin oral feeding on the 10th or 12th day, we would not institute hyperalimentation. The decision, however, may be different, as experience increases success with this technique.

This infant can receive 10 per cent dextrose in water with 20 mEq. per liter sodium chloride (or bicarbonate) and 20 mEq. per liter potassium chloride at rates of 75 to 85 ml. per Kg. initially, increasing to 110 to 120 ml. per Kg. on the fourth day. This will provide up to 50 cal. per Kg. and minimize protein catabolism.

This baby will require upper gastrointestinal decompression by nasogastric tube pre- and post-operatively until the paralytic ileus is gone. Losses by this route may be great and must be replaced ml. for ml. with normal saline and potassium as needed.

REFERENCES

1. Auld, P., Bhangananda, P., and Mehta, S.: The influence of early caloric feeding with I-V glucose on catabolism of premature infants. Pediatrics 37:592, 1966.
2. Avery, M., and Hodson, W.: The first drink reconsidered. J Pediat 68:1008, 1966.
3. Babson, S.: Feeding the low birth weight infant. J Pediat 79:694, 1971.
4. Babson, S., and Bramhall, J.: Diet and growth in the premature infant. J Pediat 74:890, 1969.
5. Barness, L.: Infant feeding. Pediat Clin N Amer 8:639, 1961.
6. Barrie, H.: Effect of feeding on gastric and esophageal pressures in the newborn. Lancet 2:1158, 1968.
7. Beard, A., Panos, T., Marasigan, B., et al: Perinatal stress and the premature neonate. 2. Effect of fluid and calorie deprivation on blood glucose. Pediatrics 68:329, 1969.
8. Churchill, J.: Weight loss in premature infants developing spastic diplegia. Obstet Gynec 22:601, 1963.
9. Cornblath, M., Forbes, A., Pildes, R., et al: A controlled study of early fluid administration on

survival of low birthweight infants. Pediatrics *38*:547, 1966.

10. Daily, W., Klaus, M., and Meyer, B.: Apnea in premature infants—monitoring, incidence, heart rate changes and the effects of environmental temperatures. Pediatrics *43*:410, 1968.

11. Dancis, J., O'Connell, J., and Holt, L., Jr.: A grid for recording the weight of premature infants. J Pediat *33*:570, 1948.

12. Davidson, M.: Formula feeding of normal term and low birth weight infants. Pediat Clin N Amer *17*:913, 1970.

13. Davidson, M., Levine, S., Bauer, C., et al: Feeding studies in low-birth-weight infants. J Pediat *70*:695, 1967.

14. Davies, P.: Feeding the newborn baby. Proc Nutr Soc *28*:66, 1968.

15. Davies, P.: Feeding. Brit Med J *4*:351, 1971.

16. Drillien, C.: *The Growth and Development of the Prematurely Born Infant.* Edinburgh and London, E. and S. Livingstone Ltd, 1964.

17. Fanaroff, A., Wald, M., Gruber, H., et al: Insensible water loss in low-birthweight infants. Pediatrics *50*:236, 1972.

18. Filler, R., Eraklin, A., Rubin, V., et al: Long-term total parenteral nutrition in infants. New Eng J Med *281*:589, 1969.

19. Fomon, S.: *Infant Nutrition.* Philadelphia, W.B. Saunders Co., 1967.

20. Glass, L., Silverman, W., and Sinclair, J.: Relationship of thermal environment and caloric intake to growth and resting metabolism in the late neonatal period. Biol Neonat *14*:324, 1969.

21. Goldman H., Freudenthal, R., Holland, B., et al: Clinical effects of two different levels of protein intake on low birth weight infants. J Pediat *74*:881, 1969.

22. Goldman, H., Liebman, O., Freudenthal, R., et al: Effects of early dietary protein intake on low-birth-weight infants: evaluation at 3 years of age. J Pediat *78*:126, 1971.

23. Gordon, H., and Levine, S.: The metabolic basis for the individualized feeding of infants, premature and full-term. J Pediat *25*:464, 1944.

24. Gordon, H., Levine, S., Deamer, W., et al: Respiratory metabolism in infancy and in childhood. XXIII. Daily energy requirements of premature infants. Amer J Dis Child *59*:1185, 1940.

25. Gryboski, J.: The swallowing mechanism of the neonate. I. Esophageal and gastric motility. Pediatrics *35*:445, 1965.

26. Gryboski, J.: Suck and swallow in the premature infant. Pediatrics *43*:96, 1969.

27. Haworth, J., and Ford, J.: Effect of early and late feeding and glucagon upon blood sugar and serum bilirubin levels of premature babies. Arch Dis Child *38*:328, 1963.

28. Holt, L., and Snyderman, S.: The feeding of premature and newborn infants. Pediat Clin N Amer *13*:1103, 1966.

29. Hubbell, J., Drorbaugh, J., Rudolph, A., et al: Early versus late feeding of infants of diabetic mothers with respiratory distress syndrome. New Eng J Med *265*:835, 1961.

30. Husband, J., and Husband, P.: Gastric emptying of water and glucose solutions in the newborn. Lancet *2*:409, 1969.

31. Kodiak, E.: Nutrition of the foetus and the newly born. Proc Nutr Soc *28*:17, 1968.

32. Lewin, P., Reid, M., Reilly, B., et al: Iatrogenic rickets in low birth weight infants. J Pediat *78*:207, 1971.

33. Olson, M.: Effects of water, 5% glucose or milk on rabbits' lungs. Pediatrics *46*:538, 1970.

34. Rabor, I., Oh, W., Wu, P., et al: Effects of early and late feeding of intrauterine fetally malnourished (IUM) infants. Pediatrics *42*:261, 1968.

35. Russell, G., and Feather, E.: Effects of feeding on respiratory mechanics of healthy newborn infants. Arch Dis Child *45*:325, 1970.

36. Sinclair, J., Driscoll, J., Jr., Heird, W., et al: Supportive management of the sick neonate: parenteral calories, water, electrolytes. Pediat Clin N Amer *17*:863, 1970.

37. Smallpiece, V., and Davies, P.: Immediate feeding of premature infants with undiluted breast milk. Lancet *2*:1349, 1964.

38. Snyderman, S., Boyer, A., Kogut, M., et al: The protein requirement of the premature infant. I. The effect of protein intake on the retention of nitrogen. J Pediat *74*:872, 1969.

39. Vengusamy, S., Pildes, R., Raffensperger, J., et al: A controlled study of feeding gastrostomy in low birth weight infants. Pediatrics *43*:815, 1969.

40. Visser, H.: Personal communication.

41. Wennberg, R., Schwartz, R., and Sweet, A.: Early versus delayed feeding of low birth weight infants: effects on physiologic jaundice. J Pediat *68*:860, 1966.

42. Wharton, B., and Bower, B.: Immediate or later feeding for premature babies: a controlled trial. Lancet *2*:969, 1965.

43. Wilmore, D., and Dudrick, S.: Growth and development of an infant receiving all nutrients exclusively by vein. JAMA *203*:860, 1968.

44. Winick, M.: Changes in nucleic acid and protein content of the human brain during growth. Pediat Res *2*:352, 1968.

45. Wu, P., Teilmann, P., Cabler, M., et al: "Early" versus "late" feeding of low birth weight neonates. Pediatrics *39*:733, 1967.

Chapter 6

TRANSPORTATION OF THE HIGH-RISK INFANT

by
AVROY FANAROFF, M.B. (Rand.), M.R.C.P.E.
and
MARSHALL KLAUS, M.D.

The development of neonatal intensive care units in the industrialized nations of the world has precipitated the growth of transportation systems for conveying the sick infant from his place of birth to specialized care centers. As early as the 1900s, Budin used warm water bottles for maintaining the baby's temperature during transport. This was followed in the early part of the century both in England and in this country by the development of containers for transport of the infants with simple but inadequate heating devices and in some cases a method for administering oxygen. In the last five years, there have been major refinements in the construction of the transport incubator, permitting the infant to be kept warm and well oxygenated while allowing the physician or nurse transporting the infant to render necessary care during transit.

A recent development, not as yet fully tested, is a mobile van equipped with intensive care facilities which goes to the infant. The infant may then be cared for in the mobile intensive care nursery while stationed at the referring hospital, or the van may convey the infant to the regional intensive care nursery (Figure 6-1).

It must be emphasized that transportation of the high-risk infant following delivery is probably not the ideal health care delivery system for the high-risk mother or infant.

Studies in Quebec Province and Arizona suggest that when the infant is delivered in a hospital with an infant intensive care unit, mortality and morbidity rates are lower (Table 6-1).

No one would dispute the fact that the possession of an intensive care unit contiguous with the place of birth of the infant represents the ideally superior situation. However, considerations of personnel, economics, and the absolute impossibility of repeating this kind of organization in every hospital in which infants are born require that the statement be analyzed much more carefully. Reference to Table 6-1 will show that, with respect to low-birth-weight infants, the mortality rate is best (i.e., lowest) in those institutions with an intramural intensive care facility, closely followed by those institutions that utilize a referral intensive care facility; institutions which neither have a facility of their own nor refer their patients are at the bottom of the list. The differences between intramural facilities and the utilization of a referral facility, however, should be analyzed a little more carefully. To begin with, in Table 6-1 the incidence of low birth weight is lower in the intramural group and some of the difference (62 per 1000 as opposed to 74 per 1000) would be accounted for by this difference in the incidence of low birth weight. Of much greater importance, however, is the difference in the time at which therapy can be undertaken. This difference depends not upon the referral facility but upon the willingness and speed with which the referring institutions transfer their infants. It is generally agreed that earlier transfer, and not just a desperation move when inept attempts at

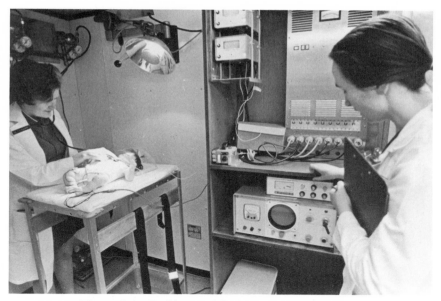

Figure 6–1 Inside a mobile intensive care nursery. (Courtesy of Dr. L. Blackmon.)

therapy in an unqualified institution have been carried out, would bring the mortality statistics for low-birth-weight infants in institutions using a referral unit even closer to that of the intramural facility itself. It should also be noted from Table 6–1 that, with respect to mortality rates for full-term infants, there are no differences between intramural and referral utilization of facilities, but that the ability to place the child either intramurally or through a referral facility in an intensive care unit results in a full-term neonatal mortality almost half that of infants in which neither facility is utilized.

L. STERN

A transport system must be considered as only one component of the larger organization required for optimal care of the fetus and newborn. It is our opinion that the uterus is the

TABLE 6–1   NEONATAL INTENSIVE CARE AND PERINATAL MORTALITY*
(PROVINCE OF QUEBEC, 1967 and 1968)[6]

NEONATAL INTENSIVE CARE FACILITY†	NO. HOSPITAL YEARS	NO. BIRTHS OVER 1000 gm.	INCIDENCE OF LBW‡ (1001-2500 gm.) *(0/1000 live births)*	LBW NEONATAL MORTALITY *(0/1000 LBW live births)*	FULL-SIZE (OVER 2500 gm.) NEONATAL MORTALITY *(0/1000 F-S live births)*	STILLBIRTH RATE *(0/1000 births)*	PERINATAL MORTALITY RATE *(0/1000 live births)*
Intramural facility	6	12,532	69	62	2.2	8.7	15.0
Referral facility utilized	13	20,962	75	74	2.0	9.8	17.2
Neither intramural nor referral facility utilized	43	73,974	75	86	3.6	10.2	19.9

*For all infants of birth weights more than 1000 gm.
†Including only metropolitan region (Montreal and Quebec City) hospitals delivering more than 1000 infants per year.
‡Low birth weight.

ideal "transport incubator" and the development of combined maternal and neonatal intensive care units, with the referral to and delivery of high-risk mothers in these special centers, would be a far better arrangement. (This has already been successfully achieved in several of the large cities of Russia.) This will not obviate the need for a transport system, for even though the majority of neonatal problems occur with high-risk pregnancies (including maternal hypertension, antepartum hemorrhage, erythroblastosis, premature ruptured membranes, and premature labor), some infants develop difficulties following a seemingly normal pregnancy and uncomplicated labor, and will require transport after delivery.

Although this chapter will discuss the transportation of the infant, this system in the future must not stand alone, but must be combined with the development of high-risk maternity infant centers.

PRINCIPLES AND PRACTICAL ASPECTS OF TRANSPORTATION

All hospitals require some transportation facilities for which the same principles apply, whether the baby is being transported from one city to another or simply within the hospital to the operating room, X-ray department, etc. The transportation of a sick, small infant is a complex act requiring the coordinated action of a number of personnel and institutions. Although in most cases each act is simple, a single omission in the intricate chain may be detrimental to the infant's health. *Communication* and teamwork are the keynotes to a successful transport system.

The following discussion and outline consider ground transportation using an ambulance for trips less than 50 to 60 miles. A slight alteration in the details can be made for longer trips using planes, helicopters, or trucks. In any transport system, plans must be made for the entire 24 hours, and alternative hospitals must be available for accepting infants when the referral center is overcrowded or closed for any reason. We have found it useful in Northern Ohio to link two large referral centers together; thus, when one unit is filled or overwhelmed, the other unit can accept all of the other infants. Our working plan is outlined in Table 6–2. The act of transporting a baby, as noted in Table 6–2, is a collaborative effort, and as in any medical endeavor, differences of opinion will arise;

TABLE 6–2 PHYSICIAN DUTIES FOR TRANSPORTATION

1. Physician controller on call receives incoming referrals and makes the decision as to which nursery can accept an infant after checking on space available.
2. The controller will require that the following essential material and information be available at time of pickup of the infant:
   A. Xerox or duplication of mother's and infants' charts.
   B. 5 ml. of mother's blood (clotted).
   C. Any X-rays of the infant.
   D. Infant's name, M.D.'s name, parents' name, address, and phone number.
   E. The father should be instructed to follow in his own car (so that he can furnish pertinent information and remain with the infant for two to three hours and report back to the mother).
   F. With great diplomacy, request that referring physician maintain infant's temperature and color (PaO_2). Tactfully give specific instructions for interim treatment.
3. A. The controller will delegate a house officer to pick up the infant. This call takes top priority and the house officer must be ready to travel in 10 minutes. This must be a person who has rotated through newborn service.
   B. The Intensive Care Nursery is informed to prepare for infant's arrival.
   C. The controller calls ambulance service and relays time of their arrival to travelling house officer. (We always use the same ambulance company.)
4. Travelling house officer collects transport incubator and emergency bag with drugs and equipment. (Check battery and O_2 cylinder.)
5. Plug incubator into ambulance during trips and use battery operation when moving in and out of hospitals. Plug in at referring hospital.
6. Prepare infant for trip, correcting acute conditions (asphyxia, metabolic acidosis, hypoglycemia, etc.) before transport. Catheterize only umbilical vein. Explain plan of action to the parents.
7. *No matter how healthy the infant looks, he must be transferred.*
8. Record procedures carried out, including drugs, problems, or complications on the information form.
9. Oxygen tank will last 80 minutes at 7 L. Battery will last for 45 minutes of constant use.

however, these must be submerged and reasonable harmony maintained, otherwise chaos may occur. The individual duties in a transportation system require that all referring hospitals, physicians, ambulance drivers, as well as the accepting hospitals with their physicians and nurses, have a clear understanding of the local organization and ground rules. In one successful center this was quickly achieved by the director having a discussion with each referring physician over a glass of wine. The responsibilities of every individual and the unit responsibilities must be clearly defined. In our system, this has been helped by having the duties of all physicians and referring hospitals clearly outlined on forms kept in their nurseries.

The transport is *initiated* by a physician requesting transfer to a regional center. His request is influenced by his experience, training, local facilities, personnel, and the overall ability to cope with the problem. (It has been our policy to accept all infants referred from outlying hospitals, even though the physician controller may have the impression that the infant is not seriously ill or is even possibly completely normal. The fact that the referring physician believes that his patient requires further specialized facilities reflects a call for help, and is justification for accepting the infant. Rarely have we collected an infant not requiring any special care.) The referring physician communicates the nature of the infant's problem and his condition to the *physician controlling* the transport system, who in turn notifies the transport team and the *nurses on the intensive care unit* of the specific nature of the problem so that a plan of action may be formulated and any special equipment prepared before setting out.

The *timing* of transport is, of course, particularly important in the premature infant. Approximately one-third of all infant deaths occur within the first 24 hours following birth, and early treatment of many conditions appears to alter outcome favorably. Therefore, for whatever reason the physician considers referring an infant, be it an illness that cannot be handled properly at his own hospital, or inadequate equipment, we recommend early transportation.

After initiating the transport, the referring physician is requested to make the following arrangements:

1. Obtain a sample of blood from the mother and copy the mother's and infant's charts and have X-rays available. (These data are invaluable in the management of the patient.)

2. The physician controller may often make helpful suggestions to the referring physician so that the infant is prepared for the trip.

These include:

   a. Increasing the environmental oxygen (if this is indicated on clinical grounds—see Chapter 8, Respiratory Problems).

   b. Administering small doses of bicarbonate through an umbilical vein catheter (if indicated).

   c. Checking the infant's hematocrit and blood sugar by means of a dextrostix.

   d. Placing the infant in the neutral thermal environment.

   e. Suctioning and decompressing the abdomen when indicated.

(The referring physician must thus warm, oxygenate, check the blood sugar on the infant before the ambulance arrives, and have patients' records prepared.)

3. The referring physician informs the parents of the reasons for transport and requests that the father be ready to accompany the ambulance in his own car.

We have often found it useful to have more than one individual on the transportation team: a physician and nurse, or physician and student/inhalation therapist. On rare occasions, it is possible to use an untrained nurse in transporting a small normal premature (greater than 1500 gm.).

It is mandatory that the transportation be carried out by a team from the receiving institution and not just by haphazard selection of a local ambulance company with unqualified personnel. Moreover, it has been our policy *always* to send a physician, together with a nurse and ambulance driver, for the transport process. The physician, in addition to being responsible for initial medical assessment of the situation and the undertaking of the procedures which are outlined below, is also an invaluable source of acquiring the information which is usually lacking when the infant arrives, unaccompanied and without documentation from a referring hospital, in a private carrier. The sources from which this information can be obtained are varied, and include case room nurses, the mother, the anesthetist, and even the referring physician, if he can be found still at the site of the delivery.

L. STERN

When the ambulance arrives at the referring hospital, the physician remains only long enough to stabilize the infant's condition so that the trip back can be accomplished without catastrophe. He must be satisfied that the infant is in reasonable condition and fit to be transported. In order for the transportation to be accomplished without damage to the infant, conditions such as asphyxia, metabolic acidosis, hypoglycemia, and hypovolemia should be promptly treated before transport. A quick clinical appraisal together with several simple laboratory tests (if necessary), such as a Dextrostix, a hematocrit on a pale infant, and a quick view of the X-rays, are carried out. If there is a history of asphyxia or the presence of respiratory distress, we make an arbitrary correction of the probable metabolic acidosis by using 3 mEq. per Kg. of sodium bicarbonate I.V. for infants greater than 2 Kg. and 4 mEq. per Kg. for infants less than 2 Kg. If the infant is gasping and pale, he may require O_2, bicarbonate, and a blood transfusion before the trip commences. Some type of assisted ventilation may have to be started in the referring hospital. For apneic episodes and severe respiratory distress, a simple mask and bag are used for assisted ventilation. (See Chapter 8, Respiratory Problems). This may be continued *during transportation,* which should be carried out in an optimally controlled environment. The interior of the ambulance should be warm and well lit so that the infant can be *closely observed* at all times. Difficulties should be anticipated and provisions made for emergency treatment. The team must be in a position to promptly relieve airway obstruction, oxygenate, assist ventilation, correct acidosis, support circulation, control seizures, and maintain temperature during the trip. Table 6–3 outlines the drugs and equipment that we use in our transport system. This checklist stays in the bag, which is replenished after each trip. The major aim is to improve the condition of the infant, and certainly the infant should arrive in no worse condition than when he started.

Detailed notes and recordings of observations made during the transport are essential for the physicians who will ultimately be caring for the infant.

The physician must have a brief discussion with the mother if at all possible, and show her the infant before leaving the referring hospital. Although it is obviously impossible to allay all her fears, a short discussion of the reasons for the transportation and the nature of the care the infant will receive in the intensive care unit (ICU) is helpful. We explain that the mother can receive information on her infant's condition by calling directly into the ICU 24 hours a day, and that she may visit as soon as she is discharged. We have observed that most mothers believe that their baby probably will not survive when it is transferred, and they need much reassurance

TABLE 6–3 CHECKLIST OF DRUGS AND EQUIPMENT

QUANTITY	ITEM
1	Laryngoscope handle with premature infant blade
	Fore-clear endotracheal tubes, sizes 3.0, 3.5, and 4.0 mm.
1	Universal endotracheal tube adaptor
1	Breathing bag
1	Set of small Bennett masks
2	Infant airway
2	10 or 12½ cc. syringes, sterile, with #20 needle
5	3 or 2½ cc. syringes, sterile, with #22 needle
5	Three-way stopcocks, sterile
1	Umbilical catheterization set and extra catheters
2	#5 F single-holed catheters
2	#5 and 8 F feeding tubes
3	Stopcock plugs (needle caps)
2	Tuberculin syringes with #26 needle
2	30 cc. amp. sterile distilled water
2	30 cc. amp. sterile saline
1	10 cc. heparin, sterile, 1000 units/cc.
2	50 cc. vials sodium bicarbonate
1	50 cc. vial 50 per cent glucose
1	1:1000 aqueous adrenalin
	Valium
	6 feet of latex tubing
1	Scissors, nonsterile
2	Hemostats, nonsterile
	Scotch tape or equivalent
3	Vial files—sharp
	Forms
	Dextrostix
	Suction catheter with rubber tubing
	Tape measure
	Disposable gloves
	Specimen tubes
	Alcohol sponges
	Preparation tray with amphyl
	Intensive Care record sheet
2	Glass 3 cc. syringes for artery sticks
2	#23 scalp needles
1	#21 scalp needle
	Rubber bands
	Lancets
2	Receiving blankets
	Stethoscope

to the contrary. Their initial comment on seeing the infant in the ICU is often: "I never thought I'd see him again." For these reasons we have found it helpful to work closely with the father, who accompanies the ambulance in his own car. He remains in the intensive care unit for several hours, learning about the condition of the infant, becoming acquainted with the physicians and nurses, and getting a better understanding of his infant's problems.

(A cup of coffee and a quiet chat are most useful.) He is encouraged to take a photograph of the infant so that the mother can see how her baby looks. We depend upon him for communicating the infant's condition and progress to his wife. She also receives a report of progress directly from her pediatrician, together with a call from the physician in the ICU.

Problems of transportation are often related mainly to the mechanical equipment. These may be minimized by careful maintenance. In our system, the intensive care nurses and inhalation therapists clean and maintain the transport incubator and equipment. We have used a battery-operated incubator which is adapted so it can be plugged into the ambulance during the trip out in order to reduce the heat loss from the incubator and conserve the battery. To maintain adequate oxygen concentrations, we carry a small plastic hood to fit over the infant's head, connected to the oxygen source. The ambulance involved in the transport comes first to the intensive care unit to pick up the equipment and incubator (which have been checked.) The chief difficulty during transport has been to maintain temperature. To overcome this, it is worth waiting at the referring hospital until the baby has started to warm up before undertaking a journey.

On arrival at the intensive care nursery, a short information form is completed by the physician who collected the infant (Table 6–4). This form is helpful in the care of the infant and in the organization and maintenance of the transportation system.

Once the infant's condition has been evaluated and diagnosis established, the referring doctor should be called and informed of the infant's condition, provisional diagnosis, etc., so that he can keep the mother up to date. When dealing with neonates, it must be remembered that there are two patients — the mother and the infant.

UNKNOWNS

1. The ideal vehicle and equipment for transporting infants over different distances are at present unknown. Many physicians have found the helicopter difficult to work in because of noise, shaking, and temperature control.

Unless under circumstances in which no other form of transport is available, we are not at all inclined towards the use of helicopters. The question of temperature loss because of the outside cold environmental temperature at such heights is critical, and relatively few helicopters are of the double-walled variety which would prevent such loss. In addition, the choice of a landing site is crucial. In most northern portions of this continent, helicopter landing pads which are not low down on the ground generally present conditions too windy to permit the helicopter to land, and although a pad on the roof may look very impressive it is rarely utilized because of adverse weather conditions. If a helicopter must be used, then an adjacent schoolyard or parking lot would appear to offer the best possibility for its regular operating capacities.

L. STERN

2. It has been difficult to completely measure the effectiveness of the transportation system in reducing mortality and morbidity. Comparisons must be made between delivery of the mothers in the high-risk unit and the transportation of the sick infant following delivery.

3. The transportation of the infant away from the mother has had a profound effect on the mother's relationship with her infant. Procedures for preventing the depression and anticipatory grief that occur in the mother at the time of transportation have not been clarified. Should the mother accompany the infant? Should she be housed with the infant two to three days later when she is discharged?

4. How does a transportation system affect care in the referring hospital?

PRACTICAL HINTS IN TRANSPORTATION OF SPECIFIC CASE PROBLEMS

1. Infants with gastrointestinal obstruction — should have indwelling nasogastric tubes and be suctioned prior to and during transportation if necessary.

2. Myelomeningocele — should be kept covered with moist sterile gauze.

3. Gastroschisis or omphalocele — the intestines should be kept covered, preferably with moist, warm, sterile, saline packs.

4. Infants with respiratory obstruction — airway to be maintained patent, either with indwelling endotracheal tube or an oropharyngeal airway (whichever method is best suited to the individual).

5. Pneumothorax, but no evidence of tension — place the infant in an enriched oxygen environment; be prepared to aspirate and

TABLE 6–4   INFORMATION FORM

Date_____

Time of call_____

Time of departure_____

Time of return_____

Referring person_____Specialty_____

Hospital_____

Referring diagnosis_____

Name of infant_____Sex_____Gest._____

Date and time of birth_____Place of birth_____

Category of patient after transfer: Staff_____Private attending_____

Parents' names_____Address_____

_____Phone: Home_____

Your diagnosis_____

What was done before leaving hospital?_____

Bicarb_____ O$_2$_____ Bag_____ I.V._____ Other_____

What, if any, Rx was given en route?_____

Baby's condition upon arrival_____

Rectal temp_____ Blood gases_____Transport temp_____

Statement of mechanical difficulties, including transport_____

_____

Statement of problems at or with ref. hospital_____

General course of Rx and baby's response in overall transport_____

Suggestions:_____

_____

_____

decompress. A tension pneumothorax should be treated before leaving the referring hospital.

6. Severe heart failure—commence therapy before leaving referring hospital (see Chapter 13).

7. Seizures—maintain airway and control seizures before leaving the referring hospital (see Chapter 16, Neurologic Problems).

There is a large variety of other technical and operational details which need to be fully understood before effective transport systems can be organized and specifically operated. For example, it is not well known, but of critical importance, that there are striking differences in amperage when AC-current-operated equipment (as used in hospitals) needs to be run from DC-battery conversion in ambulances. Failure to appreciate this difference generally results in complete breakdown of the ambulance, usually somewhere en route between the two hospitals. This and a large number of other mechanical and administrative considerations are available in a manual on infant transportation published under the aegis of the Canadian Pediatric Society, copies of which can be obtained by writing to the Society's Secretary, Dr. J. H. Victor Marchessault, at the Department of Pediatrics, University of Sherbrooke, Sherbrooke, Quebec, Canada.

The question of re-transportation of the infant back to the hospital of birth as soon as the acute illness has passed should be actively considered. While most states and provinces claim to have laws prohibiting such a move, close inspection of these regulations generally reveals this to be untrue; it merely usually reflects an administrative decision on the part of the individual hospitals, since some paper work is generally necessary to accomplish this. In most instances, the newborn infant does not have a separate existence of his own, being an appendage on his mother's hospital chart. Once she has left the hospital, re-admission of such an infant poses some administrative considerations, which, in the past, many institutions have simply not been willing to undertake. In our view, the return of the infant to the nursery (never to an older-child pediatric ward) from which he has come has been not only helpful but also of great benefit to the infant. Approximately 50 per cent of all the infants admitted to the Neonatal Intensive Care Unit at the Montreal Children's Hospital are not discharged directly home, but are returned to the hospital of birth to be cared for in that nursery until such time as they are ready for discharge. This affords two advantages. It allows the referral center to concentrate all its personnel and capabilities on the truly sick infants, and relieves the crush on beds, equipment, and personnel. Moreover, it will return the infant closer to his mother, make visiting and contact with the baby on her part much simpler and a much easier part of her daily routine, with benefits as outlined in Chapter 7.

L. STERN

REFERENCES

1. American Academy of Pediatrics' Committee on Fetus and Newborn: *Hospital Care of Newborn Infants.* Evanston, American Academy of Pediatrics, 1971, pp. 95–100.
2. Arp, L., Dillon, R., Long, M., et al: An emergency air-ground transport system for newborn infants with respiratory distress syndrome. Med Ann DC *38*:261, 1969.
3. Segal, S.: Transfer of a premature or other high-risk newborn infant to a referral hospital. Pediat Clin N Amer *13*:1195, 1966.
4. Segal, S., Ed.: *Manual for the Transport of High-Risk Newborn Infants: Principles, Policies, Equipment, Techniques.* Vancouver, Canadian Pediatric Society, 1972.
5. Shepard, K.: Air transportation of high-risk infants utilizing a flying intensive care nursery. J Pediat *77*:148, 1970.
6. Usher, R.: Clinical implications of perinatal mortality statistics. Clin Obstet Gynec *14*:885, 1971.

Chapter 7

CARE OF THE MOTHER

by

MARSHALL KLAUS, M.D.

and

JOHN KENNELL, M.D.

"Mothers separated from their young soon lost all interest in those whom they were unable to nurse or cherish."

PIERRE BUDIN, *The Nursling*

The significance of the early postpartum days to the mother-infant relationship has recently been the focus of detailed investigation. Behavioral studies in humans and a wide range of animal studies[2, 13, 15, 26] indicate that the events before and immediately following delivery may greatly influence later maternal behavior. This chapter reviews the recent human and animal studies and provides historical background which explains how mothers have been isolated from their infants in this country. Five cases are used to illustrate how presently available knowledge can be applied clinically.

HISTORY

The role of the mother in the hospital nursery for full-term and low-birth-weight infants has changed greatly during the last century. In the 1880s, rooming-in (still the popular mode in Europe) was prevalent in American hospitals.

The mother was welcomed into the premature nurseries of the Frenchman Pierre Budin (the first modern neonatologist) and was allowed to assist in her infant's care, for as Budin recognized in his book, *The Nursling*,[7] published in 1907, "Unfortunately... a certain number of mothers abandon the babies whose needs they have not had to meet, and in whom they have lost all interest. The life of the little one has been saved, it is true, but at the cost of the mother." Mothers were therefore encouraged to breast feed their premature infants and were advised in addition to nurse full-term infants to increase their milk production.

Ironically, Budin's desire to publicize his methods resulted in the exclusion of the mother from the nursery. Martin Cooney, a young pupil of Budin's, went to the Berlin Exposition of 1896, where his "Kinderbrutanstalt" (child hatchery), to which premature infants were brought and raised, became both commercially and clinically successful. After exhibiting at fairs in England and the United States, Cooney settled on Coney Island, successfully raising more than 5000 prematures during the next four decades (Figure 7–1). Mothers were not permitted to participate in their infants' care at Cooney's exhibits, and it is of significance that on some occasions Cooney experienced difficulty in persuading parents to take their infants back. In spite of the commercial aspect of Cooney's example, the early hospital nurseries in the United States adopted many of his methods of newborn care.

The high rate of morbidity and mortality of hospitalized patients in the early 1900s led to the development of strict isolation for patients with a large number of diseases.

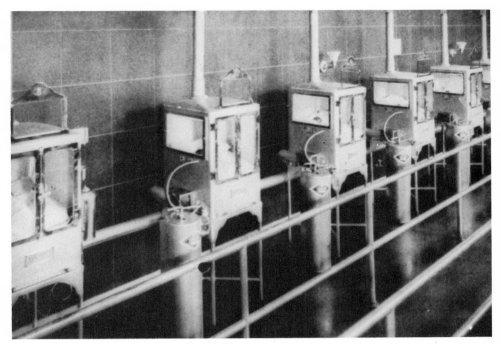

Figure 7–1 Dr. Martin Cooney's exhibit of premature infants at the Chicago World's Fair, 1933.[22]

Visitors were strongly discouraged. Unfortunately, Cooney's example and the measures introduced to prevent the spread of infection were thus combined to totally exclude the mother from hospital nurseries.

The Sarah Morris Hospital in Chicago developed the first hospital center for premature care in 1923. Following the precepts of Budin, the director, Hess, encouraged the production of breast milk at home and invited mothers' assistance in caring for the infants.

However, in premature units created after the Sarah Morris Center, a standard set of stringent regulations was followed, including only essential handling of the infants, a policy of strict isolation, and the total exclusion of visitors.

During the period after World War II, several innovative approaches to newborn care appeared. In a study of the home-nursing of prematures in Newcastle-on-Tyne, Miller[28] noted that the mortality rate was only slightly greater than that of a control group nursed in hospital. A shortage of skilled personnel was the impetus for an arrangement created by Kahn et al[17] at Baragwanath Hospital, Johannesburg, South Africa (Figure 7–2). Here mothers were able to participate in supervised care and feeding of their infants while themselves remaining in hospital. This innovation was accompanied by a sharp decline in infant mortality.

Although mothers are still not admitted into most premature nurseries, many centers have recently begun to permit them to do so.

THE HUMAN MOTHER

Since the human infant depends entirely upon his mother to satisfy all his needs, emotional as well as physical, his mother's attachment to him is absolutely necessary for his optimal growth and development. Just exactly how these affectional bonds are formed and what influences may distort them are therefore of major importance. The actual process of attachment or bond formation is not yet completely understood, but a wide diversity of observations are beginning to piece together some of the various phases. The time periods which are apparently crucial for this process are shown in Table 7–1.

PREGNANCY

Behavioral changes in the mother during this period have been described in detail.[2, 4]

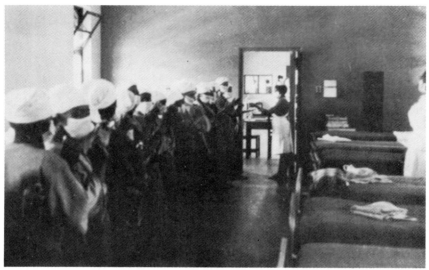

Figure 7–2   Mothers caring for their premature infants at Baragwanath Hospital.[19] (With thanks to Dr. John E. Bell, Palo Alto, California.)

Pregnancy for a woman has been considered as a process of maturation,[8] with a series of adaptive tasks, each dependent upon the successful completion of the preceding one. There are two general time periods during the pregnancy and another in the neonatal period during which a wide range of stressful factors may profoundly influence a woman's subsequent mothering behavior and ultimately the developmental outcome of her child.

Many mothers are initially disturbed by feelings of grief and anger when they become pregnant, because of factors ranging from economic and housing hardships to intrapersonal difficulties. However, by the end of the first trimester, the majority of women who initially rejected pregnancy have accepted it. This initial stage, as outlined by Bibring,[4] is the mother's identification of the growing fetus as an "integral part of herself."

The second stage is *a growing percep-* *tion of the fetus as a separate individual,* usually occurring with the awareness of fetal movement. After quickening, a woman will generally begin to have some fantasies about what the baby may be like, will attribute to him some human personality characteristics, and will develop a sense of attachment and value toward him. At this time, further acceptance of the pregnancy and marked changes in attitude toward the fetus may be observed; unplanned, unwanted infants may now seem more acceptable. Objectively, the health worker will usually find some outward evidence of the mother's preparation by such actions as the purchase of clothes or a crib, selecting a name, arranging space for the baby.

Cohen[9] suggests the following questions to learn the special needs of each mother:

1. How long have you lived in this immediate area and where does most of your family live?

2. How often do you see your mother or other close relatives?

3. Has anything happened to you in the past (or do you currently have any condition) which causes you to worry about the pregnancy or the baby?

4. What was your husband's reaction to your becoming pregnant?

5. What other responsibilities do you have outside the family?

It is important to inquire about how the pregnant woman herself was mothered—did

TABLE 7–1   STEPS IN ATTACHMENT[19]

Planning the pregnancy
Confirming the pregnancy
Accepting the pregnancy
Fetal movement
Accepting the fetus as an individual
Birth
Seeing the baby
Touching the baby
Caretaking

she have a neglected and deprived infancy and childhood or grow up with a warm and intact family life?

DELIVERY

Oddly enough, little data are available for this period. In agreement with veterinary experience, those mothers who remain relaxed in labor, who are supported and have good rapport with their attendants, are more apt to be pleased with their infants at first sight.[30] Unconsciousness during delivery does not seem to result in the rejection of the infant, as has been observed in some animals.

FIRST WEEK AFTER DELIVERY

The human mother after delivery appears to have a routine behavior pattern, as do other animal species. Filmed observations[24] show that a mother presented with her nude, full-term infant begins with fingertip touching of the infant's extremities and within a few minutes proceeds to massaging, encompassing palm contact of the infant's trunk. Mothers of premature infants also follow this sequence but proceed at a slower rate. We have observed that fathers go through some of the same routines. A strong interest in eye-to-eye contact was expressed by mothers of both full-term and premature infants

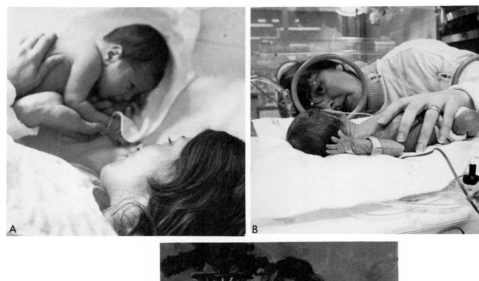

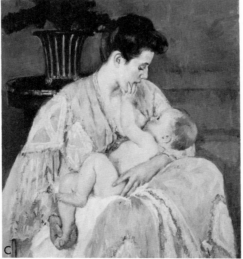

Figure 7–3 Mothers in the "en face" position. En face is defined as occurring when the mother's face is rotated such that her eyes and those of the infant meet fully in the same vertical plane of rotation.[19] *A.* A mother and her full-term infant. *B.* A mother and her premature infant. *C.* "Mother and Child," by Mary Cassatt. (Courtesy of the Art Institute of Chicago, Chicago, Illinois.)

(Figure 7–3 *A, B, and C*). It has been suggested that eye-to-eye contact appears to initiate or release maternal caretaking responses. Coinciding with the mother's interest in the infant's eyes is the early functional development of his visual pathways; the infant is alert, attentive, and able to follow during the first hour of life.

In the immediate newborn period, the maternal affectional ties which have formed during pregnancy may easily be disturbed and affected permanently[21, 32] by such minor problems as poor feeding, slight hyperbilirubinemia, and mild respiratory distress, even though the infant's problems are totally resolved before discharge.

The care of the mother at this early stage requires further study. When compulsory rooming-in was introduced at Duke University, the incidence of breast feeding increased (from 35 per cent to 58.5 per cent) and the number of anxious phone calls after discharge decreased 90 per cent. This suggests that close continual contact between mother and infant may indeed be an important factor in encouraging more relaxed maternal behavior.

Two long-term studies[2, 19, 24, 26] are underway to attempt to evaluate the results of the prolonged mother-infant separation which is a routine procedure in premature and high-risk nurseries. Shortly after birth, mothers in one group (Early Contact) are admitted into the nursery, permitted to touch their infants, and, as the infant's condition permits, perform simple caretaking duties. Another group of mothers (Late Contact) is not permitted into the nursery until after their infants reach 20 days of age. If enforced long-term separation does affect the strength of attachment, then the results of this separation might be reflected in altered maternal behavior. Results to date reveal detectable differences in mothering performance as late as six months after birth. No increase in infection or disruption of nursery procedure has been noted when parents are allowed to visit their infants in the nursery.

In another study, one group of mothers of full-term infants were given 16 additional hours with their infants during the first four days of life and compared with mothers who had routine contact with their infants (20 to 30 minutes at a feeding every four hours). Maternal behavior was measured one month later using a standardized interview, an examination of the baby, and a filmed bottle feeding.

Figure 7–4, with a posed mother, shows

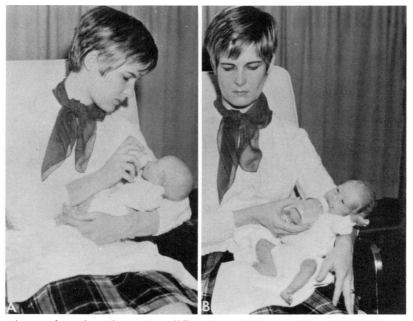

Figure 7–4 A posed mother shows two different caretaking positions.[22] *A*. Infant is held in close contact (cuddling); mother is looking at infant en face, and milk is in the tip of the nipple. *B*. Infant's trunk is held away from mother; mother is looking at infant but not en face, and there is no milk in the tip of the nipple.

TABLE 7–2 LEVELS OF INTERACTIONAL DEPRIVATION AND
COMPONENT VARIABLES[2]

LEVELS OF DEPRIVATION	DURATION OF DEPRIVATION	SENSORY MODALITIES OF INTERACTION	CARETAKING NATURE OF INTERACTION
No deprivation	Full time	All senses	Complete
Partial deprivation	Part time	All senses	Partial
Moderate deprivation	Part time	All senses	None
Severe deprivation	Part time	Visual only	None
Complete deprivation	None	None	None

an example of how the feeding films were scored. Note that on the right the mother's eyes are on the baby, but she is not in the en face position. On the left, the mother is in the en face position. Her abdomen is touching the infant's trunk, cuddling. The bottle is perpendicular to the baby's mouth and milk is in the tip of the nipple. On the right, the mother is holding the baby but not cuddling, the bottle is not perpendicular, and milk is not in the nipple.

These studies revealed that extended-contact mothers showed greater soothing behavior and engaged in significantly more eye-to-eye contact and fondling during feeding, were additionally more reluctant to leave their infants with someone else, and usually stood and watched during the examination (Figure 7–5 *A* and *B*). Interestingly enough, eleven months later the mothers were again significantly different during a physical examination. This simple modification of care shortly after delivery appeared to alter later

maternal behavior and is support for a sensitive period in the human mother. This is of additional significance when taken in light of several observations[33] which show that increased maternal attentiveness facilitates later exploratory behavior in infants. Thus, these differences in mothers may have a potent influence on the later development of their infants.

Once these and similar studies have been completed, the evidence may reveal that widespread alterations in hospital policies are required. There must be careful consideration of all the effects on the parents and babies before any changes are recommended. Most normal hospital deliveries result in several days during which the mother is deprived of many hours of contact with her healthy full-term infant; the mother of a premature must endure severe deprivation often until the 8th week of her baby's life. Using the levels of deprivation as categorized by Barnett[2] (Tables 7–2 and 7–3), it appears that

Table 7–3 DEPRIVATION LEVELS OVER TIME, RELATED TO BIRTH SITUATION[2]

BIRTH SITUATION	DEPRIVATION LEVEL. DAYS AND WEEKS POST PARTUM					
	Day 0	*Day 1*	*Day 3*	*Day 7*	*Week 8*	*Week 9*
Home, full term	Partial deprivation	No deprivation	No deprivation	No deprivation	No deprivation	No deprivation
Hospital, full term, rooming-in	Moderate deprivation	No deprivation	No deprivation	No deprivation	No deprivation	No deprivation
Hospital, full term, regular care	Moderate deprivation	Partial deprivation	Partial deprivation	No deprivation	No deprivation	No deprivation
Premature, mother allowed in nursery	Complete deprivation	Severe deprivation	Moderate deprivation	Partial deprivation	Partial deprivation (discharge nursery)	No deprivation
Premature regular care (separated)	Complete deprivation	Severe deprivation	Severe deprivation	Severe deprivation	Partial deprivation (discharge nursery)	No deprivation
Unwed mother, refuses contact	Complete deprivation	Complete deprivation	Complete deprivation	Complete deprivation	Complete deprivation	Complete deprivation

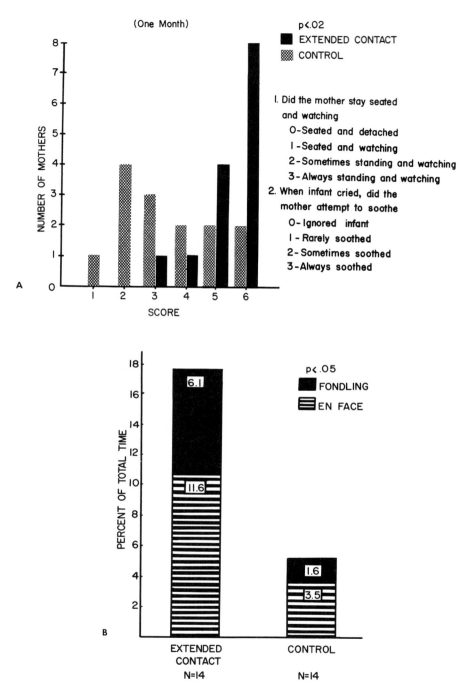

Figure 7–5 Summation of scores at one month.[23] *A.* Scores of performance from the observation of the mother during an office visit at one month post partum. *B.* Filmed feeding analysis at one month, showing percentage of "en face" and fondling times in mothers given extended contact with their infants and in the control group. (Fondling is defined as any spontaneous interaction initiated by the mother not associated with feeding, such as stroking, kissing, bouncing, or cuddling.)

only those mothers who room in or deliver at home have no period of deprivation.

The reactions of a mother to premature birth have been considered by some observers[18] as an acute emotional crisis. Four psychological tasks have been postulated, through which a mother must progress: (1) anticipatory grief, or preparing for the death of the infant, (2) the realization and acceptance of her failure to deliver an infant at term, (3) resumption of the process of relating to her infant, and (4) learning the special needs of a premature and how he differs from full-term infants. It is not known at present if these four tasks would remain the same if the mother were able to live in close contact with her infant.

A great multitude of factors influence a mother's ability to endure emotional stress, her need for solicitous care, and ultimately her maternal behavior. Some of these major influences and the resultant distortions which may occur are outlined in Figure 7–6. Some of these factors are already implanted and fixed at the time of delivery (e.g., how the mother herself was mothered as an infant, her cultural traditions, and her family relationships). Those influences which may be altered (indicated by dotted lines) include the physician's attitudes, policies, and statements; separation from the infant; and the infant himself, his personality as well as the state of his health. Obviously, one of the simplest variables to manipulate is whether or not a mother is separated from her infant after birth.

Also shown on this diagram are disorders or distortions of maternal behavior, which range from severe (the battered child syndrome) to mild (undue persistent concerns about a minor illness long since completely resolved). It is our contention that separation in the immediate newborn period may be a major component in these mothering disorders. Support for this hypothesis is the high number of premature infants who later return to the hospital with failure-to-thrive with no organic cause for the problem. Studies of failure-to-thrive infants have shown 15 to 30 per cent to have no organic disease; 25 to 41 per cent of this group were premature. Green and Solnit,[12] reporting on the vulnerable child syndrome (children whose parents expect them to die prematurely), noted that 44 per cent of these children were either born prematurely or were severely ill and separated from their mothers in the immediate newborn period.

In this country, adoptions generally take place when the infant is three to six weeks old. Perhaps if adoptions occurred at one day of life, the behavioral problems of the adopted child (which are far out of proportion to the incidence of adoption) would

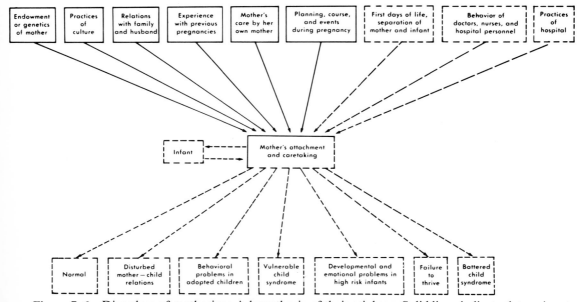

Figure 7–6 Disorders of mothering: A hypothesis of their etiology. Solid lines indicate determinants which are ingrained; dashed lines indicate factors which may be altered or changed.[22]

be decreased. In many societies, a substitute mother is ready at hand to take over when a mother dies at birth.

Probably the most dramatic manifestation of a mothering disorder is the battered child syndrome.[14] Unfortunately, authors reporting studies of the battered child usually fail to note whether or not the mothers and infants were separated following delivery. Combining two studies (totalling 44 patients) which did report birth weight or gestational age, 39 per cent of the patients were either premature or had suffered serious illness. The authors have recently learned of several cases in which battering occurred following the discharge of healthy normal prematures. These infants had been seriously ill after birth and separated from their parents for extended periods. Obviously, multiple influences are contributing to this problem, but one of the more significant factors may be separation. If prolonged separation occurs and anticipatory grief advances unduly, close affectional ties may never be securely established for the mother of a sick infant.

The relationship between prematurity, along with the question of prolonged separation of the mother from the child, and subsequent child battering has received considerable attention recently. In our own experience, we have found that the incidence of prematurity (with prolonged separation of the mother from the infant after birth) is three times as high among children who have subsequently been battered than among the general low-birth-weight incidence in the Province of Quebec. The difference is statistically highly significant and the contribution of this factor to what ultimately causes child battering should probably be taken into close consideration. It is understood that many other factors go into the ultimate relationship which results in this form of child abuse, but when viewed in this light, the early separation may play a crucial role in development of this disastrous situation.

L. STERN

It is of interest that study of behavior patterns in other cultures indicates that every society has some standard method of introducing a new member. In most cases, the mother and infant remain together, apart from other members, during the period required for the navel to heal. The mother has few if any responsibilities at this time apart from caring for her infant. There is no cultural practice except in the premature and high-risk nurseries of the Western world which routinely and completely separates a mother from her infant during the first days after birth.

ANIMAL STUDIES

As in other areas of neonatology, it has been useful to study mothers and infants of many species during the neonatal period. Although certain aspects of behavior differ from species to species, there are some overall patterns and trends which can be discerned. Despite the reluctance of many investigators to accept the concept that these patterns may apply to humans, the possibility of their extension to the human should not be neglected when they are found in a large number of species.

First, in goats, sheep, and cattle, when a mother is separated from her young in the first hour or the first few hours after delivery and then the two are reunited, the mother will show disturbances of mothering behavior, such as failure to care for her young, butting her own offspring away, and feeding her own and other babies indiscriminately.[15, 25, 29] In contrast, if the mother and infant are kept together for the first four days and are separated on the fifth day for an equal period of time, the mother quickly returns to the maternal behavior characteristic of her species when the pair is reunited. It thus appears that there is a sensitive period immediately after delivery; if the animal mother is separated from her young during this interval, deviant maternal behavior may result. (It is important to note that not all mothers are equally affected by these early separations and that the disturbed mothering performance can be modified by special handling.) Surprisingly, in spite of this sensitive period, adoptions can be arranged. Sheep and goats can be induced to adopt strange lambs and kids—between as well as within species.[16] This requires delicate arrangements to prevent the mother from destroying the strange infant. The effects of early separation vary with the species. Harlow studied rhesus monkey mothers deprived of tactile contact but allowed to see and hear their infants.[13] After two weeks without any tactile contact, these mothers rapidly decreased the amount of time they spent viewing their infants. This indicated that viewing alone is not enough stimulus to maintain maternal interest.

Secondly, clear-cut, species-specific maternal behavior patterns, such as nesting, retrieving, grooming, and exploring, have been observed in nonhuman mammalian mothers immediately after delivery. For example, in the cat during labor and just before delivery, the mother licks the genital region; then, following delivery, the mother licks the kitten completely, eats the membranes and placenta, and remains in close, almost constant physical contact through the first three to four days. This perinatal behavior may be severely distorted if the mother herself has received abnormal care as an infant,[5, 13] or if the normal sequence of behavior is altered, as shown in Birch's experiments with rats. Noting the increased amount of self-licking (especially in the anogenital region) in the pregnant rat and hypothesizing that this self-licking might extend to the pups after delivery, Birch fashioned high collars which were placed on the necks of pregnant rats to prevent self-licking.[5] The collars were removed shortly before birth. These rats subsequently exhibited abnormal maternal behavior, such as waiting a long interval before initial licking of the pups, consuming them once licking began, and in the instance of pups surviving the licking period, refusing to allow them to suckle. No offspring survived the nursing period. Control mothers and mothers wearing collars similar to those described but notched to permit self-licking did not exhibit this aberrant behavior.

Thirdly, for some period after delivery, usually weeks or even months, animal mothers have characteristic patterns and orders of behavior. For example, the rhesus monkey mother grooms her infant more at one month than at other times. At five months she spends little time retrieving, whereas at 1½ months retrieving is maximum.[13] Recurring patterns of maternal behavior within a species can be distinguished in a large number of animal species. Careful observations in Uganda suggest that repeating sequences are also found in human mothers.[1]

PRACTICAL CONSIDERATIONS FOR CARE OF THE HIGH-RISK MOTHER

We have found it useful to pick out in advance the mother who is most likely to have special difficulties in relating to her infant. Blau[6] noted that mothers who deliver premature infants have more negative attitudes toward their pregnancies, greater emotional immaturity, and more body narcissism. In our own experience, mothers who have a high incidence of severe mothering difficulties often have one of the following characteristics: (1) the previous loss of a newborn infant, including miscarriage and induced abortion; (2) a fertility problem, with no living children; (3) a previous seriously ill newborn infant; (4) primiparity if younger than 17 or older than 38 years; (5) a medical problem with which the infant may be affected, such as Rh disease, toxemia, or diabetes; and (6) the unmarried mother. Certain principles of management for obstetricians and pediatricians apply to all these situations.

1. In almost all high-risk situations, the odds are heavily in favor of the birth of a live baby who will ultimately be healthy and normal, so it is reasonable to *stress the positive and be optimistic.* This is essential for the mother's later relationship with her baby, which is in turn extremely important for his development. After a physician reads the literature or a physician's report about a woman's new or rare condition, it is tempting to tell her about the problems and pitfalls that may develop. But this will only make the course of the pregnancy more turbulent for the mother and also for the obstetrician. Mentioning the possibility of a symptom or complication is comparable to the young boy just starting to ride a two-wheeler who knows that there is one big tree in the middle of the playground.

2. The obstetrician should bring in the pediatrician early and continue to involve him in decisions and plans for the management of the mother and baby.

3. Prepare the mother for the anticipated aspects of care for her newborn. (See Case Two.)

4. Communicate with the mother about her condition and about the baby's condition. This is important before, during, and after the birth of the baby. At times, this will be brief and incomplete, but communication is essential. For example, when there is evidence of fetal distress, the mother can be told, "We have evidence that your baby should be delivered quickly, so we are proceeding with this, and we will need your full cooperation." Another example: when a baby shows stress or fails to breathe after birth, the obstetrician can say, "The baby has a problem. We will be working with the baby and will let you know more about this just as soon as we can."

Clinically, we have been impressed and disturbed by the devastating and lasting untoward effects on the mothering capacity of women who have been frightened by the physician's pessimistic outlook about the chance of survival and normal development of an infant. For example, when the newborn infant is a three-pound premature baby who is doing well, but the mother is told by a physician that there is a reasonable chance that the baby may not survive, the mother will often show evidence of mourning (as if the baby were already dead) and reluctance to "become attached" to her baby. We have repeatedly observed that such mothers may refuse to visit or will show great hesitation about any physical contact. When discussing such a situation with a physician who has spoken pessimistically with the mother, we have often been told that it is important to share all worries with a mother so that she will be prepared in case of a bad outcome. If there is a close and firm bond between the mother and infant (which occurs after an infant has been home for several months) there is no reason for the physician to withhold his concern. However, while the bonds of affection are still forming, they can be easily retarded, altered, or permanently damaged. It is not easy to keep from sharing all the problems with a mother, but with the evidence available at present, it is our conviction that both the obstetrician and the pediatrician should do their best to hold back. This does not mean that they should be untruthful, because parents will quickly sense the physician's true feelings. They must base their statements on today's situation (infant mortality rates in low-birth-weight nurseries have decreased steadily year by year), not on yesterday's high mortality figures of the period during which they were being trained. Today the vast majority of these infants will live.

During the past several years, we have made many changes in the physical arrangements for mothers and our approach to them. We find it best to describe what the infant looks like to us and how the infant will appear physically to the mother. We do not talk about chances or survival rates or percentages, but stress that most babies survive in spite of early and often worrisome problems. We do not emphasize problems which may occur in the future. We do try to anticipate common developments (e.g., the need for bilirubin reduction lights for jaundice in small premature infants). The following guidelines may be helpful:

1. A mother's room arrangements should be adjusted to her needs. Mothers are often best able to express themselves and work out their problems when they are alone.

2. If at all possible, mother and infant should be kept near each other in the same hospital, ideally on the same floor.

3. It is useful to talk with the mother and father together whenever possible. When this is not possible, it is often wise to talk with one parent on the phone in the presence of the other.

4. At least once a day we discuss how the child is doing with the parents; we talk with them at least twice a day if the child is critically ill.

5. It is necessary to find out what the mother believes is going to happen or what she has read about the problem. We move at her pace during any discussion.

6. The physician should not relieve his anxiety by adding his worries to those of the parents. If there is a possibility, for example, that the child has Turner's syndrome, it is not necessary to share this with the parents while the infant is still acutely ill with other problems and while affectional bonds are still weak. If the physician is worried about a slightly high bilirubin, it is not necessary to discuss kernicterus. Once mentioned, the possibility of death or brain damage can never be completely erased.

7. Before the mother comes to the neonatal unit, the physician should describe in detail what the baby and the equipment will look like.

8. The nurse should go into detail in describing all the equipment surrounding the infant. She should be nearby so that she may answer questions and give support during the difficult period when the mother is first seeing her infant.

9. When a mother and father come to see their infant who is under bilirubin lights, it is important to remove the eye patches so that they can see his eyes.

10. Extended visiting for the mother of a normal full-term infant when the mother is able to handle and completely care for her infant from 1 PM to 7 PM has been a useful practice.

11. The nursery should keep a record of of all phone calls and visits by parents. Our data reveal that when there are fewer than three phone calls or visits in a two-week period, there is a high incidence of subsequent severe mothering disorders.[11]

12. The nurses should feel at ease in reporting any worries or problems they have about a father and mother's behavior. To

accomplish this, there must be a good working relationship between the physician and nurses. Meetings with the nursery staff in the intensive care unit should be held every two weeks. This provides an opportunity for them to express their concerns and problems.

13. It may be possible to enhance normal attachment behavior in the human mother several days or weeks following birth by permitting a special short nesting period of close physical contact with privacy and virtual isolation during which the mother provides complete care for her small infant with help and nursing support readily available nearby. If the safety and feasibility of early discharge of premature infants, as reported by Berg in feasibility studies, is fully confirmed, we hypothesize that early discharge combined with a period of isolated physical contact with caretaking may help to normalize mothering behavior for the infants discharged from intensive care nurseries.

STILLBIRTH OR DEATH OF A NEWBORN

In spite of the advances in obstetrical and neonatal care, many mothers encounter a great disappointment with an early abortion or the perinatal loss of an infant. Until recently, it was not appreciated that a mourning reaction in both parents after the death of a newborn is universal. Whether the baby lives one hour or two weeks, whether the baby is a nonviable 500 gm. or weighs 4000 gm., whether or not the baby was planned, and whether or not the mother has had physical contact with her baby, clearly identifiable mourning will be present. Mothers and fathers who have lost a tiny newborn show the same mourning reactions as have been reported by Lindemann[27] studying the survivors of the Coconut Grove fire, or by C. M. Parkes[31] in his studies of individuals in England grieving the loss of a close adult friend or relative. Parkes reports that:

At first the full reaction may be delayed or there may be a period of numbness or blunting in which the bereaved person acts as if nothing had happened for a few hours or days up to two weeks. Thereafter attacks of yearning and distress with autonomic disturbances begin. These occur in waves and are aggravated by reminders of the deceased. Between attacks the bereaved person is depressed and apathetic with a sense of futility. Associated symptoms are insomnia, anorexia, restlessness, irritabiltiy with occasional outbursts of anger directed against others or the self, and preoccupation with thoughts of the deceased. The dead person is commonly thought to be present, and there is a tendency to think of him as if he was still alive and to idealize his memory. The intensity of these features begins to decline after one to six weeks, and is minimal by six months.

Lindemann has concluded that normal grief is a definite syndrome. It includes:

1. Somatic distress with tightness of the throat, choking, shortness of breath, need for sighing, and an empty feeling in the abdomen, lack of muscular power, and an intense subjective distress described as tension or mental pain.
2. Preoccupation with the image of the deceased.
3. Feelings of guilt and preoccupation with one's negligence or minor omissions.
4. Feelings of hostility towards others.
5. Breakdown of normal patterns of conduct.

This syndrome may appear immediately after a death, or may be delayed or apparently absent. Those who have studied mourning responses have indicated that a painful period of grieving is a normal and necessary response to the loss of a loved one, and the absence of a period of grieving is not a healthy sign but rather a cause for alarm.

With recent long-term studies focusing our attention on the family after a death, a tragic outcome for the mother has been shown in one-third of the perinatal deaths. Cullberg[10] found that 19 of 56 mothers studied one to two years after the deaths of their neonates had developed severe psychiatric disease (psychosis, anxiety attacks, phobias, obsessive thoughts, and deep depressions). Because of the disastrous outcome in such a high proportion of mothers, it is necessary to examine in detail how to care for the family following a neonatal death.

In the observations of parents who have lost newborns, the disturbance of communication between the parents has been a particularly troublesome problem. A husband and wife who have communicated well before the birth of a baby often have such strong feelings after an infant's death that they are unable to share their thoughts and therefore have an unsatisfactory resolution of their grieving. In America, it is expected that husbands will be strong and not show their feelings, so a physician should encourage a husband and wife to talk together about the loss and advise them not to hold back their responses. "Cry if you feel like crying." Unless told what to expect, their reactions may worry and perplex them and this may tend to further disturb the pre-existing husband and wife relationship.

At the time of the baby's death, it is important to tell the parents *together* about the usual reactions to the loss of a child and the length of time these last. It is desirable to meet a second time with both parents prior to discharge, to go over the same suggestions which may not have been heard or may have been misunderstood under the emotional shock of the baby's death. The pediatrician should plan to meet with the parents together again three or four months after the death to check on the parents' activities and how the mourning process is proceeding. At the same time, he can discuss the autopsy findings and any further questions presented by the parents. At this visit the pediatrician should be alert for abnormal grief reactions which, if present, may guide the physician to refer the parents for psychiatric assistance. Lindemann believes that pathologic mourning reactions represent distortions of normal grief. On the basis of his observations, he lists nine such reactions:

1) overactivity without a sense of loss; 2) acquisition of symptoms belonging to the last illness of the deceased; 3) psychosomatic reactions such as ulcerative colitis, asthma, or rheumatoid arthritis; 4) alterations in relation to friends and relatives; 5) furious hostility against specific persons; 6) repression of hostility, leading to a wooden and formal manner resembling schizophrenic pictures; 7) lasting loss of patterns of social interaction; 8) activities detrimental to one's own social and economic existence; and 9) agitated depressions.

CASE PROBLEMS

The clinical relevance of this subject can best be appreciated by the following case examples and the questions they raise. The words chosen in any discussion are dependent upon the needs and problems of individual patients at that moment. We have not given our answers as a specific formula but rather so that the reader may have an idea of how we approach parents.

Case One

Mrs. H. was happily married, had had a previous miscarriage, and had planned on having a baby for the past three years. She delivered a 3 lb. 2 oz. male infant following a normal pregnancy. The infant cried immediately but then developed moderate respiratory distress, requiring arterial catheterization and a plastic hood over his head for administration of oxygen. At 36 hours of age, in an environment of 70 per cent oxygen, the pH was 7.31; $PaCO_2$, 60 mm. Hg; and PaO_2, 73 mm. Hg.

The following questions must be answered when caring for this mother-infant dyad:

Should the mother be permitted to go into the nursery?

The mother should be permitted to enter the nursery if she wants to. With current therapy, the outlook for this baby is good. There is no evidence that the mother will have an unduly upsetting reaction if he does die; on the contrary, having already had a miscarriage, she will probably be relieved to see for herself that the baby is well formed.

Should she be in a separate room on the maternity division?

The mother should be alone in a separate room on the maternity division if she so desires, and as far away as possible from the sights and sounds of normal babies and more fortunate mothers whose healthy infants *come to them* every four hours.

What is the best method of communicating with both parents?

The best method of communicating with both parents is to have both sitting down together with you in a quiet, private room. You will be most effective if you can listen to the parents. Let them express their worries and feelings, then give simple, realistically optimistic explanations.

How should advice be given when first discussing the situation with the parents? What should they be told about their infant and his chances for survival?

When first discussing the situation with the parents, advice should be given promptly, simply, and optimistically. As soon as possible after the birth, the mother can be told that the baby is small but well formed, that you will be doing routine tests and giving the usual treatment for a premature infant, and that you will report back to her when you have had time to complete more tests and observations.

When it is clear that the baby has respiratory distress and arterial catheterization is necessary, you can explain to the mother that the child has a common problem of premature infants ("breathing difficulty") owing to the complex adjustments he must make from life in utero to life outside. Furthermore, it should be stated that because it is common you know how best to treat it; that this treatment will involve putting a tube in the blood vessel through which she fed the baby while he was inside her; that you will use this tube to obtain tiny amounts of blood on frequent occasions to guide your therapy; that the baby will be transferred to a nursery for small babies; that, prior to his transfer, her husband can see the baby and the baby will be brought to her in a special transport incubator for her to see; that babies sometimes get worse before they improve, but the outlook is good for complete recovery after several days; that you will keep her and her husband posted on the baby's progress and will tell them if problems arise; that you would like them to call at other times if they have questions; and that you would like her to come to the nursery to visit and see the baby.

At 36 hours, you have a firmer basis for an optimistic report, which should be kept simple but should include an explanation of the hood, apnea monitor, and other visible aspects of therapy. You might say, for example, "I'm pleased with your son's progress. He has responded well to our treatment, and his outlook is excellent. If you haven't been over to see him yet, I'd like to encourage you to do this today, because you will be pleased with his progress."

Can the nurses help the mother adapt to the premature infant?

The nurses can help the mother adapt to the premature infant by standing close to the mother and explaining about the equipment being used for him; by welcoming the mother by name and with personalized comments at each visit, and encouraging her to come back soon; by carefully considering the mother's concerns and feelings; by explaining to her that the baby will benefit from her visits; and by showing her how she can gradually assume more of the baby's care and do the mothering better than the nurses. An example of the nurses' encouragement to moth-

ers to continue visits later on in the patient's course is the type of note our nurses put on a baby's crib: "My mother is coming to feed me at 1:30. Boy! Will I be happy to see her!—David."

Should the mother go home before the respiratory distress syndrome has subsided?

If the mother is confident that the infant will live, she should go home before the respiratory distress has subsided. Staying in a maternity unit and only visiting her baby one or two times a day is not tolerated very long by many mothers unless they can actively care for their babies or provide breast milk. It is particularly difficult for a woman if she has young children at home. Most mothers can return daily from home to visit the baby.

If she lives far away, is unlikely to return for many days, and is greatly concerned the baby will die, the mother should not go home before the respiratory distress syndrome has subsided. It is best to reach a point where both you and the mother are confident about the baby's survival.

If the infant survives, what problems will the mother face and how can she be helped?

When the infant survives, this mother may have withdrawn some of her attachment to the baby through anticipatory grief, in spite of all the steps that have been recommended. Under the best of circumstances she will have had much less contact with her baby than a normal mother. Therefore, affectional bonds will not be as well developed as with a healthy full-term infant and she will have done relatively little caretaking. The continuation of support to the mother, so that she will visit, touch, and provide increasing care for the baby (holding, feeding, bathing, and diapering), is important during the hospital period. Detailed preparation for the care of the baby at home, the availability of support by telephone during the hospital stay, and continuing support after the baby returns home are indicated, especially during the first months at home. Through the early years of the infant's life, the pediatrician should be alert to evidence that the baby is being handled differently than other children (delay in weaning, overprotection, excessive permissiveness, or excessively regimented management). A discussion at this time with the mother about her early experiences, and her feelings and worries about the baby may be advisable. When specific questions have been answered, it may be best, if appropriate, to reassure the mother that the baby's early problems are over and will not recur, that the baby was small in the beginning but is now normal in size and development, and that for his ultimate well-being he should be handled as normally as possible.

Case Two

Mrs. J., a 22-year-old primiparous mother, delivered a full-term infant after a 12-hour uneventful labor. The infant was found to have a cleft lip and palate. The following questions should be answered in the care of this infant and mother:

Should the father be told about this before the mother has returned to her room?

Every effort should be made to tell the mother and father together about this problem. This is such an obvious defect that the father will notice it. If this is the case, the doctor should indicate that there is a problem, but that he wants to check the baby over thoroughly and he will then tell both parents about the problem and what will be done about it. It is popularly believed that the father is in much better condition to learn about difficulties right after delivery than his wife, but often a woman is able to accept news about an illness or abnormality in her baby better—in an emotional sense—than her husband. Any plan to tell one bit of news or a different shading about the prognosis to one parent and not the other interferes with the communication between husband and wife which is extremely important to support and and encourage.

When should the mother see the infant?

The infant should be brought to the mother as soon as she and the infant are in satisfactory condition and after the caring physician (obstetrician or pediatrician) has the details of the baby's problem clearly in mind and is aware of the baby's health status. It is important for the baby to be brought to the mother's bed. A cleft lip is such an obvious defect that the mother's attention will tend to be riveted to the face. With calm and positive statements about the ease and near perfection of the correction, the physician can move part of the mother's and father's attention to the many normal and healthy aspects of the infant. It is worthwhile to repeat and emphasize the general good health and well-being of the baby. In situations where the cleft lip and palate are part of a series of severe developmental abnormalities, the approach would of course be different.

Who should tell the mother: the obstetrician, the pediatrician, the nurse, or the father?

The obstetrician, whom the mother has known for many months, is usually the best person to tell the mother. He needs information from a pediatrician about the nature of the problem and the general health of the baby. Equally satisfactory is for the obstetrician and pediatrician to go together to tell the parents about the problem. If the obstetrician can speak briefly and calmly to the mother and place his mantle of acceptability upon the pediatrician's shoulders, then the pediatrician can continue with a brief explanation about the problem. Under most circumstances, neither the nurse nor the father will be in a position to provide enough reassurance to the mother to make this first encounter progress optimally.

How should the problem be presented to the mother?

It is desirable whenever possible to emphasize to the mother the normal healthy features of the baby. For example, "Mrs. Jones, you have a strong eight-pound baby boy who is kicking, screaming, carrying out all the normal functions of a healthy baby. There is one problem present which we fortunately will be able to correct so it will not be a continuing problem for the baby. As far as I can tell, the baby is completely well otherwise. I would like to show the baby and this problem to you."

Should the baby be present?

Yes. As ugly as a cleft lip and palate may appear to a mother (it never seems as grotesque to a physician who has seen the results of surgical repairs), exposure to the reality of the problem is important and is usually less disturbing than the mother's fantasies.

Should emphasis be limited to the lip?

No.

What are the normal processes that will ensue with this mother and father? Can these be modified?

It can be anticipated that the parents will focus their attention rather rigidly upon this defect, and that it will be difficult to encourage them to consider the other normal aspects of the baby. This can be enhanced by bringing the baby to the mother frequently so that she will become accustomed to the defect and gradually see more and more of the strong, normal characteristics of the baby.

As reported by Green and Solnit,[12] following the birth of a defective baby, the mother goes through a period of mourning for the loss of the perfect infant she has been expecting, and also has the difficulties of adjusting to an unusual or malformed infant. There are, with a cleft lip, additional problems of breathing and feeding that can add to the parents' concern. The period of mourning and grief is prolonged. It probably should not be suppressed and it cannot be compressed. This should be kept in mind by the attending health professionals in the ensuing months.

The reactions of mourning should be anticipated: somatic distress, intense subjective distress, preoccupation with the image of the infant, feelings of hostility, a breakdown of normal patterns of conduct, and possibly a strong and usually irrational guilt about any of the series of events that either occurred or were in the minds of the parents before or during the pregnancy. These will interfere with the parents' ability to accept fully the baby with the abnormality. A physician has to anticipate that the shock of this information will often deafen parents to what he is trying to present; therefore, he should plan to go over these items two or three times more during the hospital stay and at the first checkup of the mother. Several unhurried meetings with both parents, listening to their many questions and problems, will be most helpful.

Parental mourning responses are quite varied. For example, there may be a paternal response of intense activity—running about town, taking on extra jobs. The mother may withdraw into an apparent need to sleep for excessively long periods day and night. It will be the obstetrician's aim not to let this withdrawal occur, by encouraging longer visits between mother and baby. His further objective is to encourage the parents to talk to each other about how they feel about the problem.

What are the common reactions of physicians when anomalies are found in their patients?

Telling parents and patients about a problem is distasteful, but an integral part of a physician's responsibility. The reaction to his unfavorable report may remind him of the Greek messenger who was killed for bringing bad news to a community. It is also a common reaction for a physician to feel guilty himself about not producing a normal baby for the parents. He too can imagine that the medications he provided and permissions he gave to the parents to carry out certain activities may have had something to do with the development of the abnormality. He may feel that he can be of no help to this mother, while actually it is with this mother and infant that he can be most helpful, by appreciating her feelings and realizing his own reactions to the situation. His feelings of guilt will often make him wish to spare the parents' feelings, and the strong reactions of all concerned with the care of the mother and baby may interfere with the usual practices which are beneficial to a normal mother and infant and may be of particular importance in such a situation. For example, the usual routine of bringing the mother and baby together soon after birth and bringing the baby for regular feedings may be delayed for hours and days because of the concern of nurses and other hospital personnel about the reaction of the mother to the infant.

There is a strong tendency on the part of the house staff, attending physicians, and nurses in a maternity hospital to remove evidence of illness and failure on the part of the medical staff as soon as possible, and to transfer the baby to a facility concerned with the care of more serious diseases. Such a transfer is often made soon after birth, before the mother has had an opportunity to begin to strengthen her affectional bonds with her infant, even though the transfer to the other hospital may not really be indicated for a week or two. (For example, surgery on a lip is usually not undertaken until the baby is two weeks of age; for the palate, another year will pass.)

Case Three

Mrs. B., a 23-year-old primiparous woman, has had diabetes for 12 years. She has come to the pediatrician in the eighth month of pregnancy because a prenatal visit to the pediatrician was recommended by her obstetrician.

What items may be covered in this prenatal interview?

In the prenatal interview, it is desirable to obtain information about the backgrounds of both parents, their fears and concerns, and for the obstetrician and pediatrician to maintain as optimistic an attitude as possible. Because it is recognized that the mother's relationship with her infant will be influenced by her acceptance of the pregnancy and her appreciation of the infant within her, starting with the onset of quickening, it is important to ask how the pregnancy has been going. A helpful way to get acquainted with the parents is to obtain a thorough family history. This can be done quickly and may bring up problems that are of more concern to the parents than the effects of the diabetes. It is particularly helpful to review the health history, educational background, job experiences, and marital experiences of the parents. The pediatrician may uncover a previous illegitimate pregnancy or some other unexpected bit of information that may strongly color the mother's course during labor, delivery, and later care of her child.

With what needs, possible worries, or preparatory information should the physician be concerned?

In assessing how the mother has progressed in her acceptance of her expected infant, it is desirable to ask questions about preparations for the new baby—whether a room has been chosen, or a crib and baby-care items purchased. It is helpful to inquire what worries or concerns the mother has had. The physician can anticipate that she not only will have the wide range of questions raised by healthy women but also will have picked up a number of concerns about the effects of diabetes from reading or conversation. The wise physician will ask what she has heard and read about the course of an infant of a diabetic mother. (This holds true for any problem.) The importance of finding out what the patient has heard and just where she is in her understanding of the condition cannot be overemphasized.

As a general principle, it is valuable for the physician to prepare the mother for the events that are almost certain to occur, but to present this information in a positive manner. For example, "Mrs. B., we know from experience with many mothers with diabetes that your chances of having a normal, healthy baby are excellent, but we also know that your baby may have some temporary problems adjusting to life outside of you that will be helped by early detection and prompt treatment with the highly effective methods we now have. For example, your baby has been living in a rather unusual blood sugar environment inside of you, so we will check your baby's blood sugar, and will probably give intravenous sugar and fluid through a tube placed in one of the blood vessels through which you are feeding the baby at the present time. Your baby will be a bit premature, so we will do certain things that help premature babies. For example, your baby will be placed in a warm incubator so the metabolism of your baby will be optimal. If a breathing problem is present, we may decide it will be best for the baby to go to a part of the hospital that is set up for the management of breathing problems in babies. You will be able to visit the baby and see and feed him just as soon as you are able. If your delivery is by cesarean section, your baby will probably be in excellent health before you are, so you will be able to bring your baby back to live-in with you in your hospital room. Because of the baby's early birth, we know there will be an increased chance that the baby will develop some yellowness or jaundice. This is not a sign of disease, but another problem of adjustment to life outside. Your body has eliminated this yellow pigment for your baby during pregnancy. Once the baby is born there may be a lag in his ability to take care of this. We will keep track of the amount of yellowness by blood tests and will put the baby under some special fluorescent lights to manage this if jaundice does appear. You can be sure we will not allow the yellowness to become great enough to make the baby sick. Lastly, you can be sure your baby will not be born with diabetes."

The mother asks, "What's my chance of having a normal baby?" How should this question be answered?

"The chances of your having a normal baby are all with you. Of course, no mother can be absolutely guaranteed that her baby will be normal, but the overwhelming preponderance of babies are normal and healthy."

She asks, "Do all such babies have lung and breathing problems?" What should the physician say?

Before answering, one must find out what lies behind her question. Then, if appropriate, one may say, "By no means do all the babies of mothers with diabetes have lung and breathing problems. Unfortunately we cannot predict for you whether this will be present or not. That is why we will pay close attention to your baby from birth on, to be sure that we pick up and start treatment early for any lung problem that is present."

Case Four

The first infant of a 29-year-old mother weighed 2 lbs. 8 oz. at birth. The baby is now four days of age and is taking 6 ml. of formula every two hours.

What are the normal processes that a mother goes through when she delivers an infant this size, and how should the physician and nursing staff meet these requirements during the first four days?

When a mother delivers an infant prematurely, this means that she has been short-changed on many days or weeks of physical and mental preparation for the baby. The premature delivery often occurs before a mother is thoroughly ready to accept the idea that she is going to have an infant. Such a mother is also faced, like the mother with a malformed infant, with a baby who is thin, scrawny, and very different from the ideal, full-sized baby she has been picturing in her mind. She may have to grieve the loss of this anticipated ideal baby as she adjusts to the reality of this premature baby with all of its problems.

In most hospitals, the mother has only a fleeting glimpse of the baby who is then whisked away from her. If she has not seen the baby or has only viewed him briefly through a window, she may be picturing an infant who is fragile and much scrawnier than is actually the case. All of the equipment and activities of a premature nursery are new and may be frightening to a mother. The tubes, the flashing lights, the beepers, and other instruments used in a premature nursery are disturbing. If the functions of these items are explained to the mother, her concern will decrease. For example: "The two wires on the baby's chest and the beeping instrument tell us if the baby slows down in his respirations so we can rub his skin to remind him to keep breathing. This is frequently necessary during the first few days with a tiny infant."

There are some additional problems with a premature infant. Frequently, a mother is not able to see her infant the first day or two and other members of her family may see and even touch and hold the infant. This is often quite upsetting to a new mother, to think that others are getting an opportunity to become acquainted and enjoy the baby while she, the one who produced the infant, has been kept away. If there is a critical period for the human—and there is increasing evidence to support this—it may be important for the mother and infant to be together as much as possible in the early days. Frequently, the mother's guilt and anxiety, and the fear that touching the infant will harm it, will lead her to turn down an offer to go visit the infant. No mother should be forced to visit her infant against her wishes, but it is important for the hospital personnel to reassure her and encourage her visits. Move at the mother's pace.

It is sometimes noted that a mother wishes to avoid touching and holding her small infant because "she does not want to become attached because it would be so painful for her if the baby should die." We should consider this type of reasoning carefully. It is clear from studies[21] that mothers are already attached to their infants at the moment of birth, so mourning will be intense whether the mother visits or not. There is also evidence that it is not emotionally harmful to a mother (if she desires) to have contact with an infant who subsequently dies, although she should never be forced or pushed to touch her infant. But most important of all is the fact that the majority of babies of this weight will live, so it is extremely important for the mother and infant to be together and near each other as early as possible during the first days of life in order to develop mother-infant bonds which will sustain the mother in the days, weeks, and years ahead. If this baby is taking 6 ml. of formula every 2 hours, it is evident that this baby is in good condition and has an excellent chance for survival.

What should the mother be told when she asks, "How is the baby doing?"

It is a common reflex in physicians and nurses to prepare patients for a possible poor outcome and to think in a problem-oriented manner. Because of the great importance of providing encouragement to the mother so that mother-infant affectional bonds develop as optimally as possible, it is desirable to approach this question in an optimistic but realistic manner. For example: "Very well! We are using lights to help with the baby's yellowness, and we still have the infant on a respiration monitor which lets us keep track of the baby's respirations, but the baby is doing beautifully. We are fully confident that he will continue to improve and grow and gain. The baby is taking feedings nicely." It is often wise to start out by asking the mother how *she* thinks the baby is doing and then you know where to begin.

What arrangements should be made to keep the mother informed about the baby?

When a baby is in the excellent condition of this baby, a physician should communicate with the mother about the progress at least once a day. When the condition is more hazardous, more frequent contacts are indicated, such as morning and evening. The mother should have access to information about the baby by calling the nursery and talking to the nurses.

Should the nurses and nonprimary physicians talk with the parents?

Of course the nurses and nonprimary physicians should answer questions when asked by the parents. It is highly desirable for all who are concerned with the care of the baby to understand the general trend of the information that is being supplied to the parents. This can best be carried out if one individual takes this responsibility. The nonprimary physician and nurses can provide the parents with additional items without getting into questions of prognosis. These can usually be tactfully referred to the responsible physician. It is tempting for all physicians to show the wide range of their knowledge, but it is harmful for the parents to know that respiratory distress and its therapy can have a wide variety of unsatisfactory complications or outcomes.

What should the physician who is covering for the primary physician say?

Whenever possible, the covering physician should find out what the primary physi-cian has been saying to the family, and attempt to follow along in the same vein. There is no harm at all in his emphasizing the features that indicate improvement and a favorable outcome. Whenever possible he should avoid statements that indicate differences in approach to the prognosis or management of the patient. All who are speaking to the parents should be certain to communicate before and after conversations with the parents so that a consistent picture is presented to them. Ideally, the Weed system of problem-oriented records and problem lists should be used to record on the chart what has been discussed with the parents, so that anyone covering for another physician can immediately know just where the family is in their understanding.

When should the mother take this baby home if the baby is eating well and gaining well at 4 lbs. 4 oz.? Should there be a fixed weight at which the infant should be discharged? What factors determine the decision about the timing of discharge?

In the past, we have looked at the infant's weight, physical characteristics, and the presence of a clean bed at home. We must also look at the mother's ability to care for the infant in the hospital and her readiness and willingness to take the infant home. Her visiting pattern in the hospital and the preparations made at home have been helpful in making this decision. Preliminary observations with mothers living-in with their four-pound premature infants for three days suggest that this may be an ideal procedure to prepare mothers for routine caretaking.

If the infant has good heat control without an incubator, nipples easily, and is gaining weight, and the mother has experience in caretaking, and the home is free of infection, early discharge may be beneficial.

It is our practice never to use the infant's weight as a particular criterion of the time at which he can be discharged home. Once the baby is able to maintain his own body temperature without the application of external heat (i.e., he can come out of the incubator) and is capable of feeding on the bottle q. 4h., he is, in our view, ready for discharge. If the mother does not have other children at home and can manage, the infant will be discharged even if he is only on three-hourly feedings; however, should there be other children in the home, we feel it unmanageable for a mother to have to feed an infant every three hours and will, therefore, wait until a four-hourly feeding pattern has been established. There is no particular magic or advantage in an infant's weight, and as a criterion for discharge from hospital, it ought to be abandoned.

L. STERN

Case Five

A 2½ lb. infant of a 23-year-old primiparous mother who has been married for three years died suddenly on the second day of life. The infant was planned. The mother did not handle the infant.

What are the processes this mother and father will go through?

The parents in this situation will go through the same intense mourning reactions which have been described in the text and in Case Two. If the parents can cry together, they themselves can best help each other. The use of tranquilizers, except for a night's sleep, is therefore not indicated. Even though the mother did not handle the infant, she and her husband will be expected to show strong mourning responses which will be intense for two or three weeks and under optimal circumstances will be nearly resolved by six months. In America, where the expression of emotion is not encouraged, the husband will often force himself to hold back on emotions to provide a "strong support" for his wife. This is actually harmful because a free and easy communication between the parents about their feelings is highly desirable for the resolution of mourning. On the basis of the studies that have been carried out, the stronger the mourning reaction in the early period, the more favorable the outcome.

How can the physician help them?

It is important for the physician to explain about the details of the baby's death to both parents together within a few hours after the death of the baby. At that time, he should explain to the parents the type of mourning reaction they will go through. Then as a minimum, the physician should again meet with the parents three to four days later to go over the details once more and indicate his availability for any questions or problems. At the postpartum checkup, the obstetrician should take time to ask how the parents are managing and should evaluate the normality of their mourning and their communication. If there are other children in the family, the pediatrician should inquire about their responses. Three or four months after the death of the baby, the physician should set aside a period of time to meet with both parents to review their present status, what has occurred since the death, their understanding of the death, and the normality of their reactions. If the mourning response is pathologic, he may then refer the parents for additional assistance.

This short list of guidelines may incorrectly convey the impression of a mechanical quality of these discussions which is not at all the authors' intent. Parents appreciate evidence of human concern and reactions in a physician at times such as these, so we would encourage physicians to show the sadness they feel and to allow the parents to express their pent-up feelings by a statement such as: "I know how sad and upset you both must feel."

UNKNOWNS

The studies of maternal behavior in animals, a survey of maternal practices in other cultures, and preliminary observations in human mothers after periods of early separation from their infants force a thorough review and evaluation of our present perinatal care practices. Before any major changes should be made, the following unknowns must be answered:

1. Is there a critical or sensitive period in the human mother as there is in the animal mother?

2. What are the needs of most mothers with normal full-term infants in the first hours after delivery and during the first week?

3. Has the hospital culture, which has taken over both birth and death, produced disorders of mothering which last a lifetime?

4. Are the diseases of failure-to-thrive, the battered child syndrome, and the vulnerable child syndrome in part related to hospital care practices?

5. How should the minor problems, as well as the major problems, with which the infant is born or develops be handled with mothers of different backgrounds, cultures, and requirements?

6. Should the adopting mother receive her infant in the first hour of life? Are the problems of the adopted child a result of adoption practices and early separation? What are the needs of the biological mother who gives the baby up for adoption?

Changes in medical practices during the past 50 years have remarkably altered maternal care practices that have evolved over centuries.

Detailed observations of a wide range of mammalian mothers and babies have shown that each species exhibits recurring sequences of maternal behavior around the time of delivery and during the first days and months of life. Interference with these behavioral patterns may result in undesirable, even catastrophic, effects on the young. The knowledge that there is a sensitive period shortly after birth during which brief periods of partial or complete separation may drastically distort a mother animal's feeding and care of her infant would lead a caretaker or naturalist to be extremely cautious about any intervention in the period after birth.

Observations in human mothers suggest that affectional bonds are forming before delivery, but that they are fragile and may easily be altered in the first days of life. A preliminary inspection of fragments of available data suggests that maternal behavior may be altered in some women by a period of separation, just as infant behavior is affected by isolation from the mother.

REFERENCES

1. Ainsworth, M.: *Infancy in Uganda.* Baltimore, The Johns Hopkins Press, 1967.
2. Barnett, C., Leiderman, P., Grobstein, R., et al: Neonatal separation: the maternal side of interactional deprivation. Pediatrics 45:197, 1970.
3. Benedek, T.: *Studies in Psychosomatic Medicine: the Psycho-Sexual Function in Women.* New York, Ronald Press Co., 1952.
4. Bibring, G.: Some considerations of the psychological processes in pregnancy. Psychoanal Stud Child 14:113, 1959.
5. Birch, H.: Sources of order in the maternal behavior of animals. Amer J Orthopsychiat 26:279, 1956.
6. Blau, A., Slaff, B., Easton, K., et al: The psychogenic etiology of premature birth: a preliminary report. Psychosom Med 25:201, 1963.
7. Budin, P.: *The Nursling.* London, Caxton Publishing Co., 1907.
8. Caplan, G.: *Emotional Implications of Pregnancy and Influences on Family Relationships in the Healthy Child.* Cambridge, Harvard University Press, 1960.
9. Cohen, R.: Some maladaptive syndromes of pregnancy and the puerperium. Obstet Gynec 27:562, 1966.
10. Cullberg, J.: Mental reactions of women to perinatal death. *In* Morris, N., Ed.: *Psychosomatic Medicine in Obstetrics and Gynaecology.* New York, S. Karger, 1972.
11. Fanaroff, A., Kennell, J., and Klaus, M.: Follow-up of low-birth-weight infants—the predictive value of maternal visiting patterns. Pediatrics 49:287, 1972.
12. Green, M., and Solnit, A.: Reactions to the threat-

ened loss of a child: a vulnerable child syndrome. Pediatrics 34:58, 1964.
13. Harlow, H., Harlow, M., and Hansen, E.: The maternal affectional system of rhesus monkeys. *In* Rheingold, H., Ed.: *Maternal Behavior in Mammals.* New York, John Wiley and Sons, 1963.
14. Helfer, R., and Kempe, C., Eds.: *The Battered Child.* Chicago, University of Chicago Press, 1968.
15. Hersher, L., Richmond, J., and Moore, A.: Maternal behavior in sheep and goats. *In* Rheingold, H., Ed.: *Maternal Behavior in Mammals.* New York, John Wiley and Sons, 1963.
16. Hersher, L., Richmond, J., and Moore, A.: Modifiability of the critical period for the development of maternal behavior in sheep and goats. Behavior 20:311, 1963.
17. Kahn, E., Wayburne, S., and Fouche, M.: The Baragwanath premature baby unit—an analysis of the case records of 1,000 consecutive admissions. South African Med J 28:453, 1954.
18. Kaplan, D., and Mason, E.: Maternal reactions to premature birth viewed as an acute emotional disorder. Amer J Orthopsychiat 30:539, 1960.
19. Kennell, J., and Klaus, M.: Care of the mother of the high-risk infant. Clin Obstet Gynec 14:926, 1971.
20. Kennell, J., and Rolnik, A.: Discussing problems in newborn babies with their parents. Pediatrics 26:832, 1960.
21. Kennell, J., Slyter, H., and Klaus, M.: The mourning response of parents to the death of a newborn. New Eng J Med 283:344, 1970.
22. Klaus, M., and Kennell, J.: Mothers separated from their newborn infants. Pediat Clin N Amer 17:1015, 1970.
23. Klaus, M., Jerauld, R., Kreger, N., et al: Maternal attachment: Importance of the first post-partum days. New Eng J Med 286:460, 1972.
24. Klaus, M., Kennell, J., Plumb, N., et al: Human maternal behavior at the first contact with her young. Pediatrics 46:187, 1970.
25. Klopfer, P., Adams, D., and Klopfer, M.: Maternal "imprinting" in goats. Proc Nat Acad Sci USA 52:911, 1964.
26. Leifer, A., Leiderman, P., Barnett, C., et al.: Effects of mother-infant separation on maternal attachment behavior. Child Develop 43:1203, 1972.
27. Lindemann, E.: Symptomatology and management of acute grief. Amer J Psychiat 101:141, 1944.
28. Miller, F.: Home nursing of premature babies in Newcastle-on-Tyne. Lancet 2:703, 1948.
29. Moore, A.: Effects of modified care in the sheep and goat. *In* Newton, G., and Levine, S., Eds.: *Early Experience and Behavior.* Springfield, Charles C Thomas, 1968, pp. 481–529.
30. Newton, N., and Newton, M.: Mothers' reactions to their newborn babies. JAMA 181:206, 1962.
31. Parkes, C.: Bereavement and mental illness. Part I. A clinical study of the grief of bereaved psychiatric patients. Brit Med J Psychol 38:1, 1965.
32. Rose, J., Boggs, T., Jr., Alderstein, A., et al: The evidence for a syndrome of "mothering disability" consequent to threats to the survival of neonates: a design for hypothesis testing including prevention in a prospective study. Amer J Dis Child 100:776, 1960.
33. Rubenstein, J.: Maternal attentiveness and subsequent exploratory behavior in the infant. Child Develop 38:1089, 1967.

Chapter 8

RESPIRATORY PROBLEMS

by

MARSHALL KLAUS, M.D.

and

AVROY FANAROFF, M.B. (Rand.), M.R.C.P.E.

> *"I observed that a few days after their admission infants frequently had attacks of cyanosis. They suddenly became blue.... If assistance was not immediately rendered, they died. If, however, energetic measures were promptly taken, they usually revived, although many succumbed to subsequent attacks."*
>
> PIERRE BUDIN, *The Nursling*

The physician working in the intensive care nursery will spend the lion's share of his time caring for neonates with respiratory problems, diseases which are responsible for most of the morbidity and mortality in this period. Considering the complexity of the pulmonary and hemodynamic changes occurring after delivery, it is surprising that the vast majority of infants make the transition from intrauterine to extrauterine life so smoothly and uneventfully.

NORMAL PHYSIOLOGY

Before birth, the lung is a fluid-filled organ receiving 10 to 15 per cent of the total cardiac output. Within the first minutes of life, a large portion of the fluid is absorbed, the lung fills with air, and the blood flow through the lung increases 8- to 10-fold. This considerable increase is secondary to a decrease in pulmonary arterial tone and other physiologic changes converting the circulation from a parallel arrangement to a series circuit (Figure 8–1).

The high vascular resistance in the fetal lung is due to pulmonary arterial vasocon-striction. The pulmonary arterial vasodilation observed following delivery results in part from the increased oxygen tension, the decrease in CO_2 tension and change in pH, and only partially from the mechanical effect of the inflation.[17] Certain chemical substances, such as bradykinin, may be involved.

At the same time, an adequate functional residual capacity (FRC= volume of air in the lungs at end-expiration) is quickly attained. At 10 minutes, the FRC is the same as that found at five days. At one hour, the distribution of air with each breath in the newborn is already similar to that observed in the young adult. Specific lung compliance (lung distensibility/lung volume expressed in ml. of air per cm. of H_2O pressure change per ml. of lung volume) and vital capacity increase briskly in the first hours of life, reaching values proportional to the adult at 8 to 12 hours.

Chemical control of respiration is in general similar in the newborn infant and the adult. As the inspired CO_2 is increased, the per cent increase in ventilation is similar in the infant and adult. The ventilation of the newborn is also altered when breathing mixtures contain less than 20 per cent oxygen;

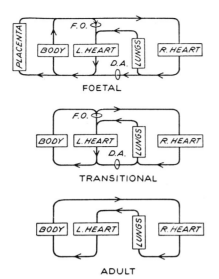

Figure 8-1 Diagrams of the fetal, transitional (neonatal), and adult types of circulation.[17]

this response as well as other evidence suggests[17] that the aortic and carotid body chemoreceptors are active at birth. If hypoxia is severe, however, respiration is depressed. Marked hypoxia depresses the medullary respiratory center and negates the hypoxic stimulation of the aortic and carotid body chemoreceptors. The response of the infant to inflation of the lung is different from the adult. In the first day or two of life, the typical response to an inflation of the lung with a pressure of 10 to 15 cm. of water is a deep gasp (Head paradoxical gasp reflex—a pressure change from 20 to 40 cm. H_2O) and a very prolonged apnea (Hering and Breuer inflation reflex). By the third and fourth day, greater pressure is required to produce the deep gasp and apnea, and a large number of infants no longer gasp. The deep gasp observed in the first day of life with low inflation pressures may explain the clinical observation that very low pressures (10 to 15 cm. H_2O) are often effective in resuscitating the apneic newborn at birth. The low pressure applied does not inflate the lung but stimulates the gasp reflex, which markedly reduces intrathoracic pressure, resulting in lung inflation.

Arterial blood gases reflect the pulmonary, cardiac, and metabolic status of the newborn. They may also give some clues as to whether the infant suffered any asphyxial episode before delivery. The partial pressure of carbon dioxide (pCO_2) measures the ability

of the lung to remove CO_2. The HCO_3 concentration is controlled by the kidney. When the pH and HCO_3 are determined, the arterial pCO_2 can be calculated by using the Henderson-Hasselbach equation:

$$pH = 6.1 + \log \frac{HCO_3}{pCO_2 \times sol.}$$

If only the pH is measured, the cause of the acidosis or alkalosis cannot be determined. With metabolic acidosis, HCO_3 is decreased. To compensate for this, the infant hyperventilates, lowering arterial pCO_2. With pulmonary disease, apnea, or hypoventilation. the arterial pCO_2 increases. The kidney attempts compensation by retaining HCO_3 and excreting hydrogen ions. Only by measuring the pCO_2 and HCO_3, as well as the pH, can the cause of an abnormality in acid-base balance be determined. The normal newborn quickly regulates his pH to near adult values. The low arterial pCO_2 of the newborn infant during the first week of life is similar to the maternal values in the last months of pregnancy.

PHYSIOLOGIC BASIS

Oxygen is carried in the blood in chemical combination with hemoglobin and also in physical solution. The oxygen taken up by both processes is dependent on the partial pressure of oxygen (pO_2).

At ambient pressures, the amount of dissolved oxygen is only a small fraction of the total quantity carried in whole blood. Most of the oxygen in whole blood is bound to hemoglobin (1 gm. of hemoglobin combines with 1.34 ml. of oxygen). The quantity of oxygen bound to hemoglobin is dependent upon the partial pressure and is described by the oxygen dissociation curve (Figure 8-2). The blood is almost completely saturated* at an arterial oxygen tension (PaO_2) of 90 to 100 mm. Hg. The dissociation curve of fetal blood

---

*The arterial oxygen saturation is the actual oxygen bound to hemoglobin divided by the capacity of hemoglobin for binding oxygen. % Saturation =

$$\frac{ml.\ O_2\ combined\ with\ Hb}{maximal\ amount\ of\ O_2\ combined\ with\ Hg}$$

1.0 gm. of hemoglobin can maximally bind 1.34 ml. of O_2.

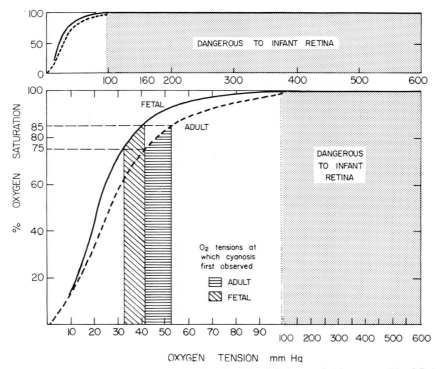

Figure 8–2   Oxygen dissociation curves of fetal and adult hemoglobins at a pH of 7.4, temperature 37° C. Cyanosis is observed at a saturation between 75 and 85 per cent, which corresponds to different arterial tensions in the adult and the infant.

is shifted to the left and at any PaO$_2$ below 100 mm. Hg binds more oxygen. The shift is the result of the lower content of diphosphoglycerate. Although this is an advantage, there is also the disadvantage that, at any partial pressure, less oxygen is given up to the tissues. The shift makes clinical recognition of hypoxia (insufficient amount of oxygen molecules in the tissues to cover the normal aerobic metabolism) more difficult, since cyanosis will be observed at a lower oxygen tension. Cyanosis is first observed by physicians at saturations from 75 to 85 per cent, which are oxygen tensions of 32 to 42 mm. Hg on the fetal dissociation curve. Cyanosis in the adult is observed at higher tensions. The flattening of the upper portion of the S-shaped dissociation curve makes it almost impossible to monitor oxygen tensions above 60 to 80 mm. Hg by following arterial oxygen saturation. The partial pressures of oxygen in various regions of the body while breathing room air are shown in Table 8–1. Note that the total pressure of gases in the tissue capillary is less than the atmospheric pressure.

The partial pressure of oxygen in arterial blood not only is dependent on the ability of the lung to transfer oxygen but also is modified by shunting of venous blood into the systemic circulation through the heart or lungs. Breathing 100 per cent oxygen for a prolonged time will correct desaturation secondary to both diffusion abnormalities and inadequate ventilation. Measurements of arterial PaO$_2$ while breathing 100 per cent oxygen are therefore useful diagnostically in determining whether arterial desaturation is caused by a right-to-left shunt, diffusion abnormalities, or inadequate ventilation. If no right-to-left shunt is present, the arterial PaO$_2$ after breathing 100 per cent oxygen is equal to the atmospheric pressure minus the partial pressures of alveolar carbon dioxide and water vapor. The right-to-left shunt of venous blood when breathing 100 per cent oxygen can then be calculated using the shunt equation:

$$\frac{\dot{Q}s}{\dot{Q}} = \frac{CaO_2 - C\dot{c}O_2}{C\dot{v}O_2 - C\dot{c}O_2}$$

where $\dot{Q}s$ is equal to the amount of cardiac output shunted from the right to left, $\dot{Q}$ is

TABLE 8-1   PARTIAL PRESSURES OF GASES IN THE ALVEOLAR AIR, ARTERIAL BLOOD, AND TISSUE CAPILLARY BLOOD IN THE NORMAL INFANT[30]

	Inspired Gas	Alveolar Gas	Arterial Blood	Capillary Blood Bathing Tissues
BREATHING ROOM AIR				
P_{O_2} mm. Hg	160	100	90	40
P_{CO_2} mm. Hg	0	40	40	50
P_{N_2} mm. Hg	600	573	573	573
P_{H_2O} mm. Hg	0	47	47	47
Total pressure mm. Hg	760	760	750	710
BREATHING 100% OXYGEN				
P_{O_2} mm. Hg	760	673	440	58
P_{CO_2} mm. Hg	0	40	40	50
P_{N_2} mm. Hg	0	0	0	0
P_{H_2O} mm. Hg	0	47	47	47
Total pressure mm. Hg	760	760	527	155

equal to the total cardiac output, CaO_2 to the arterial oxygen content, $C\dot{v}O_2$ to the mixed venous oxygen content, and $C\dot{c}O_2$ to the end pulmonary capillary oxygen content.

Immediately after birth, PaO_2 rises rapidly to between 60 and 90 mm. Hg. During the first days of life, 20 per cent of the cardiac output is shunted from right to left. It is not known whether this shunt is in the heart or lungs. When the normal adult breathes 100 per cent oxygen, PaO_2 rises to around 600 mm. Hg. The shunt from right to left is therefore about five per cent of the total cardiac output.

Figure 8–3 is a graphic representation of the shunt equation for the specified conditions. Assuming no change in oxygen consumption, cardiac output, arterial-venous oxygen differences, or right-to-left shunt with change in ambient oxygen, an estimate of the arterial oxygen tensions breathing 40 per cent and 70 per cent oxygen has been calculated. When the arterial oxygen tension breathing 100 per cent oxygen is known, the right-to-left shunt can be estimated. It can be seen that, when the right-to-left shunt is greater than 50 per cent, increasing the ambient oxygen concentration will not elevate the PaO_2 above 67 mm. Hg. Use of this graph also permits a rough estimation of what might result if the environmental oxygen is lowered. In very sick infants with the respiratory distress syndrome, the right-to-left shunt often increases when the ambient oxygen is decreased. Therefore, the actual PaO_2 will be lower than predicted from this graph.

Table 8–1 also lists the partial pressures of carbon dioxide, oxygen, nitrogen and water vapor in the normal infant after 10 minutes of breathing 100 per cent oxygen. Note the low

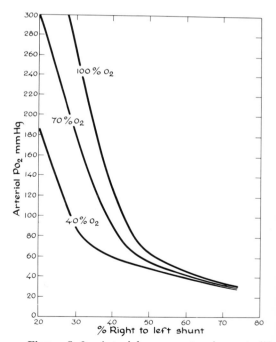

Figure 8–3   Arterial oxygen tensions at different right-to-left shunts, breathing 40 per cent, 70 per cent, and 100 per cent oxygen. Calculations assumed hemoglobin 16 g. per 100 ml., arterial pH 7.4, temperature 37° C, constant arterial-venous saturation difference 13.8 per cent, and no change in cardiac output or oxygen consumption.[29]

total pressure in the tissue capillaries when breathing 100 per cent oxygen. The large drop in oxygen tension occurs because only a small amount of dissolved oxygen is lost from the blood when the oxygen tension is decreased from 400 to 100 mm. Hg (0.003 ml. O_2/mm. Hg $\times$ 300 mm. Hg = 0.9 ml. of oxygen), but even at rest, 3 to 4 ml. of oxygen are removed from each 100 ml. of arterial blood perfusing the tissues. The arterial oxygen tension will then drop from about 400 mm. Hg to 30 to 50 mm. Hg in the tissue capillaries if the infant is breathing 100 per cent oxygen and the total pressure is reduced to 155 mm. Hg. This drop in pressure can be used therapeutically to remove gas from body cavities (gastrointestinal tract, cerebral ventricles, or the pleural cavity), as illustrated in Figure 8–4. The pressure difference is increased sixfold with 100 per cent oxygen breathing, as is the rate of absorption.

At the end of the first hour of life, perfusion of the lung is distributed in proportion to the distribution of ventilation.[3] The effects of this rapid adaptation on the blood gases are illustrated in Figure 8–5, which shows the mean arterial pH, PaO_2, $PaCO_2$, and bicarbonate in normal infants during the early hours and days of life. The speed with which pulmonary ventilation and perfusion are uniformly distributed is an indication of the remarkable adaptive capacities of the newborn infant for the maintenance of homeostasis. With this background, it is now possible to describe how disease alters function.

Present study and care of the distressed infant has in general been limited to the time following delivery. Although this discussion will center on care of the newborn, it is our belief that in the near future a major focus of study and therapy will be directed to the fetus (e.g., in some centers in Sweden and Denmark, prevention of hyperglycemia in diabetic mothers during the last ten weeks of pregnancy has been shown to reduce severly infant mortality and morbidity[34]).

PRACTICAL CONSIDERATIONS

The modern treatment required by the sick premature and full-term infant can only be administered by pooling the resources of many present-day delivery units. The treatment discussed in this section requires not only some special equipment but also more importantly, skilled nurses, a laboratory equipped for 24-hour blood gases (including PaO_2), and a physician who is readily available to the unit 24 hours a day. (The facilities and personnel are described in the 1971 edition of the Academy's "Hospital Care of Newborn Infants.") To make these facilities available financially to the largest number of infants, realistically there can only be five to six units in any large metropolitan area. We strongly urge that the present trend toward reducing the number of small delivery services be continued, and we should work toward developing perinatal centers containing a

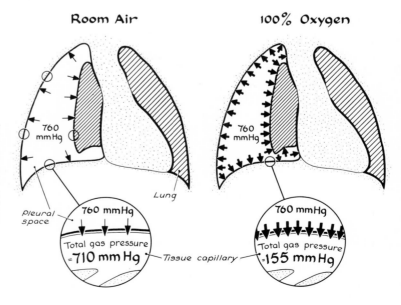

Figure 8–4 Absorption of a pneumothorax breathing air and 100 per cent oxygen. The total gas pressure in the tissue capillary is markedly reduced when breathing 100 per cent oxygen, increasing the rate of absorption.[29] (See also Table 8–1.)

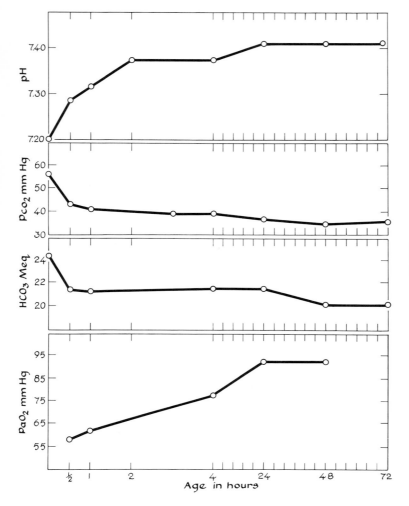

Figure 8–5 The arterial pCO_2, HCO_3, pH and pO_2 during the first hours and days of life.[29]

large delivery service (4000 to 6000) in conjunction with a neonatal intensive care nursery. In this type of unit, fetal and amniotic fluid monitoring, and prompt metabolic and ventilatory resuscitation would be economically feasible. It is with this perspective in mind for the near future that we discuss the care of the infant with respiratory distress.

Diagnosis

Even while administering emergency therapy, the initial objective is to establish an etiologic diagnosis for the respiratory symptoms. A major error in care can easily be made if other organ systems are not considered initially. *Not every cyanotic, rapidly breathing infant has hyaline membrane disease.* Hypovolemia, hypoglycemia, congenital heart dis-

ease, cerebral hemorrhage, or even the effect of drugs may all mimic primary respiratory disorders. Appropriate care depends on the diagnosis.

A working classification of some of these disorders is presented in Figure 8–6. Whenever faced with these respiratory symptoms, the next steps (following a history and physical examination) should be to obtain:

1. X-ray of chest (plate under mattress).

2. Intravascular hematocrit (peripheral hematocrits can be 25 per cent higher than intravascular hematocrits. All hematocrits should be central.)

3. Blood sugar (Dextrostix).

In our hands, the use of Dextrostix is unreliable in both directions. Hyperglycemia cannot be detected, and although it is argued that one can detect levels below 45 mg. per 100 ml. by the intelligent use of the

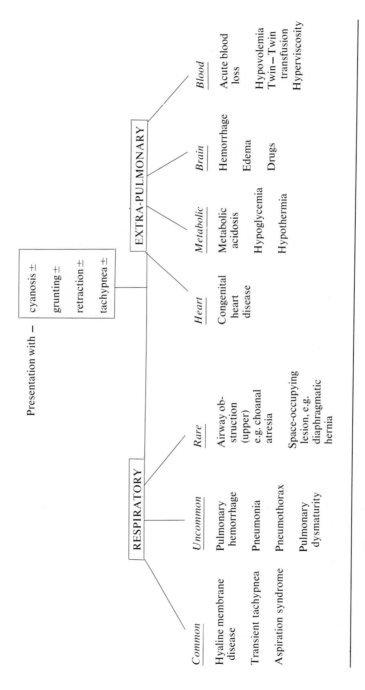

Figure 8-6 Differential diagnosis of respiratory distress in the newborn period.

Dextrostix, for us this has often proved erroneous owing to the variability not only of the batches of the dextrostix, but their tendency to degenerate in effectiveness with time of storage. They should be utilized perhaps as an emergency method only, but it is always our policy to follow them immediately with a blood glucose determination, the results of which can be available within 30 minutes at the most.

L. STERN

Editor's Comment: See Chapter 10.

In many cases, blood gases will also be required, necessitating arterial catheterization. The decision to catheterize the umbilical artery depends on the infant's condition. We catheterize the umbilical artery and vein during the first 15 minutes of life if metabolic resuscitation is required (as indicated in Chapter 1), or if the infant remains severely distressed (as defined by continued hypoxemia with or without hypotonia, and severe respiratory efforts). On the other hand, if the infant has tachypnea and grunting with retractions but is active, pink, and weighs over 2000 gm., we catheterize only if there is deterioration or if the expiratory grunting continues for longer than 45 to 60 minutes of life. (We base this on our experience and on the data of Rudolph, Desmond, and Pineda,[43] who closely observed 549 immature infants immediately after delivery. They found a high incidence of continuing respiratory disease if grunting continued after one hour of life.

At the time of arterial catheterization, a central blood pressure should be measured to check for acute blood loss. Although the newborn has a relatively larger cardiac output and a lower peripheral resistance and blood pressure than the older child and adult, measurements of blood pressure in this low-resistance circuit have been useful in diagnosing a large blood loss. (In the low-resistance circuit of the newborn kitten, the blood volume must be reduced by 40 per cent before blood pressure is observed to fall.) Hypothermia or acidemia result in severe peripheral vasoconstriction and will confound blood volume estimates from measurement of blood pressure. (In a hypovolemic infant, blood pressure often drops only when acidemia and hypoxemia are corrected.) The mean blood pressure can be measured with a strain gauge as shown in Figure 8–7. Normal mean blood pressures and ranges are found in Figure 8–8. If the initial hematocrit is below 35 or if blood pressure is reduced, we immediately start to correct the blood volume loss. We initially use saline or albumen and rush to obtain blood, doing only a major crossmatch, hopefully giving the blood within 30 minutes or earlier. We start with an infusion of 10 ml. per Kg. observing blood pressure, heart rate, and the infant's general condition.

We measure the blood pressure of infants with RDS by a noninvasive technique using the Doppler devised by Hoffman LaRoche called a premature Sonatone. This can be easily performed on a leg or arm.

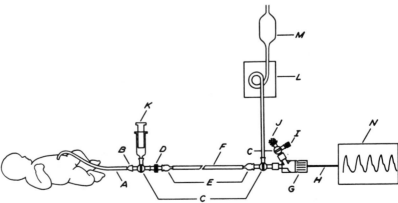

Figure 8–7 System for direct measurement of aortic pressure in newborn infants.[28] A = no. 5 Fr umbilical artery catheter with single end hole (Argyl) from which the wide proximal end has been cut off to reduce dead space. B = disposable Luer stub adaptor, 18-gauge (Intramedic). C = disposable three-way stopcocks (Pharmaseal). D = Luer double male adaptor (B-D). E = 18-gauge blunt needles. F = no. 190 polyethylene tubing, 24 inches long (PE-190). G = pressure transducer (Statham P23D series). H = cable from G to N. I = metal plug adaptor (B-D). J = sterile gauze over opening on three-way stopcock. This is opened to air (after closing system off to infant) in order to obtain a zero pressure base line for the recording system. K = syringe for flushing system. L = infusion pump. M = parenteral fluid for eight-hour period. N = electronic recorder (Model 7 Polygraph).

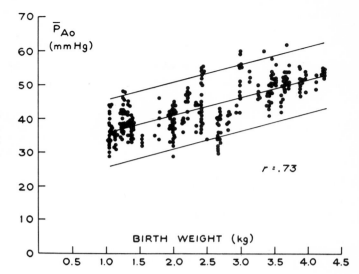

Figure 8–8 Linear regression and 95 per cent confidence limits of mean aortic blood pressure on birth weight in normal newborn infants during hours 2 to 12 of life (n = 300).[28]

We also use arterialized capillary blood from the right hand, sampling over the lateral surfaces of the fingers, particularly to obtain PaO_2. Since this blood is preductal, it will be independent of the degree of shunt through the ductus and reflects much more closely the oxygen content going to the cerebrum, whereas the sample obtained from an umbilical artery may have a significantly lower PaO_2 owing to a right-to-left shunt through the ductus. If pH is low and particularly bicarbonate, we use this as an indication of poor tissue perfusion and acutely infuse through the umbilical vein 10 to 20 cc. per Kg. of plasmanate to produce an acute expansion in blood volume and also to raise arterial pressure, which may then decrease the right-to-left shunt through the ductus, improving peripheral pulmonic perfusion. We are very impressed by the possibilities of accidents occurring on the arterial side associated with umbilical artery catheters, secondary to injection of hypertonic solutions. These produce localized hyperviscosity of the blood that will tend to produce a necrotizing medullary necrosis of the kidney or necrotizing enteritis of the gut. We have been particularly impressed by the high incidence of positive cultures of catheter tips when removed. Our limited experience with a strain gauge indicates the dynamics decrease after about four hours of catheterization owing to thrombi in the line and the necessity to calibrate the strain gauge with a mercury manometer, which introduces a contamination into the catheter line itself. We attempt to maintain the blood pressure above 45 mm. Hg.

G. ODELL

Estimating the Prognosis

Once the diagnosis has been made, it is necessary to determine if the neonatal unit has all of the facilities that might be needed during the course of the illness.

The ability to calculate the course of the respiratory disease not only satisfies our instinct for gambling, but permits the physician to determine which infant will require special respiratory therapy and must, therefore, be transferred. Several scoring systems have been adapted for infants ill with hyaline membrane disease using arterial PaO_2 breathing 100 per cent oxygen, lactic acid, pH, Apgar, and X-ray findings.[7, 45] Most useful has been PaO_2. A low PaO_2 while breathing 100 per cent oxygen usually means severe disease (Table 8–2). As others have noted, mean arterial blood pressure is also a useful indicator of prognosis (Table 8–3). If the chance of the infant surviving is less than 60 per cent using any of the scoring systems, we recommend transfer to a special center where all facilities are available while the infant is in reasonable physical condition. The use of these indicators will aid in selecting who requires care at a special respiratory center and hasten transfer before the infant is damaged or moribund.

In the following section, hyaline membrane disease (HMD) will be discussed in great depth, because not only has this problem been the primary focus of research in neonatal respiration, but also the principles of care involving approaches to management, equipment and procedures can be easily applied to other pulmonary disorders. Other neonatal pulmonary problems will be discussed later in this chapter.

TABLE 8-2   PROGNOSIS IN THE RESPIRATORY DISTRESS SYNDROME BASED ON
THE ARTERIAL OXYGEN TENSION[+]

AUTHORS	PaO_2 mm. Hg	AGE AT SAMPLING (HRS)	THERAPY[*] BEFORE SAMPLE	#	SURVIVORS	PER CENT SURVIVAL
Boston, R.W., et al.	>100 <100	1–10	variable	35 16	25 3	71 19
Stahlman, M.T., et al.	>100	<12	none	86	74	86
Roberton, N.R.C., et al.	>100 <100	....	yes	127 76	97 24	76 32
Prod'hom, L.S., et al.	<100 <50	1–92	yes	11 6	3 0	27 0
Stern, L.	<50	....	yes	60	3	5
Swyer, P.R.	<50	....	yes	16	1	6

[+]While the infant is breathing 90 to 100 per cent oxygen.
[*]Therapy is defined as the use of sodium bicarbonate, blood, or high concentration of environmental oxygen.

HYALINE MEMBRANE DISEASE (RESPIRATORY DISTRESS SYNDROME — RDS)

Hyaline membrane disease (HMD) is the most common problem in the nursery and the major cause of mortality, occurring in 0.5 to 1.0 per cent of all deliveries. The disease is observed in roughly 10 per cent of all premature infants with the greatest incidence in those weighing between 1000 and 1500 gm.

There exists a large group of infants difficult to classify who have respiratory distress from 1 to 24 hours of life. Respiratory distress is here defined as respiratory rate >60, some grunting, retractions, flaring, and cyanosis in room air. Systematical X-rays are not con-

tributory to diagnosis. There are no abnormal right-to-left shunts in these infants. In my opinion, the problem in these babies is related to delayed clearing of the alveoli of fluid, or mild aspiration with abnormal ventilation perfusion ratios. This probably makes up the largest group of respiratory problems seen in the delivery room, making the obstetrician believe HMD is an insignificant problem.

We followed 1203 consecutive deliveries in our hospital. One hundred and sixteen showed signs of respiratory distress in the first four hours of life. Table 8–4 shows distribution of diagnosis in these infants. Some physicians might classify a majority of these infants under the category of transient tachypnea. The knowledge that this group exists must be taken into account when evaluating therapy for HMD. Any babies of this group which are included will improve your results.

S. PROD'HOM

TABLE 8-3   THE PREDICTIVE VALUE OF MEAN SYSTEMIC ARTERIAL PRESSURE
IN THE FIRST 12 HOURS OF LIFE[*]

		PER CENT SURVIVED	N	PER CENT EXPIRED	N	TOTAL
Normal Blood Pressure	<1500 gm.	75.4	43	24.6	14	57
	>1500 gm.	90.5	95	9.5	10	105
Low Blood Pressure	<1500 gm.	47.1	16	52.9	18	34
	>1500 gm.	42.9	3	57.1	4	7
Total		77.3	157	22.7	46	203

[*]Observations from Babies' and Children's Hospital, Cleveland, Ohio.

TABLE 8–4 DISTRIBUTION OF DIAGNOSIS IN 116 INFANTS WITH RESPIRATORY DISTRESS IN THE FIRST FOUR HOURS OF LIFE

HMD	12
Massive aspiration syndrome	10
Bronchopneumonia	10
Cardiac malformation	2
Nasal obstruction (reserpine)	1
Pneumothorax	1
Transient respiratory problem	80

PATHOPHYSIOLOGY

The following are lists of the common early symptoms, the physiologic abnormalities, and the pathologic findings at autopsy.

Early Signs and Symptoms

1. Over half the infants have difficulty in initiating normal respiration. The disease should be anticipated in mothers who are bleeding, infants who are immature, and those with diabetic mothers.

2. Expiratory grunting or whining observed when the infant is not crying (due to partial closure of the glottis) is a most important sign which sometimes may be the only early indication of disease; a decrease in grunting may be the first sign of improvement.[43]

3. Sternal and intercostal retractions (secondary to decreased lung compliance).

4. Nasal flaring.

5. Cyanosis in room air (often).

6. Respirations—rapid or often slow when seriously ill.

7. Auscultation—diminished air entry.

8. Extremities edematous—after several hours (altered vascular permeability).

9. X-ray—reticulogranular, ground-glass appearance with air bronchograms.

10. Pulsation of the umbilical cord after the age of 20 minutes is frequently an early sign of HMD.

Physiologic Abnormalities[3, 14]

1. Lung compliance is reduced to as much as one-fifth to one-tenth of normal (see Figure 8–9).

2. Large areas of lung are not perfused (up to 50 to 60 per cent).[36, 39]

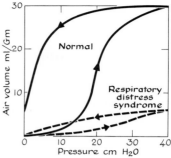

Figure 8–9 Air pressure volume curves of a normal and abnormal lung. Volume is expressed as milliliters of air per gram of lung. The lung from an infant with respiratory distress syndrome accepts a smaller volume of air at all pressures. Note also that the deflation pressure volume curve follows closely the inflation curve.[29]

3. Large right-to-left shunt of blood (30 to 60 per cent).[46]

4. Pulmonary capillary blood flow decreased.[13]

5. Alveolar ventilation decreased although minute ventilation and the work of breathing are increased.

6. Lung volume reduced.

These changes result in hypoxemia, often hypercarbia, and, if hypoxemia is severe, a metabolic acidosis.

A fixed heart rate early in the disease is always associated with a severe course. (This is also noted by the obstetrician regarding fetal asphyxia.)

S. PROD'HOM

Pathologic Findings (Anatomical, biophysical, and biochemical)

1. Gross—the lung is collapsed, firm, dark red, and liver-like.

2. Microscopic—alveolar collapse, with overdistention of the dilated alveolar ducts, pink-staining membrane on alveolar ducts (composed of products of the infant's blood and destroyed alveolar cells). Muscular coat of pulmonary arteriolar walls thickened, lumen small. Distended lymphatic vessels.

3. Electron microscopic—
   A. Damage and loss of alveolar epithelial cells.
   B. Swelling of capillary endothelial cells.
   C. Disappearance of lamellar inclusion bodies.

4. Biophysical—
   A. Altered, deficient, or absent pulmonary surfactant.[2]
   B. Abnormal air pressure volume curve as shown in Figure 8–9.[23]
   C. Perfusion studies of vascular tree reveal severly reduced arterial bed with blockage near the pulmonary arterioles.

5. Biochemical—the lung contains decreased phospholipid and surface-active lipoprotein fractions.[8]

ETIOLOGY

In the past twenty years, numerous theories to explain the respiratory distress syndrome (hyaline membrane disease) have been proposed and rejected.[35, 44] At present, two theories are under active exploration, examination, and debate.

I. An attractive proposal is that the disease is the result of a primary absence, deficiency, or alteration of the highly surface-active alveolar lining layer (the pulmonary surfactant). The surfactant, a lipoprotein, binds to the internal surface of the lung and markedly lessens the forces of surface tension at the air water interphase, thereby reducing the pressure tending to collapse the alveolus. By equalizing the forces of surface tension in units of varying size it is a potent antiatelectasis factor and is essential for normal respiration. Alteration or absence of the pulmonary surfactant would lead to a sequence of events shown in Figure 8–10; starting with position 'S,' resulting in decreased lung compliance (stiff lung), and thus an increase in the work of breathing. The additional work would soon tire the infant, leading to a sequence of reduced alveolar ventilation, atelectasis and both asphyxia and alveolar hypoperfusion. Asphyxia would induce pulmonary vasoconstriction and blood would bypass the lung through the fetal pathway (patent ductus, foramen ovale) lowering pulmonary blood flow, and a vicious cycle would be promoted. The resulting ischemia would be an added insult and further reduce lung metabolism and surfactant production.

Favoring this theory are the following findings:

1. Avery and others have demonstrated an absence or alteration of pulmonary surfactant in infants dying with HMD. This correlates with the inability of the diseased lung to retain a normal volume of air at a low

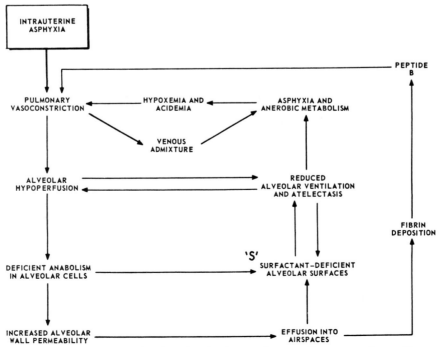

Figure 8–10   Alveolar function in the respiratory distress syndrome.[29]

transpulmonary pressure (abnormal air pressure volume curves—see Figure 8–9), thus explaining the deranged mechanical properties of the lungs.

2. The increased incidence of the disease in prematures weighing 1000 to 1500 gm., a stage when surfactant may not have developed.

3. The observation that mechanisms for producing surfactant are not fully developed early in gestation.

4. The ease of inducing with asphyxia a model of the disease in immature animals, when surfactant is minimal or absent.

5. Biochemical measurements showing a deficiency of the probable surface-active lipid in infants dying with HMD.

6. The exciting and important observation of Gluck[22] that a deficiency of saturated lecithins in amniotic fluid (the component that conveys the unusual surface activity) can be neatly correlated with the development of the disease in the newborn.

7. The early induction of surfactant in an immature animal fetus following an injection of steroid. The length of survival is also increased if delivered early. With this as a background, Liggins,* in a carefully controlled study, injected betamethasone in one-half of a group of women with premature onset of labor. He found a statistically reduced incidence of HMD in the infants of treated mothers. This striking finding is under active exploration and emphasizes again a trend toward treating the fetus.

The studies of Liggins and Howie* are not entirely convincing as to the possible role of steroid protection against hyaline membrane disease in premature delivery. It should be pointed out that the animal experimentation upon which this is based stems from the original observation by Liggins that when steroid was given to experimental animals (it induces early labor), the lungs of these animals were noted to be more mature than one would otherwise have expected. In the group of women studied by Howie and Liggins, the difference in survival rates is entirely due to enhanced survival of infants under 32 weeks' gestation, in which the numbers are relatively small. Infants with greater than 32 weeks' gestational age did not appear to have any benefit from such therapy administered to the mothers; thus, although the data are encouraging, more solid confirmation will be required before this can be accepted as an effective preventative measure. It

should also be pointed out that the fact that steroids are capable of inducing lung maturation does not necessarily make them the endogenous maturational controllers of pulmonary maturity since, as has been shown for other induction phenomena (i.e., glucuronyl-transferase in the liver), multiple agents may be capable of doing the same thing. Evidence now exists that thyroxin, and possibly heroin, are also capable of producing pulmonary maturation in animals, and while heroin cannot be considered a naturally occurring endogenous substance, thyroxin most certainly is.

L. STERN

Evidence against this hypothesis comes from a therapeutic trial in sick infants using an aerosol of dipalmityl lecithin (a synthetic surfactant whose properties as a surface film closely resemble those of pulmonary surfactant). Although lung compliance doubled, pulmonary gas exchange either did not improve or even worsened. Improved lung elasticity was not associated with any clinical improvement. Also, the higher incidence in the infants of diabetic mothers cannot be explained by this theory.

This argument seems irrelevant, because the aerosol of DPL was given quite late in the course of the disease.

S. PROD'HOM

The dipalmityl lecithin administration studies cannot be considered strong evidence against the surfactant hypothesis for two major reasons. It has been shown that DPL, while it is similar, is not as effective a surfactant as the naturally occurring substance. In addition, the administration of the material by aerosol once the baby already has the disease would be of relatively limited value, since not only is there an excellent chance that the material would be digested by tracheal enzymes before it ever reached the lung but also those portions of the lung which are already collapsed could not be reached by the material in any event. Finally, there is serious doubt as to whether even its administration into expanded alveoli and lying free in the alveolar space would be helpful, since in the normal course of the synthesis and utilization of surfactant, it is synthesized in the alveolar lining layer and then extruded onto the surface of this layer for its action to be effective.

L. STERN

II. An alternative hypothesis is that the primary and crucial lesion is pulmonary hypoperfusion secondary to asphyxia, possibly associated with the release of a vasoactive peptide rather than surfactant deficiency.[13] The cycle would begin with intrauterine asphyxia (Figure 8–10), which results in increased vascular resistance and shunts

*Liggins, G., and Howie, R.: Prevention of respiratory distress by antepartum corticoids. Pediatrics 50: 515, 1972.

much of the cardiac output away from the lung. (The kidney and gastrointestinal tract may also become ischemic.) Pulmonary ischemia would damage the alveolar lining cells that produce surfactant and increase alveolar-wall permeability and lead to an effusion into the airspace and membrane formation. When fibrinogen is transformed to fibrin, peptides A and B are formed. Peptide B is a potent pulmonary vasoconstrictor, and its presence in this area of the lung would potentiate and continue the vasoconstriction.

Findings lending support to this are:

1. The marked increase in pulmonary vascular resistance observed in the fetal lung with asphyxia, a frequent prenatal occurrence in infants with the disease.

2. The large areas of the diseased lung that are ventilated with air but not perfused with blood.

3. The intense pulmonary arteriolar vasoconstriction observed when perfusion studies are performed on autopsied hyaline lungs.

4. The increase in effective pulmonary flow, gas exchange, and clinical improvement following therapeutic measures that dilate the pulmonary arteriole.

5. The abnormally large mass of pulmonary arteriolar muscle found in infants delivered from diabetic or latent diabetic mothers.

Factors against this theory are:

1. The smaller medial thickness of the pulmonary arteriole in the immature neonate, who is most susceptible to the disease.

2. An inability to demonstrate larger right-to-left shunts at four hours in infants who subsequently die with HMD than in infants dying of other pulmonary causes. If an early reduction in pulmonary blood flow was severe enough to cause loss in surfactant, this would possibly be true.

It is possible that, in some immature infants, the primary disorder is surfactant deficiency, while in larger infants who suffer intrauterine asphyxia the primary trigger could be pulmonary vasoconstriction intensified by a vasoactive peptide. An alternative proposal is that in each infant the etiology could be differing proportions of surfactant deficiency and pulmonary vasoconstriction. In any case, the vicious cycle outlined in Figure 8–10 is useful to inspect when considering various therapeutic measures.

From our studies of the early stages of HMD, it appears that asphyxia is not a condition sine qua non

for initiating the process. HMD is related to gestational age, but perinatal asphyxia aggravates the natural course of the disease. Arguing against pulmonary hypoperfusion is the fact that there is only a slight increase in right-to-left shunt early in the disease. It may play a role later in the disease.

S. PROD'HOM

These two theories are not really self-contradictory or mutually exclusive. It has been clearly shown that synthesis of surfactant is in fact dependent upon pulmonary blood flow and that in the experimental preparation, surfactant synthesis as measured by incorporation of C^{14} tagged lipid fractions can be influenced by either increasing or reducing the blood flow to the animal lung preparation. In this view, the pulmonary vasoconstriction induced by hypoxia could well set off the chain of events resulting in reduced surfactant synthesis with failure to keep up with normal surfactant turnover, thereby setting in motion the chain of events outlined in Figure 8–10 and providing a unifying base for both the surfactant and pulmonary blood flow theories.

L. STERN

Actual Clinical Management

Although much of the pathophysiology of the respiratory distress syndrome has been described and a multitude of treatments suggested and in some cases partially studied, the following approach appears most reasonable during this period of continuing research:[35, 44] for infants not moribund with the disease, the treatment should be of minimal risk for the infant and based on physiologic principles that are known to increase survival. Therapeutic regimens with increased risk (namely respirator therapy and continuous positive airway pressure) should only be used with infants whose chances of surviving are severely diminished.

Most infants with either hyaline disease or severe aspiration syndrome will survive if treated with a similar plan. A somewhat similar approach can also be used for other neonatal pulmonary problems such as a small pneumothorax or transient tachypnea.

The clinical care can be divided into the acute and recovery phases. The acute phase lasts until it is reasonably certain the infant will survive. During the acute phase, every maneuver is directed at increasing the chance of recovery. The infant is placed in a neutral thermal environment (see Chapter 4) to reduce oxygen requirements and CO_2 production. For an infant with severe pulmonary involvement, this step alone may be life saving. To meet fluid and partial caloric requirements, the infant is given 65 to 150 ml. per Kg. per 24 hours of 10 per cent glucose by I.V.; because of poor gastric motility he is not fed orally. To meet the immediate and changing oxygen, metabolic, and ventilatory requirements of the infant, we monitor color, activity, heart rate, and skin or rectal temperature every hour and pH, $PaCO_2$, PaO_2 and HCO_3 at a minimum of every four hours. Respiration and heart rate are monitored continuously to prevent a long apneic period.

Most important in the prescription is skilled nursing and physician management. Vital signs and observations must be made in such a fashion as not to disturb the infant continually, yet the patient must always be observed. In many English units an essential part of the recipe is gentle, gentle care. Many students of the disease have noted definite clinical worsening with simple maneuvers, such as (1) a rectal temperature, (2) vigorous oral and pharyngeal suctioning, and (3) cleaning or positioning the face with a change in environmental oxygen lasting two to three minutes. The real skills of a unit can be tested by closely noting the care given an infant with HMD. Is the environmental oxygen at the correct percentage, temperature and flow rate? Is the arterial oxygen permitted to go too high or too low for a prolonged period? Is the unit anticipating the future needs of the infant or always treating complications? As an example, if, during the acute phase, an infant with HMD has an apneic episode, it usually signifies that the infant's condition will worsen and death will probably occur during the next one to six hours. Waiting for a PaO_2 of 10 to 20 mm. Hg and a severe respiratory and metabolic acidosis before beginning ventilatory therapy is not adequate anticipation. Once the basic care has been arranged (metabolic rate minimized, fluid and electrolyte needs met), the essentials of care involve maintaining an adequate PaO_2 and pH, and closely observing for a change in the infant's state.

Our general plan is to maintain the PaO_2 in the abdominal aorta between 60 and 90 mm. Hg, and the pH above 7.25 (with alkali if metabolic acidosis is present). To prevent the toxic effects of hyperosmolar solutions we are cautious about using $NaHCO_3$ and limit the total amount of alkali administered to 8 to 10 mEq. per Kg. every four to six hours. (The amount of HCO_3 is calculated from the Astrup nomogram—Figure 8–11.) In only rare instances do we administer this amount. (For more complete discussion of oxygen and alkali therapy, refer to "Therapeutic Tools," the next section, and Cases Two to Four.)

An alternative to the use of bicarbonate is to reduce the pCO_2 with assisted ventilation by manual bagging. It is also a common observation that whenever the pCO_2 is elevated in infants with hyaline membrane disease, the bicarbonate concentration is usually above 17 mEq. per liter; that is, in the presence of high pCO_2's, organic acidemia is not common unless there is severe hypoperfusion secondary to hypovolemia.

G. ODELL

Around 10 to 30 per cent of infants with HMD will require further care in the form of either continuous positive airway pressure (CPAP) or ventilatory treatment (see pp. 153–157).

There is general agreement that assisted ventilation should be used only when supportive measures as outlined earlier have little chance of being successful. Table 8–5 outlines a scoring procedure we use in determining if assisted ventilation should be used. The most valuable prognostic laboratory measurement appears again to be the arterial oxygen tension. An arterial oxygen tension below 30 to 40 mm. Hg with the infant breathing 100 per cent oxygen is an indication for ventilatory therapy; at this oxygen tension, the chance of survival without ventilatory assistance is probably less than 10 per cent.

In our experience, the chances of survival with a PaO_2 less than 40 mm. Hg in a 100 per cent ambient oxygen atmosphere are considerably less than the

TABLE 8–5 A SCORING SYSTEM USED TO SELECT INFANTS FOR ARTIFICIAL RESPIRATION*

	0	1	2	3
PaO_2 (100% O_2) (mm. Hg)	>70	50–70	*	* <50
pH	>7.30	7.20–7.29	7.0–7.19	<7.0
$PaCO_2$ (mm. Hg)	<60	60–70	71–80	>80

*Indications for artificial ventilation are: (1) a total score of three or greater, (2) an arterial oxygen tension less than 50 mm. Hg, or (3) two apneic episodes greater than 45 seconds.

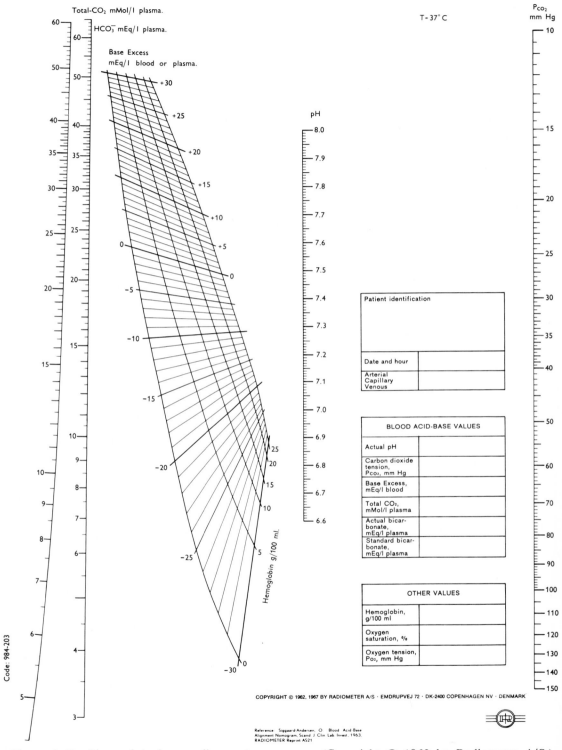

Figure 8–11 Siggaard-Andersen alignment nomogram. (Copyright © 1962 by Radiometer A/S.)

stated figure of 10 per cent. In effect, it is extremely important for each unit to establish what its own limits and levels of probability are, since they will depend on a multiplicity of factors (including the accuracy of the determinations, the efficiency of the personnel, etc.). Only once this is done for any individual department can a universally applicable confidence level *(for that department alone)* be utilized as a guide to when ventilatory assistance is indicated.

L. STERN

We use CPAP whenever more than 70 per cent oxygen is required to maintain PaO_2 above 50 to 60 mm. Hg (See pp. 153–157). For a complete discussion of mechanical ventilation and continuous positive airway pressure, see Chapter 9.

Between 60 and 90 hours of age, most infants will start the recovery phase. Respiratory rate and retractions will decrease and PaO_2 will rise.

One needs to be careful about interpreting on a clinical basis alone a decrease in respiratory rate and retractions. While it is correct that this may often herald improvement of the infant, it is equally correct that with elevations of $PaCO_2$ both the respiratory rate and the retractions will decrease as a result of the CO_2 depression. This may indeed signal a serious deterioration on the part of the infant, and we would therefore prefer never to depend upon these clinical signs without the supportive evidence of arterial blood gases to confirm them.

L. STERN

During this phase, expertise in oxygen management is required. PaO_2 should be kept below 90 mm. Hg, but if environmental oxygen is dropped too rapidly and PaO_2 is not closely monitored, a condition termed "flip-flop" can occur. (Flip-flop is a larger than expected drop in PaO_2 when the ambient oxygen is lowered and the PaO_2 does not return to the original level when the ambient oxygen is again raised.) From Figure 8–3 the anticipated PaO_2 can be determined as the oxygen is lowered, assuming that the right-to-left shunt, A-V difference for oxygen, hemoglobin, and so forth, are fixed. We rarely drop faster than 10 per cent every hour, checking PaO_2 before each drop in ambient oxygen.

It should be noted that during the recovery phase of HMD (especially if the infant is on a respirator), some infants reopen their ductus, resulting in a right-to-left shunt. Hence, the PaO_2 in the abdominal aorta is much lower than the right radial. In this case, your judgment should be based on the radial values.

S. PROD'HOM

We start oral feedings only during the recovery phase, when bowel sounds are present and the ambient oxygen is 40 per cent or below. During the recovery phase, the umbilical arterial catheter is removed when PaO_2 has been adequate for several hours at an ambient concentration of 40 per cent. It should be emphasized that an ambient concentration of 25 to 40 per cent oxygen can be toxic to the retina if maintained for a prolonged period. We continue to lower ambient oxygen in five per cent increments, monitoring closely the infant's clinical state (i.e., respiratory rate, heart rate, color, and observing for abdominal distention). A few infants appear to require small amounts of additional oxygen for prolonged periods (six to eight days). As the infant recovers, apneic periods are now observed, but they do not have the ominous significance as when observed in the acute phase. (For further details, see Table 8–6.) The case problems and questions further illustrate the care of these infants.

THERAPEUTIC TOOLS— OXYGEN AND ALKALI THERAPY

Oxygen Therapy

Although high concentrations of oxygen at atmospheric pressures can affect the stability of the red cell membrane and possibly alter the neonatal brain, obvious toxicity has been observed in the lung and retina.

The Retina. The effect of oxygen on the retinal vessels is dependent upon (1) the stage of development of the retinal vessels, (2) the length of the exposure to oxygen, and (3) the concentration of oxygen in the arterial blood. (If just the eyes of susceptible young animals are exposed to oxygen by cupping the eye, no toxic effects are observed.) The vasoconstricting effects of short periods of high oxygen are reversible. If the vasoconstriction (first stage) lasts longer than several hours, it may not be reversible. Pronounced vasoconstriction is not observed when the retina is fully vascularized. In the full-term human neonate, the temporal portion of the retina is still sensitive at birth, but no lasting damage has been observed.

The second stage is the proliferative phase, in which new vessels grow from the capillaries and sprout through the retina into

TABLE 8-6   ESSENTIALS OF CARE FOR INFANTS WITH RESPIRATORY DISTRESS

TREATMENT	LOGIC
1. A. Trained nurses (ratio of at least 1/1–3) and monitoring equipment. B. Available physician.	1. Early management of complications and notification of change in course (i.e., apnea, bleeding from catheter).
2. Precise temperature control to maintain infant in neutral temperature (includes oxygen hood — see Chapter 4).	2. Maintain minimal oxygen consumption and carbon dioxide production.

3. A. pH, PaO_2, $PaCO_2$, and HCO_3 measurement every 4 hours (night and day). Maintain PaO_2 60–100 mm. Hg.
   B. Attempt to keep pH > 7.25. If $PaCO_2$ > 75, consider changing treatment.
   C. Lower environmental oxygen slowly when RDS infant is still ill. Drop 10% every hour with monitoring if PaO_2 > 110 mm. Hg.
   D. Limit $NaHCO_3$ to 10 mEq./Kg./4 hrs.
	3. A + B. To determine requirements for oxygen and additional HCO_3. Permits continual assessment of infant's condition and limits toxic effects of oxygen.
	
	   C. Prevents "flip-flop" (greater than expected drop in $PaCO_2$ when environmental oxygen is reduced. (R-L shunt etiology?)
	   D. Prevents hypernatremia with brain damage.

4. No oral feeding (see Chapter 5).	4. Prevents aspiration in a sick infant; gastrointestinal motility reduced.
5. I.V. glucose 65 ml./Kg. 1st day, 100 ml./Kg. 2nd day with body wt. determ. for small infants to calculate if larger amounts of H_2O required. May require 150–200 ml./Kg.	5. Meets a portion of the large caloric requirements. Reduces hyperbilirubinemia.
6. Controlled oxygen administration: warmed and humidified, using a hood.	6. Prevents large swings in environmental oxygen and decreases water requirements. Prevents "flip-flop."
7. Continually monitor respiration and heart rate.	7. Prevents hypoxemia and acidemia with apneic episodes.
8. Frequent determinations of blood sugar and Hct. (Na, K, and Cl every 24–48 hrs.)	8. Necessary for calculating general metabolic requirements.
9. Transfuse if initial central Hct <35 or if Hct <35 during acute phase of illness.	9. For adequate oxygen-carrying capacity.
10. Record all observations (lab., nurse notes, etc.) on single form (see Figure 8–12).	10. Permits immediate correlation of many variables.
11. Urinary pH, output, osmolality.	11. Evaluation of blood flow to the kidney. An increase in output occurs as the infant starts to improve.
12. Frequent blood smears.	12. Checking for first signs of infection.

the vitreous. These vessels are usually permeable, and hemorrhages and edema sometimes follow. Organization of the hemorrhages that enter the vitreous can produce traction on the retina and may result in detachment and blindness.

In the human, infant retinal damage is observed when the gestational age is less than 36 weeks. The collaborative study[27] revealed changes in only a small number of infants if the ambient oxygen is below 40 per cent. To prevent retinal damage, the arterial oxygen tension must be kept below the level that stimulates vasoconstriction. The exact concentration that is toxic is unknown, however, if the PaO_2 is kept below 90 mm. Hg, obvious and lasting retinopathy is negligible.

Levels of PaO_2 that cause retrolental fibroplasia are not known at the present time. Repeated referrals to a "safe" level are unwarranted. I see no reason to keep pO_2 at 90 if, at a pO_2 of 60 mm. Hg, you can

get almost a 90 per cent saturation of hemoglobin. Thus, a range of pO_2 from 60 to 90 mm. Hg may not be a "safe" range, as suggested.

G. ODELL

The collaborative study referred to here is presumably the one carried out in the 1950s, in which the selection of the ambient oxygen figure at 40 per cent was made purely by chance in order to contrast it with high oxygen (which was obviously assumed to be 100 per cent). A more recent study currently underway has obtained evidence that even with such restriction, significant retrolental fibroplasia appears in some extremely immature infants; indeed, the suspicion has arisen for some infants that even the oxygen concentration of room air itself is sufficient to produce the retinopathy of prematurity. While it is not disputed that oxygen is the responsible agent for the retinal arterial vasoconstriction, which, if allowed to progress, will ultimately result in full-scale retrolental fibroplasia and blindness, the equal partner in the equation is the degree of immaturity of the retinal vessels. Also unknown are what, if any, other factors predispose towards the interaction of these two to produce the damaging end result. It needs to be stressed, however, that since oxygen is not absorbed directly through the sclera of the eyeball, the reliance on inspired oxygen concentration is inappropriate. The risk for retrolental fibroplasia, therefore, becomes a powerful motive towards obtaining arterial oxygen tension measurements, which in the end are the only levels that one should consider when evaluating the risk for eye damage.

The more recent study now in progress has also shown that the infant most at risk is not the premature with hyaline membrane disease in the first few days of life but rather the small premature infant who is repeatedly resuscitated for a period beyond that time for apneic spells, usually with a bag and mask into which a 100 per cent oxygen concentration is flowing. It is, therefore, recommended by the Fetus and Newborn Committees of both the Canadian Pediatric Society and the American Academy of Pediatrics that a self-inflatable (ambu-type) bag be kept in the incubator of such a child, and that when resuscitation is necessary it be carried out at the same oxygen concentration in which the infant is being kept at that time.

L. STERN

Pulmonary Oxygen Toxicity (Bronchopulmonary Dysplasia). The use of assisted ventilation for some infants with respiratory distress in conjunction with high concentrations of oxygen has resulted in a new clinical syndrome first described by Northway, Rosan and Porter[37] and called bronchopulmonary dysplasia. Their patients had been on respirators using greater than 70 per cent oxygen for longer than five to six days. During the prolonged recovery, the infants had tachypnea, subcostal retractions, rales bilaterally, and persistent cyanosis. As the infants improved, their X-rays followed the characteristic sequence outlined in Table 8–7. Increased concentrations of oxygen were required for

TABLE 8–7   COMPARISON OF PULMONARY DYSMATURITY AND BRONCHOPULMONARY DYSPLASIA[29]

	PULMONARY DYSMATURITY (MIKITY WILSON)	BRONCHOPULMONARY DYSPLASIA (OXYGEN TOXICITY)
Birth weight	Usually under 1500 gm.	Not specific.
Etiology	Unknown (Occurs in very immature infants, some of whom have received no additional O_2).	Probably oxygen toxicity. Preceded by severe respiratory distress syndrome, usually treated for a minimum of 4–6 days in an environment containing greater than 70% O_2.
Chest radiograph	Often normal in the first few days of life. Small cyst-like foci with diffuse coarse and lace-like pattern of infiltrates noted throughout the lung (similar to those seen in cystic stage of bronchopulmonary dysplasia). Usually complete clearing in 2–12 months; base of the lung clearing before apex.	Following four stages are observed: Typical ground-glass appearance of the respiratory distress syndrome. Marked opacity of the lungs. Small rounded areas of radiolucency distributed throughout the lung (similar to the cystic stage of pulmonary dysmaturity). Strands of increased pulmonary parenchymal density which often clear completely.
Pulmonary pathology		
a. Gross	Hyperaerated foci, separated by depressed gray-blue areas at atelectasis, often has a cobblestone appearance.	
b. Light microscopy		
1. Bronchiolar mucosa	Sometimes contains a few mononuclear cells.	Necrosis and metaplasia with patchy loss ciliated cells. Later irregular peribronchiolar muscular thickening.
2. Bronchiolar lumen	Normal.	Partially blocked with eosinophilic exudate and patchy squamous metaplasia.
3. Alveolar region	Normal, or on occasion mild to moderate fibrosis.	Early there is necrosis and repair of alveolar epithelium; later an increase in alveolar macrophages with alveolar coalescence. Focal thickening of the basement membrane and remnants of hyaline membrane with sheet-like masses of histiocytes.

several weeks before slow improvement was noted. In those infants who expired, autopsy revealed their lungs were diffusely involved (Table 8–7). Because these infants were also ill with HMD and on respirators with endotracheal intubation, it was not possible to implicate solely the toxic effects of high oxygen. Studies necessary for space flight, however, clarified the pathogenesis. Most informative among these are the precise descriptions and measurements of Kaplan, Robinson, Kapanci, and Weibel,[25, 26] who exposed monkeys to one atmosphere of 100 per cent oxygen for varying periods of time. After 48 hours of breathing 100 per cent oxygen, only equivocal histologic changes were noted. When oxygen was continued for a longer period, a specific sequence of morphologic changes was observed: after four days, the alveolar epithelium was almost completely destroyed (exudative phase); after seven days of high oxygen, Type One epithelial cells were replaced exclusively by Type Two cells (proliferative phase). Figures 8–12 and 8–13 illustrate the changes in the lung dimensions with differing lengths of exposure and recovery. The vascular endothelium appears to constitute the target tissue in the early

reaction. The blood-air barrier becomes progressively thickened. After 12 days of 100 per cent oxygen, the animals required gradual weaning back to room air, similar in many ways to infants with supposed pulmonary oxygen toxicity. Eighty-four days after the weaning, the lungs appeared surprisingly normal, but exact measurements revealed that a remodeling had occurred with a large increase in the capillary bed but only a slight enlargement in the air-blood-tissue barrier.

In experimental animals, obvious and striking pulmonary pathology is observed whenever the partial pressure of oxygen is greater than 500 mm. Hg (70 per cent at 1 atm.). Clinically, if the environmental oxygen concentration is above 70 per cent for longer than four or five days, obvious and severe pulmonary disease often results. Although there are some similarities between pulmonary dysmaturity and oxygen toxicity (e.g., second stage X-rays of pulmonary dysmaturity with third stage oxygen toxicity), they appear to have completely different etiologies.

An especially disturbing observation to the physician using oxygen in the nursery is the altered developmental pattern observed in

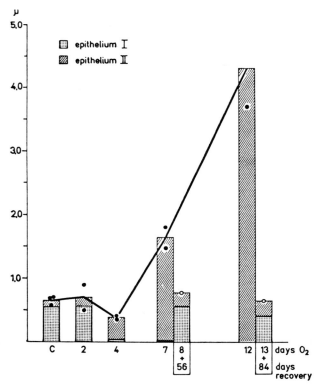

Figure 8–12 Change in epithelial thickness with exposure to pure oxygen (arithmetic mean thickness). Closed circles = animals sacrificed immediately after exposure. Open circles = animals allowed to recover. C = control animals.[25]

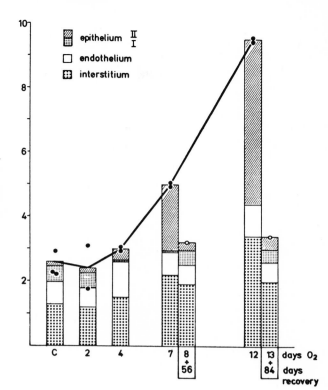

Figure 8–13 Change in the thickness of air-blood tissue barrier with exposure to pure oxygen (arithmetic mean thickness). Closed circles = animals sacrificed immediately after exposure. Open circles = animals allowed to recover. C = control animals.[25]

the infant rat lung when given as little as 46 per cent oxygen to breathe for 15 days.[5, 6] This early data suggests that the growing lung may be more sensitive to oxygen than was previously believed.

With the rapid development that is observed in lung growth in early life and the known remodeling that occurs in the experimental animal following a prolonged period of high oxygen, the final anatomical resolution of the infant lung poisoned by oxygen is at present only speculation.

The evidence that oxygen toxicity is in fact the sole guilty party in the occurrence of so-called bronchopulmonary dysplasia (respirator lung disease) is in our view most unconvincing. Pathologically, the changes described for this condition do not seem to us to be different from those of chronic infection, obstruction, fibrosis, and compensatory emphysema in the lung. Moreover, while there are clear and definite pathologic features of pulmonary oxygen toxicity, they are quite different from those originally described by Northway, Rosan, and colleagues. The strongest evidence against this view comes from our own experience with the use of negative pressure respirators (see Chapter 9) in which ventilation is accomplished without the use of intratracheal tubes. We have not seen any evidence of bronchopulmonary dysplasia in any of the survivors (who now number in excess of 125), or pathologic

evidence of its occurrence in any of the deaths of infants so treated, despite the use of concentrations of oxygen up to 100 per cent for periods as long as four weeks. Like others, we have seen it occur in infants managed on positive pressure respirators with the use of intratracheal tubes. It is, therefore, our contention that if oxygen should in some measure be responsible for these changes, it requires the presence of either an intratracheal tube and/or the use of a positive pressure respirator for the full expression of its harmful effects in this regard.

L. STERN

Oxygen Administration. Use a small hood or plastic cover to prevent fluctuation when opening the incubator (Figure 8–14). The temperature of the oxygen must be warmed to that of the incubator and checked hourly. The flow into the hood must be at least five liters per minute to prevent CO_2 accumulation. Improper oxygen administration can be disastrous for the small infant and result in death, or brain, lung, or eye damage.[41]

1. Peripheral cyanosis may be present in a neonate with a normal or high arterial oxygen tension.

2. The environmental oxygen should be monitored hourly in all infants receiving supplementary oxygen. The oxygen analyzer

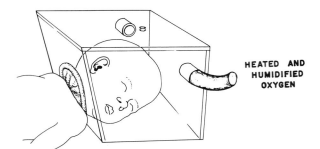

HEATED AND HUMIDIFIED OXYGEN

Figure 8–14 A plastic hood for oxygen administration.

should be calibrated at least once a day with high and low concentrations.

3. We measure PaO$_2$ every four hours (night and day) if the infant is receiving >40 per cent oxygen.

4. An infant with a low cardiac output or a reduced hemoglobin concentration may require slightly higher PaO$_2$'s for a short time (less than 60 minutes) to maintain adequate oxygen delivery. Additional hemoglobin is often helpful.

5. Arterial oxygen tensions greater than 110 mm. Hg for longer than one to two hours have been associated with permanent eye damage in a number of infants.

6. Small infants with respiratory problems cannot usually maintain adequate tissue oxygenation for a prolonged period if PaO$_2$ falls to between 30 and 40 mm. Hg, and they require some form of assistance.

7. Long periods of time (3 to 10 days) at 25 to 40 per cent environmental oxygen can result in retrolental fibroplasia in the normal small immature infant.[24]

8. When the infant with HMD is improving (PaO$_2$ >90 mm. Hg), we lower environmental oxygen in five per cent increments and repeat PaO$_2$ before each drop in concentration.

9. A partial pressure of environmental oxygen >500 mm. Hg (70 per cent at 1 atm.) can be damaging to pulmonary tissue if maintained longer than four to five days. It may be harmful before this time. Oxygen at this level is only continued if absolutely necessary.

10. Some infants recovering from respiratory disease (severe HMD, pulmonary dysmaturity) may require slightly increased oxygen concentrations (25 to 30 per cent) for prolonged periods. These infants should have a PaO$_2$ determination at least every other day. When the environmental oxygen is to be lowered, observe these infants closely for pallor, tachycardia, tachypnea, abdominal distention, and a fall in body temperature, all of

which are due in part to chemoreceptor stimulation secondary to hypoxia. If any of the symptoms appear, obtain blood gases and slightly raise the ambient oxygen concentration.

11. Management of oxygen therapy without arterial oxygen tension determinations is dangerous. If the infant is kept in greater than 40 per cent oxygen for more than four hours, periodic arterial samples (at least every six hours) should be obtained by radial or brachial puncture to demonstrate that the PaO$_2$ is not at toxic levels.

Alkali Therapy

Correction of a severe metabolic acidosis with alkali has many physiologic benefits. With normalization of pH, myocardial contractility is increased, pulmonary vascular resistance is reduced, and the length of survival with asphyxia is prolonged. However, the rapid injection of hypertonic solutions of NaHCO$_3$ or Tham is associated with a marked change in osmolality.[19] (It is sometimes forgotten that although Tham does not contain Na, there is an equivalent cation — the amine — which has the same osmolal effect.) A brisk change in serum osmolality will alter many parameters. As water moves into the plasma, the vascular volume increases and intracellular water is decreased. The rapid infusion of hypertonic solutions produces a sudden rise in cerebrospinal fluid pressure and venous pressure followed by a steep fall in CSF pressure. As the plasma volume and venous pressure are increased, profound effects on the brain may result, including fatal hemorrhage. We use the following general rules for alkali therapy:

1. We exclusively use NaHCO$_3$ because of the possibility of hypoglycemia with Tham.

2. To reduce the corrosive effects of hypertonic solutions we dilute with equal

parts one-half distilled H_2O and inject the solution into either a peripheral vein, the fast-flowing arterial stream by way of an arterial catheter, or into the umbilical venous catheter if it is known to be above the liver.

3. We use the Astrup nomogram (Figure 8–11) to calculate the alkali correction, usually giving only three-fourths of the calculated amount.

4. To prevent the toxic effects from large changes in osmolality, we limit alkali to 10 mEq. per Kg. every five to six hours. In practice we usually use a much smaller dose.

5. We do not correct a respiratory acidosis with alkali.

We would strongly support this recommendation. Respiratory acidosis is due to retention of CO_2 and its relief can be accomplished only by reduction of the CO_2 levels, usually with some form of controlled or assisted ventilation.

L. STERN

6. When an infant is severly asphyxiated, we administer alkali before the pH and HCO_3 measurements have been completed (4 mEq. per Kg. $NaHCO_3$ for infants <2000 gm. and 3 mEq. per Kg. for those >2000 gm.).

Use of base deficit to calculate the amount of HCO_3 to be given in a mixed type of acidosis is fallacious (see Pediat Res 5:523, 1971). Chances are that it is overestimated, and if CO_2 can be effectively blown off, it will not do any good to correct pH (see J Pediat 80:671, 1972).

G. ODELL

NEONATAL PULMONARY PROBLEMS

MECONIUM ASPIRATION

Meconium is present in the amniotic fluid of 10 per cent of all births, and its presence suggests that the infant may have suffered some asphyxial episode in utero. It is doubtful that amniotic fluid alone can produce any airway obstruction. However, pulmonary disease is definitely observed in infants who have aspirated meconium. While meconium can be aspirated from the tracheas of 60 per cent of all infants who are born covered with meconium, only 20 to 25 per cent of these infants will develop symptoms of respiratory distress or pulmonary radiographic changes.

Clinical Findings

Because asphyxia is often the basis for the presence of meconium in the amniotic fluid, the infant who aspirates meconium at birth is often depressed and requires some resuscitation. Positive-pressure resuscitation should be avoided in these infants until adequate laryngotracheal toilet has been performed to prevent pushing meconium further into the small airways.

Gasping respirations are sometimes observed, the chest is enlarged, especially in the anterior posterior diameter, respirations are rapid, and rales may or may not be heard. A chest X-ray is helpful diagnostically and shows areas of increased density and areas of overexpansion irregularly distributed throughout the lung.

It is of interest that the lung can remove meconium rapidly. Marked recovery is usually noted after 48 hours of life. It has been observed that a small number of infants with meconium aspiration recover over a prolonged period of time, One complication of the partially blocked overexpanded areas of lungs, occurring in 10 per cent of meconium-covered infants, is rupture with pneumothorax. This should be suspected if the clinical status of the infant deteriorates suddenly.

In our experience, the meconium aspiration syndrome is a frequent finding, and in referral intensive care units, it combines respiratory distress with impairment of cardiovascular function. There are transient cardiomegaly, murmurs, poor peripheral perfusion, and cerebral irritation. This condition is related to primary hypoperfusion of the lung, as suggested by repeated determinations of right-to-left shunt at an early age, and angiocardiographic studies. There is a significant relationship between the pH and the degree of shunting. Correction of the pH early in the course is followed by a decrease in shunting. (See Huntingford, P., Beard, R., Hytten, F., et al: Perinatal Medicine, 2nd Congress, 1971.)

S. PROD'HOM

TRANSIENT TACHYPNEA OF THE NEWBORN

This syndrome usually follows an uneventful term pregnancy and is first detected in the transitional care nursery, because the infant is noted to have a persistently high respiratory rate.[4] Cyanosis is not prominent, although a few infants require 35 to 40 per cent oxygen to remain pink. Air exchange is good with no rales or rhonchi, an expiratory grunt is not heard, intercostal retractions are minimal, and arterial pH and $PaCO_2$ measurements should be within normal limits. The chest X-ray reveals central perihilar streaking, and often the cardiac silhouette is slightly enlarged. The X-ray can usually be distinguished from meconium aspiration or the respiratory distress syndrome.

In most cases, respirations slow gradually during the first five days of life, and the infants are usually able to go home when their mothers are discharged from the hospital. The pathogenesis has not been clarified; however, it has been suggested that this syndrome may be secondary to slow absorption of lung fluid. Fluid remaining in the periarterial tissue would explain the X-ray findings, and lung compliance would be decreased owing to the additional fluid. The infant's increased respiratory rate would then minimize respiratory work. The syndrome appears to be self-limited and there have been no reported complications.

MASSIVE PULMONARY HEMORRHAGE AND HEMORRHAGIC PULMONARY EDEMA
by E. O. R. Reynolds, M.D., M.R.C.P.

Massive pulmonary hemorrhage has been judged to be the principle cause of death in about nine per cent of neonatal autopsies.[21]

The illness occurs most commonly on the second to fourth days of life and is almost always fatal. It may present in infants who have previously appeared well, or, more often, in those who are already suffering from other life-threatening abnormalities or illnesses. A large number of predisposing factors have been implicated in the causation of the illness, including intrapartum asphyxia, low birth weight, infection, aspiration of gastric contents, hypothermia, severe rhesus iso-immunization, congenital heart disease, and defective coagulation of the blood.[15, 18, 21, 42]

The usual mode of presentation is that the infant develops bradycardia, apnea or slow gasping respirations, and evidence of peripheral vasoconstriction. Bloodstained fluid is then seen welling from the trachea. Once resuscitative measures have been undertaken, the flow of liquid usually ceases, although it sometimes continues or recurs.

Cole et al[15] have analyzed the composition of the lung effluent in infants with massive pulmonary hemorrhage and found that, although it looked like blood, in most cases it was edema fluid with a comparatively small admixture of whole blood. These authors postulate that the outpouring of hemorrhagic edema fluid is due to acute left heart failure, often resulting from hypoxia and acidosis

caused by, for example, a severe apneic spell. Increasing left atrial pressure is then followed by a rise in pulmonary capillary pressure with edema formation and rupture of the pulmonary capillaries and alveolar membranes. Such a hypothesis would account for the fact that, in most cases of massive pulmonary hemorrhage, the bleeding is confined to the lung.[21]

An acute rise in left atrial pressure may be expected to have far more serious consequences in newborn infants than in adults. An adult with a failing left heart filters excess fluid into the bases of the lungs, but ventilation can proceed normally at the apices. In a newborn infant, however, the height of the column of blood in the lung is by comparison very small, and a similar rise in left atrial pressure will cause increased filtration into the whole lung more or less simultaneously. Factors identified by Cole et al[15] which might have predisposed infants in their series to develop massive pulmonary hemorrhage (or hemorrhagic pulmonary edema) if they sustained an episode of acute left heart failure included those favoring increased pulmonary capillary pressure (hypoproteinemia, overtransfusion, increased surface tension at the alveolar air-liquid interface) and those causing damage to lung tissue (infection, hyaline membrane disease, oxygen breathing, mechanical ventilation). Abnormalities of coagulation were present in some of the infants, but it was concluded that these abnormalities probably did not initiate the hemorrhage but could exacerbate it by allowing continued bleeding through ruptured capillaries.

Treatment. The treatment of massive pulmonary hemorrhage is very unsatisfactory. Fresh blood transfusions and mechanical ventilation are often employed, usually to little purpose. Probably of more importance is the prevention of asphyxia at birth and subsequently by suitable monitoring and resuscitative techniques, together with proper management of the underlying illnesses or abnormalities which appear to predispose infants to develop the "hemorrhage."

PNEUMOTHORAX

An asymptomatic pneumothorax is found in about one per cent of all routine newborn chest radiographic examinations. Considering the very high intrathoracic pressures recorded during the first minutes of life, it is surprising that pneumothorax is not a more frequent occurrence. Macklin[32] described the path of the air after rupture: air from the ruptured alveolus dissects up the vascular sheath into the mediastinum and from there into the pleural cavity. In some series, as high as one-half of the symptomatic patients aspirated meconium or blood. This suggests that obstruction with a ball-valve action may be the basis for the rupture.

Pneumothorax should be suspected in any newborn with respiratory distress, and a chest radiograph should be quickly taken, since adequate therapy is available.

It is our practice never to rely on AP and lateral films alone when a pneumothorax is suspected. These will often fail to reveal the presence or true extent of the extrapulmonary collection of air. A lateral decubitus horizontal beam film should be done on the suspected side or sides, which will show the free air in its most advantageous position radiographically and allow for true assessment of the size of the pneumothorax.

L. STERN

Clinical Findings. Cyanosis, tachypnea, grunting, and flaring of the alae nasae are often observed. Percussion is sometimes helpful, but shift of the apical impulse is usually more easily noted. Auscultation may be misleading because of wide referral of breath sounds. The sudden onset of a tense, distended abdomen is often a useful clinical feature signifying a pneumothorax.

Treatment. If the pneumothorax is asymptomatic, no specific therapy is necessary, but the infant's color, heart rate, and respiratory rate should be closely observed. If severe respiratory distress is noted, a catheter should be placed in the pneumothorax and a continuous suction of 10 to 20 cm. of water placed on the catheter. Usually only 24 hours of suction are necessary. Because the air in the pneumothorax is absorbed by the pleural capillaries, breathing 100 per cent oxygen will markedly hasten the absorption of the pneumothorax and can be lifesaving (see Figure 8–4). Since the pressure in the pneumothorax is always close to 760 mm. Hg, the very low capillary pressure produced with oxygen breathing hastens the absorption considerably, because gas flows from a high to a low pressure. A sixfold increase in the rate of absorption of a pneumothorax has been observed with 100 per cent oxygen breathing. However, because of the toxic effects of oxygen on the retina and lung, the complete effects of this mechanism cannot be utilized.

SPECIAL PULMONARY PROBLEMS IN THE IMMATURE NEONATE

PULMONARY DYSMATURITY (MIKITY-WILSON)

Pulmonary dysmaturity is a pulmonary disease of premature infants first described by Wilson and Mikity in 1960.[48] The usual clinical course is marked by an insidious onset of mild respiratory symptoms, usually after the first week of life. It is most commonly noted around three weeks of age. Most of the affected infants have birth weights below 1500 gm. The first signs are usually tachypnea, periods of apnea, and slight cyanosis. X-rays at this time usually appear far more abnormal than is apparent from the clinical findings. Chest radiographs show a diffuse, bilateral, coarse, and lace-like pattern of infiltrates with alternating cyst-like foci of hyperaeration (Figure 8–15). There is usually no fever and the blood count is within normal limits. Moderate osteoporosis with rib fractures are sometimes found. In infants with severe disease, arterial blood gases reveal an elevated $PaCO_2$ (60 to 80 mm. Hg) with cyanosis in 20 to 40 per cent oxygen, and right heart failure may supervene. Pulmonary function studies show a reduced functional residual capacity and vital capacity, an increased resistance to air flow especially during expiration, and an increased work of breathing.[1, 47] Symptoms become increasingly severe and reach a maximum intensity usually four to eight weeks after onset. In the reported series, the fatality rate varies between 25 and 50 per cent. In surviving infants, the symptoms gradually disappear over weeks and months. During the recovery phase hyperaeration is first observed by X-ray at the lung bases.[24] By six months to two years, the chest X-ray becomes normal. The cystic phase of this disease is sometimes confused with bronchopulmonary dysplasia (a chronic pulmonary disease that develops following respirator therapy with high oxygen). Table 8–7 compares the X-ray findings, pathology, and etiology in both diseases. In our experience, most of these infants will survive.

Pathology

Surprisingly, light and electron microscopic studies from lung biopsies and autopsy specimens have not shown any characteristic

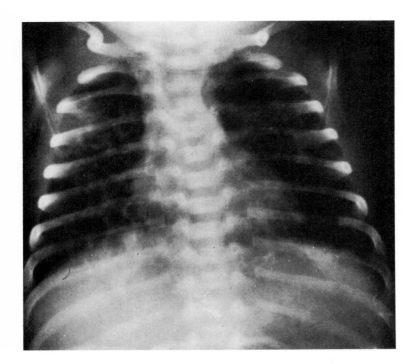

Figure 8–15 Radiogram of an infant with pulmonary dysmaturity (Wilson-Mikity syndrome) showing typical cystic appearance.[29] (Courtesy of Dr. Harold Goldman.)

cellular changes. Mild pulmonary fibrosis has been noted on occasion. Sections taken of inflated and fixed lung specimens show an uneven pattern of aeration with overexpansion in some areas (Figure 8–16).

Etiology

The studies of Burnard[9, 11] have suggested a working hypothesis. He demonstrated an increased distensibility of the bronchial tree with decreasing gestational age. During any respiratory effort, transpulmonary pressures developed by the small premature infant could easily collapse the airways. The small radius of the bronchi of the premature infant in conjunction with the increased collapsibility would make the small premature infant prone to unequal distribution of air. Partial airway obstruction might, therefore, more easily occur following the aspiration of a small quantity of milk as a result of an undeveloped gag reflex.

APNEA IN THE IMMATURE INFANT

Periodic breathing (short pauses in respiration) is common in the immature infant and should be differentiated from apnea, which has been defined as either (1) a given time period with complete cessation of respiration (15 to 30 seconds); or (2) the time without respiration after which functional changes are noted in the infant, such as cyanosis, hypotonia, or metabolic acidosis. Although the use of a standard, set time period appears to simplify routine nursery management, some small infants (usually <1200 gm.) appear to suffer if the apneic period extends beyond as little as 5 to 10 seconds.

Hypoglycemia, mild dehydration, hypocalcemia, sepsis, and severe brain lesions can be heralded by apneic spells and should be ruled out when apneic episodes first begin.[10] However, the vast majority of apneic periods occur in infants who are immature and have no organic disease. An exception is an apneic episode in an infant ill with severe HMD, which usually indicates the presence of hypoxia and acidemia, and is a notice that death will occur in several hours if there is no special intervention, such as assisted ventilation.

When respirations and heart rate are closely monitored, it has been noted that about 30 per cent of all infants below 1750 gm. birth weight will have an apneic period, commonly in the beginning of sleep immediately after eating.[16] These spells are usually limited to the first 12 days of life. In 90 per cent of these infants, heart rate

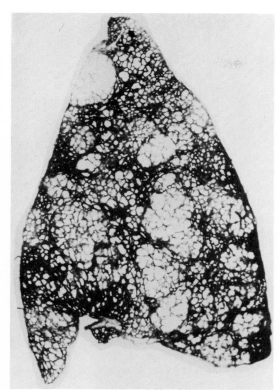

Figure 8–16 A section of lung from an infant dying with pulmonary dysmaturity. The lung was inflated at 15 cm. of water and fixed in formalin for 48 hours. Note the uneven aeration.[24]

the first 12 days of life. Since heart rate does not regularly drop in all infants with apnea, respiration monitors should not depend solely upon a change in heart rate to signal an alarm. We recommend diffuse cutaneous stimulation rather than painful stimuli to reinstitute breathing. Stimulation alone will stop 80 to 90 per cent of apneic spells if begun early. However, a mask and bag should be set up near every monitored infant, to be used if breathing does not begin promptly after stimulation. (Room air or 30 to 40 per cent oxygen may be used in the bag.)

We would stress again that the use of a mask and bag in resuscitating a premature infant from apnea needs to be carried out within the oxygen concentration limits in which the infant has previously been kept. It is the view of the present collaborative study on retrolental fibroplasia that the practice of resuscitating

starts dropping within 10 to 15 seconds after the onset of apnea and is usually below 100 beats per minute within 30 seconds (Figure 8–17).

No good physiologic or chemical explanation completely describes these spells. However, several observations suggest that changes in the excitatory state of the immature respiratory center can remarkably alter breathing. As examples, either restraining the extremities of a small premature (thus changing sensory input from bones and joints) or increasing incubator temperature (thus altering skin temperature receptors) will often induce or increase the number of apneic episodes.[16, 40] In certain infants, apneic spells may be the equivalent of a convulsion.

If undetected, the first apneic episode can result in catastrophe. Therefore, because these spells occur so commonly, we suggest that all premature infants below 1750 gm. be routinely and continuously monitored during

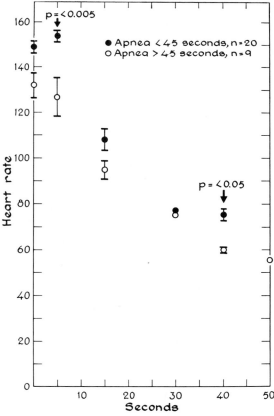

Figure 8–17 The heart rate response of infants having prolonged apnea is compared to the response of infants having apnea of lesser duration. Brackets represent one standard error of the mean.[16]

such an infant, who may indeed have been in room air all alone, episodically with 100 per cent oxygen directly from a wall source may indeed be responsible for the increased re-appearance of retrolental fibroplasia in such infants.

L. STERN

Miller[33] noted a decreased frequency of apneic episodes but an increase in the length of apnea when environmental oxygen was increased. (The memory of the recent medical disaster in using oxygen to regularize respirations is strong evidence for not increasing oxygen concentration to prevent or reduce apnea in a normal premature infant.)

Clinical observations have noted metabolic acidosis at times following short repeated episodes of apnea. This may be the result of slightly reduced oxygen delivery secondary to altered perfusion or a short period of hypoxemia.

Apnea Monitors. Because heart rate does not always drop with apnea, we monitor respiration; we favor mattress monitors developed in England* which require no attachments on the infant, although we still use impedance monitoring as well. (Impedance measures the electrical resistance across the chest which changes with respiration.) If the infant has a gestational age less than 34 weeks or weight less than 1750 gm., we monitor for 12 days and until no apneic episode has occurred for three days.

In our department, the nurses prefer the use of heart rate meters to apnea monitors which are respiration-dependent. The latter are extremely unreliable in terms of giving false alarms on numerous occasions. Even with the proper use of the air-filled mattress (which should be kept only very minimally filled), this still occurs and results in unnecessary attempts at resuscitation, as well as in serious interference with routine and time patterns in the nursery. By contrast, the intelligent use of heart meters, whose sound is far more pleasing and comforting to the ears of the attending personnel, has, in our department, afforded ample warning of a serious apneic spell, and their use is, therefore, preferred on these grounds.

L. STERN

Editors' Comment: Our nurses prefer combination heart rate-respiration monitors with attendant oscilloscope. Unfortunately, these are too expensive to have available for each infant who requires monitoring.

---

*Codman Apnea Alarm, Codman & Shurtleff Inc., Randolph, Massachusetts 02368.

PRACTICAL HINTS

1. Prompt resuscitation possibly prevents respiratory disease.

2. Grunting or whining is a most valuable clinical sign in diagnosing HMD. It is not normally heard 50 minutes after delivery.

3. Although close observation of temperature control, respiration, and acid-base balance are necessary, frequent handling and manipulation of a sick infant may be harmful.

4. When using high concentrations of oxygen (>40 per cent), arterial oxygen tension measurements should be made at least every four hours. Environmental concentrations of oxygen between 25 and 40 per cent (atm. pressure) for prolonged periods (3 to 10 days) can damage the eyes of small immature infants.

5. Do not start early feeding in an infant with respiratory distress. Gastrointestinal motility is reduced and there is a risk of aspiration. We start feeding when the respiratory rate is below 60 and bowel sounds are present.

6. Repeated apneic episodes in the small premature sometimes result in metabolic acidosis. Unrecognized apneic episodes may produce permanent neurologic sequelae.

QUESTIONS

True or False

As long as the arterial PaO$_2$ remains below 130 mm. Hg, there will be no retinal damage when using high concentrations of oxygen (greater than 40 per cent) for the treatment of the respiratory distress syndrome.

When PaO$_2$ is measured every four hours and is less than 130 mm. Hg, a small number of infants have been observed with retinal damage. There are several possible explanations: (1) large right-to-left shunt directed to sampling site in lower aorta while retinal vessels received blood with a higher PaO$_2$, (2) PaO$_2$ actually varied between measurements, and (3) increased sensitivity of retinal vessels to oxygen. The statement is false.

Sensory stimulation in the form of multiple examinations and routine nursing measurements of pulse, rectal temperature, heart rate, and so forth, may be harmful to an infant with severe RDS.

Striking changes have been recorded in heart rate and PaO$_2$ with standard nursing manipulations. Several English physicians strongly recommend minimal handling. It is the authors' personal belief, without adequate supporting data, that this may be true.

While we would agree that minimal handling is desirable, it has in too many institutions become a euphemism for simply doing nothing for the infant. Gentleness and avoidance of unnecessary trauma is mandatory, but it should not and must not be allowed to become an excuse for failure to initiate and carefully apply adequate therapy when indicated.

L. STERN

Adequate experimental and clinical data now support the thesis that Mikity-Wilson (pulmonary dysmaturity) and bronchopulmonary dysplasia are probably the result of oxygen toxicity.

Although the lungs of infants with Mikity-Wilson resemble grossly and by X-ray some stages of lungs poisoned with oxygen, the light and electron microscopic appearance of the lungs of infants with Mikity-Wilson are completely different. Therefore the statement is false.

B. W. is a two-day-old, 1200-gm. male infant with moderate hyaline membrane disease. During the first two days of life he has not been apneic and has maintained a reasonable pH, PaCO₂, and PaO₂ in 40 per cent oxygen. However, the most recent PaO₂ has dropped to 35 mm. Hg (breathing 40 per cent oxygen). This environmental oxygen concentration should be left the same, since raising the concentration may be harmful to the retina.

A drop to 35 mm. Hg suggests worsening of the infant's condition. He may deteriorate rapidly if he remains in 40 per cent oxygen. If the arterial oxygen is monitored closely (every four hours), raising the inspired oxygen concentration to maintain the PaO_2 between 60 and 90 mm. Hg does not result in retinal disease. Therefore the statement is false. The oxygen concentration should be raised.

The occurrence of 20 apneic periods (no respiration >20 to 30 seconds) during the first 10 days of life in a premature infant without respiratory distress is commonly associated with brain damage.

In years past, when respiration was not closely monitored and apneic episodes were not promptly terminated with either stimulation (90 per cent) or short-term mask and bag ventilation (10 per cent), frequent apneic periods were associated with brain damage.

Today this should not occur. Although there may be a slightly increased incidence of damaged infants, most of them do quite nicely. Therefore the statement is false.

If apneic periods are noted after several feedings, it is recommended that oral feeding be stopped.

Apneic periods are more commonly noted after feedings and are not an indication to stop feedings. Therefore the statement is false.

It is our impression that in a certain percentage of apneic infants, the apnea occurs in response to swallowing and distension of the stomach, as well as with passage of stool. This appears to be a vaso-vagal response, producing first bradycardia and subsequently apnea, and is the equivalent of a Stokes-Adams attack. This should be decided before the decision to feed or not is made.

G. ODELL

Maintaining the arterial PaO₂ between 50 and 90 mm. Hg will prevent pulmonary oxygen toxicity.

Pulmonary oxygen toxicity is related to the inspired concentration of oxygen, not the arterial oxygen concentration. Therefore the statement is false.

CASE PROBLEMS

(When studying each case, refer to the blood gas sheet, pages 148 and 149.)

Case One

A. B. is a 1500-gm. female with aspiration pneumonia. At eight hours of age, she is in an oxygen concentration of 70 per cent. She has meconium-stained nails, and a good urine output.

At 12 hours, the left leg turns white. What should be done?

Gently pull the catheter back 1 to 2 cm. If the blanching does not quickly disappear, remove the catheter. Sometimes no problems arise when another catheter is inserted into the same artery. Otherwise, attempt to catheterize the other umbilical artery.

If you decide to remove the catheter, how do you manage the infant's environmental oxygen concentration?

There is no substitute for arterial blood

sampling. This infant is quite ill and only 12 hours old; therefore, repeated brachial artery sampling is not practical. Repeated sampling from the radial and temporal arteries is a possible solution. These routes have been successful in skilled hands. Digital arterial samples may also be utilized. Heel blood from young infants (1 to 3 days old) is not reliable. Venous blood sampling cannot be used to control ambient oxygen.

BLOOD GAS RECORD SHEET (to be used in conjunction with Cases One through Four)

Start _____
Date _____ Time _____
Finish _____
Date _____ Time _____

ACTIVITY
++ = ACTIVE
+ = ACTIVE (STIMULATED)
− = LIMP
A = IRRITABLE
S = TWITCHY

COLOR
P = PINK
W = PALE
D = DUSKY
B = BLUE

S = SKIN
R = RECTAL
M = MEAN

	Time	Age (Hrs.)	O₂ conc.	TEMPERATURE (°C) Hood / Inc.	TEMPERATURE (°C) S / R	B.P. (M)	P.	R.	Hct. / Hgb.	Dext. / Sug.	Bil.	#	pH	pO₂	pCO₂	Act. HCO₃
Case One		8	70	34 / 34	36⁵ / 37¹							5	7.28	50	60	27.3
		12	70	34 / 34	36⁵ / 37²		160	50				6	7.29	40	62	29
Case Two		½	40	33⁵ / 33⁵	33 / 32	39			43	>90		1	7.14	30	35	11.4
		1		33⁵ / 33⁵	34 / 33	22			43				7.28	90	36	16.4
Case Three		8	40	32 / 34	36² / 36⁵	38			50	>90		6	7.40	60	32	19.5
		11	40	32 / 34	36¹ / 36	39						7	7.40	30	38	23.2
		13		32 / 34	36 / 36⁵	39						8	7.40	60	42	25.6
		18	50	32 / 34	36 / 35	48						10	7.20	25	50	18.8
		25	100	32 / 34	36 / 35							13	7.21	35	58	22.4
Case Four		3	70	33⁵ / 33⁵	36⁴ / 36⁶	40			54	>90		2	7.36	280	40	22.2
		4½	60	33⁵ / 33⁵	36⁴ / 36⁶	39						4	7.35	250	42	22.8

(Record sheet continued on opposite page.)

BLOOD GAS RECORD SHEET (to be used in conjunction with Cases One through Four) *Continued*

Start _____
   Date   Time

Finish _____
   Date   Time

ACTIVITY

++ = ACTIVE
+ = ACTIVE (STIMULATED)
− = LIMP
A = IRRITABLE
S = TWITCHY

COLOR

P = PINK
W = PALE
D = DUSKY
B = BLUE

S = SKIN
R = RECTAL
M = MEAN

Time	Age (Hrs.)	O_2 conc.	TEMPERATURE (°C) Hood / Inc.	TEMPERATURE (°C) S / R	VITAL SIGNS B.P. (M)	VITAL SIGNS P.	VITAL SIGNS R.	LAB. WORK Hct. / Hgb.	LAB. WORK Dext. / Sug.	LAB. WORK Bil.	BLOOD GASES #	BLOOD GASES pH	BLOOD GASES pO_2	BLOOD GASES pCO_2	BLOOD GASES Act. HCO_3
	5	40	33^5 / 33^5	36^5 / 37	39						5	7.36	30	43	23.9
	5½	60	33^5 / 33^5	36^4 / 37^1	38						6	7.37	70	33	18.7

SP 346-REV. 11/68

Case Two

C. D. is a 2100-gm. male, grunting since birth. X-ray shows no pneumothorax, but is technically of poor quality.

What are this infant's obvious problems?

(a) Hypothermia, (b) hypoxemia, and (c) metabolic acidosis. He may have been resuscitated without good thermal control, which hastened his drop in body temperature. Infants with prenatal asphyxia have been noted to have a greater drop in body temperature during the first hours of life. His $PaCO_2$ is not elevated, but he is not making a respiratory adjustment for the metabolic acidosis as one might expect in the "normal" infant.

How should they be handled?

Provide an increased concentration in the oxygen environment and treat with bicarbonate (4 mEq. per Kg.) and repeat the pH and HCO_3.

Our response would have been to initially provide an acute expansion of blood volume with 10 cc. per Kg. with either blood or plasma to improve tissue perfusion and oxygenation, which would provide improvement in the infant's circulation and pH simultaneously.

G. ODELL

What problem is noted at one hour?

The blood pressure has dropped (but the hematocrit has not).

How do you explain what happened?

Hypoxemia or acidemia alone or in combination may result in an elevation of blood pressure. Partial correction of the metabolic acidosis and raising the PaO_2 probably reduced the increased peripheral vascular resistance. The low blood pressure suggests a severely reduced blood volume. Blood volume should be expanded.

Case Three

E. F. is an 1100-gm. female. Her Apgar at one minute $= 1$. She was bagged at 10 minutes, and has been grunting since that time. The chest X-ray was compatible with the diagnosis of respiratory distress syndrome.

Should NaHCO₃ be given one hour after Blood Gas #6?

No. Her pH, $PaCO_2$ and HCO_3 are within the normal range.

Should anything else be changed?

Yes. The hood temperature is too low. At this level, metabolic rate (oxygen consumption) is increased. It should be raised to her neutral temperature (incubator temperature).

At 11 hours, should anything be changed?

Yes. The hood temperature is still ignored. Also, the environmental oxygen should be increased. At this low oxygen tension, metabolic acidosis and death often quickly ensue.

At 18 hours, after Blood Gas #10, should anything be changed?

Yes. Hood temperature, environmental oxygen, and a dash of bicarbonate.

It is quite obvious that the patient is suffering from CO_2 retention. Why not bag her rather than give a "dash of hypertonic HCO_3," which will only further increase pCO_2?

G. ODELL

Check X-ray for pneumothorax; repeat the hematocrit.

At 25 hours, what is the prognosis? What next?

As things stand, she will probably not survive without some additional treatment. We would have started continuous positive airway pressure using nasal CPAP when greater than 70 per cent oxygen was required to maintain PaO_2 above 50 to 60 mm. Hg.

Case Four

G. H. is a 2000-gm. male, grunting since birth. His X-ray reveals questionable respiratory distress syndrome. He has been placed in 70 per cent oxygen and given NaHCO₃.

At three hours, what would you do, if anything?

Decrease environmental oxygen to 60 per cent and repeat the PaO_2 in 30 minutes. This is a dangerous level of oxygen.

At four and one-half hours, what should be done next?

Decrease environmental oxygen concentration to 50 per cent and repeat PaO_2 in 30 minutes.

What happened at five hours? What now?

This patient demonstrated the "flip-flop" phenomenon which sometimes occurs when environmental oxygen is decreased. First, return the baby to an oxygen concentration of 60 to 70 per cent. Second, obtain a chest X-ray to rule out the possibility of pneumothorax. Determine another blood oxygen tension in 15 or 20 minutes after the environmental oxygen has been increased.

What is the explanation for what happened between four and one-half and five and one-half hours of life?

There is not a complete physiologic explanation underlying the "flip-flop" phenomenon. It is assumed that in some infants the pulmonary vessels are particularly sensitive to changes in oxygen tension, and lowering the environmental oxygen results in pulmonary vasoconstriction and an increased right-to-left shunt. Under these circumstances, the PaO_2 will drop out of proportion to what might ordinarily be expected when the environmental oxygen is reduced.

REFERENCES

1. Aherne, W., Cross, K., Hey, A., et al: Lung function and pathology in a premature infant with chronic pulmonary insufficiency (Wilson-Mikity syndrome). Pediatrics 40:962, 1967.
2. Avery, M., and Mead, J.: Surface properties in relation to atelectasis and hyaline membrane disease. Amer J Dis Child 97:517, 1959.
3. Avery, M., Frank, N., and Gribetz, I.: The inflationary force produced by pulmonary vascular distention in excised lungs. The possible relation of this force to that needed to inflate the lungs at birth. J Clin Invest 38:456, 1959.
4. Avery, M., Gatewood, O., and Brumley, G.: Transient tachypnea of newborn. Amer J Dis Child 111:380, 1966.
5. Bartlett, D., Jr.: Postnatal growth of the mammalian lung. Influence of exercise and thyroid activity. Resp Physiol 9:50, 1970.
6. Bartlett, D., Jr.: Postnatal growth of the mammalian lung. Influence of low and high oxygen tensions. Resp Physiol 9:58, 1970.

7. Boston, R., Geller, F., and Smith, C.: Arterial blood gas tensions and acid-base balance in the management of the respiratory distress syndrome. J Pediat 68:74, 1966.

8. Brumley, G., Hodson, W., and Avery, M.: Lung phospholipids and surface tension correlations in infants with and without hyaline membrane disease. Pediatrics 40:13, 1967.

9. Burnard, E.: The pulmonary syndrome of Wilson and Mikity and respiratory function in very small premature infants. Pediat Clin N Amer 13:999,1966.

10. Burnard, E., and Grauaug, A.: Dyspnoea and apnoea in the newborn: Some results of investigation. Med J Aust 1:445, 1965.

11. Burnard, E., Grattan-Smith, P., Picton-Warlow, C., et al: Pulmonary insufficiency in prematurity. Aust Paed J 1:12, 1965.

12. Campiche, M., Jaccottet, M., and Juillard, E.: La pneumonose à membranes hyalines. Observations au microscope électronique. Ann Pediat 199:74, 1962.

13. Chu, J., Clements, J., Cotton, E., et al: The pulmonary hypoperfusion syndrome. Pediatrics 35: 733, 1965.

14. Chu, J., Clements, J., Cotton, E., et al: Neonatal pulmonary ischemia. Pediatrics 40:709, 1967.

15. Cole, V., Normand, I., Reynolds, E., et al: Pathogenesis of hemorrhagic pulmonary edema and massive pulmonary hemorrhage in the newborn. Pediatrics 51:175, 1973.

16. Daily, W., Klaus, M., and Meyer, H.: Apnea in premature infants: monitoring, incidence, heart rate changes, and an effect of environmental temperature. Pediatrics 43:510, 1969.

17. Dawes, G.: Foetal and Neonatal Physiology. Chicago, Year Book Medical Publishers, 1968.

18. Esterley, J., and Oppenheimer, E.: Massive pulmonary hemorrhage in the newborn. I. Pathologic considerations. J Pediat 69:3, 1966.

19. Fanaroff, A., and Reiter, E.: Personal communication.

20. Fanaroff, A., Aladjem, S., France, F., et al: Identification of the high-risk infant from placental phase microscopy. Pediat Res 5:411, 1971.

21. Frederick, J., and Butler, N.: Certain causes of neonatal death. IV. Massive pulmonary hemorrhage. Biol Neonat 18:243, 1971.

22. Gluck, L., Kulovich, M., and Borer, R., Jr.: Diagnosis of the respiratory distress syndrome by amniocentesis. Amer J Obstet Gynec 109:440, 1971.

23. Gribetz, P., Cook, C., O'Brien, D., et al: Studies of respiratory physiology in the newborn infant. II. Observations during and after respiratory distress. Acta Paediat 43:397, 1954.

24. Hodgman, J., Mikity, V., Tatter, D., et al: Chronic respiratory distress in the premature infant: Wilson-Mikity syndrome. Pediatrics 44:179, 1969.

25. Kapanci, Y., Weibel, E., Kaplan, H., et al: Pathogenesis and reversibility of the pulmonary lesions of oxygen toxicity in monkeys. II. Ultrastructural and morphometric studies. Lab Invest 20:101, 1969.

26. Kaplan, H., Robinson, F., Kapanci, Y., et al: Pathogenesis and reversibility of the pulmonary lesions of oxygen toxicity in monkeys. I. Clinical and light microscopic studies. Lab Invest 20: 94, 1969.

27. Kinsey, V., Jacobus, J., and Hemphill, F.: Retro-

lental fibroplasia: Cooperative study of retrolental fibroplasia and the use of oxygen. AMA Arch Ophthal 56:481, 1956.

28. Kitterman, J., Phibbs, R., and Tooley, W.: Aortic blood pressure in normal newborn infants during the first 12 hours of life. Pediatrics 44:959, 1969.

29. Klaus, M.: Respiratory function and pulmonary disease in the newborn. In Barnett, H., Ed.: Pediatrics. New York, Appleton-Century-Crofts, 1972. 15th Edition, pp. 1255–61.

30. Klaus, M., and Meyer, B.: Oxygen therapy for the newborn. Pediat Clin N Amer 13:731, 1966.

31. Lauweryns, J.: Pulmonary arterial vasculature in neonatal hyaline membrane disease. Science 153:1275, 1966.

32. Macklin, C.: Transport of air along sheaths of pulmonic blood vessels from alveoli to mediastinum. Arch Intern Med 64:913, 1939.

33. Miller, H., Behrle, F., and Smull, N.: Severe apnea and irregular respiratory rhythms among premature infants. Pediatrics 23:676, 1959.

34. Möller, Eva-Brita: Studies in Diabetic Pregnancy. Lund, Dept. of Obstetrics and Gynecology, Central Hospital, Boras, Sweden, 1970.

35. Nelson, N.: On the etiology of hyaline membrane disease. Pediat Clin N Amer 17:943, 1970.

36. Nelson, N., Prod'hom, L., Cherry, R., et al: Pulmonary function in the newborn infant. II. Perfusion—Estimation by analysis of the arterial-alveolar carbon dioxide difference. Pediatrics 30:975, 1962.

37. Northway, W., Rosan, R., and Porter, D.: Pulmonary disease following respirator therapy. New Eng J Med 276:357, 1967.

38. Oski, F., and Naiman, J.: Hematologic Problems in the Newborn. Philadelphia, W. B. Saunders Co., 1966.

39. Prod'hom, L., Levison, H., Cherry, R., et al: Adjustment of ventilation, intrapulmonary gas exchange and acid-base balance during the first day of life: Infants with early respiratory distress. Pediatrics 35:662, 1965.

40. Perlstein, P., Edwards, H., and Sutherland, J.: Apnea in premature infants and incubator-air temperature changes. New Eng J Med 282:461, 1970.

41. Roberton, N., Gupta, J., Dahlenberg, G., et al: Oxygen therapy in the newborn. Lancet 1:7556, 1968.

42. Rowe, S., and Avery, M.: Massive pulmonary hemorrhage in the newborn. II. Clinical considerations. J Pediat 69:12, 1966.

43. Rudolph, J., Desmond, M., and Pineda, R.: Clinical diagnosis of respiratory difficulty in the newborn. Pediat Clin N Amer 13:669, 1966.

44. Sinclair, J.: Prevention and treatment of the respiratory distress syndrome. Pediat Clin N Amer 13:711, 1966.

45. Stahlman, M., Battersby, E., Shepard, F., et al: Prognosis in hyaline membrane disease. New Eng J Med 276:303, 1967.

46. Strang, L., and MacLeish, M.: Ventilatory failure and right-to-left shunt in newborn infants with respiratory distress. Pediatrics 28:17, 1961.

47. Swyer, P., Delivoria-Papadopolous, M., Levison, H., et al: The pulmonary syndrome of Wilson and Mikity. Pediatrics 36:374, 1965.

48. Wilson, M., and Mikity, V.: A new form of respiratory disease in premature infants. Amer J Dis Child 99:489, 1960.

Chapter 9

ASSISTED VENTILATION

by
ANN LLEWELLYN, M.D., M.R.C.P. (London)
and
PAUL SWYER, M.B., M.R.C.P. (London)

"But that life may, in a manner of speaking, be restored to the animal, an opening must be attempted in the trunk of the trachea, into which a tube or reed or cane should be put; you will then blow into this so that the lung may rise again and the animal take in air. Indeed, with a single breath in the case of this living animal, the lung will swell to the full extent of the thoracic cavity and the heart become strong and exhibit a wondrous variety of motions . . . when the lung long flaccid has collapsed, the beat of the heart and arteries appears wavy, creepy, twisting, but when the lung is inflated, it becomes strong again and swift and displays wondrous variations . . . and as I do this, and take care that the lung is inflated at intervals, the motion of the heart and arteries does not stop."

ANDREAS VESALIUS, *De Humani Corporis Fabrica,* 1543

The primary objective of assisted ventilation is to undertake gas exchange until there is recovery from the potentially reversible pathologic process which has caused respiratory failure. Hence, it follows that prior to instituting therapy the following facilities must be available: continuous expert nursing and medical care; a suitable mechanical ventilator and inhalation therapy support; and a means of monitoring therapy, i.e., blood gas estimations.

This chapter is only intended as an introduction to assisted ventilation. Before undertaking mechanical ventilation or continuous positive airway pressure (CPAP), it must be recognized that the techniques require experienced personnel, suitable equipment, and are demanding on time and resources. It is advised that before introducing a program of assisted ventilation in a unit, the supervising physician and nurse spend at least 14 days observing in a center where these techniques have been well established.

BACKGROUND

The following conditions may be associated with respiratory failure in the newborn infant (Table 9–1) which may be treated with assisted ventilation. Infants with respiratory distress syndrome (RDS) constitute the greatest number of patients receiving mechanical ventilation.

Definition of Respiratory Failure

1. Rising arterial pCO_2.

2. Falling arterial pO_2 despite increased concentration of inspired oxygen.

3. Increasing acidosis, i.e., falling pH —

TABLE 9–1 CONDITIONS ASSOCIATED WITH RESPIRATORY FAILURE IN THE NEWBORN

PULMONARY	EXTRAPULMONARY
Respiratory distress syndrome	Cerebral hemorrhage or edema
Aspiration syndrome	Effect of drugs
Pulmonary hemorrhage	Extreme immaturity
Pneumonia	Tetanus neonatorum
Pneumothorax	
Diaphragmatic hernia	
Mikity-Wilson syndrome	
Bronchopulmonary dysplasia	

partly respiratory due to high pCO_2; partly metabolic due to hypoxemia.

Clinical Manifestations of Respiratory Failure in the Newborn

1. Fall in respiratory rate or periods of apnea.

2. Cyanosis unrelieved by high concentration of inspired oxygen.

3. Falling blood pressure and tachycardia progressing to pallor, evidence of peripheral circulatory failure, and bradycardia.

CONTINUOUS POSITIVE AIRWAY PRESSURE

The application of continuous positive airway pressure (CPAP) throughout the respiratory cycle constitutes a major break-through in the treatment of severe RDS in infancy.

Gregory's exciting studies demonstrate that gas exchange in RDS can be significantly improved by applying a constant positive pressure to the airway. CPAP is now the first method we use to assist ventilation of the infant severely ill with RDS. Because of surfactant deficiency in RDS, alveoli tend to collapse easily. The resulting atelectatic areas of lung are the sites of shunting from right to left. When alveoli are prevented from closing by maintaining a continuous positive transpulmonary pressure throughout the respiratory cycle, functional residual capacity (FRC) increases and there is improved ventilation of perfused areas of lung, resulting in a marked decrease in intrapulmonary shunt. We start CPAP whenever more than 70 per cent oxygen is needed to maintain a PaO_2 greater than 50 to 60 mm. Hg. Continuous positive transpulmonary pressure may be achieved by either applying continuous positive airway pressure (CPAP) or applying continuous negative pressure to the body wall (CNP). *CPAP is useful only in infants with decreased lung compliance. In other pulmonary conditions it can be harmful.*

The technique for applying CPAP has been developed primarily by Gregory et al.[4] and a modification of their technique is shown in Figure 9–1.

1. A suitable air/oxygen mixture (total flow not exceeding 5 liters per minute) passes through a humidifier. Gas passes to the elbow, which is attached to an endotracheal tube.

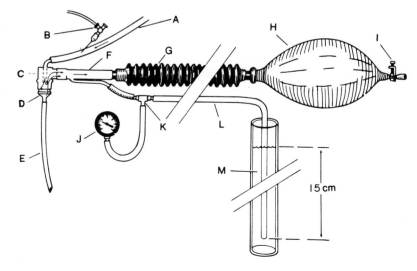

Figure 9–1 System for applying continuous positive airway pressure (CPAP) through an endotracheal tube. (Adapted from Gregory et al.[4]). A = gas flow. B = oxygen sampling port. C = Normal elbow (modified T piece). D = endotracheal-tube connector. E = endotracheal tube. F = Sommers T piece. G = corrugated anesthesia hose. H = reservoir bag (500 ml.) with open tail piece. I = screw clamp. J = aneroid pressure manometer. K = plastic T connector. L = plastic tubing (1 cm. internal diameter). M = underwater "pop-off." Arrows indicate direction of gas flow.

The screw clamp on the reservoir bag is used to control the flow of gas and maintain a constant positive pressure within the system, as indicated on the pressure manometer. The side-arm ends under a column of water (15 cm). This acts as an underwater safety valve.

2. An endotracheal tube initially was the most successful when using CPAP, but alternative methods have now been developed which avoid the risks of intubation (see below).

3. Initially 6 cm. H_2O of continuous airway pressure is used. If this fails to produce an improvement in 20 minutes, 8, 10, and 12 cm. of H_2O are then tried. The highest level of continuous airway pressure used is +15 cm. H_2O. These positive pressures at the airway are not completely transmitted to the pleural space because of the severely reduced pulmonary compliance. Hence, venous return and cardiac output are not compromised.

4. An initial improvement in arterial oxygen tension usually occurs on applying CPAP. Priority should be given to reducing environmental oxygen by decrements of five per cent until reaching 40 per cent. Then the level of CPAP may be slowly reduced 1 cm. H_2O at a time. Total weaning from CPAP may take several days.

5. Recurrent apnea is not a contraindication to a trial of the use of CPAP. Indeed, apnea sometimes ceases on applying CPAP. The mechanism is not well understood, but may be related to activation of sensory stretch receptors in the lung or improvement in brain oxygenation.

Nursing and medical management, tube care, etc., are as exacting as during mechanical ventilation.

Other methods of applying continuous positive airway pressure have been developed which avoid the use of an endotracheal tube. A head box designed by Gregory may be useful, although it can be difficult to obtain an effective neck seal. Barrie[1] has described the use of a "head bag" in which a large plastic bag is used to maintain constant positive pressure at the airway.

A method of providing continuous positive transpulmonary pressure has been devised using a negative pressure respirator. Constant negative pressure to the infant's body, with the head at atmospheric pressure, achieves the same beneficial physiologic effect as endotracheal CPAP. The technique is effective in both RDS and the management of very small (<1200 gm.) premature infants with recurrent apnea and progressive atelectasis. In the latter group, maintenance of these infants at 3 to 5 cm. H_2O constant negative pressure for prolonged periods has occasionally been effective.

We recently completed a sequential controlled trial* of continuous negative pressure (CNP) versus oxygen in severe respiratory distress syndrome (PaO_2 <60 mm. Hg in environmental oxygen concentrations —FiO_2— of 70 per cent or greater). CNP was applied by means of a newly designed, inexpensive, plastic chamber. Twenty-nine infants with similar birth weights, sexes, gestational ages, and ages and blood gases at the time of admission to the trial were studied. Study failure was defined as a PaO_2 <50 mm. Hg in 100 per cent oxygen, or the onset of apnea. Sequential analysis revealed CNP was superior to the oxygen-control group (p<.05). CNP improved oxygenation in RDS, and significantly reduced duration of exposure to high oxygen concentrations and the need for respirator therapy.

CPAP or CNP has thus been successfully applied via endotracheal tube (Gregory), sealed head chamber (Gregory), pressurized plastic bag enclosing the head of the infant (Barrie), nasal mask (Harris), modified negative pressure respirator (Vidyasagar), and plastic body chamber (Fanaroff). All of these methods are associated with potentially undesirable complications. The endotracheal tube is irritating to the airway, eliminates much of the normal ciliary activity of the trachea, and may easily become occluded or dislodged. The positive pressure hood, plastic head bag, or CNP body chamber all tend to isolate the infant and prevent accessibility without temporary interruption of therapy. Potentially harmful effects of positive pressure to the eyes, cooling of the face, high sound levels, and fluctuations of oxygen concentration are problems presented by several of the systems. All of these methods appear to be associated with a significant incidence of pneumothorax. We are, therefore, using nasal tubes for the application of CPAP, and have found this method very successful.

Agostino and associates in Italy have designed an apparatus which cannulates both nares and thus provides CPAP without violating the lower airway. Thus, the infant is easily accessible without interruption of therapy, and the complications mentioned above are avoided. We have modified this apparatus.**

The nasal piece (Figure 9–2 A and B)*** is moulded from Silastic and strapped to the infant's head in

*Fanaroff, A., Cha, C., Sosa, R., Crumrine, R., et al: Controlled trial of continuous negative external pressure in the treatment of severe respiratory distress syndrome. J Pediat, 1973 (in press).

**Adapted from G. Duc, Zurich.

***Dr. David Fleming, Biomedical Engineering Department, Case Western Reserve University.

the same manner as oxygen prongs in older children (see Table 9–2). The small tubes have an outer diameter of 4.5 mm. and enter the nares for a distance of approximately 1 cm. Additional dead space is minimal. At steady flow rates of less than 3 liters per minute through the nasal unit, the resistance also was found to be small (pressure drop of less than 1 cm. H_2O). This value is about half of that produced by an endotracheal tube of 3.0 mm. inner diameter with similar flow rate. This size unit is adequate for use on infants with birth weights from about 1100 to 2100 gm., but is slightly too tight or loose for the small group of infants who fall outside of that weight range. (We are presently designing units for use in very small and large infants.) With the exception of the substitution of the nasal device for the endotracheal tube and the insertion of an orogastric tube, the rest of the apparatus is essentially identical to that described by Gregory et al.

To date, 37 infants have been treated with nasal CPAP when PaO_2 <60 mm. Hg in FiO 70 per cent or greater, and there have been minimal complications. Two infants had mild ulceration of the external nares secondary to pressure necrosis from the device. Both have healed completely, and this complication has not recurred since the unit has been redesigned by changing the angle of the nasal prongs (Figure 9–2 A). No pneumothoraces have been encountered, in contrast to the significant incidence of this complication in other series. Perhaps the absence of this complication in the present series is a result of the physiologic "blow-off" at high pressures provided by the infant's unrestricted mouth.

CPAP significantly improves arterial oxygenation

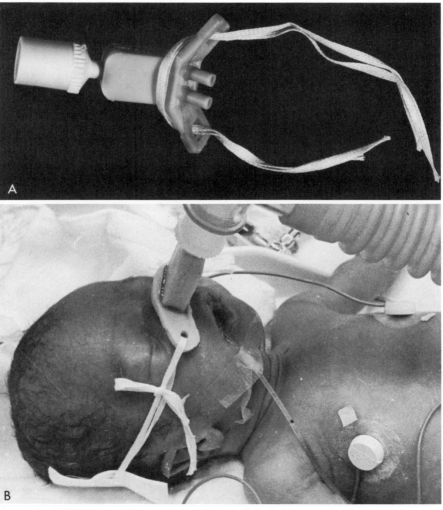

Figure 9–2 Nasal CPAP. *A*. Silastic device for administration of nasal CPAP. *B*. Nasal CPAP unit in place on infant.

TABLE 9-2   GUIDELINES FOR THE USE OF NASAL CPAP* AT RAINBOW BABIES' AND CHILDREN'S HOSPITAL, CLEVELAND, OHIO (Refer to the Gregory apparatus, Fig. 9–1, for diagram of the apparatus proximal to the nasal piece.)

1. Consider CPAP therapy when PaO_2 <60 mm. Hg with FiO_2 >70%.
2. Insert orogastric tube. This is left open to atmosphere or intermittently suctioned to allow for stomach decompression. It is not necessary to tape the mouth closed.
3. Before connecting the nasal piece to the system, check the following:
   A. Nebulizer is warm and adequately filled with water;
   B. Safety valve is in place and set at about 20 cm. H_2O;
   C. Pinch clamp on anesthesia bag is completely open;
   D. Oxygen concentration is equal to that of FiO_2 prior to initiation of CPAP;
   E. Flow rate from nebulizer is between 6 and 12 liters per minute.
4. Apply 1% hydrocortisone cream to nasal prongs. Prongs should be cut to a length of 1 cm.
5. Connect nasal piece to system and insert in infant's nares. (Manometer pressure should be reading zero.)
6. Secure device to infant's head as shown in Figure 9–2 B.
7. Gradually increase the pressure in the system by tightening the pinch clamp on the anesthesia bag until the desired pressure is achieved.
8. After stabilization (10–20 minutes), obtain a blood gas determination.
9. Try various pressures (e.g., 6, 8, 10, 12) to achieve the best PaO_2 without significant elevation of $PaCO_2$. (Final pressure is usually 8–10 cm. H_2O. At pressures between 7 and 12 cm. H_2O, the blow-off through the mouth becomes evident.)
10. Adjust FiO_2 to keep the PaO_2 between 60 and 90 mm. Hg.
11. Lower FiO_2 gradually as blood gases dictate, but by no greater than 5% decrements.
12. Bag breathe the infant for 3 minutes every 30 minutes by holding the mouth closed, using pressures from 25–35 cm. H_2O.
13. Always check to be sure there is sufficient flow coming from outflow of anesthesia bag. If flow at this point is too low:
    A. There is a leak in the system at the wall, nebulizer, or tubing; in which case the infant may be rebreathing his own expired gas.
      OR
    B. The nasal device is too loose in the infant's nose, so that there is a large flow through the nasal unit. If this is so, the resistance of the unit is significant and actual nasopharyngeal pressure may be considerably lower than is indicated by the system manometer.
14. When FiO_2 has reached 40%, begin to lower CPAP by 1 to 2-cm. decrements, with a blood gas determination after each change.
15. When CPAP = 0 and FiO_2 = 40%, remove the device and place the infant in an oxygen hood.

*Kattwinkel, J., Fleming, D., Cha, C., et al: A device for administering continuous positive airway pressure by the nasal route. Pediatrics, 1973 (in press).

in RDS, shortens the exposure time to high concentrations of oxygen, and arrests the downhill progression of the disease, thus lessening the need for mechanical assisted ventilation. We believe that application of the principle by the nasal technique renders the treatment effective, simple, inexpensive, safe, and readily available to any nursery involved with intensive care of the sick neonate.

If CPAP fails (i.e., adequate arterial gases cannot be maintained, or if the infant becomes apneic), mechanical ventilation or intermittent bagging using the CPAP set-up is required. It is sometimes desirable to apply the principle of continuous positive airway pressure after initating mechanical ventilation. During the expiratory phase, the gas in most ventilators is vented to the atmosphere and circuit pressure dropped to atmosphere. If expired gas is passed through a resistance or under a column of water (Figure 9–3), positive circuit pressure may be maintained. The technique of CPAP may also be usefully applied during weaning from mechanical ventilation.

EDITORS

There is concern about the early administration of continuous positive airway pressure, for, if the lungs are compliant, this pressure will be translated to the pulmonary circulation and reduce cardiac output. If the lungs are stiff, this pressure is not going to interfere with cardiac output. As a rule, we place the infant on continuous positive pressure if arterial PaO_2 cannot be maintained above 45 mm. Hg at ambient oxygen concentrations greater than 60 per cent or if the infant is apneic. We prefer the use of nasal catheters rather than endotracheal tubes for administering positive pressure, and we also place a feeding tube in the stomach and close the mouth to prevent inflation of the gastrointestinal tract.

G. ODELL

When establishing guidelines for the use of equipment, it is extremely important to allow for flexibility; rigid rules applied from one institution may not necessarily be equally applicable in another. In our experience, we have been able to use successfully

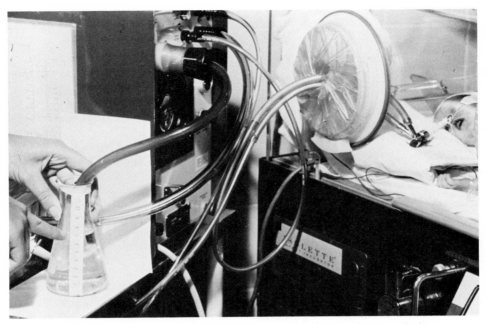

Figure 9–3 Positive expiratory pressure during mechanical ventilation.

intermittent negative pressure ventilation in infants well below 1500 gm. Although the survival rate is not nearly as high as it would be in infants greater than 1500 gm., we have nevertheless successfully carried infants on such equipment, with our smallest survivor in the range of 1100 gm. We have not been successful with its use below 1000 gm., but nevertheless do believe that it affords a number of advantages over the use of positive pressure respirators and is, therefore, in our department, when feasible, the mechanism of choice following an initial attempt at the use of continuous negative pressure (CNP). The success rate with any ventilator is heavily dependent on the facility with which the personnel in any individual department use it and their experience with it. It is, therefore, our belief that any institution should and must use whatever equipment it finds most appropriate and efficacious in the management of these infants. For ourselves, we prefer the negative pressure ventilators for a number of reasons, prime among which is the lack of an intratracheal tube. It is our contention that this avoids the occurrence of bronchopulmonary dysplasia or respirator lung disease, irrespective of the length of time that the infant needs to be kept on the ventilator, and irrespective of the use of high concentrations of oxygen even for prolonged periods. We consider this to be a major advantage and, although we recognize some of the shortcomings, particularly with regard to the difficulty of feeding an infant on prolonged ventilator therapy, we prefer it as an initial attempt when possible. No single means of mechanical ventilation is most efficacious for every infant; indeed, various permutations

and combinations of different respirators and alterations in their usage with any individual infant should not only be tried and explored but applied when deemed appropriate. Thus, we have utilized both continuous negative pressure alone, intermittent negative pressure alone, positive pressure using a residual end expiratory pressure (PEEP), as well as a combination of intermittent positive pressure and continuous negative pressure as a residual phenomenon, all of which have under different circumstances yielded efficacious results in a number of cases. Finally, we should stress that our own use of intermittent negative pressure has always involved the maintenance of a residual negative pressure during expiration so that when a pressure swing of 40 mm. Hg is desired, the equipment is usually set to operate between −44 mm. Hg and −4 mm. Hg. It is highly possible that this type of usage of INPV may well have accounted for the apparent greater success with this equipment in our department than has been reported from other institutions in which the equipment has been used.

L. STERN

INDICATIONS FOR INITIATING MECHANICAL VENTILATION

These depend on the facilities available at a center, the attitudes of the medical attendants towards a potentially hazardous therapy, their previous experience with the technique, and on reported experience in other units. Indications in current usage include:

1. pO_2 less than 40 mm. Hg in 100 per cent oxygen in two consecutive arterial samples (see Table 8–3).

2. Apnea not responding to usual resuscitative measures.

3. Prognostic scoring systems derived from data of large numbers of infants and incorporating multiple factors (e.g., age, gestation, birth weight, temperature, as well as blood gas status).[7, 12] (See Table 8–5.)

VENTILATORS*

PRINCIPLES OF MECHANICAL VENTILATION

The principle of all mechanical ventilators is to achieve a pressure gradient producing flow of gas into the lung. This may be by intermittently building up a positive pressure in the airway or by intermittently creating a negative pressure around the chest wall.

Innumerable mechanical ventilators are commercially available. The clinician should learn to understand one or two ventilator circuits available to him.

INTERMITTENT POSITIVE PRESSURE VENTILATORS

The two types of intermittent positive pressure ventilators currently in use are the flow generator and the pressure generator. The *pressure generator* determines the pressure pattern at the airway and the flow changes are determined by the compliance and resistance of the patient's lungs.

The *flow generator* determines the pattern of flow in the lungs and the pressure changes depend on the physical characteristics of the lungs. *Constant flow generators* (e.g., Bird, Blease, Bourns) produce a steadily rising volume and pressure with an abrupt fall to atmospheric pressure at the onset of expiration. Flow remains constant even in the face of increased airway resistance and a reduction in compliance. *Variable flow generators* (e.g., Engström) generate an accelerating gas flow pattern with an increase in flow rate to mid-inspiration with a falling-off at the end of inspiration. This may be helpful in providing optimal distribution of gas.

*For a listing of mechanical ventilators and their suppliers, see Appendix 18.

Cycling

Ventilators may be:

Pressure-cycled—the end of inspiration is determined by a pre-set pressure being attained. The advantage of pressure-cycling is that small leaks in the circuit (e.g., around the endotracheal tube) will be adequately compensated for without loss of tidal volume. Examples of this type of ventilator include Cyclator, and Bird Mark VII and Mark VIII.

Volume-cycled—inspiration ends when a pre-set volume is delivered by the pump. Although tidal volume is lost in the presence of leaks, this type of cycling is advantageous in the presence of some types of lung disease. Even with severe reduction of lung compliance or a varying lung compliance, tidal volume will remain adequate. Examples of this type of ventilator include Beaver Mark III, Starling pump, and Bourns "Pediatric."

Time-cycled—the exact duration of inspiration is predetermined. Examples are the Amsterdam Infant Ventilator, Engström, East Radcliffe.

Flow-cycled—inspiration ends when gas flow falls below a critical level, as on all models of Bennett ventilators.

Mixed—utilizing more than one form of cycling. For example, a volume-cycled ventilator may have a pressure-relief valve, so that when a maximum pressure is reached, inspiration ends, regardless of the volume delivered.

Special Considerations for Infant Ventilators

The ventilators should deliver a suitable gas volume (tidal volume = 5 ml. per Kg. body weight) and compensate for loss of gas volume by compression, dead space, and leaks.

In a large ventilator circuit, compression volumes may be prohibitively high with high inflation pressures. Hence, keep circuit volumes low, use nondistensible tubing, and calculate actual compression loss prior to using the ventilator.

High cycling frequencies and sensitive patient triggering may be required. There should be provision for a wide range of air/oxygen mixtures, and the ability to vary I:E ratios to as high as 4:1. Remember that the airway resistance is high (approximately 30 cm. H_2O/1-second); hence, a large pressure drop occurs down the small airways.

Intermittent positive pressure. It may be

applied using a tracheostomy or an endo-tracheal tube.

Use of Tracheostomy. For prolonged mechanical ventilation of the newborn, the use of tracheostomy has been superseded in most centers by nasotracheal tubes, as it is fraught with the hazards of tube displacement, infection, and an inability to extubate because of the development of stenosis.

Use of Endotracheal Tubes. Naso-tracheal tubes (NTT) are generally used for prolonged ventilation, so they must be biologically safe.

1. Size.
   If b.w. < 1250 gm. = 2.5 mm. int. diam.
   1250 to 2000 gm. = 3.0 mm. int. diam.
   2000 gm. = 3.5 mm. int. diam.

2. *Insertion of a naso-endotracheal tube* should be performed as a sterile procedure. Intubation should be performed under a radiant heat lamp. Use a laryngoscope with Miller 0 or 1 blade, visualize the glottis by slight extension of the head and pressure on the glottis.

Insert the lubricated NTT through the nares until visualized in the oropharynx. McGill forceps may be needed to guide it into the glottis. It is helpful if the plastic endotracheal tube has been previously curved.

Do not use a stylet during intubation.

Do not make repeated attempts at intubation without allowing the infant to "recover" with manual ventilation with O_2.

3. The tip of the NTT should be midway between the carina and the glottis. (See Figure 9–4.) Check the air entry bilaterally after insertion. It is easy to allow the NTT to pass into the right main stem bronchus. The position should be checked radiologically at the completion of the procedure.

4. The NTT should be secured so that movement of the head and neck will not dislodge the tube (Figure 9–5). Use lightweight plastic connectors in order to avoid kinking the tube.

5. Suctioning is potentially dangerous because it may introduce infection; it may result in an anoxic episode by discontinuing ventilation and extracting gas from small airways producing atelectasis; and it may produce traumatic lesions in the trachea at the site of the suction catheter tip.

Hence, suction only when necessary, and briefly, using a strict sterile technique with disposable gloves and suction tubes. The infant must be allowed to "recover" between episodes of suctioning.

Routine instillation of saline to facili-

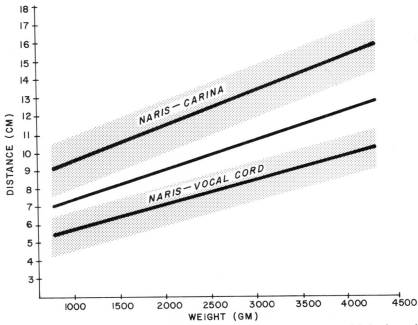

Figure 9–4 The relation of naris-carina and naris-glottis distance with body weight.[3]

tate removal of secretions is used in some centers. However, if adequate nebulization is used, this is not necessary.

6. Changing of an endotracheal tube is indicated if the tube becomes dislodged or blocked. Routine changing of the NTT is probably not indicated.

Setting Up the Positive Pressure Ventilator

It is essential that the clinician understand the circuit, the capabilities, and the principles of one ventilator. Prior to starting mechanical ventilation:

1. *Check that the circuit to be used is leakproof.* This may be done by cycling the ventilator with a finger over the patient outlet. At this time you may set a pressure relief valve at the maximum pressure to be achieved.

2. *Ensure that the nebulization of inspirated gas is adequate* — that the ultrasonic nebulizer or conventional heated nebulizer is functioning.

Temperature gradients between the air outside the infant's incubator and inside the incubator will tend to result in condensation of water in respirator tubing. Hence, keep the volume of tubing outside the incubator minimal and maintain the temperature of the nebulizer to just avoid condensation in tubings inside the incubator. Inspired gas at body temperature will then be approximately 70 per cent saturated.

3. *Select ventilator settings suitable for patient.* There are no absolute rules for selection of tidal volume, etc. Although there has been very little assessment of the effect of altering ventilator settings on gas exchange, we recommend the following:

If volume-cycled. The tidal volume as delivered by the ventilator must be adequate to normalize arterial oxygen and carbon dioxide, and consists of: (1) infant's tidal volume (5 ml. per Kg.); (2) compression loss in the ventilator tubings (if ventilator tubing volume is large, this may be appreciable—

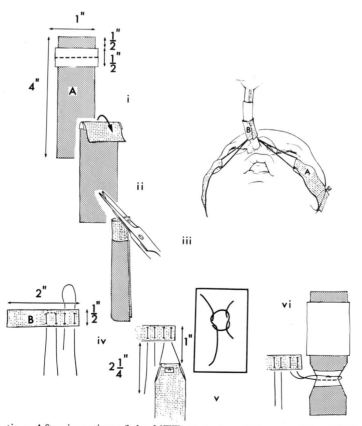

Figure 9–5 Method of attachment of endotracheal tube.

1. Place 1″ long piece of polyethylene tubing about ½″ from one end of a 4″ × 1″ piece of adhesive nonelastic tape (A) on the adhesive surface as shown in (i) and roll over the short end-portion to enclose the tubing as shown in (ii).

2. Trim the edges of the folded portion so as to taper to a width of approximately ½″ (iii). Cover the adhesive surface of the remainder of the tape with waxed paper strip, leaving bare a small portion near the folded end extending a little beyond the other free end.

3. Place two loops of linen thread close to each other in one end of a 2″ × ½″ strip (B) of adhesive nonelastic tape as shown in (iv).

4. Thread one arm of the loop through the polyethylene tubing—enclosed in the folded end of (A)—and close the loop with a knot so as to have a distance of about 1″ between the two adhesive tape pieces (A and B) (v).

5. Application procedure: prepare the skin with benzoin application. After insertion of the NTT, wrap tape (B) around the NTT, close to the nostril. Holding the tube in situ, remove the wax paper strip from (A) and stick firmly to the skin, keeping the linen thread taut. For quick removal of the tube, cut the linen thread. Subsequent NTT may be fixed by a new set of tapes applied over the old.

these volumes must be known prior to using the ventilator, from either manufacturer's instructions or preferably from direct measurement[10]); and (3) volume losses by leaks from the tubing system and around the NTT.

If pressure-cycled. The peak inflation pressure will depend on the compliance of the lungs. In most infants, a pressure of 25 cm. H_2O is a reasonable starting point. Current evidence is that increasing airway pressure improves oxygenation[2, 6, 12] but increases the risk of a pneumothorax.

4. *Assisted (patient-triggered) vs. controlled ventilation.* Assisted ventilation may be desirable and more physiological than controlled ventilation if the ventilator has a rapid response time and high sensitivity and the infant has good respiratory efforts. *Controlled ventilation* is more appropriate if the infant is apneic or has poor respiratory effort, or you wish to control cycling frequency and I:E ratio.

5. *Cycling frequency of controlled ventilation.* Current evidence is that very high (80+) cycling frequencies may be associated with lower PaO_2 than low cycling frequencies (30 per minute).[12] Frequency is closely associated with inspiratory-expiratory (I:E) ratio. The latter is also related to inspiratory flow rate. Optimal I:E ratio would seem to vary from patient to patient depending on the condition of the lung.[9] Reynolds,[12] however, has found that progressive increase in inspiratory phase (i.e., I:E ratio up to 4:1) results in a progressive rise in PaO_2 in infants with hyaline membrane disease (HMD). This is a most significant observation, since these high ratios and low frequencies permit ventilation of infants with HMD at much lower pressures, thereby decreasing the risk of a pneumothorax.

6. *Concentration of inspired oxygen* should initially correspond to the oxygen necessary to maintain adequate PaO_2 during spontaneous ventilation. Effective mechanical ventilation may result in sudden reduction in O_2 requirements; hence, watch for a high PaO_2 after starting IPPV.

We would reinforce the comment regarding the need to monitor PaO_2 while an infant is on a ventilator. This is not as critical for low levels, for these may truly be apparent on visual inspection if the infant remains cyanosed. There are, however, no clinical guidelines to hyperoxia, since once full saturation is achieved at a PaO_2 in the region of 80 mm. Hg, the infant's color will not change even if the PaO_2 rises to 500 mm. Hg. The risk for retrolental fibroplasia, therefore, becomes

enormous; particularly in situations where sudden improvement on the ventilator occurs, the arterial oxygen tension may take dramatic rises without the awareness of the personnel unless such monitoring is carried out. It needs to be carried out frequently, therefore, and all attempts must be made to establish and maintain an arterial source for the effective adjustment of the ventilator itself and for the prevention of the serious effects of artificial hyperoxygenation.

L. STERN

Maintaining the Infant During Mechanical Ventilation

When you initiate mechanical ventilation you undertake the responsibility for the infant's gas exchange. Hence, monitoring the patient is vital and requires ideally one nurse per patient for continuous observation.

Frequent arterial blood gas estimations should be performed: (1) within 30 minutes of initiating mechanical ventilation; (2) within 30 minutes of altering any ventilator setting; or (3) immediately, if the infant's condition changes markedly; otherwise every four hours. The goal shoud be to maintain PaO_2 between 60 and 90 mm. Hg, $PaCO_2$ between 35 and 45 mm. Hg, and pH between 7.30 and 7.45.

Changes in Blood Gas Status

SUDDEN FALL IN PaO_2 ACCOMPANIED BY RISE IN $PaCO_2$ ASSOCIATED WITH RAPID CLINICAL DETERIORATION OF THE INFANT. This may be due to a problem with the ventilator or with the infant. These may be separated by disconnecting the ventilator from the infant and by manually inflating the lungs.

If the infant improves clinically there is a *ventilator problem.* Check:

1. Concentration of inspired O_2 going to ventilator.

2. Presence of leaks, e.g., slipped tubing.

3. Mechanical or electrical failure.

4. Ineffective patient triggering due to condensation of water in tubing, etc.

If no clinical improvement occurs with manual inflation there is an *infant problem.* Check air entry bilaterally by auscultation, listen over stomach, and determine the position of the heart and trachea.

If air entry diminished *bilaterally:*

1. *Tube displaced* into nasopharynx. There may be air entry heard over stomach, and air may be visibly escaping at the mouth. ACTION — Replace nasotracheal tube.

2. *Tube blocked.* This occurs especially from the third day of ventilation onwards owing to increased secretions.

ACTION – Suction NTT briefly. If no effect, replace the tube. (With good humidity and adequate suction there is no need to replace the endotracheal tube. This will markedly reduce injuries to the larynx.)

3. *Bilateral pneumothorax.* Results in abdominal distension and an easily palpable liver and spleen; clinically, the condition is usually critical.

ACTION – Emergency relief of tension pneumothorax by inserting a No. 18 needle attached to a three-way tap and a 20 ml. syringe into the third intercostal space at the midclavicular line. Remove air until the condition improves. A chest drain is then inserted.

If air entry diminished *unilaterally:*

1. *Tube in main stem bronchus.* This is usually into the right main stem bronchus producing diminution of air entry on the left.

ACTION – Withdraw NTT 0.5 cm. to 1 cm. Immediate improvement in air entry will result. Recheck position by X-ray.

2. *Unilateral pneumothorax.*

ACTION – same as for bilateral pneumothorax. Check for displacement of the heart and trachea. Although air entry may be diminished unilaterally, a bilateral pneumothorax may account for failure to improve with relief of tension on one side only.

Radiological confirmation of clinical diagnosis is obtained if the condition of the infant warrants a delay in initiating therapy.

Pneumothorax is frequently associated with pneumomediastinum, which gives a classic butterfly appearance to the thymus on the AP projection and can often be seen as a collection of air on the lateral X-ray film. The pneumomediastinum is rarely responsible for any of the debility, but does reflect the usual associated presence of the pneumothorax. Of interest also is the occasional occurrence of pneumoperitoneum as a result of forcing of air through the diaphragm in the periaortic spaces. This can seriously mislead the clinician into the assumption that a ruptured viscus has occurred and abdominal surgery is indicated. When pneumoperitoneum is associated with pneumothorax in the course of hyaline membrane disease, we have found it useful to exclude the presence of a ruptured viscus by the installation of a small amount of contrast material into the stomach. If the material does not leak out of the GI tract, then we have assumed that the pneumoperitoneum is merely an extension of the pneumothorax and unnecessary surgery in a desperately ill infant has been avoided. Another rare but potentially fatal complication is the occurrence of pneumopericardium, which presents as sudden collapse due to tamponade. Its immediate recognition both on clinical grounds and with X-ray confirmation can be life saving if the pneumopericardium is immediately drained.

L. STERN

If air entry is not *diminished* and the *infant does not improve* with manual lung inflation, this suggests cerebral hemorrhage, convulsion, hypoglycemia, or overwhelming sepsis. (It may also be pneumopericardium.)

GRADUAL FALL IN PaO_2 ACCOMPANIED BY A RISE IN $PaCO_2$ AND ASSOCIATED WITH GRADUAL CHANGE IN CLINICAL CONDITION. This suggests inappropriate ventilator settings, although the factors outlined above should be considered. A fall in PaO_2 suggests increasing intrapulmonary shunting due to progressive atelectasis.

If *pressure-cycled* ventilation – increase peak inflation pressure by 5 cm. H_2O.

If *volume-cycled* ventilator – increase tidal volume by 3 to 5 ml. (hence increasing peak inflation pressure). Both these maneuvers will probably increase minute volume.

Consider:

1. Altering cycling frequency, decreasing the rate to 28 to 32.

2. Altering I:E ratio to a longer inspiratory phase: 3:1 or 4:1

3. Changing to assisted or controlled ventilation as appropriate.

The responses to these three maneuvers are variable, and repeat blood gases must be obtained.

CHANGES IN $PaCO_2$ WITHOUT GROSS CHANGES IN PaO_2.

A rise in $PaCO_2$ is due to increased ventilation of dead space, in either the ventilator tubings and connectors, "anatomical" dead space of the infant, or "physiological" dead space of the infant (i.e., nonperfused but ventilated alveoli).

It is an indication for an increase in overall minute volume by increasing peak inflation pressure if pressure-cycled, increasing tidal volume if volume-cycled, or by increasing cycling frequency slightly.

A fall in $PaCO_2$ is due to overventilation. It is potentially dangerous, as it will produce a respiratory alkalosis and rise in pH. Alkalosis is associated with a fall in cardiac output and cerebral blood flow. Hence, it is an indication for a reduction in overall minute volume (providing oxygenation is adequate), or the insertion of artificial dead space to increase "dead space ventilation."

RISE IN PaO_2 ACCOMPANIED BY CHANGES IN PaO_2.

This suggests a fall in intrapulmonary shunting and reduction in degree of atelectasis. Because of the toxic effect of oxygen on lung tissue it is generally believed that the concentration of inspired oxygen should be reduced to below 70 per cent prior to attempting to reduce any ventilator parameter.

We would once again reiterate that while it is desirable to be able to reduce the inspired oxygen concentration as a first step, we believe that in very small infants the danger of pneumothorax from high pressures is such that our first maneuver would be to attempt to reduce the pressure in the ventilator itself. This, while it will not lower the inspired oxygen concentration, will immediately reduce the PaO_2. We accept the increased risk of pulmonary toxicity with inspired oxygen concentrations for a limited period of time and would, therefore, attempt to reduce inspired oxygen concentration as soon as ventilatory pressures are below the level at which pneumothoraces are usually produced. We should additionally point out that when negative pressure ventilators are used without intratracheal tubes, the risks of lung damage from the ventilation procedure are not nearly as high as they may be with positive pressure equipment; therefore, we have felt it appropriate to delay reduction in inspired oxygen concentration for perhaps longer periods than we would with a positive pressure ventilator.

L. STERN

Routine Care of Infant During Mechanical Ventilation

Remember that monitoring of blood gases is only one aspect of supportive treatment. Due attention must also be paid to temperature control, caloric and fluid intake, and metabolic balance, etc. (See Table 8–6.)

Avoid excessive and unnecessary handling of infant.

Care of NTT	1. Suction p.r.n. (at least q. 2h.).
	2. Culture suction catheters daily.
Posture	Turn infant every four hours.
Ventilator	1. Change ventilator and nebulizer tubings every 24 hours.
	2. Use bacterial filters if available.

Weaning from Ventilator

This should be attempted when the concentration of inspired oxygen is 50 per cent or lower, and the peak inflation pressure does not exceed 30 cm. H_2O. Initially, the infant is placed in a concentration of oxygen 10 per cent higher than on the ventilator and allowed to breathe spontaneously through the endotracheal tube.

Do not suction or distress the infant just prior to weaning.

Allow short periods (5 to 10 minutes) of spontaneous breathing initially. Slowly decrease the time on the ventilator, keeping the duration of spontaneous breathing constant. This may be more useful than increasing the duration of the periods of spontaneous breathing. During periods of spontaneous breathing, it is helpful to use continuous positive airway pressure, which appears to prevent progressive airway closure during this critical period.

Extubate when breathing spontaneously for several hours without significant changes in blood gases or clinical condition.

After extubation, brief periods of manual inflation with a face mask or mask ventilation may be helpful.

Editors' Comment: When weaning any infant from assisted ventilation—respirator, bagging, or CPAP—change one variable at a time and check blood gases. For example, do not reduce oxygen concentration and respirator pressure at the same time. Our practice is to reduce environmental oxygen until it is 40 per cent, and then reduce pressure.

Care of Ventilator

After use, ensure:

1. Adequate sterilization (ideally by soaking detachable tubings in bactericidal solution, and gas autoclaving of ventilator unit.)

2. Maintenance by experienced technician.

3. Routine cultures prior to usage to check sterilization and mode of storage.

INTERMITTENT NEGATIVE PRESSURE VENTILATOR (INPV)

The negative pressure ventilator consists of an incubator divided into two compartments. The head compartment is independently ventilated and heated at atmospheric pressure. The body compartment is isolated from the head compartment by an iris diaphragm sealing around the neck; it is cycled to subatmospheric pressure by venting intermittently to a vacuum reservoir maintained by a pump. Development of an intermittent negative pressure around the chest wall results in an intermittent gas flow down the airway. Inspiratory and expiratory times are independently variable and the settings determine the cycling frequency.

Some patients require intubation during NPV. This may be due to some glottic obstruction by the cuff. The airtight seal of the respirator must be broken at times to permit access for nursing and other procedures. During these periods, the infant will not be ventilated unless some other method is applied (e.g., positive pressure by face mask or tube.)

The same principles of mechanical ventilation apply to the negative pressure respirator as well as to positive pressure ventilators. This technique appears especially useful in infants with HMD who weigh over 1500 gm.

The main problems especially related to the negative pressure respirator are:

1. Infants less than 1500 gm. are difficult to manage for technical reasons (e.g., fixation of cuff, and movement of the infant's body).

2. Access for nursing procedures, radiographic studies, blood sampling, etc., is difficult.

3. Abdominal distension occurs with INPV and may require orogastric tube decompression.

COMMENTS

A large number of centers have used mechanical ventilation as part of the supportive management of newborn infants with respiratory failure. Results and experience vary from center to center. Controlled studies assessing the efficacy of the therapy are few and indicate the apparent lack of success in the lower weight groups (i.e., less than 1500 gm.).

It would seem that by utilizing mechanical ventilation, mortality from RDS may be reduced by 13 per cent.[16] The early use of continuous positive airway pressure may reduce this further.[4]

It is encouraging that most survivors of mechanical ventilation appear intact neurologically[14] and have normal pulmonary function at the age of five years.[7] The incidence of neurologic deficit is no higher than in infants of similar weight and gestation who had no respiratory problems.

QUESTIONS

True or False

The reduction in mortality resulting from the use of mechanical ventilation has been far more dramatic in management of tetanus neonatorum than of RDS.

It is estimated that mortality in tetanus neonatorum has dropped from 80 per cent to 20 per cent by the use of IPPV, whereas RDS is 13 per cent. The statement is therefore true.

If you set a pressure-limited safety valve on a volume-cycled ventilator at 40 cm. H_2O, a pneumothorax will not occur.

Although pneumothorax is particularly associated with high inflation pressures, it can occur at any time either during mechanical or spontaneous ventilation. Therefore the statement is false. The fine airways of the infant lung reduce the pressure applied to the lung tissue. Also, the noncompliant lung of the infant with RDS reduces the possibility of a pneumothorax at this pressure.

The larger the volume of ventilator tubings, the less the compression volume at any given pressure.

During positive pressure ventilation, a proportion of the gas delivered by the pump ("compression volume") does not reach the alveoli. The larger the volume of ventilator tubings, the greater the compression volume. Hence, ventilator tubings should be low-volume and nondistensible. The statement is false.

Condensation of water in ventilator inspiratory tubings can be reduced by placing as much tubing as possible inside the incubator.

A temperature gradient exists between air outside and inside the incubator. Water tends to condense out at lower temperatures and droplets will appear in tubing outside the incubator (not reaching the baby). Therefore the statement is true. In addition, care must be taken to avoid an excessive water load to the infant during humidification. Water intoxication has been described following the use of an ultrasonic nebulizer.

If a small leak develops in a ventilator, there will be adequate compensation, provided the ventilator is volume-cycled.

A volume-cycled ventilator delivers a pre-set volume regardless of the pressure developed in the system. Recycling will occur even if no pressure is developed and all the gas is lost through a leak. Therefore the statement is false. A pressure-cycled ventilator delivers gas until a pre-set pressure is attained. Hence, it is possible to compensate for a small leak (e.g., around the endotracheal tube); a large leak causes failure of cycling.

During IPPV in 80 per cent oxygen (for RDS), it is possible to achieve an increase in PaO_2 of 200 mm. Hg by increasing peak inflation pressure, without altering $PaCO_2$ significantly.

When breathing a high concentration of oxygen, a low PaO_2 is indicative of venous admixture or shunting (a disturbance in diffusion or ventilation-perfusion balance is corrected by the high alveolar pO_2). This shunting is thought to occur primarily through areas of atelectatic lung. Effective positive pressure ventilation may open some of these atelectatic areas, reducing the degree of shunting, with an ensuing increase in PaO_2. However, a large right-to-left shunt will not alter $PaCO_2$, as the A-V difference for CO_2 is only 6 mm. Hg. Therefore $PaCO_2$ will not rise, so the statement is true.

During mechanical ventilation, providing the $PaCO_2$ does not change, pH will remain constant.

pH depends on both $PaCO_2$ and bicarbonate levels. Metabolic and respiratory factors are often closely associated (e.g., a period of apnea is associated with both a rise in $PaCO_2$ and a fall in PaO_2, the latter leading to tissue anoxia and anaerobic metabolism). However, they may operate quite independently. Therefore the statement is false.

(The following paragraph pertains to the next three questions.)

Prior to mechanical ventilation using a pressure-cycled ventilator, the PaO_2 is 30 mm. Hg and the $PaCO_2$ is 60 mm. Hg in 100 per cent oxygen. Thirty minutes after initiating therapy, a blood gas estimation is performed.

1. The PaO_2 has risen to 140 mm. Hg. This is a dangerous level and the concentrations of inspired oxygen should be reduced at once.

In immature infants, arterial oxygen tensions in that range have been associated with retrolental fibroplasia. As the infant is breathing 100 per cent oxygen, the lung may also be affected. Therefore the statement is true. Priority should be given to reducing the concentration of inspired oxygen in this situation rather than altering other ventilator settings. However, beware of reducing inspired oxygen concentrations too suddenly and quickly. This can result in a sudden deterioration in the infant's condition possible due to pulmonary vasoconstriction. We drop environmental oxygen 5 to 10 per cent every hour, and obtain a blood gas measurement before each drop.

2. PaO_2 has risen to only 35 mm. Hg and pCO_2 is still 60 mm. Hg. It is advisable to switch to a volume-cycled ventilator, as the lungs are too stiff to be adequately ventilated by a pressure-cycled machine.

The statement is false. The initial ventilator settings were probably quite arbitrary and should now be adjusted to the infant's requirements. The high pCO_2 indicates hypoventilation and an attempt should be made to increase minute ventilation by increasing peak ventilation pressure. At the same time, PaO_2 may rise. Adjustments should be made every 15 minutes, checking blood gases until $PaO_2 > 60$ mm. Hg and $PaCO_2$ is normal.

3. PaO_2 is only 35 mm. Hg and $PaCO_2$ is 35 mm. Hg. It might be helpful to try adding positive expiratory pressure before increasing peak inflation pressure further.

A positive expiratory pressure of 5 to 8 mm. Hg will help to prevent small airway closure. This may prevent atelectasis and hence reduce the degree of right-to-left shunt. Therefore the statement is true.

(The following paragraph pertains to the next three questions.)

A blood gas estimation is performed during mechanical ventilation in 80 per cent oxygen. There has been no change in the clinical condition of the infant since the previous estimation.

1. It is found that $PaCO_2$ has changed from 36 to 24 mm. Hg and pH has risen from 7.38 to 7.56. This is a sign that the infant is recovering and ventilator settings should remain unchanged.

A $PaCO_2$ of 24 mm. Hg suggests overventilation. The resulting alkalosis is dangerous, as it causes a reduction in cardiac output and cerebral blood flow. The $PaCO_2$ should be brought back to a more physiologic range by reducing minute volume (i.e., by reducing peak inflation pressure, tidal volume, or cycling frequency), or by inserting a dead space if oxygenation is precarious. The statement is therefore false.

2. The arterial oxygen tension is 39 mm. Hg, pH is 7.36, and pCO₂ is 35 mm. Hg. The ventilator should not be changed.

At a pH of 7.36 and an arterial oxygen tension of 39 mm. Hg., fetal hemoglobin is approximately 80 per cent saturated. There is no evidence of tissue hypoxia at present. The infant must be watched carefully because of the precarious PaO_2, and blood gases repeated in one hour.

We believe that despite the fact that a pH of 7.36 and a $PaCO_2$ of 35 mm. Hg are quite acceptable, the arterial oxygen tension of 39 mm. Hg is too low and represents a marginal level of operation. In our view there is a need here to increase the inspired oxygen concentration or, if this is not possible, to increase ventilator settings. If under the latter circumstances, $PaCO_2$ falls further, then an increase in dead space can be placed in the equipment to compensate for this. We would prefer not to leave an arterial oxygen tension at this level, since even the minutest change could seriously decompensate the infant at this point with disastrous results from which recovery may be difficult if not impossible.

L. STERN

3. The arterial oxygen tension is 46 mm. Hg, pH is 7.30, and pCO₂ is 26. Although pH is within normal range, there is some degree of metabolic acidosis which should be corrected with intravenous sodium bicarbonate.

Hyperventilation on the ventilator is compensating for a metabolic acidosis. Correction of metabolic acidosis is indicated with intravenous bicarbonate and the measures outlined above to handle the low pCO_2. Therefore the statement is true. A search should be made for the etiology of the acidosis, such as reduced cardiac output.

(The following sentence pertains to the next three questions.)

During mechanical ventilation, an infant becomes cyanosed.

1. He is noted to be making very vigorous respiratory efforts with considerable intercostal and sternal recession out of phase with the ventilator. This is a good indication for sedation and attempting to adjust the ventilator to accommodate the infant's respiratory pattern.

Although "out of phase" respiration could account for this clinical picture, an obstructed airway must first be excluded. Vigorous respiratory efforts with cyanosis suggest an obstructed endotracheal tube. Therefore the statement is false.

2. Air entry is diminished over the left lungfield. The diagnosis is pneumothorax, which should be relieved immediately.

Diminution of air entry over the left lungfield may be due to:
1. The endotracheal tube slipping into the right main stem bronchus.
2. Pneumothorax.

The procedure should be to withdraw the endotracheal tube slightly. If this fails to improve the infant, a chest X-ray is indicated unless the infant's condition is deteriorating rapidly and the left side of the chest is tympanitic and the heart displaced. Emergency relief of a pneumothorax is then indicated.

3. A blood sample for gaseous estimation is taken immediately and resuscitative measures started. When the blood sample is estimated one hour later, the results show pO₂ to be 127 mm. Hg and pCO₂ to be 8 mm. Hg. This suggests that the infant has been crying prior to this cyanotic spell.

The most likely explanation for these bizarre blood gas findings is that an air bubble was left in the syringe and equilibration has occurred between gas in the blood and gas in the air. In the ensuing one hour, the values tend to approximate the pO_2 and pCO_2 of room air. (Samples drawn for blood gases must be bubble-free, capped and iced, and analyzed immediately.) The statement is false.

After extubation following prolonged IPPV, an infant may have some stridor and copious secretions. The stridor usually decreases spontaneously.

Despite the use of nontoxic nasotracheal tubes, there is almost always some laryngeal edema. This together with large quantities of secretions and lack of tracheal cilia may lead to some degree of upper airway obstruction. This will decrease in two to three days. Therefore the statement is true.

Negative pressure during the expiratory phase of the ventilatory cycle may be useful,

as it will overcome the high expiratory resistance of small airways and of narrow bore endotracheal tubes in infants.

Negative pressure during the expiratory phase of the ventilating cycle promotes airway closure and is contra-indicated during IPPV for RDS. Therefore the statement is false. Indeed, positive pressure during expiration is now advocated as a means of maintaining small airways open in the absence of surfactant.

During intermittent negative pressure ventilation, if abdominal distension occurs, the best solution is to pass an orogastric tube and leave it open to the atmosphere.

If an orogastric tube is left open in this situation, the lower end is at negative pressure and the upper end at atmospheric pressure, and air will tend to be sucked into the stomach. Hence, an orogastric tube must be closed off and aspirated intermittently. The statement is false.

REFERENCES

1. Barrie, H.: Simple method of applying continuous positive airway pressure in respiratory distress syndrome. Lancet *1*:776, 1972.
2. Cave-Smith, P., Daily, W., Fletcher, G., et al: Mechanical ventilation of newborn infants. I. The effect of rate and pressure on arterial oxygenation of infants with respiratory distress syndrome. Pediat Res *3*:244, 1969.
3. Coldiron, J.: Estimation of naso-tracheal tube length in neonates. Pediatrics *41*:823, 1968.
4. Gregory, G., Kitterman, J., Phibbs, R., et al: Treatment of the idiopathic respiratory distress syndrome with continuous positive airway pressure. New Eng J Med *284*:1333, 1971.
5. Gregory, G., Kitterman, J., Phibbs, R., et al: Continuous positive airway pressure as treatment in the idiopathic respiratory distress syndrome. Unpublished data.
6. Harrison, V., Heese, H., and de V. Klein, M.: The effects of intermittent positive pressure ventilation on lung function in hyaline membrane disease. Brit J Anaesth *41*:908, 1969.
7. Levison, H., Featherby, E., Weng, T., et al: Pulmonary function 6–8 years after recovery from respiratory distress syndrome. Programme and Abstracts Canadian Pediatric Society, 1969, p. 5.
8. Llewellyn, M., Hardie, M., Bryan, M., et al: The use of positive expiratory pressure during mechanical ventilation of newborn infants with respiratory distress syndrome. In preparation.
9. Murdock, A., Corey, P., and Swyer, P.: An objective multifactorial linear discriminant scoring system for neonates with the respiratory distress syndrome. Biol Neonat *18*:263, 1971.
10. Okmian, L.: Direct measurement of pulmonary ventilation in newborns and infants during artificial ventilation with the Engstrom respirator. Acta Anaesth Scand *7*:155, 1963.
11. Owen-Thomas, J., Ulan, O., and Swyer, P.: The effect of varying inspiratory gas flow rate on arterial oxygenation during IPPV in the respiratory distress syndrome. Brit J Anaesth *40*:493, 1968.
12. Reynolds, E.: Effect of alterations in mechanical ventilator settings on pulmonary gas exchange in hyaline membrane disease. Arch Dis Child *46*:246, 1971.
13. Saklad, M., and Paliotta, J.: A nomogram for the correction of needed gases during artificial ventilation. Anesthesiology *29*:150, 1968.
14. Stahlman, M.: What evidence exists that intensive care has changed the incidence of intact survival? Proceedings of the 59th Ross Conference on Pediatric Research, 1969, p. 17.
15. Stahlman, M., Battersby, E., Shepard, F., et al: Prognosis in hyaline membrane disease. Use of a linear discriminant. New Eng J Med *276*:303, 1967.
16. Swyer, P.: An assessment of artificial respiration in the newborn. Report of the 59th Ross Conference on Pediatric Research, 1969, p. 25.
17. Vidyasagar, D., and Chernick, V.: Continuous positive transpulmonary pressure in hyaline membrane disease: a simple device. Pediatrics *48*: 296, 1971.

Chapter 10

PROBLEMS IN CHEMICAL ADAPTATION

by

MICHAEL K. WALD, M.D.

"These infants are remarkable not only because like foetal versions of Shadrach, Meshach and Abednego, they emerge at least alive from within the fiery metabolic furnace of diabetes mellitus, but because they resemble one another so closely that they might well be related. They are plump, sleek, liberally coated with vernix caseosa, full-faced and plethoric.... They convey a distinct impression of having had such a surfeit of both food and fluid pressed upon them by an insistent hostess that they desire only peace so that they may recover from their excesses. And on the second day their resentment of the slightest noise improves the analogy while their trembling anxiety seems to speak of intra-uterine indiscretions of which we know nothing."

JAMES W. FARQUHAR, "The Child of the Diabetic Woman"*

———————
*Farquhar, James: The child of the diabetic woman. Arch Dis Child *34*:76, 1959.

Throughout fetal life, plasma levels of glucose and calcium are closely regulated by placental exchange. Perhaps in consequence, the newborn infant's regulatory mechanisms for both these substances are immature. The healthy newborn shows, as evidence of this immaturity, rapid changes in plasma calcium and glucose during the first days of life, with a delay of one to two weeks before levels characteristic of maturity are attained. An infant born prematurely, one subjected to an abnormal intrauterine environment because of maternal diabetes or hyperparathyroidism, or one with postnatal illness additionally straining his homeostasis, frequently develops a profound metabolic disturbance which can be symptomatic and may directly threaten survival.

HYPOGLYCEMIA

THE METABOLIC BACKGROUND[3, 6–8, 14, 20, 22]

Glucose is continuously transferred across the placenta during pregnancy, moving down a concentration gradient, with the umbilical vein glucose ranging from 70 to 80 per cent of the maternal venous level. It represents a major source of energy for the fetus.

168

Hepatic gluconeogenesis probably does not occur in utero, although the necessary enzymes are present in the liver at birth. Plasma free fatty acids remain at low levels, and fat catabolism is not a significant energy source.

Glycogen is stored in the liver and heart as term approaches, reaching three to seven per cent by weight in liver and two to four per cent in heart muscle. This stored, rapidly available energy is essential to survival during labor and immediately after birth. These stores are labile, however, and with intrauterine malnutrition or anoxia they may fail to accumulate or may be catabolized before birth.

It is of interest that newborn animals killed instantly at birth show the presence of these glycogen stores in the heart muscle, whereas those which have been asphyxiated prior to death do not. These changes are not similarly seen in the liver, suggesting that it is the heart glycogen rather than the liver glycogen which participates in the defense against asphyxia at birth.

L. STERN

Insulin appears in the fetal pancreas by 12 weeks' gestation and can be detected at low levels in fetal serum. However, glucose loads presented to a fetus at this time evoke no additional insulin secretion. Even close to term, the insulin response to a glucose load is sluggish and blunted.[20, 22]

It may be correct that under normal circumstances the amount of glucose which reaches the fetus is insufficient to evoke fetal insulin secretion. Infants of diabetic mothers, however, show both pancreatic hyperplasia of the islet cells and hyperinsulinism; it is seriously suspected that the etiology of this is a reflection of an intrauterine stimulation of insulin secretion as a response to the much higher levels of maternal glucose presented to the fetus than under normal circumstances.

L. STERN

At birth, energy demands suddenly increase, but the glucose supply is cut off. The newborn, with scant carbohydrate stores, must radically alter his handling of energy substrates in order to defend his blood glucose. The first response is rapid glycogenolysis, utilizing almost all the hepatic glycogen in the first two to three hours. During this time, free fatty acid levels treble in plasma and subsequently remain elevated. The respiratory quotient drops progressively over two to three days, as most tissues switch to

burning fat. Gluconeogenesis, commencing in the first few hours, becomes increasingly important as a source of glucose for the brain.

Insulin levels during this period of rapid adjustment remain low. Adequate catecholamine secretion and the usually high plasma growth hormone levels in the newborn may participate in the switch to fat catabolism. Adequate adrenocortical function is necessary for the establishment of gluconeogenesis.

Blood glucose at birth is 60 to 70 per cent of the simultaneous maternal level. A rapid decline ensues, terminating at one to two hours of age, after which a slight rise occurs (see "normal" curve—Figure 10–1). At four to six hours of age, healthy full-term infants show average blood glucose levels of 50 to 60 mg. per 100 ml; 40 to 50 mg. per 100 ml. if hypothermia has occurred. Low-birth-weight infants have average levels about 40 mg. per 100 ml. Levels below 30 mg. per 100 ml. in full-term infants or 20 mg. per 100 ml. in low-birth-weight infants during the first three days of life occur in less than four percent of all glucose determinations. After three days of age, all glucose values should be above 40 mg. per 100 ml.

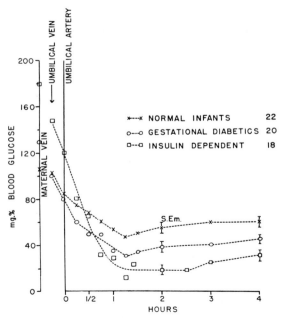

Figure 10–1 Serial changes in the concentration of glucose in the blood of infants immediately following delivery. Mothers with gestational diabetes had abnormal intravenous glucose tolerance tests during pregnancy but received no insulin therapy.[6]

Hypoglycemia is defined, chemically, as a true blood glucose below 30 mg. per 100 ml. in full-term infants, and 20 mg. per 100 ml. in low-birth-weight infants on two sequential samples obtained at least one hour apart during the first three days of life. After this period, 40 mg. per 100 ml. is the diagnostic level.[6-8]

We would take exception to this definition of hypoglycemia, since it is based not on any risk or physiologic status, but on incidence. Once the term hypoglycemia is applied to such a level it tends to propagate the view that because the incidence of levels somewhat higher than those defined may be relatively common, they are therefore not dangerous. In our view, such thinking is incorrect. We have seen symptoms relievable by glucose infusion at levels between 30 and 40 mg. per 100 ml. in full-term infants and similarly at the same levels in low-birth-weight infants. It is, therefore, our policy to correct blood glucose levels below 40 mg. per 100 ml. for any infant, and we would urge that the definition as stated above be disregarded in terms of clinical usefulness. It can be retained only as an index of incidence, but it is not of physiologic importance. Such a view would tend to indicate that hypoglycemia (and concomitantly attempts to correct it) is considerably more common in the newborn than would otherwise be noted. We do not feel that the therapy needed to compensate for this is difficult and therefore are of the view that all levels below 40 mg. per 100 ml. are worthy of attention.[*]

L. STERN

METHODOLOGY[8-9]

Glucose is labile in biological samples, and the available methods present several pitfalls. These must be avoided or results may be grossly misleading.

1. Capillary blood glucose may underestimate the venous level as a result of stasis unless the extremity is warmed.

2. If blood is allowed to stand, glycolysis will lower blood glucose up to 18 mg. per 100 ml. per hour at room temperature. Preservation with sodium fluoride, immediate cooling in ice, protein precipitation, or centrifugation with separation of serum from the clot is required.

3. Nonglucose reducing substances range to 60 mg. per 100 ml. in newborn blood. Methods specific for glucose or true sugar must be used. Somogyi-Nelson, ortho-toluidine, glu-

cose oxidase, or autoanalyzer methods are appropriate.

4. Alkaline zinc salts (Somogyi) are preferable as protein precipitants. They remove most nonglucose reducing substances, and also reduced glutathione, which can cause the glucose oxidase method to underestimate true glucose.

5. Plasma glucose levels exceed whole blood glucose by 15 per cent.

6. Dextrostix (Ames), especially in inexperienced hands, are not a satisfactory screening device. A modification of the technique[30] improves results, as does use of a reflectance meter (Ames),[18] but neither eliminates the possibility of falsely high readings. Dextrostix are useful in following an infant on treatment.

Thus, ideally, venous or warmed heel-stick blood should be preserved with fluoride, precipitated with Somogyi reagents, and analyzed for true hexose.

SYMPTOMS

There are no symptoms specific for hypoglycemia. It has been associated with jitteriness, cyanosis, convulsions, apnea, apathy, high-pitched or weak cry, limpness, refusal to feed, and temperature instability (Table 10–1). Infants of diabetic mothers may be asymptomatic despite glucose levels below 20 mg. per 100 ml. in the first four hours of life. Low-birth-weight infants may be tran-

*Pogliara, A., Kerl, I., Haymond, M., et al: Hypoglycemia in infancy and childhood. J Pediat 82:365, 1973.

TABLE 10–1 NEONATAL SYMPTO-MATIC HYPOGLYCEMIA IN 56 INFANTS[6]

CLINICAL MANIFESTATIONS	NO.	PRESENTING SIGN
Tremors ("jitteriness")	42	20
Cyanosis	43	19
Convulsions	29	9
Apnea, irreg. resp.	23	6
Apathy	16	2
Cry, high pitched or weak	10	1
Limpness	13	4
Refusal to feed	5	1
Eye rolling	2	2

AGE OF ONSET (HOURS)

<6	6–24	24–48	48–72	>72
8	6	18	18	6

siently hypoglycemic without symptoms,[3, 12] but symptoms appear as low levels persist.

The differential diagnosis of infants with typical hypoglycemic symptoms is extensive (Table 10–2). Ninety per cent of such infants are *not* hypoglycemic. Thus, a chemical diagnosis and confirmation by response to treatment are necessary to exclude other problems.

SYNDROMES AND PATHOGENESIS

Transient Symptomatic Neonatal Hypoglycemia[3, 6, 8, 23, 24]

This syndrome typically affects low-birth-weight infants who are undergrown-for-gestational-age. Two-thirds of cases are male. The smaller of discordant twins is frequently affected. Incidence reflects these risk factors (Table 10–3). Of this group of hypoglycemic infants, 50 per cent have toxemic mothers, 20 per cent are polycythemic, 15 per cent have CNS anomalies or injury, and seven per cent are hypocalcemic. Hypoglycemia may occur by four hours of age

TABLE 10–2 DIFFERENTIAL DIAGNOSIS IN NEONATE WITH EPISODES OF TREMORS, CYANOSIS, CONVULSIONS, APNEA, IRREGULAR RESPIRATION, APATHY, HIGH-PITCHED OR WEAK CRY, LIMPNESS, REFUSAL TO FEED, EYE ROLLING[6]

Central nervous system
  Congenital defect
  Birth injury, anoxia
  Infection
  Kernicterus

Sepsis

Heart disease
  Congenital
  Acquired
  Arrhythmias

Iatrogenic
  Drugs to mother
  Overheating

Adrenal hemorrhage

Polycythemia

Metabolic
  Hypocalcemia
  Hyponatremia
  Hypernatremia
  Pyridoxine dependency
  Magnesium deficiency
  Uremia
NEONATAL SYMPTOMATIC HYPOGLYCEMIA

TABLE 10–3 INCIDENCE OF TRANSIENT SYMPTOMATIC NEONATAL HYPOGLYCEMIA

PATIENT GROUP	PER CENT INCIDENCE
Full-term infants	0.13
All live births	0.29
Low birth-weight infants (<2500 gm.)	5–6
Birth weight <2500 gm.; <50th percentile for gestational age. Symptomatic.	15
Twin. Birth weight <2000 gm. Other twin weight >2700 gm.	70

but usually presents between 24 and 72 hours (See Table 10–1).

The relationship between hypoglycemia and hypocalcemia is also common in our experience. Both are frequently associated with asphyxia, but the two will occur together even without such evidence. One proposed mechanism for this interdependence may lie in the fact that glucagon is known to promote excretion of calcium by the kidney; its increase under hypoglycemic conditions may be the mediator of the hypocalcemia which often accompanies low blood glucose levels.

L. STERN

The pathogenesis is multifactorial. In small-for-dates infants, glycogen stores are reduced. Gluconeogenesis in an undergrown liver may be inadequate to support a relatively well-grown brain.[7] In appropriately grown prematures, increased energy consumption caused by hypothermia, anoxia, acidosis, and respiratory distress may simply exhaust substrate.

Infants of Diabetic Mothers[3, 6, 10]

Hypoglycemia occurs in at least 50 per cent of infants of diabetic mothers, usually at two to four hours of age. Less than 10 per cent show symptoms, however, and by six hours most have stabilized their blood glucose at acceptable levels (Figure 10–1). Babies who show symptoms, who remain hypoglycemic at six to eight hours, or who become hypoglycemic thereafter, need treatment.

These infants have islet cell hyperplasia and probably hyperinsulinism, although direct support for this is lacking. Both exogenous and endogenous glucose are rapidly disposed of, in contrast to the slow glucose disposal of the normal newborn. Low catecholamine secretion has been demonstrated in these infants, and may explain why some of them fail to rebound successfully from their initial hypoglycemia.[29]

Hypoglycemia is not observed in infants whose mothers have had rigid control of blood glucose during the last two months of pregnancy (<120 mg. per 100 ml. with five blood samples per day).

Infants of gestational diabetic mothers have a less dramatic fall in blood glucose at two to four hours and less likelihood of symptoms (Figure 10–1). Since the maternal condition may be undiagnosed, any infant over 4 Kg. birth weight should be screened at two hours of age with Dextrostix. Early hypoglycemia in the infant may be a clue to prediabetes in the mother.

Other Less Common Hypoglycemic Syndromes[6]

Failure of glycogen storage or release: glycogen synthetase deficiency; glycogen storage disease, type I.

Failure of hepatic gluconeogenesis or conversion: fructose intolerance; galactosemia; hepatitis; adrenal insufficiency — adrenogenital syndrome, adrenal hemorrhage; hypopituitarism.

Increased peripheral glucose utilization: insulin excess. (1) Islet cell tumors,[11] (2) islet cell hyperplasia or hyperfunction. (a) Erythroblastosis — hypoglycemia may occur postexchange,[2] (b) hyperplastic fetal visceromegaly (Beckwith)[5] — macroglossia and umbilical hernia usual; (c) maternal chlorpropamide therapy.[35]

Unknown pathogenesis: hypoglycemia accompanying sepsis.[34]

Idiopathic spontaneous recurrent hypoglycemia: with or without leucine sensitivity; with or without catecholamine deficiency.

TREATMENT[3, 6, 8]

All symptomatic infants with hypoglycemia deserve immediate treatment, the objective of which is to maintain blood glucose over 30 mg. per 100 ml. Hypoglycemia accompanying other serious problems (CNS bleeding, sepsis) should be treated, as it may be an important secondary cause of CNS damage. Asymptomatic infants with demonstrated hypoglycemia on repeat sampling should be treated also. However, the asymp-

tomatic infant of a diabetic mother may be managed expectantly for the first four hours with careful monitoring.

"Standard" Treatment[3, 8]

a. STAT infusion: 50 per cent D/W 1 to 2 ml. per Kg. I.V. or 20 per cent D/W 2 to 3 ml. per Kg. I.V.

b. Maintenance infusion: 15 per cent D/W 75 to 85 ml. per Kg. per 24 hours first 48 hours, thereafter 10 per cent dextrose in 0.2 per cent saline (100 to 110 ml. per Kg. per 24 hours).

c. Steroids: If blood glucose is still below 30 mg. per 100 ml. after 6 to 12 hours of treatment with intravenous glucose, add: hydrocortisone (5 mg. per Kg. q. 12h) or ACTH (4 units per Kg. q. 12h).

Whenever glucose infusions are given in our department, we would prefer the use of a constant infusion pump rather than a hand regulated I.V. This allows for a constant rate of infusion thereby eliminating fluctuations in blood glucose which will result from variations in the rate of the insulin response to the glucose infusion, where the infusion is hand-regulated often at irregular intervals. The latter is much more serious when the rates of infusion are slow, and constant hand-regulation thereby is considerably more difficult to maintain.

L. STERN

Glucose levels must be *monitored* during therapy at intervals of one to two hours initially. Either persistent hypoglycemia or hyperglycemia can occur.

Glucose infusion must be *tapered* slowly after oral feedings have been tolerated. Infusion should never be allowed to terminate abruptly, since rebound hypoglycemia may occur.

Other Measures

1. Early feeding: Asymptomatic infants who are at risk for hypoglycemia may receive glucose-water, followed by formula feedings beginning at two to four hours of age. Small or distressed infants should receive caloric support intravenously.[28]

2. Glucagon: Mobilizes glycogen reserves in the liver and is an effective emergency treatment for infants of diabetic mothers or hypoglycemic, erythroblastotic infants.[6] Glucagon is not effective in infants with transient neonatal hypoglycemia, since hepatic glycogen is deficient. The dose is 300 μg. per Kg. I.M.

3. Contraindicated or not yet proven:[3] fructose—must be converted to glucose in the liver. Blood glucose falls initially during fructose infusion.

Epinephrine—in infants of diabetic mothers, epinephrine suppresses insulin release and mobilizes glycogen and fat. However, lactic acidosis has accompanied its use. It is still under investigation.

PROGNOSIS[3, 7]

Hypoglycemia is a serious event in the neonate which, if untreated, can result in all degrees of central nervous system damage, including death. Long-term follow-up of infants with transient symptomatic neonatal hypoglycemia shows a 30 to 50 per cent incidence of neurologic impairment and a 10 per cent incidence of recurrent hypoglycemia. However, in vigorously treated infants, average IQ scores and growth were not significantly different from matched nonhypoglycemic controls. Asymptomatic hypoglycemic infants fare well. Hypoglycemic infants of diabetic mothers also do well, almost without exception. When hypoglycemia accompanies an inborn metabolic error, however, or occurs with the Beckwith syndrome, prognosis is extremely poor.

HYPOCALCEMIA

THE METABOLIC BACKGROUND[13, 16, 21, 25, 27, 31, 33]

Throughout pregnancy, the fetus is supplied transplacentally with both calcium and maternal parathyroid hormone. Calcium is actively transported by the placenta and accumulated by the fetus at a progressively increasing rate towards term, so that 75 per cent of the calcium in a full-term newborn is acquired after the 28th gestational week. The active transport of calcium maintains fetal plasma concentrations higher than maternal, and allows fetal calcification to proceed normally despite poor maternal nutrition, and even with placental insufficiency and fetal malnutrition. Therefore, small-for-dates infants usually have normal calcium stores at birth, while the true premature, who has missed the period of most rapid intrauterine calcium accumulation, is born relatively calcium deficient. The role of maternal para-

thyroid hormone in fetal calcification is unknown, but the transfer of hormone across the placenta helps to suppress fetal parathyroid function.

At birth, the rapid supply of calcium is cut off, as is maternal parathyroid hormone. The neonate is left with his accumulated calcium stores in bone (deficient if he is premature), with parathyroid glands capable initially of only a sluggish response, and with kidneys which respond poorly to parathyroid hormone and have a very low capacity to excrete phosphorus. Not unexpectedly, the serum calcium falls and phosphorus rises in the first days after birth. A number of factors can accentuate this fall in serum calcium, and occasionally precipitate symptomatic hypocalcemia:

1. The degree of prematurity and calcium deficiency in bone.

2. Maternal hyperparathyroidism—the cutoff of hormone at birth is accentuated and fetal parathyroid suppression more profound.

3. Stress secondary to obstetrical difficulty or asphyxia—endogenous corticosteroid production tends to drive the serum calcium downward.

In addition to the possibility that enhanced corticosteriod production would tend to lower the serum calcium, asphyxia has also been demonstrated to be a powerful stimulus to calcitonin release, which in turn will also operate to lower the serum calcium.

L. STERN

4. Treatment of acidosis with bicarbonate—a common situation in premature infants which acts to decrease the physiologically important ionized fraction of the serum calcium (see below).

5. Dietary factors—hypocalcemia is potentiated by diets which are low in calcium and relatively high in phosphorus. Breast milk has a phosphorus content of 150 mg. per liter and a calcium:phosphorus ratio of 2.3:1. In contrast, formulas derived from cow's milk have higher phosphorus content (362 to 1000 mg. per liter) and a calcium:phosphorus ratio of 1.3:1. Low doses of vitamin D, such as are added to all commercial formulas, encourage calcium transport into bone and potentiate hypocalcemia.

6. Special factors—such as citrate load in exchange transfusion, which can precipitate tetany by complexing calcium.

It should be pointed out that citrate complexes not only with calcium but also with magnesium which, like calcium, is a divalent cation. The latter is not measured nearly as often as calcium is, but relatively simple means for its ionic determination do exist, and reports of depletion with symptomatology following exchange transfusion with citrated blood have appeared, suggesting that both its measurement and possible replacement post-transfusion may be worthwhile.

L. STERN

At birth, serum calcium exceeds maternal calcium by about 1 mg. per 100 ml. The level begins to fall in the first few hours and normally stabilizes on the second day at an average of 7.5 mg. per 100 ml. Over the next one to two days there is a considerable rise towards normal adult levels, followed in some infants by a second fall at five to six days, related to feeding. After 7 to 10 days, most newborns achieve normocalcemia (Figure 10–2). At six days of age, breast-fed babies show a serum calcium about 1 mg. per 100 ml. higher than bottle-fed babies, and a serum phosphorus 1 to 2 mg. per 100 ml. lower.

It is frequently difficult to correlate hypocalcemia with symptoms in the newborn, and no solid guidelines exist defining a "significantly" low level. Surveys defining hypocalcemia chemically (and arbitrarily) as a serum calcium below 7 to 7.5 mg. per 100 ml. report incidence rates of 1.2 per cent of all births, and as high as 50 per cent in high-risk infants. On the other hand, the incidence

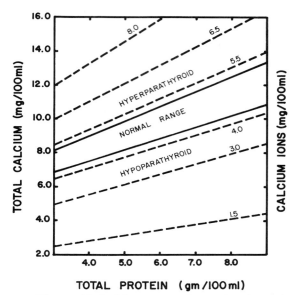

Figure 10–3 Nomogram for estimation of serum ionized calcium from total calcium and total protein values. (Adapted by L. I. Gardner from McLean and Hastings.[19])

of true hypocalcemic tetany has been reported as 0.14 per cent of live births.[27]

METHODOLOGY

Serum calcium, as routinely measured, includes protein-bound calcium and calcium complexed to small organic molecules such as citrate, in addition to the physiologically crucial ionized calcium. The nomogram of McLean and Hastings (Figure 10–3)[19] was developed to allow for variations of the protein-bound fraction. A recently developed calcium electrode, not in general clinical use, is capable of determining ionized calcium directly. Studies with this electrode have revealed surprising variations in total and ionized calcium in certain clinical situations. For example, during an exchange transfusion with citrated blood using calcium gluconate in recommended dosage, total calcium rises while ionized calcium abruptly falls (Figure 10–4).[17, 26] Such phenomena may explain the poor correlation noted between calcium levels and clinical symptoms.

It should be stressed that the usual hospital laboratory measurement of serum calcium measures total serum calcium and not the ionized fraction. Therefore, the infant with symptoms suggestive of hypocalcemia

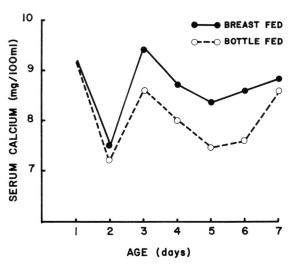

Figure 10–2 Mean calcium levels in the first week of life. (Adapted from Harvey et al.[13])

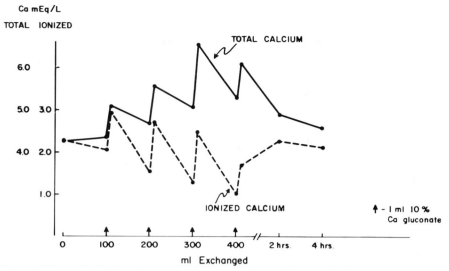

Figure 10–4 Effect of added calcium gluconate on total and ionized calcium (ACD blood).[17]

following exchange transfusion who has his serum calcium measured will generally have a normal level, since the problem is not one of calcium loss but of complexing with the citrate in the transfused blood. If hypoglycemia can be excluded, then either hypocalcemia or hypomagnesemia should be suspected and calcium and/or magnesium administered despite the normal levels which are apparent from the routine laboratory under such situations.

L. STERN

SYMPTOMS

The symptoms of hypocalcemia, like those of hypoglycemia, are nonspecific in the newborn. Twitching, jitteriness, and convulsions are most frequently described, followed in order by cyanosis and vomiting.[27] The Chvostek and Trousseau signs, typically present in older children with hypocalcemia, occur in only 20 per cent of hypocalcemic neonates, and the former sign is present in many normal infants. A recent survey of a low-birth-weight population showed that typical symptoms of hypocalcemia were widely prevalent in normocalcemic infants.[31] Symptoms such as twitching of the extremities and a high-pitched cry were relatively specific for hypocalcemia but present in less than one-fifth of cases. The electrocardiogram may show prolonged QT interval, but in practice is rarely helpful in diagnosis in the newborn period. Obviously, then, hypocalcemia may only be *suspected* on clinical

grounds. It must subsequently be *confirmed* by chemical analysis and by response to specific therapy.

SYNDROMES AND THEIR PATHOGENESIS

The classification of hypocalcemic syndromes presented is that of Mizrahi, London, and Gribetz who point out that all syndromes except the first two are rare.[21]

"First-Day" Hypocalcemia[21, 27, 31]

Hypocalcemia occurring in the first two days of life represents an accentuation of the normal fall in serum calcium seen at this time. Two-thirds of affected infants are males. The incidence is highest in the late winter and early spring. Eighty per cent of cases have one or more of the following associations:

a. Obstetrical trauma including breech delivery, midforceps rotation, precipitate delivery, cesarean section occasioned by hemorrhage, or abnormal presentation.

b. Prematurity with appropriately low birth weight.

c. Maternal diabetes: the risk of symptomatic hypocalcemia is increased 25-fold in these infants.

d. Initially low Apgar scores.

e. Metabolic and/or respiratory acidosis corrected with intravenous bicarbonate.

The pathogenesis involves several factors: cutoff of maternal calcium and para-thormone, parathyroid immaturity, and possibly corticosteriod excess due to the stress of obstetrical difficulties. In the infant of the diabetic mother, the pathogenesis is unknown. Iatrogenic factors clearly obtain in the post-acidotic infant. Poor calcium stores in bone may partly explain the susceptibility of premature infants. In contrast to classical alimentary hypocalcemia, described below, serum phosphorus is frequently normal in these infants.

Classical Neonatal Tetany[21, 27]

A second peak incidence of hypocalcemia is seen at five to seven days of age occurring almost exclusively in infants fed formulas derived from cow's milk. The high phosphorus and low calcium-phosphorus ratios in such formulas have already been mentioned. Interestingly, about half of these babies also have the clinical associations of the "first-day" group, suggesting that the stress imposed by the diet selects out some infants already susceptible to hypocalcemia for other reasons. In classical neonatal tetany, the serum phosphorus is elevated.

Maternal Hyperparathyroidism[15]

By 1966 there were eight case reports with the association of maternal parathyroid adenoma and neonatal tetany. The maternal condition was frequently silent. Tetany is early and severe, unduly prolonged, and may occur during breast feeding. A history of previous abortions or stillbirth, a previous baby with tetany, or any vague symptoms make a check of the mother's serum calcium and phosphorus mandatory.

Accompanying Hypoproteinemia

If this is the only reason, ionized calcium will be normal and tetany absent.[19]

Exchange Transfusion

Ionized calcium is dramatically depressed by exchange transfusion using citrated blood, whether or not calcium gluconate is given.[17, 26]

Other Syndromes[21]

Hypocalcemia can accompany lactic acidosis, hypernatremia, and uremia, and has been described with severe maternal rickets. The parathyroids may be congenitally absent, and there may frequently be absent thymus and immunologic deficiency.

PRACTICAL CONSIDERATIONS

Treatment[21, 27]

Parenteral therapy of hypocalcemia is hazardous and should be reserved for symptomatic infants. However, in the presence of seizures or extreme irritability, a trial of therapy is indicated while awaiting confirmation of hypocalcemia from the laboratory.

Immediate Therapy. Ten per cent calcium gluconate is injected slowly into an established intravenous line with continuous monitoring of the electrocardiogram or of the apical pulse. The maximal dose should be 10 ml. for a full-term infant or 6 ml. for a premature. Inject no faster than one ml. per minute, avoiding extravasation. Stop as soon as clinical improvement occurs.

Continued Therapy

a. Intravenous maintenance: Calcium gluconate 1 to 2 gm. (10 to 20 ml. of 10 per cent solution) per 24 hours by steady infusion with frequent monitoring of pulse. Parenteral calcium is rarely needed for more than 24 to 48 hours.

b. Oral maintenance: This is usually given for two to four weeks and then tapered. Oral treatment alone may be used for asymptomatic hypocalcemia.

Calcium chloride (27 per cent calcium) at a dose of 1 to 2 gm. per day. The *concentration* fed must not exceed one per cent or gastric mucosal necrosis can occur. Metabolic acidosis may appear if this salt is used for more than two or three days. Nonetheless, this may be the most effective oral form of calcium.

Calcium lactate (13 per cent calcium) two to three gm. per day and calcium gluconate (nine per cent calcium) two to four gm. per day are effective for long-term treatment, are nonirritating orally, and do not cause acidosis. Calcium glubionate (calcium content 92 mg. per 4 ml.; dosage two to four gm. per day) is available commercially as Neo-Calglucon Syrup (1.395 gm. per 4 ml.).*

c. Low phosphorus formula: The best commercial formula for this purpose is PM 60/40 (Ross) which has a phosphorus content of 172 mg. per liter and a calcium-phosphorus ratio of 2.0:1.

Prognosis

Hypocalcemia with seizures may present an immediate threat to life in an infant who frequently has other problems with which to contend. However, unlike hypoglycemia, there seems to be no structural damage to the central nervous system. Thus, hypocalcemia has an excellent prognosis. If hypocalcemia is complicating other serious conditions, such as asphyxia, respiratory distress, or CNS injury, the prognosis is dominated by the other problems.

Treatment is rarely required after one month of age, but may need to be prolonged in an occasional infant with severely depressed parathyroid function.

HYPOMAGNESEMIA[1, 27, 32]

This metabolic defect has occasionally been noted in tetanic infants, usually in association with hypocalcemia. The pathogenesis is not known, although serum magnesium levels are to some extent supported by parathyroid function. The typical hypomagnesemic infant has been defined by surveys as low birth weight, undergrown-for-gestational-age, and showing signs of placental insufficiency. Thus, hypomagnesemia usually seems to be an index of fetal malnutrition. Serum magnesium levels average 1.4 to 1.7 mEq per liter (2.8 to 3.4 mg. per 100 ml.) in the neonate and tend to rise with postnatal age.

With symptoms of tetany unresponsive to calcium therapy and a demonstrated hypomagnesemia, treatment is indicated as follows: 50 per cent magnesium sulfate (0.2 ml. per Kg. q. 4h I.M.), or oral magnesium sulfate (30 mEq. per day).

QUESTIONS

True or False

There is a seasonal variation in the incidence of neonatal hypocalcemia.

---
*Sandoz.

The incidence is highest in the late winter and early spring. The pathogenesis is believed to be increased maternal parathyroid activity at this time of year to compensate for vitamin D deficiency due to lack of sunlight.[27] Therefore, the statement is true.

Since hypoglycemia is transient in infants of diabetic mothers, a single intravenous injection of glucose (1 gm. per Kg.) at two hours of age may be effective treatment.

The infant of the diabetic mother has pancreatic islet-cell hyperplasia and hyperinsulinemia, and responds to a rapid glucose infusion with an exaggerated insulin output. Disposal of endogenous or exogenous glucose is rapid. Rebound hypoglycemia is almost certain unless sustained glucose infusion is given.[6] Therefore, the statement is false.

While it is true the Dextrostix range does not extend below 40 ml. per 100 ml., at least a positive result is reassuring in a symptomatic infant and obviates the need for a quantitative blood glucose.

Dextrostix can show positive reactions with blood glucose values below 20 mg. per 100 ml. The likelihood of error is increased by poor light and inexperienced personnel. Therefore the statement is false.

In a convulsing neonate, a response to intravenous calcium gluconate does NOT prove that the seizure was due to hypocalcemia.

Intravenous calcium gluconate has a nonspecific anticonvulsant action. It is necessary to prove hypocalcemia chemically in pretreatment serum. Therefore the statement is true.

All hypoglycemic infants are at risk of serious sequelae, regardless of whether they are symptomatic or asymptomatic.

The infant of the diabetic mother who has hypoglycemia without symptoms in the first four to six hours of life has an excellent prognosis. Therefore the answer is false. Low-birth-weight infants with transient neonatal hypoglycemia have a much worse prognosis if they are symptomatic, but all such infants should be treated.[3]

An asymptomatic premature infant with

hypocalcemia (serum calcium 6.7 mg. per 100 ml.) may be treated with oral calcium.

Of course this level may not be significantly low if the infant also has hypoproteinemia (see Figure 10–3). Oral treatment may be started with PM 60/40 (Ross) and added calcium gluconate or calcium chloride (see page 176 for dose and precautions). Asymptomatic hypocalcemic infants should be managed orally because of the hazard of intravenous calcium infusion. Therefore the statement is true.

A symptomatic infant with transient neonatal hypoglycemia may be treated orally.

Oral treatment has been proved ineffective in hypoglycemic infants. Parenteral treatment is required. The statement is therefore false. Dr. Stern in his comment on p. 170 has suggested treatment of any infant whose blood glucose falls below 40 mg. per 100 ml. Other investigators (see footnote, page 170) support this view, for the reasons he has expressed. Many infants with glucose levels between 20 and 40 mg. per 100 ml. will be asymptomatic and should be managed by early, frequent oral glucose feedings and careful monitoring.

Hypocalcemia can occur as a result of magnesium deficiency.

Although the mechanism is not known, in the presence of severe magnesium deficiency there may be hypocalcemia which is resistant to treatment with calcium. Since hypocalcemia and hypomagnesemia may coexist in both low-birth-weight infants and infants of diabetic mothers, it is important to check serum magnesium in any hypocalcemic infant who does not respond to treatment.[4] The statement is true.

Even with effective therapy, symptoms due to hypoglycemia may not respond promptly.

With severe or prolonged hypoglycemia, there may be a protracted recovery period. Therefore the statement is true.

Neonatal hypocalcemia can be expected less frequently in infants who receive vitamin D supplemented formulas.

Small doses of vitamin D encourage calcium movement into bone and potentiate hypocalcemia. In one study,[27] addition of 600 units vitamin D per quart to cow's milk increased the incidence of hypocalcemia from 10 per cent of infants to 30 per cent. The statement is false.

Match the remaining statements appropriately and state reasons.
   A. Hypoglycemia.
   B. Hypocalcemia.
   C. Both.
   D. Neither.

A maternal history of three miscarriages.

A history of excessive fetal wastage can mean maternal gestational diabetes with a propensity for neonatal hypoglycemia. Fetal wastage is also seen with chronic hyperparathyroidism. Therefore the answer is C.

An infant, birthweight 1200 gm, 29-week gestation, early respiratory distress with mixed acidosis treated with intravenous bicarbonate, 22 hours old.

This infant has multiple risk factors for hypocalcemia. His risk of hypoglycemia is not great, especially if he is receiving intravenous fluid and caloric support, as he should be with prematurity and respiratory distress. Therefore the answer is B.

Severe erythroblastosis following exchange transfusion.

Hypoglycemia may occur following exchange transfusion in erythroblastosis as a rebound effect precipitated by the glucose (300 mg. per 100 ml.) in ACD blood. The ACD solution also causes a severe drop in serum ionized calcium, even if calcium gluconate is given. Therefore the answer is C.

Apneic spells, extreme lethargy, and decreased tone.

Although there is considerable overlap in symptomatology of these two metabolic problems, symptoms of depressed neuromuscular function are more likely in hypoglycemia. Hypocalcemia usually causes increased tone. Therefore the answer is A.

Irritability, jitteriness, and convulsions.

These symptoms may mean either hypocalcemia or hypoglycemia. Therefore the answer is C.

May be a clue to significant undiagnosed disease in the mother.

A hypoglycemic infant weighing over 4 Kg. requires a glucose tolerance test to rule out asymptomatic diabetes in the mother. Neonatal hypocalcemia may be a clue to a maternal parathyroid adenoma. Therefore the answer is C.

May be precipitated by medication taken during pregnancy.

Hypoglycemia of the newborn may be severe and prolonged if a mother is treated with oral hypoglycemics. Exchange transfusion may be necessary to remove the drug from the infant.[35] Although much less likely, a mother with the milk-alkali syndrome and hypercalcemia could have a hypocalcemic infant. Therefore the answer is C.

A 2600-gm. newborn with a hemoglobin of 26 gm. per 100 ml.

Hypoglycemia is frequently seen in plethoric infants. Infants of diabetic mothers and those with hyperplastic fetal visceromegaly[5] are frequently polycythemic. Pildes, Forbes, and Cornblath describe a set of parabiotic twins in which the larger and more plethoric twin had hypoglycemia while his sibling did not.[23] Therefore the answer is A.

A 3400-gm., 53-cm. long infant with desquamation and meconium-stained nails and cord, estimated gestation 43 weeks.

Classically postmature infants show neither of these metabolic problems in excess frequency. Therefore the answer is D.

We would take some exception to this statement since we have seen a number of classically postmature infants who do show hypoglycemia, presumably on the basis of exhaustion of their liver supplies of glycogen. Despite their large birth weight, their clinical appearance does give them away, and some of them do remain at risk for serious hypoglycemia which should be both measured and corrected if present.

L. STERN

A jittery and twitchy 4200-gm. infant two hours old.

This infant is too young to be hypocalcemic. He is at a typical age for the early hypoglycemia of an infant of a diabetic mother. Of course, the problem might also be an anoxic insult at birth or CNS injury. The answer is A.

CASE PROBLEMS

Case One

You are called to see a five-day-old infant because of irritability and jerking movements of the left arm and leg. He was the product of a full-term pregnancy, birth weight 2892 gm. Pregnancy was complicated by second and third trimester bleeding. Delivery was by cesarean section because of placenta previa. One-minute Apgar was 6; five-minute Apgar was 9. Enfamil formula was begun at 16 hours of age and he did very well until a few hours ago when he became tremulous, began to cry constantly, and fed poorly; intermittent convulsions were noted. Examination reveals irritability. No abnormalities are found, but as the examination ends, the child convulses.

What diagnostic tests and procedures would you perform initially?

The symptoms shown by this baby are, of course, nonspecific. CNS hemorrhage or infection should be immediately considered, and a lumbar puncture must be done. There is nothing in the case history to suggest hypoglycemia as a *probable* cause of the seizures, but some of the less common hypoglycemic syndromes may present this way (leucine sensitivity, islet-cell tumor, etc.), and Dextrostix should be performed. Serum for electrolytes, calcium, total protein, BUN, and glucose should be drawn.

Several features of this case suggest the possibility of hypocalcemia, notably: stormy obstetrical course, milk feedings, age of onset of symptoms after initially benign course, and irritability and tremulousness as cardinal symptoms. These features would justify a therapeutic trial with calcium after initial studies are completed.

Subsequent to immediate evaluation and treatment, the laboratory reports a calcium of 5.8 mg. per 100 ml. and phosphorus 11.5 mg. per 100 ml.

What factors may be important in pathogenesis of the hypocalcemia?

The features outstanding in this case have been mentioned above. The high serum phosphorus suggests that dietary factors are predominant. Relative hypoparathyroidism and renal immaturity have combined to aggravate phosphate retention.

What further tests are indicated?

Subclinical maternal hyperparathyroidism should be ruled out by a careful history and serum calcium and phosphorus determinations on the mother.

What management would you institute?

The therapeutic trial utilizes 10 per cent calcium gluconate, up to 10 ml. by slow infusion with EKG monitoring. The infusion should be stopped when the seizures cease. Maintenance therapy may begin as follows:
Low phosphorus milk, PM 60/40.
Calcium gluconate, 20 ml. 10 per cent solution per 24 hours added to I.V. OR
Calcium chloride, 2 to 3 gm. per day in three to four doses added to feedings (concentration must not exceed one per cent). OR
Calcium lactate or calcium gluconate, 3 to 4 gm. per day in four to six doses.

What is the prognosis?

Excellent. Supplemental calcium may be tapered and withdrawn at three to four weeks of age. Serum calcium should be monitored at this time to be sure hypocalcemia does not recur. There should be no long-term sequelae.

Case Two

You attend the delivery at 36 weeks by cesarean section of a 24-year-old juvenile-onset diabetic. The infant boy weighs 3700 gm. and is plethoric, appears cushingoid, and has moderate hepatomegaly and splenomegaly, and a respiratory rate of 60 without retractions or grunting. His Dextrostix at 15 minutes of age reads 90 mg. per 100 ml. At two hours of age, all seems well. A capillary blood glucose is obtained. An hour later, the laboratory reports a value of 12 mg. per 100 ml.

How would you proceed at this point?

Coolly. As many as 50 per cent of infants of diabetic mothers will reach levels as low as 12 mg. per 100 ml. in the first two hours, and most will rebound satisfactorily (see Fig. 10–1). Check the baby. If he is symptomatic, treat after drawing another sample. If symptoms are doubtful or absent, draw a sample

and wait. Dextrostix are now of no help. (The laboratory reported the second sample as 27 mg. per 100 ml. At four hours, blood glucose was 34 mg. per 100 ml.) Early feeding may be considered if clinical condition is good.

At 24 hours of age, the baby is reported as irritable. Feedings have been started and are taken very slowly. Examination reveals Moro and tone are reduced. Color is good, pulse = 120 per minute, and respiratory rate = 65 per minute without retractions. Chvostek sign is elicited. Blood glucose is 35 mg. per 100 ml. Serum calcium is 7.8 mg. per 100 ml.

Management?

This behavior is typical of the infant of a diabetic mother and calls for the usual careful evaluation and observation for complications found in these babies (venous thromboses, anomalies). There is no indication of hypoglycemia or hypocalcemia sufficient to cause the baby's symptoms. The mother should be told that everything is going well with the infant.

Case Three

A 39-year-old mother of six delivers at 38 weeks' gestation. Pregnancy has been complicated by recurrent pyelonephritis and mild hypertension. Membranes ruptured 18 hours prior to delivery. There has been some fetal bradycardia with contractions. At birth the infant is cyanotic and limp, but responds after two minutes of assisted ventilation with mask and bag. One-minute Apgar = 3, five-minute Apgar = 7.

Physical examination in the nursery at 20 minutes shows a thin, malnourished male infant. Temperature is 35.2° C. Pulse is 115 per minute. Respirations are 34 per minute without retractions or grunt. Weight is 2100 gm. Length is 47 cm. Head circumference is 33 cm. He shows good activity and color, and has a good cry and a fair suck. No other abnormalities are found.

What diagnostic and therapeutic steps are indicated for this infant? What problems might you anticipate, and why?

This baby boy is at serious risk of hypoglycemia both because he is undergrown and malnourished and because his meager energy stores have been compromised by intrauterine asphyxia and significant hypothermia. He needs to be promptly warmed. Immediate plans should be made to (a) monitor his condition and his blood glucose frequently (hourly vital signs, blood glucose at four-hour intervals), and (b) start feedings as early as possible, even immediately. The physician in this case elects to start glucose water at four hours of age, and orders a Dextrostix at six hours.

At five hours of age, the baby is noted to be apneic, florid, and unresponsive. Immediate ventilatory resuscitation is begun, the umbilical vein is cannulated, blood drawn for glucose, and 5 ml. of 20 per cent glucose injected, effecting an immediate and gratifying improvement. An infusion of 10 per cent dextrose in water is started at 60 ml. per Kg. per 24 hours. The laboratory reports the pretreatment sample as "too low to read."

What additional diagnostic steps should now be taken?

A repeat blood sugar should be done immediately, and if satisfactory, repeated one to two hours later to ensure effective treatment. An X-ray should be ordered to check catheter position.

A Dextrostix determination immediately after treatment is started reads 130 mg. per 100 ml. Two hours later the baby again becomes unresponsive. The Dextrostix is unreactive.

What next? Why has treatment been ineffective?

Another quantitative blood glucose should be sent to the lab and the infant should be treated immediately with hypertonic glucose 0.5 to 1.0 gm. per Kg. by push (the baby immediately improved).

The sustaining infusion of glucose given this baby would supply 6 gm. glucose (24 calories) per Kg. per 24 hours. This is much too low for this dysmature baby, who has basal requirements over twice this value. Note that the recommended maintenance infusion of 15 per cent glucose at 80 ml. per Kg. supplies twice as much glucose per unit time, and even this amount may be insufficient in some infants.

Recognizing this, the infusion is increased to 15 per cent dextrose in water at 80 ml. per Kg. per 24 hours. Plans are made to monitor blood glucose at four-hour intervals. On revised treatment, blood glucose is initially 130 mg. per 100 ml. However, four hours later it is 27 mg. per 100 ml. and the infusion is speeded. At 18 hours of age, blood glucose is 23 mg. per 100 ml. with the infusion running 110 ml. per Kg. per 24 hours. The infant again shows poor tone and refuses to suck.

What should be the next therapeutic step?

Further increases in intravenous glucose risk fluid overload or venous thrombosis. Hydrocortisone therapy should be started, with the aim of establishing gluconeogenesis and reducing the glucose requirement. The dose is 5 mg. per Kg. every 12 hours I.V.

The blood sugar subsequently remained between 40 and 70 mg. per 100 ml. Oral feedings were begun 24 hours later and gradually advanced. As soon as basal requirements (50 to 60 calories per Kg.) were tolerated orally, the intravenous glucose was decreased stepwise over 36 hours, with frequent blood determinations. Intravenous glucose was discontinued at five days of age, along with cortisone.

REFERENCES

1. Anast, C., and Folvell, J.: Interrelationship of magnesium metabolism and parathyroid activity. Proc Soc Pediat Res, Atlantic City, New Jersey, 1969.
2. Barrett, C., and Oliver, T.: Hypoglycemia and hyperinsulinism in infants with erythroblastosis fetalis. New Eng J Med 278:1260, 1968.
3. Beard, A., Cornblath, M., Gentz, J., et al: Neonatal hypoglycemia: a discussion. J Pediat 79:314, 1971.
4. Clarke, P., and Carre, I.: Hypocalcemia, hypomagnesemic convulsions. J Pediat 70:806, 1967.
5. Combs, J., Grunt, J., and Brandt, I.: New syndrome of neonatal hypoglycemia. New Eng J Med 275: 236, 1966.
6. Cornblath, M., and Schwartz, R.: Disorders of Carbohydrate Metabolism in Infancy. Philadelphia, W.B. Saunders Co., 1966.
7. Cornblath, M., Segal, S., and Smith, C., Eds.: Energy metabolism in the newborn—an international exploration. Pediatrics 39:582, 1967.
8. Cornblath, M., Joassin, G., Weisskopf, B., et al: Hypoglycemia in the newborn. Pediat Clin N Amer 13:905, 1966.
9. Ek, J., and Daae, L.: Whole blood glucose determination in newborn infants, comparison and evaluation of five different methods. Acta Paediat Scand 56:461, 1967.
10. Farquhar, J.: Metabolic changes in the infant of the diabetic mother. Pediat Clin N Amer 12:743, 1965.
11. Garces, L., Drash, A., and Kenny, F.: Islet cell tumor in the neonate—studies in carbohydrate metabolism and therapeutic response, Pediatrics 41:789, 1968.
12. Guthrie, R., Van Leeuwen, G., and Glenn, L.: The

frequency of asymptomatic hypoglycemia in high-risk newborn infants. Pediatrics *46*:933, 1970.

13. Harvey, D., Cooper, L., and Stevens, J.: Plasma calcium and magnesium in newborn babies. Arch Dis Child *45*:506, 1970.

14. Haworth, J.: Carbohydrate metabolism in the fetus and the newborn. Pediat Clin N Amer *12*:573, 1965.

15. Hertenstein, H., and Gardner, L.: Tetany of newborn associated with maternal parathyroid adenoma. New Eng J Med *274*:266, 1966.

16. Hohenauer, L., Rosenberg, T., and Oh, W.: Calcium and phosphorus metabolism in the newborn infant. Proc Soc Pediat Res, Atlantic City, New Jersey, 1969.

17. Maisels, M., Li. T-K., Piechocki, J., et al: Effect of exchange transfusion on serum ionized calcium. Proc Amer Pediat Soc, Atlantic City, New Jersey, 1971.

18. McCann, M.: Screening for neonatal hypoglycemia with reagent strips. Proc Amer Pediat Soc, Atlantic City, New Jersey, 1971.

19. McLean, F., and Hastings, A.: The state of calcium in the fluids of the body. I. The conditions affecting the ionization of calcium. J Biol Chem *108*:285, 1935.

20. Mintz, D., Chez, R., and Harger, E., III: Fetal insulin and growth hormone metabolism in the subhuman primate. J Clin Invest *48*:176, 1969.

21. Mizrahi, A., London, R., and Gribetz, D.: Neonatal hypocalcemia: its causes and treatment. New Eng J Med *278*:1163, 1968.

22. Obenshain, S., Adam, P., King, K., et al: Human fetal insulin response to sustained maternal hyperglycemia. New Eng J Med *283*:566, 1970.

23. Pildes, R., Forbes, A., and Cornblath, M.: Studies of carbohydrate metabolism in the newborn infant. IX. Blood glucose levels and hypoglycemia in twins. Pediatrics *40*:69, 1967.

24. Pildes, R., Forbes, A., O'Connor, S., et al: The incidence of neonatal hypoglycemia—a completed survey. J Pediat *70*:76, 1967.

25. Radde, I., Shaml, Y., and Parkinson, D.: The placental calcium pump. Proc Amer Pediat Soc, Atlantic City, New Jersey, 1971.

26. Radde, I., Parkinson, D., Hoffken, B., et al: Ionized calcium in infants treated with exchange transfusions. Proc Soc Pediat Res, Atlantic City, New Jersey, 1970.

27. Saville, P., and Kretchmer, N.: Neonatal tetany: a report of 125 cases and review of the literature. Biol Neonat *2*:1, 1960.

28. Sinclair, J., Driscoll, J., Heird, W., et al: Supportive management of the sick neonate—parenteral calories, water, and electrolytes. Pediat Clin N Amer *17*:863, 1970.

29. Stern, L., Ramos, A., and Ledue, J.: Urinary catecholamine excretion in infants of diabetic mothers. Pediatrics *42*:598, 1968.

30. Swiatek, K., Lueblen, G., and Cornblath, M.: Screening method for determining glucose in blood and cerebrospinal fluid. Amer J Dis Child *117*:672, 1969.

31. Tsang, R., and Oh, W.: Neonatal hypocalcemia in low-birth weight infants. Pediatrics *45*:773, 1970.

32. Tsang, R., Light, I., and Oh, W.: Serum magnesium levels in pre-term infants and infants small-for-gestational-age. Proc Soc Pediat Res, Atlantic City, New Jersey, 1970.

33. Widdowson, E., and McCance, R.: The metabolism of calcium, phosphorus, magnesium and strontium. Pediat Clin N Amer *12*:595, 1965.

34. Young, C.: Hypoglycemia in neonatal sepsis. J Pediat *77*:812, 1970.

35. Zucker, P., and Simon, G.: Prolonged symptomatic neonatal hypoglycemia associated with maternal chlorpropamide therapy. Pediatrics *42*:824, 1968.

Chapter 11

NEONATAL HYPERBILIRUBINEMIA

by

GERARD B. ODELL, M.D.,

RONALD L. POLAND, M.D.,

and

ENRIQUE M. OSTREA, JR. M.D.

"In this simple form of icterus neonatorum, scarcely any treatment is required. Mild, laxative medicines, such as syrup of rhubarb, and, if necessary, a small dose of calomel with magnesia...."

F. T. FRERICHS, *A Clinical Treatise on Diseases of the Liver, 1879.*

To understand neonatal jaundice one must consider the sources, hepatic clearance, and intestinal excretion of bilirubin in normal newborns (Figure 11–1). Bilirubin is formed from the catabolism of heme pigments, primarily (80 to 85 per cent) hemoglobin. The catabolism of other heme-containing molecules, such as myoglobin and the enzymes tryptophane pyrrolase, cytochromes, and catalases, constitute the remaining sources of bilirubin; these are known as shunt bilirubin formation.[47] The major sites of bilirubin production are the spleen and liver. However, all tissues of the body have macrophages that can form bilirubin from hemoglobin because they contain microsomal heme-oxygenase and biliverdin reductase, which are the two enzymes necessary for the degradation of heme into bilirubin.[30] The catabolism of 1 gm. of hemoglobin results in the formation of 35 mg. of bilirubin, which is transported in the circulation bound to albumin. In the sinusoidal circulation of the liver, that small fraction of bilirubin which is dissociated from albumin can diffuse into the hepatocyte where it is bound by receptor-carrier proteins (Y and Z anion-binding proteins) that remove it

from the aqueous phase of the cytosol.[46] Within the hepatocyte, the lipid-soluble bilirubin is conjugated primarily with glucuronic acid to its acylglycoside which is water soluble. This conjugation is done by the microsomal enzyme bilirubin-UDP-glucuronyl transferase. The conjugated pigment is secreted from the hepatocyte through the canalicular apparatus into the biliary tree and eventually excreted as a component of bile into the intestine.[3]

The lumen of the small bowel in fetuses and newborns contains the enzyme, β-glucuronidase, which can hydrolyze the conjugated bilirubin to yield the lipid-soluble unconjugated bilirubin and glucuronic acid.[9] This deconjugated bilirubin can be reabsorbed into the circulation of the fetus and newborn. In utero, the placental circulation can clear the bilirubin from the fetal circula-

From the Department of Pediatrics, Johns Hopkins University School of Medicine and the Harriet Lane Service of the Children's Medical and Surgical Center of the Johns Hopkins Hospital. These studies have been supported by U.S. Public Health Service Grants HD–00091 and HD–02268.

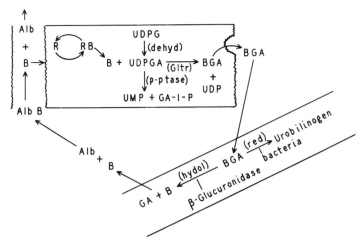

Figure 11–1 The hepatic clearance of bilirubin. The bilirubin enters the sinusoidal circulation of the liver attached to albumin (Alb B), as illustrated at the left. That small fraction of the bilirubin (B) which is in the aqueous phase of plasma, dissociated from albumin (Alb), can penetrate the plasma membrane of the hepatocyte and is bound by receptor-carriers (R) in the cytosol of the hepatocyte. The bilirubin is subsequently conjugated to its acyl glycoside, bilirubin glucuronide (BGA), and secreted from the hepatocyte at the canaliculus into the biliary tree, as shown on the right. The conjugation of bilirubin requires the microsomal enzyme bilirubin-UDP-glucuronyl transferase (Gltr), and the additional substrate uridine-diphospho-glucuronic acid (UDPGA). The latter is derived from the precursor, uridine-diphospho-glucose (UDPG), which is oxidized to UDPGA by a soluble dehydrogenase (dehyd) enzyme. Competing reactions for the UDPGA which are involved in bilirubin conjugation are shown as microsomal pyrophosphatases (p-p tase) and sugar hydrolases that form uridine-mono-phosphate (UMP) and glucuronic acid-1-phosphate (GA-1-P).

In older children and adults, the conjugated bilirubin, BGA, is excreted into the intestinal tract where it undergoes reduction (red) to urobilinogen by the bacterial flora. In the fetus and newborn, the BGA can be hydrolyzed to bilirubin and glucuronic acid (GA). Some of this unconjugated bilirubin can be reabsorbed into the portal circulation and requires hepatic clearance again.

tion, but after birth this reabsorbed bilirubin contributes to the overall load of bilirubin which requires hepatic clearance.[44]

PHYSIOLOGIC JAUNDICE

"Physiologic jaundice" during neonatal life can be operationally characterized by a rise in the serum bilirubin to 7.5 to 8.0 mg. per 100 ml. by the fourth day of life and a gradual fall to concentrations <1.5 mg. per 100 ml. by 10 days of age. The appearance of visible jaundice (serum concentration >8 mg. per 100 ml.) before 48 hours or levels which exceed 12 mg. per 100 ml. are considered of pathologic origin and warrant diagnostic investigation. Also, persistence of icterus beyond 10 days of age requires laboratory study.

The reasons for "physiologic jaundice" during neonatal life are controversial and multiple.[34] Almost every phase of bilirubin

metabolism has been implicated. The normal newborn produces 6 to 8 mg. of bilirubin per Kg. per 24 hours, which is approximately two and one-half times greater than the adult.[29] One reason for this greater production of bilirubin is that the life span of red cells in newborns is only 90 days in contrast to the 120 days of adult erythrocytes, and the shunt bilirubin from nonhemoglobin pigments is believed to be greater in infancy.[42, 50] The perfusion of the liver is also reduced in some infants owing to a persistent patency of the ductus venosus through which portal blood is shunted and consequently by-passes the sinusoidal circulation.[40] The uptake of bilirubin by the hepatocyte may also be impaired, because low concentrations of anion-binding proteins in the hepatocytes have been found in other mammals including primates.[28]

The enzyme required for bilirubin conjugation (bilirubin-UDP-glucuronyl transferase) has also been claimed to be deficient in the newborn;[10] however, the more recent measurements of this enzyme have demonstrated greater activity and therefore fail to account for physiologic jaundice.[17] The formation of UDPGA has also been suggested to be rate-limiting because of low activity of the UDPG-dehydrogenase of the liver.[10]

Finally, enterohepatic circulation of bilirubin from the gut after its deconjugation has been demonstrated to contribute to physiologic jaundice.[44] The meconium in normal fetuses and newborn infants contains between 0.5 and 1.0 mg. of bilirubin per gm. Thus, any condition that delays the passage of meconium is frequently associated with the early appearance of jaundice and abnormally high serum concentrations of bilirubin. Experimental interruption of this intestinal reabsorption of bilirubin in normal infants has reduced the degree and duration of neonatal hyperbilirubinemia.[44]

PATHOLOGIC JAUNDICE

The causes of neonatal jaundice due to underlying disease in the infant involve many disorders but operate by means of only two mechanisms: overproduction and/or underexcretion of bilirubin (Table 11–1).

Significant jaundice within the first 36 hours of life is usually due to overproduction, since the hepatic clearance of bilirubin is rarely so severely reduced that the serum bilirubin would exceed 10 mg. per 100 ml. Although categorized under overproduction, reabsorption of bilirubin from the intestinal tract and conversion of extravasated blood to bilirubin are gradual processes and rarely lead to obvious jaundice in the first 36 hours of life. Thus, early icterus is primarily associated with hemolytic diseases.

A hemoglobin destruction rate that would lower the whole blood concentration by 1 gm. per 100 ml. per day represents about four times the normal daily production of bilirubin (28 mg. per Kg. per day), and such a hemolytic process can, in some infants, exceed their capacity for the hepatic clearance of bilirubin.

Diagnosis of Hyperbilirubinemias Due to Overproduction

The recognition of hyperbilirubinemia due to overproduction should be suspected by the clinical appearance of jaundice before 48 hours of life. With Rh incompatibility there is usually both hepatic and splenic enlargement. The latter is rare in ABO disease. Diagnostic work-up (Table 11–1, Group A) requires blood typing of mother and baby and a Coombs test of the infant's cells for the presence of an abnormal antibody. In ABO disease, a very high anti-A or anti-B antibody titer is often found, but it is not necessarily diagnostic. A low acetylcholinesterase activity of the infant's erythrocytes is a better discriminator.[25] In Rh disease, the mother's serum will have anti-Rh antibody to the infant's cells that can be demonstrated by the indirect Coombs test.

Hematologic study should include reticulocyte counts in addition to serial hematocrits. After the third day of life, a reticulocyte count in excess of six per cent usually signifies the presence of a hemolytic process. The blood smear is probably the most useful examination. The presence of microspherocytes, polychromatophilia, acanthocytes and/or anisocytosis are all indicative of a hemolytic disturbance (Table 11–1, Groups A to C). Bizarre-shaped cells and clumped hemoglobin and Heinz bodies are seen in the hereditary anemias (Table 11–1, Groups B and C); examination of the parents' smears is important as well as the appropriate erythrocyte enzyme and hemoglobin analyses. The infants with excessive red cell destruction and consequent hyperbilirubinemia due to extravasated blood (Table 11–1, Group D) rarely show significant anemia or reticulocytosis, but careful physical examination will indicate the presence and location of extravasated blood.

The hyperbilirubinemias associated with polycythemias (Table 11–1, Group E) appear after 48 hours and show only the elevated hematocrits. Presumably the normal destruction of one per cent of the circulating erythrocytes per day in an infant with a hematocrit of 80 per cent would result in twice the rate of formation of bilirubin than when the hematocrit is 40 per cent, and could overwhelm the infant's capacity for hepatic clearance. A maternal-fetal transplacental bleed may be suspected if the infant has more than 30 per cent adult hemoglobin and if the serum contains an elevated level of IgA. Differential agglutination, if the baby's and mother's blood types differ, will demonstrate two cell types in the infant's circulation. Feto-fetal transfusion in twins is common when the infants are discordant in size; the larger twin

TABLE 11–1 CAUSES OF NEONATAL HYPERBILIRUBINEMIA

OVERPRODUCTION	UNDERSECRETION	MIXED

A. Fetal-maternal blood group incompatibility — Rh, ABO, others	G. Metabolic-Endocrine
	  1. Familial nonhemolytic jaundice types 1 and 2
	  2. Galactosemia
	  3. Hypothyroidism
	  4. Tyrosinosis
	  5. Hypermethioninemia
	  6. Drugs and hormones
	    a. Novobiocin
	    b. Pregnanediol
	    c. Certain breast milks
	    d. Lucey-Driscoll syndrome
	  7. Infants of diabetic mothers
	  8. Prematurity
	  9. Hypopituitarism and anencephaly
		I. Sepsis
		
		J. Intrauterine infections
		  1. Toxoplasmosis
		  2. Rubella
		  3. CID
		  4. Herpes simplex
		  5. Syphilis
		  6. Hepatitis (HAA)
		
		K. Respiratory distress syndromes

B. Hereditary spherocytosis		

C. Nonspherocytic hemolytic anemias
  1. G6PD deficiency and drug.
  2. Pyruvate kinase defic.
  3. Other red-cell enzyme def.
  4. α-thallassemia
  5. β-δ thallassemia
  6. Vitamin K_3 induced hemolysis		

D. Extravascular blood — petechiae, hematomata, pulmonary, cerebral, or occult hemorrhage	H. Obstructive
	  1. Biliary atresia*
	    a. Trisomy 18
	  2. Dubin-Johnson and Rotor's syndromes*
	  3. Choledochal cyst.*
	  4. Cystic fibrosis* (inspissated bile)
	  5. Tumor or *band**
	    (extrinsic obstruction)
	  6. α_1 antitrypsin deficiency*	

E. Polycythemia
  1. Maternal-fetal or feto-fetal transfusion
  2. Delayed clamping of the umbilical cord		

F. Increased enterohepatic circulation
  1. Pyloric stenosis*
  2. Intestinal atresia or stenosis including annular pancreas
  3. Hirschprung's Disease
  4. Meconium ileus or meconium plug syndrome
  5. Fasting and/or other cause for hypoperistalsis
  6. Drug-induced paralytic ileus (hexamethoniums)
  7. Swallowed blood		

*Jaundice not usually seen in neonatal period.

usually exhibits polycythemia and the smaller twin is often anemic.

The jaundice due primarily to enterohepatic circulation is not infrequent (Table 11–1, Group F). Abdominal distention and bile-stained vomitus, as well as a history of polyhydramnios, are the hallmarks of intestinal obstruction. It is important to review carefully the nurses' observations of the infant for the time of passage of meconium and number of stools. A saline enema to relieve a meconium plug should always be followed by testing the meconium for high protein content in order to identify the baby with cystic fibrosis.[11] This is most simply done by mixing 1 gm. of meconium in 4 vol. of water. After centrifugation, a few drops of 20 per cent trichloroacetic acid are added to the supernatant fluid; a white precipitate will develop if abnormal amounts of protein are present. The albustix can also be used but the fluid tested must be clear in order to avoid bile-staining, which gives falsely positive readings.

Patients with the swallowed blood syndrome are often jaundiced because some of the adult hemoglobin is catabolized by the intestinal mucosa, resulting in the formation and release of bilirubin to the circulation.[31]

Undersecretion

The recognition and identification of the diseases which interfere with the hepatic clearance of bilirubin and result in its undersecretion (Table 11-1) are often difficult, and require primarily a high index of suspicion on the part of the physician and a determination to discover the cause of the hyperbilirubinemia, because examinations for the presence of hemolytic diseases are negative. The familial nonhemolytic jaundices of infancy (Table 11-1, Group G, 1) are due to a deficiency of the UDP-glucuronyl transferase in the endoplasmic reticulum of hepatic microsomes, and all of the serum bilirubin is nonconjugated. Type 1 (the Crigler-Najjar syndrome) is the more serious, for the deficiency is complete and the hyperbilirubinemia more severe (serum bilirubins exceed 25 mg. per 100 ml.). It has an autosomal recessive pattern of inheritance and both parents can usually be demonstrated to be hemizygous when tested for their ability to excrete a number of aglycones as glucuronides.[13] The type 2 patients have a partial deficiency of UDP-glucuronyl transferase, which can be induced to greater activity by carcinogenic hydrocarbons as well as phenobarbital. The hyperbilirubinemia is not as severe as in type 1 (serum bilirubins <25 mg. per 100 ml.), and the inheritance is more consistent with an autosomal dominant, for only one of the parents exhibits a partial deficiency for glucuronidization.[4] These latter patients are comparable to a severe form of Gilbert's syndrome, but the latter has not been diagnosed in infancy.

Patients with galactosemia (Table 11-1, Group G, 2) often have only nonconjugated hyperbilirubinemia during the first week of life, and urine analysis will reveal a non-glucose reducing substance. Specific assay for erythrocyte uridyl transferase is necessary for the diagnosis of galactosemia, and if suspected, a lactose-free formula should be used for the infant's feedings.[23]

The neonatal hyperbilirubinemia of hypothyroidism (Table 11-1, Group G, 3) not only exceeds 12 mg. per 100 ml., but, like galactosemia, is persistent beyond the first 10 days; unlike galactosemia, however, it remains as a nonconjugated hyperbilirubinemia.[2] The hyperbilirubinemia is often the only significant sign (i.e., macroglossia, acrocyanosis, or hoarse cry may not be present). A serum BEI or T_4 should be determined on any suspicion, and the absence of a distal femoral epiphysis by X-ray in a term infant is highly suggestive of hypothyroidism. The jaundice of hypopituitarism and anencephaly (Table 11-1, Group G, 9) are most likely the result of hypothyroidism secondary to the deficiency of TSH stimulation for thyroid secretion.[19]

In addition to hyperbilirubinemia, the disorders of amino-acid metabolism, tyrosinosis and hypermethioninemia (Table 11-1, Group G, 4, 5) frequently exhibit hypoglycemia, and hypophosphatemia and phosphaturia. The amino-acidemia and amino-aciduria are diagnostic if performed, and elimination dietary therapy can prevent or delay the otherwise progressive hepatic insufficiency in these disorders.[21, 43]

The exact mechanism by which hepatic clearance of bilirubin is delayed is not precisely known in the diseases of Group G, 2-5 (Table 11-1), but initially either hepatic uptake or conjugation is primarily involved because the hyperbilirubinemia is nonconjugated. With the diseases of Group G, 2, 4, 5 (Table 11-1), hepatic necrosis and fibrosis eventually develop. With the development of hepatic necrosis, regurgitation of some of the conjugated bilirubin from the hepatocyte into the circulation results, and a significant fraction of the total serum bilirubin is conjugated (>2 mg. per 100 ml.). Bilirubinuria is also found when conjugated bilirubin concentrations exceed 2 mg. per 100 ml; it is filtered at the renal glomerulus because of its greater water solubility and weaker protein binding.

It should be mentioned that conjugated hyperbilirubinemia and bilirubinuria are also found in severe hemolytic diseases, but there is usually no intrinsic liver disease. In these latter instances, the uptake and conjugation of the bilirubin exceed the capacity of the canalicular secretion of the conjugated bilirubin because of the very high loads of bilirubin being cleared by the hepatocytes.[3] Occasionally, infants with severe Rh disease do have hepatic injury and will also show regurgitation jaundice.[18]

The drugs and hormones that are associated with neonatal hyperbilirubinemia (Table 11-1, Group G, 6 a and b) appear to interfere primarily with conjugation of bilirubin, but may also secondarily delay the hepatic uptake from the sinusoids because the receptor-carriers of bilirubin in the liver cytosol are already partly saturated with bilirubin.[22] In addition to the breast milk jaundice (Table 11–1, Group G, 6 c) associated with the presence of pregnane-3α, 20β-diol,[5] there are other mothers whose milk is inhibitory to the conjugation of bilirubin where this latter progesterone derivative is not found.[1] In both groups of breast-fed jaundice, the hyperbilirubinemia develops on the third day of life and becomes exaggerated and persistent (>12 mg. per 100 ml.) after the fifth day of life. The most direct diagnosis can be made by in vitro assay of the milk for its inhibitory effect on the conjugation of bilirubin in rat liver microsomes. Temporary substitution with alternate feedings of formula will prevent the bilirubin from rising to toxic levels. Most of the hyperbilirubinemias found in infants who are breast fed are not related to an inhibitor in the milk, but can be ascribed to fasting (Table 11–1, Group F, 5). The infants, unless supplemented with water or formula, have fewer and smaller bowel movements, because the volume of colostrum before the milk comes in is too small to prevent greater dehydration than in formula-fed babies. Once lactation is established, the hyperbilirubinemia promptly clears.

Dr. Odell's proposal that some of the so-called breast milk hyperbilirubinemia may indeed be due to insufficient intake of food with subsequent effects on the enterohepatic circulation certainly has considerable merit. We have never considered it likely that hyperbilirubinemia occurring within the first few days of life in an infant of a woman who is attempting to breast-feed is related to the breast milk, since very little breast milk has actually been received at this point by the baby.

Finally, there is a small group of infants in whom either the inhibitor is sufficiently strong in the mother's breast milk or the hepatic conjugating system is sufficiently immature to allow for repeated elevations of bilirubin level each time breast milk is re-introduced with the fall, after it has been discontinued. We have seen a number of infants who have persisted with this situation for up to three or four months of life. The bilirubin elevations under these circumstances are, however, not very great and if the baby is otherwise healthy, we have allowed the mothers to continue the breast feeding, advising a change to ordinary formula only if the icterus proves disturbing or disquieting to the parents.

L. STERN

By the in vitro assay for bilirubin conjugation, Arias[6] found that the serum of a group of infants described by Lucey and Driscoll was markedly inhibitory to the conjugation of bilirubin, as was the serum of their mothers. The hyperbilirubinemia in some of these infants was of sufficient severity to have been associated with bilirubin encephalopathy. The identity of the inhibitor is not known but disappears from the circulation of both the mother and infant during the postnatal period. Diagnosis can be suspected from the family history but ascertained only by serum assay.

The jaundice frequently encountered in infants of diabetic mothers is multifactoral (Table 11–1, Group G, 7). In some, enterohepatic circulation is prominent, for it can be reduced by early feeding. In others, premature delivery by cesarean section may contribute because hypotension and respiratory distress occur and are associated with intestinal ileus and consequent delayed passage of meconium.

The hyperbilirubinemia of prematurely born infants (less than 37 weeks' gestation) is also multiple in its etiologies. All of the factors which were previously discussed that are ascribed to physiologic jaundice in term infants have been invoked to explain the jaundice of prematures by *assuming* that the hepatic clearance mechanisms are even further deficient. In addition, these infants often have a persistent patency of their ductus venosus if hyaline membrane disease is present.[40] Excessive production of bilirubin due to extravascular hemolysis (Table 11–1, Group D) is often contributory because petechial and ecchymotic lesions of the skin and subcutaneous tissues are frequent in premature infants.

The obstructive jaundice associated with the diseases in Group H of Table 11–1 is rarely recognized as pathologic during neonatal life, but in all the diseases of this group a significant fraction of the total serum bilirubin is conjugated and is therefore "direct-reacting" in the Evelyn-Malloy modification of the van den Bergh test (> 2 mg. per 100 ml.).[36] Patients with trisomy 18 are usually identified by suggestive physical anomalies and chromosomal karyotype. The patients with either Dubin-Johnson or Rotor's syndrome cannot be diagnosed without special liver function tests and liver biopsy. The infants with choledochal cyst usually have acholic stools, and in some, a right upper quadrant mass can be palpated which trans-illuminates. The liver scan after injection of ^{125}I-rose bengal can localize this obstruction as an extrahepatic lesion.

Patients with mucoviscidosis often present with obstructive jaundice at three weeks of age, and may have a history of a meconium-plug syndrome. The elevation of the chloride concentration in the sweat is diagnostic in these patients. If they are edematous, it may be falsely low.

Although usually associated with pulmonary emphysema, some of the patients with the deficiency in the α_1 antitrypsin activity of the serum have initially presented with obstructive jaundice, and they characteristically show a deficiency of the α_1 globulins on the electrophoretic pattern of their sera.

Combined Overproduction and Undersecretion

In many instances, neonatal jaundice of pathologic origin represents disturbances which involve both excessive formation of bilirubin and simultaneous depression in its hepatic clearance. The diseases most frequently associated with these mixed causes of neonatal jaundice are recorded in Table 11–1 (Groups I to K).

The infants with neonatal sepsis frequently show anemia that may be related to the hemolysins elaborated by the bacteria, which would reduce red cell survival. The septicemia may simultaneously prevent erythrocyte replacement from marrow depression. There is also bile stasis at the canaliculus of the hepatocyte, and infants beyond one week of age often show a significant fraction of the total serum bilirubin as conjugated (>1.5 mg. per 100 ml.). In contrast to the diseases of Group J, the liver shows little evidence, either histologically or by serum chemistries, of inflammatory disease.[27] Patients with sepsis often become lethargic and feed (suck) poorly. Hypo- or hyperthermia is not infrequent, and neutropenia is as frequently found as leucocytosis of the peripheral blood. Urine analysis and culture, as well as culture of the blood and spinal fluid, should be performed if bacterial sepsis is suspected. The selection of antibiotics for therapy will depend upon the organism, but we employ methicillin and kanamycin and injection of fresh plasma (10 cc. per Kg.) intravenously to enhance the opsonophago-cytic activity of the infant's leucocytes.[20]

The infants with the infections of Group J (Table 11–1) are difficult to distinguish from one another clinically. Their hyperbilirubinemia is noteworthy, for a significant fraction of the total serum bilirubin is conjugated (>1.5 mg. per 100 ml.) and may constitute as much as half of the total. These infants are often of low birth weight for their gestational age, and malformations of the eyes and heart may be coexistent. The peripheral blood smear characteristically exhibits thrombocytopenia, and pathologic calcification is frequently found in the X-rays of the long bones (celery-stalking in Group J, 1 to 4, and metaphysitis in Group J, 5). Intracranial calcifications are frequent in Group J, 1 to 3, and either microcephaly or hydrocephalus may be found in all.[41]

The diagnosis is most readily made by serologic examination of the peripheral blood or cord blood if it was saved from the time of delivery. An elevated IgM level is very suggestive of an intrauterine infection. Specific virologic culture of freshly passed urine can be diagnostic in Group J, 1 to 4, as well as culture of skin lesions in herpes simplex and dark-field examination for treponemes if syphilis is suspected. Viral isolation of CID can occur before any rise in serologic titer is encountered. Determination of the mother's titer in relation to the infant's is necessary for proper interpretation unless specific testing for antibody in the infant's circulating IgM can be done. The infant's titer may simply reflect the passively acquired IgG from the mother by way of the placental circulation. Neonatal hepatitis due to Australia antigen can now be identified by specific testing of the infants and maternal serum for the hepatitis antigen activity. In contrast to the diseases in Group J, 1 to 4, occurrence in a previous child is not uncommon in syphilis and hepatitis. Also, a history of drug addiction of the mother is more likely.

In all of the diseases of Group J, giant cell hepatitis on liver biopsy[36] associated with elevation of the serum transaminases and alkaline phosphatase is frequently found and accounts for the regurgitation of the conjugated bilirubin into the circulation from the diseased hepatocytes. The etiologic diagnosis is very important, for antimicrobial therapy is quite different in these disorders.

Those premature infants with idiopathic respiratory distress syndrome have a combined cause of their jaundice from overproduction and undersecretion. These infants frequently have intracranial and pulmonary hemorrhages, and the extravasated blood undergoes a more rapid catabolism to bilirubin similar to that already discussed under Group D of Table 11–1.[16]

BILIRUBIN TOXICITY

The mechanism of bilirubin toxicity in vivo is not precisely known, but in vitro studies have shown its toxicity to intact cells as well as intracellular organelles. Bilirubin, when dissociated from albumin, can readily diffuse into plasma membranes of cells and mitochondria. It can uncouple oxidative phosphorylation, accelerate glycolysis, and reduce protein syntheisis at concentrations which exceed 0.5 mg. per 100 ml.[15]

The clinical toxicity of bilirubin during neonatal life is known as kernicterus, which pathologically shows yellow staining in nuclear areas of the brain. The basal ganglia and hippocampus are the most frequently affected areas. The clinical manifestations are initially seen by the third or fourth day of life and rarely after two weeks of age.[35] The syndrome, however, has been documented as late as 14 years of age in the Crigler-Najjar syndrome.[7]

We must take issue with the statement that there is some time-limiting element in the possibility that kernicterus may or may not occur. The documentation as pointed out in the above paragraph that kernicterus has occurred as late as 14 years of age in the Crigler-Najjar syndrome further supports the contention that the relationship to time has little to do with bilirubin toxicity itself but rather with the likelihood that previously high levels will fall or that levels sufficient to result in kernicterus will not, under the usual course of events, be attained.

L. STERN

The Moro response is first diminished and characterized by incomplete flexion of the extremities. A startling stimulus may produce cervical extension with absence of flexion of the arms and legs. The sucking behavior becomes weak, and feeding is difficult. Vomiting, hypotonia, and a high-pitched cry are frequent. In advanced cases, paresis of extra-ocular muscles associated with a constant downward gaze ("setting-sun" sign), or intermittent oculogyric crises can occur. These initial signs of central nervous depression are followed by irritability, and the infant's musculature becomes rigid with opisthotonic posturing. The arms are pronated and alternately extended and flexed at the elbows with the fists tightly clenched. Hyperpyrexia and convulsions are seen in severely affected infants. Terminal gastric and pulmonary hemorrhages frequently occur.

While all of the physical signs above are present either singly or in combination in older infants, it has been our experience that kernicterus in very small premature infants can occur (and subsequently be identified pathologically at autopsy) without any of these signs, the only clinical warning being the onset of unexplained apneic spells with a rapid downhill course and death. Because of this, we have viewed such occurrences in small prematures (particularly those who have been subject to acidosis, asphyxia, and hypothermia) with the utmost concern and, subject to findings on estimations of free bilirubin (see below), would recommend a policy of early exchange transfusion in such instances.

L. STERN

Editors' Comment: Dr. Odell wonders if this is not bilirubin staining of dead tissue which had been injured during the period of asphyxia.

Late sequelae in surviving infants include choreo-athetosis, spasticity, sensory and perceptual deafness, mental retardation, and visual-motor incoordination. Deficiency of short-term memory and abstract reasoning, and short attention spans are also found in less severely involved infants. Thus, hyperbilirubinemia during neonatal life can produce anything from severe cerebral palsy with deafness to the syndrome of "minimal brain damage."[39] The more subtle forms of neurotoxicity are not clinically manifested in the newborn period. Since the toxicity of bilirubin to the CNS is largely irreversible after clinical signs become manifest, the identification of infants at risk to bilirubin encephalopathy is required before symptomatology occurs. Until recent years, management of hyperbilirubinemia was directed at keeping the serum bilirubin below 20 mg. per 100 ml., based on the observations of Hsia et al[24] that kernicterus in term infants with Rh disease was unlikely to occur if the serum bilirubin did not rise above that level. However, neurologic impairment has been found in premature infants at levels significantly less than 20 mg. per 100 ml.[8] More recently, it has been appreciated that protein-bound bilirubin is innocuous but that free bilirubin is toxic since it can penetrate cells.[33] In vivo bilirubin is primarily bound to albumin, and 1 mole of albumin can effectively bind an equimolar amount of bilirubin. The normal albumin concentration in newborns is 3.0 to 3.5 gm. per 100 ml. and one might anticipate that the infant could tolerate bilirubin concentrations of 25 to 30 mg. per 100 ml. before the aqueous phase concentration reaches toxic concentrations; however, in vivo, not all of the primary sites of albumin are available for binding bilirubin because of the presence of other organic anions. Such anions as hematin, some synthetic penicillins, sulfonamides, salicylates, benzoates, and non-esterified fatty acids reduce the ability of albumin to bind bilirubin.[32] The high affinity of bilirubin for albumin can be further compromised by the low pH of body fluids associated with acidemia of both respiratory or metabolic origins.[32]

There is no convenient method for the direct determination of tissue bilirubin levels. Currently, indirect methods to measure free bilirubin are employed that quantitate the relative saturation of the serum albumin with bilirubin.[26, 45] The principle underlying these tests is based on the mass action equation which governs the binding of bilirubin to albumin:

$$Alb + B \rightleftarrows AlbB$$

From this equation, it can be seen that the amount of free bilirubin varies inversely with the concentration of albumin available to bind it. When the available albumin becomes saturated with bilirubin, any new bilirubin formed will directly increase the concentration of free bilirubin. However, as this occurs, the bilirubin is no longer restricted to the aqueous phases of the albumin space but will diffuse into intracellular spaces. Consequently, even though the albumin is virtually saturated, one would not expect the aqueous phase concentration of free bilirubin in plasma to rise very much, for it will continually diffuse from the plasma into cells. Thus, the methods which attempt to measure free bilirubin in plasma do not lend themselves to meaningful quantitative measurement.[26]

The methods devised to measure the degree of saturation of albumin with bilirubin are more easily quantitated. In addition, they not only can predict whether the free bilirubin concentration is likely to be high but also can quantitate the margin of reserve present before the free bilirubin concentration will reach the critical concentration at which metabolic damage to cells is likely to occur.

In principle, two methods for measuring the reserve of albumin binding capacity for bilirubin in serum are possible. One method, developed by Porter and Waters,[45] involves the addition of a dye which is normally bound by albumin. In their studies, hydroxybenzeneazo benzoic acid (HABA) was used. When bilirubin is previously bound by albumin, the binding of HABA is decreased; the decrease in HABA-binding is directly proportional to the bilirubin previously present on the serum albumin. This assay, however, only measures the interference of the dye-binding capacity of albumin, for the dye added and many organic anions other than bilirubin can block this binding. Also, this dye-binding test is not pH-sensitive, whereas the albumin binding of bilirubin is strongly influenced by pH changes within the physiologic range.

The second method which we have used[38] involves the addition of salicylate to the serum from jaundiced infants. The salicylate anion can compete with bilirubin for protein binding and will displace some of the previously bound bilirubin. The amount of bilirubin displaced can be quantitated spectrophotometrically and is directly proportional to the relative saturation of the infant's serum albumin with bilirubin. Thus, as the infant's circulating albumin becomes more saturated with bilirubin, its displacement by added salicylate is proportionately greater. The advantage of this method is that it directly measures the relative saturation of circulating albumin for bilirubin itself. This method also accurately reflects the saturation at the actual pH of the infant's blood. The major disadvantage of this technique is that it requires spectrophotometric methodology, which is beyond the quantitative capabilities of hospital laboratories.

In the HABA saturation test, a decrease of more than 50 per cent binding capacity is considered a high saturation; therefore bilirubinemia should be treated. In the salicylate saturation test, a saturation index which exceeds 8 on a scale of 0 to 14 is interpreted as excessive saturation and the infant is at risk to bilirubin encephalopathy. (This value was based on the subsequent psychologic performances of the children at five years of age.[39])

Another simple assessment of serum saturation of bilirubin can be obtained by determining the concentrations of the serum bilirubin and total proteins if one has previously established that the hyperbilirubinemia is due to undersecretion and that no hemolytic disease is present.[38] *There is a good correlation between the concentration ratio of the serum bilirubin in mg. per 100 ml. divided by the total serum proteins in gm. per 100 ml. and the salicylate saturation index of the serum albumin with bilirubin. If the numerical value of this concentration ratio exceeds 3.7,* then the infant's salicylate saturation index is likely to be greater than 8 and *the albumin is sufficiently saturated with bilirubin to endanger the infant* to bilirubin encephalopathy; immediate therapy is necessary.

Other techniques for measuring serum saturation with bilirubin which are based on the principles described above will be developed in the future. Gel-filtration to separate protein-bound and free bilirubin in serum is currently being popularized,[12] but as discussed above, the concentration of free bilirubin will never be very high, so this technique can only provide information as to whether the infant's serum is already saturated. The rate of dissociation of bilirubin from albumin and its adsorption on cholestyramine is another means of quantitation,[37] but cannot be performed rapidly enough to be clinically useful.

We would agree with Dr. Odell that the present gel-filtration technique, if used simply by itself, does not offer much predictive value as to reserve; moreover, the equilibration phenomenon described by him allows for only relatively small amounts of the free material to be recovered from any in vivo suspected plasma. We have, however, developed in our department a predictive method which consists of the in vitro addition of graded amounts of bilirubin to the plasma of any individual infant whereby the capacity of that plasma (with its own known level of serum bilirubin) to accommodate additional bilirubin can then be demonstrated. When utilized in this fashion, the Sephadex gel-filtration technique can afford an index as to when one is approaching the danger level for kernicterus and at what point appropriate measures to lower serum bilirubin ought to be introduced.*

L. STERN

---

*Schiff, D., Chan, G., and Stern, L.: Sephadex G-25 quantitative estimation of free bilirubin potential in jaundiced newborn infants' sera: A guide to the prevention of kernicterus. J Lab Clin Med *80*:455, 1972.

CLINICAL MANAGEMENT

TREATMENT

Because of the multiple causes of neonatal hyperbilirubinemia, all efforts should be made to identify the etiology of the infant's jaundice *before* treatment is initiated.

This involves the following determinations:

1. Blood type and Coombs test.
2. Retype the mother and cross-match the infant's cells in maternal serum to detect abnormal antibodies when infant and mother have the same blood type.
3. Hematocrit and reticulocyte count.
4. Examination of the peripheral blood smear for platelets, leucopenia, and abnormally shaped erythrocytes.
5. Review of the medications and the feeding and stool history of the infant.
6. Culture of urine, blood, if sepsis is suspected.
7. Urine analysis for protein, cells, and reducing substances.

In infants whose hyperbilirubinemia is due to hemolytic disease, an exchange transfusion is performed to replace the sensitized erythrocytes with that of a donor cell which is compatible with both the infant's and maternal serum. (See Table 11–2.) The amount of cell replacement is a function of the volume of the donor blood used (not its hematocrit). An 80 per cent replacement of the infant's circulating erythrocytes can be be expected if the volume of the donor unit is twice that of the infant's blood volume.

TABLE 11–2   INDICATIONS FOR
EXCHANGE TRANSFUSION

INDICATIONS FOR EXCHANGE TRANSFUSION IN HEMOLYTIC DISEASE

Anemia (Hct. <45%), positive Coombs test and a rate of rise in the serum bilirubin >0.5 mg. per hour.
In ABO disease a rate of rise in the serum bilirubin >1.0 mg. per hour.
Whenever the salicylate saturation index is ≥8.0 or the HABA binding <50%.
Whenever the serum bilirubin exceeds 20 mg. per 100 ml. in the absence of a previous exchange transfusion.

INDICATIONS FOR EXCHANGE TRANSFUSION IN HYPERBILIRUBINEMIA NOT RELATED TO ISO-IMMUNE HEMOLYTIC DISEASE

A salicylate saturation index ≥8.0 or HABA binding <50%.
A total bilirubin: total serum protein concentration ratio ≥3.7.
A serum bilirubin >18 mg. per 100 ml. in prematures or >15 mg. per 100 ml. if acidosis and anoxia present (if the infant was not previously exchanged).

The choice of donor blood obviously depends upon the cause of the hemolytic disease. In Rh incompatibilities, Rh negative cells are to be used. If the blood bank is very good, ABO type-specific cells that will cross-match with maternal serum are appropriate. O-negative cells resuspended in the plasma of an AB donor are always satisfactory. In ABO incompatibilities, O Rh specific cells should be used with a low titer of anti-A and anti-B antibody; otherwise, the cells should be resuspended in plasma of an AB donor. Fresh blood is always desirable; however, bank blood which is less than four days from the time it was collected can be used.

The type of anticoagulant to be used is important. If the infant exhibits evidence of acidosis or hypocalcemia, fresh heparinized blood should be used and 0.4 mg. of protamine sulfate can be given at the completion of the exchange for each mg. of heparin that was present in the donor unit. In the absence of acidosis or hypocalcemia, we prefer the ACD-preserved blood, for the increase in fatty acid concentration associated with heparin is avoided and the albumin is better able to bind bilirubin.[48] Also, if islet-cell hyperplasia is present, as with Rh incompatibilities, hypoglycemia will not occur during the exchange. When ACD-preserved blood is used, calcium gluconate may be required.

Editors' Comment: Acidosis is observed during and shortly after an exchange with ACD blood. Then, as the citrate is metabolized, the infant develops a very mild alkalosis. To decrease the morbidity of the exchange transfusion for infants with cardiopulmonary insufficiency, we therefore buffer each unit of blood with 10 mM. of 1.0 to 1.2M. Tham.* This reduces or prevents the acidosis. Dr. Odell points out, however, that this does increase the alkalosis after the citrate is metabolized and increases the risk of ionic hypocalcemia, while Tris increases the risk of hypoglycemia and hyperosmolality (the latter producing acidosis).

The packed-cell exchange is used for severely sensitized infants who require immediate correction of anemia and anoxia at the time of birth. In these circumstances, the obstetrician will have notified the nursery service of the sensitized mother's imminent delivery. Fresh O-negative blood should have

*Pierson, W., Barrett, C., and Oliver, T.: The effect of buffered and non-buffered acid blood on electrolyte and acid-base homeostasis during exchange transfusion. Pediatrics *41*:802, 1968.

TABLE 11–3 TYPES OF EXCHANGE TRANSFUSION

Packed cell
Whole blood
Albumin-Primed

been obtained and cross-matched with the mother's serum. The cells should be sedimented or packed; these are brought to the delivery floor. Upon delivery of the infant, anemia is immediately assessed by the color of the infant and the cord-blood hematocrit. The presence or absence of edema and ascites, as well as hepatosplenomegaly, is noted. If edema, anemia, and hepatomegaly are present, an umbilical catheter is inserted into the vein to the inferior vena cava above the diaphragm and the venous pressure noted. If elevated, blood is withdrawn to reduce it to 10 cm., and exchange of packed cells for the infant's blood is performed in isovolumetric aliquots of 10 to 20 ml. until 100 ml. has been exchanged in term infants, or 50 to 75 ml. in prematures.

The infant can usually then be moved to an intensive care nursery and allowed to establish thermal stability and readjustment of his cardiopulmonary circulation and ventilation. A whole blood exchange transfusion can subsequently be carried out some four to six hours later. We believe it is a greater risk to try to accomplish a complete exchange transfusion right after birth. Cord blood will have been saved and the blood bank can then cross-match another unit which is compatible with the original donor unit, the blood of the baby, and the maternal serum.

Whole-blood exchange transfusions are employed for the replacement of the infant's sensitized erythrocyte population, and can simultaneously remove circulating antibodies. The exchange transfusion will also remove bilirubin. With a 2-volume exchange, the post-exchange bilirubin concentration will be half the value of the pre-exchange concentration.

Albumin-primed exchange transfusions are used to facilitate the removal of bilirubin when the red cell population of the infant is normal and there is no evidence of anemia or cardiac failure. One gm. per Kg. of albumin is given intravenously as 25 per cent albumin solution through a peripheral vessel about 60 minutes before the exchange is begun. The serum bilirubin usually rises in response to the albumin injection. An additional 10 mg. of bilirubin can be removed in both premature and full-term infants by this technique, which improves the efficiency of the exchange by 50 per cent.

A number of workers have proposed the addition of albumin to the exchange blood itself rather than priming the infant with albumin prior to the transfusion. The data on the amount of bilirubin removed by such procedures has varied depending on the formula used for calculating the bilirubin extracted.

L. STERN

TECHNIQUE OF EXCHANGE TRANSFUSION

The properly identified donor unit should be removed from the refrigerator about an hour before the exchange and allowed to warm to room temperature. Exogenous heat should not be applied, for the erythrocytes closest to the surface are likely to be over-heated (tanned) and will produce an intra-vascular hemolysis. Long warming coils are not used because they increase the possibility of mechanical trauma.

The infant should be fasted for at least three hours prior to the procedure and, if there is doubt, nasogastric aspiration can be performed. Hydration should be maintained by parenteral glucose infusion.

The infant is restrained by gauze bandages in a warm environment. We prefer an overhead heating unit with a servo control unit operated from the thermistor on the infant's skin. Additional materials should include a source of oxygen, and suction and appropriate resuscitation equipment. A single channel oscilloscope for cardiac monitoring is applied. At least three people are required to perform an exchange transfusion safely: (1) the physician who actually performs the exchange; (2) a physician who is skilled in resuscitation, who stands at the head of the infant and actually monitors the infant by recording pulse, respiration, volumes exchanged, and venous pressures; and (3) a circulating nurse who is available for obtaining necessary equipment, sample tubes, etc.

The exchange unit is disposable, and a surgical prep and cut down set is needed. Determine the length of the catheter from Figure 1–7. (See pages 15–16 for the procedure of catheter placement.) For exchange transfusion, we use a larger sized catheter (5 to 8 French).

Once blood return is obtained, the venous pressure is measured with the ruler provided. The pressure should remain between 4 and 9 cm. of blood during the procedure. A deficit of 8 to 10 cc. per Kg is established with the first withdrawal; this blood is saved for bilirubin, hematologic, serologic, and miscellaneous studies. Passes of 10 to 20 cc. are then used until a total of 170 cc. per Kg. body weight is exchanged. A comfortable rate of exchange is 2 to 4 cc. of donor blood per Kg. per minute. After each 100 cc. of exchanged blood, the venous pressure should be measured and the patient should be evaluated for signs of hypocalcemia. If there is irritability, tachycardia, or prolongation of the Q-T segment, then 1 ml. of 10 per cent calcium gluconate may be infused slowly. Bradycardia should be watched for during the calcium infusion; saline should be used to wash the catheter before and after the calcium infusion. In the absence of symptoms, the hazards of calcium infusion outweigh its theoretical usefulness.

When performing an exchange on a hydropic infant, the venous pressure must be measured after each 50 ml. of exchange. This is essential because the plasma protein concentration of the hydropic infant is low and is gradually raised as the exchange progresses. The infused plasma from the donor unit will increase the intravascular oncotic pressure and the extravascular edema fluid will shift into and expand the infant's plasma volume. This will be associated with greater demands for cardiac output on a cardiac musculature which may not be able to respond because of anoxia, and the venous pressure will rise. Repeated deficits may have to be established in order to prevent this vascular overload.

We would reinforce the concept expressed in the preceding paragraph. The failure to appreciate this has often resulted in death from cardiac overload in the hands of an inexperienced though well-meaning house officer.

L. STERN

The final aliquot of blood withdrawn can be used for determination of bilirubin and hematocrit, and for future cross-matching.

The infant's vital signs should be monitored every 15 minutes for the first hour, every thirty minutes in the next three hours, and feedings resumed by four hours post-exchange if the infant is stable. Blood glucose should be checked one and two hours after an ACD exchange and immediately after a heparin exchange.

Other complications to be alert for during and after exchange transfusion are listed in Table 11–4. The six-hour mortality risk in all infants after exchange transfusion by pediatric house officers was under one per cent[51] over a six-year period.

If the infant's umbilical area is believed to be infected or the catheter cannot be inserted, a supra-umbilical cutdown can be performed 1 cm. above the umbilical stump. Also, a cutdown can be performed on the anterior tibial vein and donor blood administered through it. By extending the incision posteriorly, the tibial artery can be used for withdrawal of blood from the infant either by cannulation or by free bleeding into a medicine glass. Some centers have used the umbilical artery, but we have had insufficient experience with this method to comment.

Antibiotic prophylaxis is not routinely used after exchange transfusions, and the parents are encouraged to visit and feed their infants as soon as medically feasible.

Because of the morbidity and mortality risk of exchange transfusion, an alternative form of management of hyperbilirubinemia has been sought. The most successful has been administration of Rhogam.[14] Postnatal administration of this antibody has sharply reduced the necessity for exchange transfusions for Rh incompatibility, by eliminating the sensitization of the mother. Recently, prenatal and neonatal administration of phenobarbital and neonatal phototherapy have been advocated for hyperbilirubinemia. However, these are not really treatments but are used as prophylactic agents to prevent hyperbilirubinemia. If generally applied, they will mask the hyperbilirubinemia, a characteristic early sign of the many diseases listed in Table 11–1, which leads one to the early diagnosis of diseases for which specific therapy already exists. It is also important to recognize that only about one per cent of live births will develop serum bilirubin levels for which exchange therapy is necessary, and of this group, less than one per cent would succumb to exchange mortality. Thus, prophylactic treatment with phenobarbital or phototherapy would be required in 10,000 infants to avoid the one exchange mortality. However, in hemolytic diseases, these prophylactic agents would eliminate the need for exchange transfusions in only a small number of infants with isoimmune hemolytic disease. These infants will actually require more frequent follow-up and multiple supportive transfusions, since the hemolytic disease will continue.

Because of his concern for the potential dangers of phototherapy, Dr. Odell has not included any discussion of the clinical use of phototherapy for hyperbilirubinemia. He believes it is still too experimental a procedure to warrant either recommendation or condemnation. To add controversy, we suggest that there is a place for the use of phototherapy.

As background to therapy, the concentration of indirect-reacting unconjugated bilirubin present in an in vitro solution of human albumin and bilirubin decreases when exposed to light of wavelengths between 300 and 600 nm. The water soluble, in vitro oxidation products of bilirubin, when injected into the circulation of Gunn rats, do not enter the central nervous system or produce injury, and are excreted primarily in the urine. However, the products formed by the in vivo photo-oxidation of bilirubin are excreted primarily in the bile. Thus, the products formed in vitro and in vivo are not the same; we know nothing of the toxicity of those formed in vivo. However, in vivo, 50 to 60 per cent of the products excreted in the bile appear to be bilirubin. In jaundiced infants exposed to lights, the presence of icterus in shielded areas of skin suggests that oxidation occurs in the skin, not in the plasma. The exact chemical nature of the breakdown products are unknown.

It has been demonstrated that phototherapy can significantly reduce serum indirect bilirubin levels in human premature infants and in adult Gunn rats. It is not known how light affects bilirubin metabolism. It might alter metabolism at several points. Light may affect the microsomal hemoxidase system, which would increase the amount of bilirubin carried in the serum

TABLE 11–4 COMPLICATIONS OF EXCHANGE TRANSFUSIONS

Vascular	Embolization with air or clots
	Thrombosis
Cardiac	Arrhythmias
	Volume overload
	Arrest
Electrolyte	Hyperkalemia
	Hypernatremia
	Hypocalcemia
	Acidosis
Clotting	Overheparinization
	Thrombocytopenia
Infections	Bacteremia
	Serum hepatitis
Miscellaneous	Mechanical injury to donor cells
	Perforation
	Hypothermia
	Hypoglycemia

presented to the liver. It might alter albumin-binding of bilirubin, or affect protein receptors, etc.

There are a number of other biological effects that are less well known, and are a potential concern in making any judgment about the management of small infants, using phototherapy. For example, in animals, altering the light may affect the onset of puberty, gonadal weight, and the timing of ovulation.

In addition to the photo-oxidation of bilirubin, albumin is also altered by light. The imidazole ring may be destroyed with loss of histidine. This photo-sensitization of albumin decreases the capacity of albumin to bind bilirubin. If this occurred in vivo, the decreased serum bilirubin levels secondary to photo-therapy may only reflect the increased tendency of bilirubin to escape outside the vascular system. At this time, there is no good evidence that the binding capacity for bilirubin or the serum proteins are altered with phototherapy.

Although it has been demonstrated that there is a decrease in neurologic abnormalities and damage to neurons in light-treated adult Gunn rats, there are no long-term organized follow-up studies in human infants, even though there has been extensive use of phototherapy. It might be argued that the absence of serious effects in reported and unreported clinical experiences provides data to outweigh the unknown risks, and therefore it is not proper to wait many years before accepting phototherapy. However, it is important to appreciate the extreme sensitivity of developing organisms. Thus, though we believe light therapy is useful, it is our general belief that photo-therapy should only be used when the risks of treating a patient are less than treating the jaundice by any other procedure. Dr. Odell points out that Ballowitz, when initially using lights, found an increased mortality and a decrease in weight gain in survivors.

Cool white or blue lamps with blue wavelengths from 400 to 500 nm. are the most effective in rapidly photo-oxidizing bilirubin. It is important to cover the eyelids so that the light does not reach the eyes, since it has been demonstrated that in young animals the retina can be damaged. We suggest that blue lights not be used because the unusual color of the infants makes recognition of cyanosis difficult and is also very frightening to parents. Phototherapy should be used for infants in whom the risks of hyperbilirubinemia outweigh the risks of phototherapy. It can be used in infants for whom an exchange transfusion is not yet indicated but when there is a reasonable chance that a transfusion will have to be considered because of (1) the clinical condition of the infant, (2) the bilirubin level, or (3) the rate of increase in the serum concentration of bilirubin.

There is no ideal formula as to when to intervene. Figure 11-2 is a rough guide to our management of hyperbilirubinemia in the absence of blood-group incompatibility where the binding capacity is unknown. *This figure is only to be used when there has been no asphyxia, hypoxemia, metabolic acidosis, or hypo-thermia.* For example, if the infant weighs less than 1200 gm. and has a bilirubin level between 5 and 9 mg. per 100 ml. the bilirubin reduction lights should be commenced prophylactically before the serum bilirubin is markedly elevated. Thus, lights should be used even though the level is 5 mg. per 100 ml. It is very difficult in these small infants, when the bili-rubin level is between 10 and 12 mg. per 100 ml. to decide whether albumin infusion should be given or an exchange performed. Measurement of albumin-binding capacity will help in the future to define the management of these difficult points. (The case problems at the end of the chapter will highlight this area.)

EDITORS' COMMENT

Our own views regarding phototherapy can be summarized as follows. While there is little question regarding the efficacy of phototherapy in lowering serum bilirubin, the question of its safety is open to a good deal of discussion and controversy. Had photo-therapy been a drug, it would never have been permitted for use in humans on the basis of the evidence presented concerning its safety. The only institu-tions which should be using phototherapy are those that are equally equipped to use all of the other skills and complicated approaches necessary to the management of a sick, newborn infant. As pointed out later in this chapter, its use in relatively unsuper-vised nurseries bears the immediate risk of deceiving the physician regarding the infant's true condition, since the light leaches the color from the skin (the re-action occurs in the skin); therefore it is impossible to tell what the serum bilirubin level is from looking at the infant. This error has often resulted in serious trouble, with the serum bilirubin level continuing to rise (usually from causes which have not been investi-gated because the symptoms seemed so easy to treat) despite the fact that the baby does not look jaundiced at all. Therefore, its use demands strict control of bili-rubin levels in addition to investigations aimed at determining the etiology, rather than a simplistic approach towards the bilirubin itself.

Our own policy, therefore, is to adopt a risk/benefit ratio approach to the problem. It is our feeling that an otherwise healthy, full-term infant should not have his hyperbilirubinemia treated with phototherapy. We would prefer to take our chances with the possibility that we may have to do an exchange transfusion in a small number of these infants when the need arises. Similarly, unless other circumstances make it imperative, infants with any form of hemolytic disease are not, in our view, appropriate candidates for such therapy; here again, however, caution must be introduced, in that the risks of exchange transfusions with respect to morbidity and mortality must be known for any in-dividual institution before such a judgment is made. We prefer, however, not to run the risk of prolonged future anemia or indeed to confuse the picture by subjecting infants with hemolytic disease to photo-therapy in any kind of routine fashion (this includes ABO incompatiblity as well as that due to Rh and the other auto-immune subgroups).

In our department, phototherapy has been re-served generally for the small, otherwise ill infant who is either badly asphyxiated or is suffering from hyaline membrane disease, and in whom the perform-

Serum Bilirubin mg/100 ml	< 24 hrs		24–48 hrs		49–72 hrs		< 72 hrs	
	<2500g	>2500g	<2500g	>2500g	<2500g	>2500 g	<2500 g	>2500 g
<5								
5–9	Phototherapy if hemolysis							
10–14	Exchange if hemolysis		Phototherapy					
15–19	Exchange				Phototherapy			
20 and +	Exchange							

Use phototherapy after any exchange ▢ Observe ▨ Investigate Jaundice

*Consider immediate phototherapy but exchange if bilirubin continues to rise
†Consider exchange, particularly if previous phototherapy not effective

In presence of:
1. Perinatal asphyxia
2. Respiratory distress
3. Metabolic acidosis (pH 7.25 or below)
4. Hypothermia (temp below 35° C)
5. Low serum protein (5g./100 ml or less)
6. Birth weight 1500 g
7. Signs of clinical or CNS deterioration

} Treat as in next higher bilirubin category

Figure 11–2 Guidelines for the management of hyperbilirubinemia taking age, birth weight, and bilirubin into consideration. (Usage of phototherapy lights in clinical icterus as employed at University Hospitals, Cleveland, Ohio. Courtesy of Dr. M. J. Maisels.)

ance of an exchange transfusion represents an actually greater physical hazard to his very existence than what we would at present consider the unknown long-term risks of phototherapy. Depending on the situation, we have begun light exposure in such infants sometimes immediately after admission to the department in anticipation of a rise in bilirubin which, because of the other attendant conditions in the baby, we would prefer to avoid.

L. STERN

Editors' Comment: Dr. Odell points out that other centers treat hyaline membrane disease by exchange transfusion, to take advantage of fibrinolysis and adult blood oxygen dissociation curves.

REFERENCES

(for Editors' Comments)

1. Ballowitz, L., Heller, R., Natzschka, J., et al: Effects of blue-light on infant Gunn rats. Birth Defects: Original Article Series 6:106, 1970.
2. Behrman, R., and Hsia, D.: Summary of a symposium on phototherapy for hyperbilirubinemia. J Pediat 75:718, 1969.
3. Broughton, P.: The effectiveness and safety of phototherapy. Birth Defects: Original Article Series 6:71, 1970.
4. Cremer, R., Perryman, P., and Richards, D.: Influence of light on the hyperbilirubinemia of infants. Lancet 1:1094, 1958.
5. Johnson, L., and Schutta, H.: Quantitative assessment

of the effects of light treatment in infant Gunn rats. Birth Defects: Original Article Series 6:114, 1970.

6. Lucey, J., Gerreiro, M., and Hewitt, J.: Prevention of hyperbilirubinemia of prematurity by phototherapy. Pediatrics *41*:1047, 1968.

7. Oski, F., and Naiman, J.: *Hematologic Problems in the Newborn.* Philadelphia, W.B. Saunders Co., 1972. 2nd Edition.

8. Ostrow, J., and Branham, R.: Photodecay of bilirubin in vitro and in the jaundiced (Gunn) rat. Birth Defects: Original Article Series 6:93, 1970.

9. Sisson, T., Kendall, N., Davies, R., et al: Factors influencing the effectiveness of phototherapy in neonatal hyperbilirubinemia. Birth Defects: Original Article Series 6:100, 1970.

QUESTIONS

True or False

The administration of 1 gm. per Kg. albumin one hour before an exchange transfusion significantly influences the amount of bilirubin removed with an exchange.

The administration of albumin just before the exchange will result in the removal of about 40 per cent more bilirubin. Therefore the statement is true. The albumin must be given with caution, as it increases the blood volume.

In a full-term infant with Rh sensitization, if the serum indirect bilirubin remains below 18 mg. per 100 ml., there is no need to worry that there has been any brain damage secondary to bilirubin.

Although it would be unlikely that kernicterus has occurred, the upper limit of safety cannot be defined. Studies of Odell and Johnson suggest that present criteria using indirect bilirubin levels alone are not adequate in determining whether an infant requires an exchange. The degree of saturation of the albumin molecule must be considered. Therefore the statement is false.

The eyes of the infant should be covered when using bilirubin reduction lights because light may affect the retina.

In piglets, Sisson* has demonstrated that similar lights will permanently damage the

retina and produce blindness when the eyelid is raised. Therefore the statement is true.

Phenobarbital appears to be a safe drug for lowering the serum indirect bilirubin, and it can be administered either to the mother or to the infant.

Although phenobarbital does lower the bilirubin, its actions are complex. Full effects of large doses of phenobarbital on the infant are not known. Brazelton demonstrated that phenobarbital in the mother or infant markedly alters the infant's sucking and activity for three to four days. In rats, neonatal mortality is increased following the use of phenobarbital in the mothers. Phenobarbital also activates a large number of enzymes in the liver, and it is not known whether all of these effects are favorable. Therefore the statement is false.

Any level of bilirubin greater than 9 mg. per 100 ml. may be damaging to some infants.

Boggs,[8] using data from the collaborative study, found an increased percentage of low motor and mental scores at eight months when the serum bilirubin was greater than 16 to 19 mg. per 100 ml. This was a preliminary study, and later follow-up of these infants will be necessary. The statement is possibly true.

Kernicterus has been observed with levels as low as 9 mg. per 100 ml.

Several studies of small premature infants have demonstrated kernicterus at autopsy. Most of these infants had been acidotic, asphyxiated at birth, or on respirators during their acute hospital course. All had low serum albumin levels. The statement is true.

Hypoglycemia is a complication which is sometimes noted following an exchange transfusion for erythroblastosis.

This is a real entity in Rh-affected infants. Some of these infants are hypoglycemic. Pathologic studies have noted islet-cell hypertrophy in infants with erythroblastosis, and there is suggestive evidence of increased insulin levels in the hypoglycemic infants. The statement is true.

Severe erythroblastosis often has hypoglycemia as a complication irrespective of whether an exchange

---

*Sisson, T., Glauser, S., Glauser, E., et al: Retinal changes produced by phototherapy. J. Pediat. 77:221, 1970.

transfusion is being carried out or not. This is due to the islet-cell hyperplasia which has been demonstrated in such infants associated with the large elevations in serum insulin. The precise reasons for this hyperinsulinism in the severely erythroblastotic infant is uncertain, but it may be that glutathione produced as a result of broken down red cells may act as a stimulus to insulin production in utero, with subsequent islet-cell hyperplasia and hyperinsulinism. The relationship to exchange transfusion is independent of erythroblastosis, although it will clearly be greater in the erythroblastotic infant who is already hypoglycemic. In brief, heparinized blood which contains no added glucose and which, in addition, will raise serum free fatty acid levels can result in hypoglycemia both by its own lack of glucose and by the inverse relationship between free fatty acids and glucose (elevations of free fatty acid usually result in a depression of glucose). When ACD blood is used, there is a good deal of glucose in the transfusing blood (average for the usual acid/citrate/dextrose mixture gives donor blood with blood glucose levels about 300 mg. per 100 ml.). This high glucose load, however, provokes a reactive insulin response which will persist once the exchange is completed. In this situation, the glucose infusion (i.e., the exchange) has been discontinued, but the persistent levels of insulin provoked in response to it may result in a surprising fall in blood glucose some two hours after the exchange transfusion. For this reason, we always recommend concomitantly an I.V. infusion of glucose when heparinized blood is used for the exchange transfusions and careful control of blood glucose in the post-exchange period when ACD blood is used; greater surveillance for both is necessary if the infant is also either severely erythroblastotic or the infant of a diabetic mother, both of whom can be hyperinsulinemic and therefore already hypoglycemic before the procedure is even begun.

L. STERN

Physiologic jaundice seen in newborns and prematures is secondary to a decreased amount of glucuronyl transferase.

At the present time, it is not clear why newborn infants are jaundiced on the third or fourth day of life. It may be the result of decreased amount of carrier proteins (Y) in the liver cell. The statement is false.

Immediately following an exchange with ACD blood, infants are slightly acidotic. The normal infant becomes slightly alkalotic two to three hours later.

Usually during and immediately following an exchange, the infant is acidotic secondary to the acidity of the blood used in the exchange. For a short period of time after the citrate infusion, the infant becomes alkalotic.

The reason the infant becomes alkalotic is that the citrate is metabolized more rapidly than the Na is excreted. Therefore, citrate is metabolized to H_2CO_3, which under normal circumstances would dissociate to $CO_2 + H_2O$; however, because of excess Na, the H_2CO_3 reacts with Na $\rightarrow$ Na$^+$ + HCO$_3^-$ to maintain electrical equivalence. Therefore the statement is true.

With proper techniques, the mortality from exchange transfusions should be less than one per cent.

With an experienced physician who attends to minute details such as temperature control, mixing of the blood, record-keeping, and close monitoring of the infant during the exchange, mortality is low. Therefore the statement is true.

If a full-term infant with Rh disease is treated with bilirubin lights on the fourth day of life, and serum bilirubin is dropped from 12 mg. per 100 ml. to 8 mg. per 100 ml. and then on the following day to 4 mg. per 100 ml., the infant can be discharged with no further worries if he is eating well.

Bilirubin light treatment is only covering one aspect of this infant's problem. Rh antibody can continue to destroy red cells and the infant can easily develop a severe anemia. This infant should be followed closely. Small transfusions may well be needed at two to five weeks of age. Therefore the statement is false.

For precisely this reason and as pointed out above, we would not have treated this baby with phototherapy to begin with.

L. STERN

When lights are used, it is necessary to do a blood bilirubin level even if the infant does not appear jaundiced.

Bilirubin lights have an effect on the bilirubin in the skin. When an infant is under the lights, serum bilirubin can be quite high with no visible jaundice of the skin. Therefore the statement is true.

It is best with a small premature weighing 1000 to 1500 gm. to start the bilirubin lights before the bilirubin has risen to 10 or 12 mg. per 100 ml.

This has been our own policy (Editors),

adopted from the studies of Lucey. Because the bilirubin lights lower the bilirubin only about 2 mg. per 100 ml. every 24 hours, we have found it useful to reduce bilirubin levels by using early light treatment. This is especially true in the small premature, who shows damage from bilirubin at a much lower level. Therefore the statement is true.

Editors' Comment: Dr. Odell observes that Lucey found no difference in neurologic outcome in light-treated and control patients.

Some infants become gray-black following the use of bilirubin lights.

This is a very upsetting experience, when the infant becomes a grayish-to-black color, often a death-like blue. It appears to be due to one of the breakdown pigments produced by the lights. It is not known what specific pigment produces this color. The statement is true. This is seen more often if there has been some initial elevation of the direct-acting fraction before therapy.

Many compounds should not be given to the small infant (such as Gantrisin, etc.) because they compete for binding sites on albumin, and may result in kernicterus.

In a trial using Gantrisin and penicillin in one group and penicillin and streptomycin in another group, Silverman observed that there was a higher mortality secondary to kernicterus in the Gantrisin-penicillin group. Therefore the statement is true.

Other compounds, such as salicylates, caffeine sodium benzoate, and the injectable form of Valium (diazepam) are also capable of uncoupling bilirubin from albumin. The latter does so not by virtue of its principal (diazepam), but because of the sodium benzoate. Unfortunately, sodium benzoate is a rather commonly used solubilizer and stabilizer for many parenteral preparations, and in testing such compounds attention needs to be paid not only to the compound itself but also to the vehicle in which it is carried. The elevations of free fatty acids resulting from hypothermia and from heparin can, if high enough, also uncouple bilirubin from albumin.

L. STERN

A mother who is Group O Rh negative has a newborn infant, also blood group O Rh negative, who develops a Coombs positive hemolytic disease accurately diagnosed as erythroblastosis fetalis. How is this possible?

The maternal Rh antibody is on all the Rh positive sites of the infant's cells, and therefore the typing sera cannot reach the Rh positive antigen sites, so the baby is called Rh negative. A possible alternative explanation is that since the routine terminology of Rh negative refers solely to the D antigen, in this situation, erthyroblastosis could occur as a result of blood group incompatibilities in the systems involving Cc, Ee, Kell, Duffy, etc.

There are many factors placing the premature at greater risk. Can you name some of them?

a. Lower total serum albumin.

b. Increased frequency of acidosis with decreased binding of bilirubin to albumin.

c. Increased frequency of anoxia.

d. Increase in free fatty acids with cooling.

A girl who is blood type O negative has two boyfriends, one O positive and one A positive. Which one should she marry?

a. The one with the most money.

b. Prior to Rhogam, the answer would be the boyfriend who is A positive, since A is a better antigen than Rh and one might expect development of ABO erythroblastosis which could be expected to be less severe though more frequent. Since the development of Rhogam, however, a better choice would be the boyfriend who is O positive.

CASE PROBLEMS

Case One

Baby Frank is a full-term infant, the product of a normal first pregnancy and easy delivery. The infant cried and breathed spontaneously. On physical examination at one hour of life, he was completely normal. Jaundice was noted on the first day of life. The mother was O, Rh positive, and the infant was Coombs positive, Rh positive, type A.

This is most probably what disease?

The most likely diagnosis is an ABO blood-group incompatibility, in which the baby's A cells have traversed the placenta and the mother has developed a hyperimmune anti-A antibody which in turn traversed the placenta, causing sensitization of the infant's circulating red cell mass. In actuality, despite its relative infrequency, an O mother with a B baby is much more likely to produce clinical disease than an O mother with an A baby.

How could you check this?

This may easily be checked by screening the mother's serum for hyperimmune anti-A, but more importantly by looking at the blood smear of the baby for spherocytes in the first 24 hours of life. If available, the red cell cholinesterase activity can be determined, for in ABO disease it is distinctly low.

At this time, should the infant be left alone, receive a replacement transfusion, be placed under bilirubin lights, or be given an injection of albumin?

At 36 hours of life, the bilirubin has risen to 12 mg. per 100 ml. Should this infant at this time be given a replacement transfusion, albumin, or continued under bilirubin lights?

Our therapy at both these times consists of observing the baby. When the bilirubin achieves 10 mg. per 100 ml., we do a saturation test to determine whether his circulating albumin is completely competent to bind bilirubin. If it is not, then we would do an exchange transfusion at 36 hours. We would otherwise follow the course of the baby's bilirubin.

Editors' Comment: At this time, the bilirubin is higher than that which was seen normally, certainly not at a level necessary for an exchange. We at Cleveland believe the bilirubin lights would seem a reasonable choice at this time.

At 36 hours, if one plots these two points on the curve of Allen and Diamond (Figure 11–3), it can be seen that the bilirubin will probably not rise to the zone of obligatory exchange transfusion. It must be remembered that these curves were constructed before the use of bilirubin lights. It seems reasonable at this time to continue the use of bilirubin lights; however, the bilirubin should be rechecked in six to eight hours.

At 48 hours, the bilirubin has risen to 13.5 mg. per 100 ml. with 2.0 direct. At this time, should we (a) perform an exchange transfusion, (b) continue the lights, or (c) give an albumin infusion?

The conversion of some of the baby's serum bilirubin to the direct-reacting fraction in the absence of light therapy is usually a good prognostic sign, for it means that now the baby is conjugating at a rate greater than his capacity to secrete bilirubin. This usually means that there will be an abrupt fall in the bilirubin in the next 24 hours. However, if this baby were treated with bilirubin lights, the rise in conjugating bilirubin could be secondary to the light therapy.

Editors' Comment: We would continue the lights.

In this instance, we would agree with Dr. Odell and treat this child like any other child with hemolytic disease. In our department, such an infant, otherwise healthy, would *not* be treated with phototherapy.

L. STERN

At 96 hours of life, the infant's total bilirubin had risen to 16 mg. per 100 ml., with 3 direct. On the seventh day, the bilirubin level (after the lights had been removed on the fifth day) had dropped to 4 mg. per 100 ml. The infant can be discharged.

Three weeks after discharge, what should be followed in this infant?

We should check this infant every two to three weeks, because the hemoglobin will drop, hemolysis will continue, and a small transfusion may be required. The lowest level is reached at about 6 to 10 weeks.

Case Two

T. A. is the product of a 21-year-old mother suffering from diabetes who has been under good control for the past two years. During the pregnancy there was no ketosis or hypoglycemia; however, the mother did gain 35 lb. At delivery, the infant weighed 3.8 Kg., was 35 to 36 weeks' gestation, and mildly asphyxiated. During the first 48 hours of life, the infant suffered from moderate respiratory distress, requiring environmental oxygen concentrations up to 60 per cent. On the third day, the infant was in 40 per cent oxygen, with a PaO_2 of 85 mm. Hg, a $PaCO_2$ of 50 mm. Hg, a pH of 7.31, and a total bilirubin of 6 mg. per 100 ml.

At this time, should the infant be treated with bilirubin lights, an injection of albumin, or no treatment at all?

The baby of a diabetic mother who develops mild respiratory distress and has a mild elevation of bilirubin probably represents hypoperfusion of the liver due to the well-

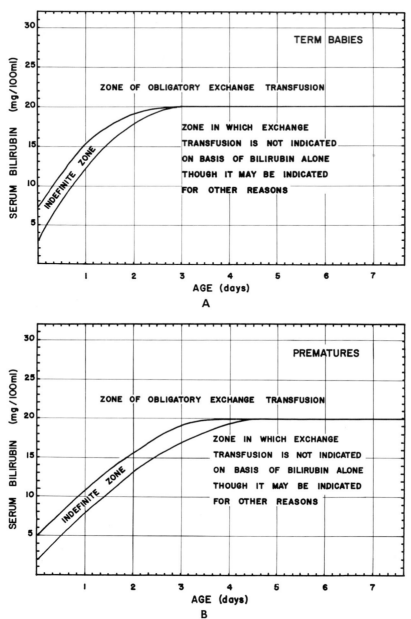

Figure 11–3 Bilirubin chart for newborns.[7] Please note that this chart was constructed before the use of bilirubin lights. *A*. Bilirubin chart for term newborns. *B*. Bilirubin chart for premature newborns.

established shortage of extracellular water; this infant would need circulatory support. The studies of Mogans Osler have been particularly revealing in documenting the shortage of total body water and the high risk for for possible stasis and thrombosis in these infants. Aside from an acute expansion of extracellular volume with a Ringer's lactate solution, we would not provide any additional treatment.

At six days of age, the bilirubin has risen to 9 mg. per 100 ml. This infant should:
a. Receive a replacement transfusion.
b. Be left under the lights.
c. Receive an albumin infusion.
d. Be left alone with no treatment for this bilirubin level.

The modest elevation of bilirubin to a level of 9 mg. per 100 ml. at day 6 would not be of concern, for by this time I would hope the infant would be on an oral intake and no longer have disturbances in ventilation. Continued hydration seems the most obvious answer.

Case Three

T. W. is a 1600-gm. premature infant, born in Cleveland, the product of a 32-week pregnancy complicated by some bleeding during the early weeks of the pregnancy. On physical examination, the infant was completely normal at birth, although he did require mask and bagging and bicarbonate. Sustained normal respiration began at 10 minutes of age. Grunting was noted immediately after he started to breathe, with increasing respiratory distress which required the use of a respirator at 48 hours. At 60 hours of age, the PaO_2 had risen to 120 mm. Hg, with a respirator pressure of 30 cm. H_2O and an environmental oxygen inspired concentration of 50 per cent. The infant was about to be weaned from the respirator when a total bilirubin of 12.0 mg. per 100 ml. was returned from the laboratory.

> At this time, the infant should
> a. Be placed under the lights.
> b. Receive an exchange transfusion.
> c. Be left alone.
> d. Receive an albumin infusion.

The baby with acute respiratory distress and respirator therapy who develops hyperbilirubinemia is a matter of acute concern. We will often perform the saturation test on the baby at the pH of the baby's blood to determine if he is in the "high-risk" category of above 8 mg. per 100 ml. These infants also have hypoalbuminemia, and we frequently have given either small infusions of plasma or whole blood. If the baby's saturation is high and his albumin is particularly low, we would perform an exchange transfusion which would do four things: (1) reduce the bilirubin level; (2) increase the baby's circulating plasma proteins to provide more protection; (3) expand the baby's blood volume, increase his blood pressure, and decrease shunting; and (4) provide adult hemoglobin which would release oxygen to the tissues at much lower saturations. Indeed, it may even provide fibrinolysins to help dissolve the hyaline membranes. If the baby were

acidotic, we would use heparinized rather than ACD preserved blood.

Editors' Comment: It is our impression that early use of lights might have prevented this elevation of bilirubin.

In this case, we would agree with the editors — phototherapy would, in such a sick infant, be our method of choice, too.

L. STERN

REFERENCES

1. Adlard, B., and Lathe, G.: Breast milk jaundice: Effect of 3α 20β -pregnanediol on bilirubin conjugation by human liver. Arch Dis Child *45*:186, 1970.
2. Akerren, Y.: Early diagnosis and early therapy in congenital cretinism. Arch Dis Child *30*:254, 1955.
3. Arias, I., Johnson, L., and Wolfson, S.: Biliary excretion of injected conjugated bilirubin and unconjugated bilirubin by normal Gunn rats. Amer J Physiol *200*:1091, 1961.
4. Arias, I., Gartner, L., Cohen, M., et al: Chronic nonhemolytic unconjugated hyperbilirubinemia with glucuronyl transferase deficiency. Amer J Med *47*:395, 1969.
5. Arias, I., Gartner, L., Seifter, S., et al: Prolonged neonatal unconjugated hyperbilirubinemia associated with breast feeding and a steroid pregnane-3(α), 20 (β)-diol in maternal milk that inhibits glucuronide formation in vitro. J Clin Invest *43*:2037, 1964.
6. Arias, I., Wolfson, S., Lucey, J., et al: Transient familial neonatal hyperbilirubinemia. J Clin Invest *44*:1442, 1956.
7. Blumenschein, S., Kallen, R., Storey, B., et al: Familial non-hemolytic jaundice with late onset of neurological damage. Pediatrics *42*:786, 1968.
8. Boggs, T., Jr., Hardy, J., and Frazier, J.: Correlation of neonatal serum total bilirubin concentrations and developmental status at age eight months. J Pediat *71*:553, 1967.
9. Brodersen, R., and Herman, L.: Intestinal reabsorption of unconjugated bilirubin: a possible contributing factor in neonatal jaundice. Lancet *1*:1242, 1963.
10. Brown, A., and Zuelzer, W.: Studies on the neonatal development of the glucuronide conjugating system. J Clin Invest *37*:332, 1958.
11. Buchanan, D., and Rapoport, S.: Chemical comparison of normal meconium and meconium from a patient with meconium ileus. Pediatrics *9*:304, 1952.
12. Chan, G., Schiff, D., and Stern, L.: Competitive binding of free fatty acids and bilirubin to albumin: differences in HBABA dye versus sephadex G-25 interpretation of results. Clin Biochem *4*:208, 1971.
13. Childs, B., Sidbury, J., and Migeon, C.: Glucuronic acid conjugation by patients with familial nonhemolytic jaundice and their relatives. Pediatrics *23*:903, 1959.
14. Combined study from centers in England and Baltimore: Prevention of Rh-haemolytic disease:

final results of the "high-risk" clinical trial. Brit Med J 2:607, 1971.

15. Cowger, M., Igo, R., and Labbe, R.: The mechanism of bilirubin toxicity studied with purified respiratory enzyme and tissue culture systems. Biochem 4:2763, 1965.

16. Craig, W.: Intracranial hemorrhage in the newborn, a study of the diagnosis and differential diagnosis based upon pathological and clinical findings in 126 cases. Arch Dis Child 13:89, 1938.

17. DiToro, R., Lupi, L., and Ansanelli, V.: Glucuronation of the liver in premature babies. Nature 219:265, 1968.

18. Dunn, P., and Chir, D.: Obstructive jaundice, liver damage and Rh haemolytic disease of the newborn. Jewish Mem Hosp Bull 10:94, 1965.

19. Gartner, L.: The hormonal regulation of hepatic bilirubin excretion. In Bouchier, I., and Billing, B., Eds.: Bilirubin Metabolism. Oxford, Blackwell, 1967, p. 175.

20. Gluck, L., and Silverman, W.: Phagocytosis in premature infants. Pediatrics 20:951, 1957.

21. Halvorsen, S., Pande, H., Løken, A., et al: Tyrosinosis. A study of 6 cases. Arch Dis Child 41:238, 1966.

22. Hargreaves, T.: The Liver and Bile Metabolism. New York, Appleton-Century Crofts, 1968, p. 125.

23. Holzel, A., and Komrower, G.: A study of the genetics of galactosaemia. Arch Dis Child 30:155, 1955.

24. Hsia, D., Allen, F., Jr., Gellis, S., et al: Erythroblastosis fetalis. VII. Studies of serum bilirubin in relation to kernicterus. New Eng J Med 247:668, 1952.

25. Kaplan, E., Herz, F., and Hsu, J.: Erythrocyte acetyl cholinesterase activity in ABO hemolytic disease of the newborn. Pediatrics 37:205, 1964.

26. Kaufmann, N., Kapitulnik, M., and Blondheim, S.: The adsorption of bilirubin by Sephadex and its relationship to the criteria for exchange transfusion. Pediatrics 44:543, 1969.

27. Kenny, J., Medearis, D., Jr., Klein, L., et al: An outbreak of urinary tract infection and septicemia due to Escherichia Coli in male infants. J Pediat 68:530, 1966.

28. Levi, A., Gatmaitan, B., and Arias, I.: Deficiency of hepatic organic anion-binding protein, impaired organic anion uptake by liver and "physiologic" jaundice in newborn monkeys. New Eng J Med 283:1136, 1970.

29. Maisels, M., Pathak, A., Nelson, N., et al: Endogenous production of carbon monoxide in normal and erythroblastotic infants. J Clin Invest 50:1, 1971.

30. Marver, H., and Schmid, R.: The porphyrias, In Stanbury, J., Wyngaarden J., and Frederickson, D., Eds.: The Metabolic Basis of Inherited Disease. New York, McGraw-Hill Book Co., 1972. 3rd Edition.

31. Nelson, T.: The relationship between melena and hyperbilirubinemia in mature neonates. Biol Neonat 8:267, 1965.

32. Odell, G.: The dissociation of bilirubin from albumin and its clinical implications. J Pediat 55:268, 1959.

33. Odell, G.: The distribution of bilirubin between albumin and mitochondria. J Pediat 68:164, 1966.

34. Odell, G.: "Physiologic" hyperbilirubinemia in the neonatal period. New Eng J Med 277:193, 1967.

35. Odell, G.: Postnatal care. In Cooke, R., and Levin, S., Eds.: The Biologic Basis of Pediatric Practice. New York, McGraw-Hill Book Co., 1968, p. 1500.

36. Odell, G., and Boitnott, J.: Conjugated hyperbilirubinemias of infancy. In James, E., Jr., Ed.: Pediatric Nuclear Medicine. (In press.)

37. Odell, G., Brown, R., and Holtzman, N.: Dye-sensitized photo-oxidation of albumin associated with a decreased capacity for protein-binding of bilirubin. Birth Defects: Original Article Series VI:31, 1970.

38. Odell, G., Cohen, S., and Kelly, P.: Studies in kernicterus. II. The determination of the saturation of serum albumin with bilirubin. J Pediat 74:214, 1969.

39. Odell, G., Storey, G., and Rosenberg, L.: Studies in kernicterus. III. The saturation of serum proteins with bilirubin during neonatal life and its relationship to brain damage at five years. J Pediat 76:12, 1970.

40. Ogawa, J.: Post-natal circulatory observations of liver and intestine in newborn infants. In: Proceedings of the XI International Congress of Pediatrics, 1965, p. 87.

41. Overall, J., Jr., and Glasgow, L.: Virus infections of the fetus and newborn infant. J Pediat 77:315, 1970.

42. Pearson, H.: Life-span of the fetal red blood cell. J Pediat 70:166, 1967.

43. Perry, T., Hardwick, D., Dixon, G., et al: Hypermethioninemia: a metabolic disorder associated with cirrhosis, islet cell hyperplasia and renal tubular degeneration. Pediatrics 36:236, 1965.

44. Poland, R., and Odell, G.: Physiologic jaundice: the enterohepatic circulation of bilirubin. New Eng J Med 284:1, 1971.

45. Porter, E., and Waters, W.: A rapid micromethod for measuring the reserve binding capacity in serum from newborn infants with hyperbilirubinemia. J Lab Clin Med 67:660, 1966.

46. Reyes, H., Levi, A., Gatmaitan, Z., et al: Studies of Y and Z. Two hepatic cytoplasmic organic anion-binding proteins. Effect of drugs, chemicals, hormones and cholestasis. J Clin Invest 50:2242, 1971.

47. Robinson, S.: Increased bilirubin formation from non-hemoglobin sources in rats with disorders of the liver. J Lab Clin Med 73:668, 1969.

48. Schiff, D., Aranda, J., Chan, G., et al: Metabolic effects of exchange transfusion. I. Effect of citrated and of heparinized blood on glucose, non-esterified fatty acids, 2-(hydroxybenzeneazo) benzoic acid binding, and insulin. J Pediat 78:603, 1971.

49. Strebel, L., and Odell, G.: Bilirubin uridine diphosphoglucuronyl transferase in rat liver microsomes: genetic variation and mutation. Pediat Res 5:548, 1971.

50. Vest, M., Strebel, L., and Hauenstein, D.: The extent of "shunt" bilirubin and erythrocyte survival in the newborn infant measured by the administration of (^{15}N) glycine. Biochem J 95:11C, 1965.

51. Weldon, V., and Odell, G.: Mortality risk of exchange transfusion. Pediatrics 41:797, 1968.

Chapter 12

NEONATAL INFECTIONS

by
AVROY FANAROFF, M.B., M.R.C.P.E.
and
MARSHALL KLAUS, M.D.

> *"Epidemic is fatal to these frail little creatures, scarcely able to exist outside an incubator. Congenital feebleness... greatly diminishes an infant's power of resistance."*
>
> PIERRE BUDIN, *The Nursling*

Historically, infection has played a dominant role in the determination of nursery design and admission policies. The high mortality and morbidity of infants in the early 1900s (usually resulting from epidemic diarrhea, respiratory infection, and inadequate equipment) led to strict isolation techniques in some cases, and to the development of separate wards for all patients who were free from infection. Standard textbooks on newborn care from 1945 to 1965[20, 32] recommend minimal handling, strict isolation, and the exclusion of all visitors from the nursery. While every effort was made to reduce the incidence of contamination and cross-infection, no provisions were made for the mother-infant dyad, and we are only now learning about the deleterious effects of early separation on the subsequent maternal relationship.

We now recognize that babies with suspected infection require more intensive observation than they would usually receive in the isolation or "observation units" which are legally required in some areas. Intensive care means *more and closer supervision.*

Today the incubator is regarded as the equivalent of an isolation room; therefore, with some exceptions, all infants may be admitted to intensive care nurseries. Rigorous handwashing is the infant's major protection from his environment, and allowing visitors under close supervision does not increase the incidence of infection in nurseries.[4, 40]

The fetus and newborn are vulnerable to most common bacterial, viral, fungal, and parasitic infections. In addition, some organisms not usually pathogenic for humans have been the cause of hospital-acquired infection in the newborn, such as some gram-negative bacilli, and listeria.

Whereas both mother and infant were formerly at risk from infection, over the past two decades penicillin has eradicated the streptococcus as the main cause of infection in the maternity units. Consequently, the mother is no longer at a significant risk, but the infant is now the chief victim of the staphylococcus and gram-negative organisms.

As a result of impaired local inflammatory response, systemic invasion by pathogens frequently complicates infection in the neonatal period. The symptomatology is often subtle and is usually similar, irrespective of the offending organisms, whether bacteria, virus, fungus, or parasite. A high index of clinical suspicion is needed for early diagnosis so that prompt and appropriate management may be instituted and morbidity and mortality reduced. Because of the high mortality (13 to 45 per cent),[19] the physician is forced to a decision before all the evidence is available.

The manifestations of congenital and acquired infections in the newborn period (e.g., syphilis, rubella, septicemia), together with the diagnosis and therapy, have been documented in detailed monographs, textbooks, and review articles. The aims of this chapter are to present a working diagnostic approach to infections in the perinatal period, and to consider the predisposing features and peculiarities of the immune response, laboratory work-up, and therapy of the commonly encountered situations in the nurseries, as well as policies in nursery procedure directed at preventing infection. No attempt will be made to systematically cover the entire field.

BASIC CONSIDERATIONS

INCIDENCE

The incidence of infection within the nursery will vary with the strictness of handwashing and infectious disease control, the type of hospital, local socioeconomic conditions, the number and types of problems admitted from referring hospitals, and the number of surgical patients on the unit. The incidence of septicemia in New Haven was 2 per 1000 live births from 1958 to 1961, and 1.8 per 1000 from 1962 to 1965, following the establishment of the neonatal intensive care unit.[18] A collaborative study involving 54,535 deliveries revealed that the incidence of neonatal meningitis was only 0.46 per 1000 births.[29] Therefore, even a large referral unit will not see many severe infections (usually 10 to 25 annually). The approximate frequency of virus infections in the mother during pregnancy and in the newborn are summarized in Table 12–1.

SIGNIFICANCE

The role of intrauterine infection as a cause of birth defects or disease of the newborn has been established for syphilis, rubella, cytomegalic inclusion body disease, and toxoplasmosis.[5, 13, 25]

The important role of infection in the perinatal area is emphasized by the evidence of Naeye and Blanc,[25] who showed that in-

TABLE 12–1   APPROXIMATE FREQUENCY OF VIRUS INFECTIONS IN THE MOTHER DURING PREGNANCY AND IN THE NEWBORN INFANT[30]

Infection	APPROXIMATE FREQUENCY	
	Mother No./1000 pregnancies	Neonate No./1000 live births
Cytomegalovirus	30–50	6–15
Rubella	1–22	0.7–7
Herpesvirus hominis (simplex)	0.5–25	Uncommon*
Coxsackie B	90	Uncommon*
Mumps	1.0	Rare*
Varicella-zoster	0.5	Rare*
Rubeola	0.06	Rare*

*There are insufficient data to permit numerical estimates.

fection commonly antecedes premature labor. In a study of 1044 consecutive autopsies on stillborn and newborn infants, 36 per cent showed anatomic evidence of antenatal infection in the placenta, membranes, umbilical cord, or newborn organs. In 77 per cent of the infected cases, infant organs were involved, and in the majority of cases, infection appeared to antedate labor and membrane rupture.

The precise contribution of viruses to abortion, stillbirth, congenital malformations, neonatal infections, and the long-term sequelae remains incompletely defined.[30] Although five per cent of 30,000 pregnancies were complicated by at least one definite or presumed virus infection (excluding the common cold),[36] viruses do not play a major role in neonatal morbidity or mortality, except during epidemics such as rubella in 1964. Then, despite the widespread practice of therapeutic abortion for rubella in the first trimester of pregnancy, a conservatively estimated 30,000 children developed rubella-associated birth defects.[7]

SPECIAL FEATURES OF DEFENSE IN THE NEONATAL PERIOD

Although defense mechanisms of the newborn infant are imperfectly understood,

TABLE 12-2 COMPARISON OF IMMUNOGLOBULIN CONCENTRATIONS OF HEALTHY PREMATURE INFANTS WITH NORMAL NEWBORN INFANTS[34]

GROUP	NO. OF INFANTS	DAY	IgG* Mean	IgG* Range	IgA* Mean	IgA* Range	IgM* Mean	IgM* Range
1500–1899 Gm.	5	Birth	970	695–1290	0		8	< 7–25
		7	1084	747–1330	0		23	9–44
		14	844	560–1025	10	5–16	33	31–48
		21	749	500– 980	16	10–22	29	22–37
1900–2250	7	Birth	1007	795–1150	0		4	<7–17
		7	1060	795–1350	0		24	18–41
		14	937	730–1200	7	0–19	30	24–52
		21	714	600– 900	19	10–24	32	24–55
Full-term infants[15, 25]	10	Birth	1080	810–1390	0		18	13–20
		7	940	700–1290	0	0– 6	30	18–40
		14	830	690–1120	3	0–10	37	20–60
		21	750	600–1100	8	0–18	36	20–58

*Mg. per 100 ml. of serum.

impaired cellular and humoral responses have been demonstrated.[2] The cellular response after the first 24 hours of life is limited by a reduced (in number) and inefficient population of leukocytes. Newborn infants are unable to concentrate their inflammatory cells selectively at the site of inflammation. The neonate's polymorphonuclear leukocytes demonstrate less ameboid movements and reduced ability to phagocytose particulate matter. This can be corrected in vitro by the addition of opsonins, normally present in 19S gamma globulin provided there is complement available. The impairment of opsonic activity in neonatal serum involves a functional deficiency of the fifth component of serum complement (C_5).[24] (Restoration can be brought about by infusion of fresh plasma, which contains functionally active C_5. This is the rationale for use of fresh plasma/blood in therapy of neonatal septicemia). Limited phagocytosis together with the delay in appearance of inflammatory exudates probably permits rapid invasion and spread and multiplication of offending organisms, especially in premature infants. Thus, poor localization with minimal inflammatory response are features in both the very young and the aged.

In the neonate, there is a lower enzyme content in leukocytes (glycolytic and pentose shunt pathways). Does this also impair the newborn's ability to combat infection?

S. PROD'HOM

The normal immunoglobulin values in the newborn are seen in Table 12-2.[34] The immunoglobulin G (IgG, 7S) is acquired from the mother transplacentally, and the concentration varies with the duration of the gestational period. Immunity from certain infections is thus conferred (see Table 12-3).[35] Immunoglobulin A (19S) and M (IgM 19S), containing the specific bactericidal antibodies to gram-negative organisms, which are largely IgM molecules, are not transferred. This deficiency has been postulated as the factor responsible for the high incidence of gram-negative septicemia in the newborn. Some observers[19] argue, however, that all newborns have this deficiency; therefore, neonatal

TABLE 12-3 ANTIBODIES PASSIVELY ACQUIRED BY THE FETUS[35]

ANTIBODIES IN CORD BLOOD EQUAL TO OR HIGHER THAN THOSE IN MATERNAL BLOOD	ANTIBODIES IN CORD BLOOD LESS THAN THOSE IN MATERNAL BLOOD, AT TIMES ABSENT
Tetanus antitoxin	Streptococcus agglutinins
Diphtheria antitoxin	H. influenzae antibodies
Smallpox hemagglutinins	Blood group isoagglutinins
Antistreptolysins	Shigella antibodies
Antistaphylolysins	Poliomyelitis antibodies
B. pertussis antibodies	Salmonella somatic (O) antibodies
Toxoplasma (complement-fixing and neutralizing)	E. coli (H and O) antibodies
Salmonella flagellar (H) antibodies	Rh complete antibodies
Rh blocking antibodies	Heterophile antibodies

sepsis should be more common. They feel that other host defenses play a more important role in protecting the newborn from invasion by infecting organisms. Normal cord blood levels of IgM are <20 mg. per 100 ml. and of IgA, 0 mg. per 100 ml. IgM globulin elevations may occur in a wide sprectrum of neonatal illness associated with chronic infections acquired in utero. IgA starts appearing in secretions shortly after birth, (e.g., tears—particularly in the presence of conjunctivitis) even before it appears in the blood.

For a long time it was erroneously believed that newborns were totally immunologically incompetent; however, following antigenic stimulation they do demonstrate a limited humoral response with initial production of IgM. In contrast to the child or adult who then readily produces specific gamma G antibody, in the neonate IgM persists for 20 to 30 days before quantities of gamma G antibody appear. (The passively acquired maternal antibody may be suppressing the immune response.)

In summary, the newborn demonstrates limited cellular and humoral responses to invading organisms. He acquires gamma G antibodies passively from the mother. The finding of elevated gamma M levels in the cord blood suggests intrauterine infection;

however, normal gamma M does not rule out the presence of infection. Although colonization occurs far more commonly than does the incidence of infection, there is a close parallel between the incidence of colonization with a particular organism and infection in the nursery (e.g., Staphylococcus aureus).

PREDISPOSING FEATURES, PATHOGENESIS, AND ETIOLOGY OF NEONATAL INFECTION

The predisposing features and pathogenesis of perinatal infection are summarized in Table 12–4. Many factors may all operate in the same infant, increasing the risk of infection. For example, labor may be induced *prematurely* because of *prolonged ruptured membranes,* resulting in an *asphyxiated* infant requiring *resuscitative procedures* including *assisted ventilation* and *catheterization.*

Blood-borne transplacental infection is encountered in association with maternal infection. Unfortunately, even asymptomatic infections in the mother may have devastating sequelae on the developing fetus.[26] Thus, a mother who acquires toxoplasmosis during pregnancy may remain asymptomatic yet deliver an infant with hydrocephalus.

A documented history of maternal in-

TABLE 12–4 THE INFANT AT RISK FOR INFECTION: ROUTES AND FACTORS FACILITATING INVASION BY ORGANISM AND ASSOCIATED DISEASE

TRANSPLACENTAL WITH MATERNAL INFECTION	ASCENDING INFECTION	PASSAGE THROUGH BIRTH CANAL	THE INFANT	THE NURSERY

Virus
  rubella, herpes
  cytomegalovirus
Protozoa—toxoplasmosis
	Prolonged rupture of membranes
	Prolonged labor and fetal distress
		Gonococcus
		Monilia
		Herpes
		Listeria
		Colonization with vaginal flora
			Prematurity
			Males >Females
			Congenital malformations (meningomyelocele)
				Equipment—incubators, respirators e.g. Pseudomonas
				Personnel—poor handwashing

Spirochete—syphilis	Prematurity	Trauma—with abrasions	Surgical problems	Other infected infants—β-streptococcus, rubella, E. coli, staphylococcus
Bacteria—e.g., urinary tract, gastroenteritis		Obstetrical manipulation Asphyxia (probably secondary to multiple procedures)	Catheterization of arteries and veins	
Congenital infections—usually present within first 48–72 hours (early or primary septicemia)			Late or secondary septicemia Present after 48–72 hours	

fection is helpful in suggesting the etiologic agent, and, when her bacterial cultures are available, they are used in initiating therapy. For example, in a mother with *Escherichia coli* urinary tract infection, appropriate therapy for *E. coli* will be included in the coverage for the infant if he manifests features of sepsis.

The infant is protected from ascending infection by the intact membranes. Premature rupture of membranes may be complicated by amnionitis, and the risk of infection is great, with the infant bathed in infected or contaminated amniotic fluid. Aspiration of this amniotic fluid or meconium into the lungs under conditions of fetal distress and asphyxia may lead to neonatal pneumonia. The fluid may reach the eustachian tubes and the middle ears, inducing an infection and meningitis.

Colonization with organisms from the vagina occurs during passage through the birth canal. Normal vaginal commensals such as β-hemolytic streptococcus may be acquired by the baby in this way and result in either local or generalized disease, including septicemia.

The invasion of pathogenic organisms is facilitated by skin and mucosal abrasions or defects seen following prolonged labor, difficult obstetrical manipulation, and vigorous resuscitative measures. The devitalized tissue is an ideal nidus for bacterial growth, while major congenital malformations, such as myelodysplasia, provide ready pathways for the bacteria.

The hazards of infection are increased by the use of indwelling venous and arterial catheters, which have become an integral part of intensive care management and are used for monitoring of vital signs, blood sampling, and infusions.

Sepsis is more commonly associated with venous catheterization than with arterial. *Staphylococcus albus* and Candida are potent pathogens when hypertonic solutions are infused via an indwelling catheter in the superior vena cava, while gram-negative organisms, particularly Klebsiella, complicate major surgery, such as small bowel resections or manipulative procedures of the genitourinary tract.

The risk of infection from prolonged venous catheterization has led us to avoid, wherever possible, the use of the umbilical vein as a source for infusion. Granted, infection can also occur in peripheral veins; however, this is generally locally around the infusion site and can be readily and easily treated. Infections through the umbilical vein itself have resulted in hepatic abscesses, splenic and portal vein thromboses, and systemic septicemias and are, therefore, in our view, best avoided. Wherever possible, therefore, a peripheral vein should be used for intravenous infusions of all kinds.

L. STERN

Admission to the intensive care nursery is not synonymous with arrival in a nonhostile environment with regard to risk of infection. This is an area in which exposure to infection can be minimized in part by the use of incubators, careful handwashing, exclusion of infected personnel, and use of sterile equipment.

In summary, organisms may reach the fetus transplacentally or be introduced directly into the bloodstream. They may be swallowed, inhaled, or gain entrance via abraded skin or denuded mucous membranes. Males are more often infected than females, and immature infants more often than full-term.

Etiology

The most common bacterial pathogens encountered in the nursery are listed in Table 12–5; the viral and other important infections in Table 12–6. Whereas before 1953, gram-positive organisms (particularly β-streptococcus) were the most common, at present the gram-negative bacilli are more prominent. In septicemia occurring after surgery, Klebsiella is the chief offending organism. Pseudomonas thrives in a moist environment and is a serious threat to infants on mechanical ventilators or those requiring prolonged oxygen therapy with humidification. Because

TABLE 12–5 ETIOLOGY OF NEONATAL SEPTICEMIA (Summary of some reported series.[11, 17, 19, 22, 27, 37, 38]

	1927–1957	1953–1968
NUMBER OF CASES	170	240
β-hemolytic streptococcus	28.2%	6.6%
Staphylococcus	15.8%	11.3%
Enterococcus	--	7.4%
E. coli	34.0%	33.3%
Klebsiella, Aerobacter	<1%	17.9%
Pseudomonas	7.6%	9.2%
Proteus	--	2.0%
Mixed	3.5%	1.6%
Other	9.4%	10.8%

TABLE 12-6 EFFECTS OF MATERNAL INFECTION ON FETUS AND NEONATE*

	EFFECTS ON FETUS AND NEONATE	ASSOCIATED FACTORS	PROGNOSIS OF INFANT
Coxsackie virus	? congenital malformations in first trimester. Transplacental meningoencephalitis and/or myocarditis. Acquired infections.	Maternal infection mild.	Depends on the extent of the disease.
Cytomegalic inclusion body disease	Intrauterine death. Premature delivery. Severe generalized disease — jaundice, hemolytic anemia, thrombocytopenia, hepatosplenomegaly, central nervous system disease including cerebral calcification and chorioretinitis), microcephaly, and undergrowth.	Half the women in early childbearing years show no immunologic response to this virus. Mothers are asymptomatic.	Early death in majority of severely affected infants. Severe mental and motor retardation in some survivors.
Hepatitis (serum)	Abortion. Neonatal hepatitis.	Circumstantial evidence incriminates hepatitis virus.	
Herpes simplex	Mild infection with a few skin lesions; infant does not appear ill. Viremia, severe generalized disease, CNS involvement. ? congenital malformations.	Maternal herpetic vulvo-vaginitis usually present. Transplacental infection of fetus may occur.	Mild disease — recovery. Severe disease — usually fatal.
Influenza	Increased incidence of abortion and premature labor. Occasional association of congenital malformations, especially anencephaly and meningomyelocele.	Active immunization by an attenuated vaccine should not be given during pregnancy for fear of fetal damage.	
Listeriosis	Infants infected either through direct invasion or from birth contamination. Generalized disease, skin rash, meningitis, pneumonia, etc. Fetal involvement with scattered foci of necrosis (granulomatosis infantiseptica). Delayed infection of the newborn infant, usually listerial meningitis.	4% of pregnant women harbor *Listeria monocytogenes* in the cervix or vagina. Occasionally influenza-like symptoms in the mother. Amniotic fluid noted to be dirty brown.	Mortality and morbidity high, especially from CNS complications.
Malaria	Direct transmission of *P. falciparum* occurs rarely. Diminished growth with placental involvement.	Placental involvement 10 times more frequent than fetal involvement.	
Mumps	Abortion, premature birth or stillbirth not unusual. ? cause of endocardial fibroelastosis.		
Mycoplasma	Chronic reproductive failure. Interstitial pneumonia or generalized sepsis.	Mycoplasma isolated from genital and lower urinary tracts of women and men.	Abortion in early pregnancy. Neonatal death common, generally from respiratory involvement.
Poliomyelitis	Abortion. Rare congenital or acquired poliomyelitis. Growth retardation in chronic, severe, maternal, paralytic poliomyelitis.	Widespread use of immunization procedures has all but eliminated this disease as a pregnancy problem. Use of Sabin live virus vaccine during pregnancy is contraindicated. May safely administer Salk vaccine.	Fetal and neonatal loss — 33%.

*Adapted by Rudolph from data of Desmond.[9]

TABLE 12–6 EFFECTS OF MATERNAL INFECTION ON FETUS AND NEONATE (*Continued*)

	EFFECTS ON FETUS AND NEONATE	ASSOCIATED FACTORS	PROGNOSIS OF INFANT
Rubella	Abortion. Congenital malformations of heart, eye, ear, brain; dermatoglyphic abnormalities. Systemic involvement with or without malformation, anemia, thrombocytopenia with purpura, jaundice, hepatosplenomegaly, bone changes, myocarditis, encephalitis, pneumonia, etc.	Maternal infection usually mild, occasionally arthritis and/or encephalitis. Strict isolation for neonates with congenital rubella as long as virus is present in pharynx or urine.	Residua and sequelae for the neonate depend on time during pregnancy when mother acquires the disease, virulence of the virus, and extent of the infectious process. Incidence of malformation in the infant is 35% in first month, 25% in second month, and 16% in third month of gestation. After 4th month, abnormalities are uncommon.
Rubeola (measles)	Interruption of pregnancy. Congenital or neonatal measles, with or without bronchopneumonia (typical dermal lesions are in same stage as those in mother).	Measles vaccine should be given to all nonimmune women prior to but not during gestation.	Maternal rubeola at any time during pregnancy is responsible for increased perinatal death rate. Great majority of infants are normal.
Smallpox and vaccinia	Increased fetal wastage in all stages of pregnancy. Congenital malformations not more frequent, but congenital infections with skin lesions reported.	Primary vaccination and revaccination against smallpox must be deferred until after delivery because vaccinia often causes fatal widespread fetal visceral and cutaneous lesions.	
Syphilis	Major cause of mid-trimester abortion, fetal death in utero, or premature labor and delivery. Early congenital syphilis (septicemia, skin lesions, anemia, jaundice, periostitis). Late congenital syphilis.	If maternal infection occurs less than 1–2 years prior to gestation, fetus probably will be affected seriously. When onset of disease occurs in early pregnancy, congenital infection usually occurs. Transmission of infection is rare before the 5th month of gestation.	40–50% of infants affected in untreated mothers. 40% of above show clinical signs at birth.
Toxoplasmosis	High incidence of abortion. Premature delivery. Generalized disease — hepatosplenomegaly, jaundice, chorioretinitis, microphthalmia, convulsions. Later manifestations — hydrocephalus or microcephaly, mental retardation, cerebral calcifications.		Poor
Tuberculosis	Small infants born to mothers with active disease. Congenital tuberculosis — rare. Acquired infection readily contracted.	Severe maternal disease and malnutrition. Essential to segregate mother with pulmonary tuberculosis from her infant to avoid neonatal infection.	Great majority of infants unaffected.
Varicella (chickenpox)	Premature delivery. Congenital varicella.	Low maternal immunity; most mothers have had the disease and developed immunity in childhood; therefore, congenital varicella is rare.	Mortality high.

of the large variety of pathogenic bacteria in the neonatal period, the establishment of a bacteriologic diagnosis is essential for optimal management.

PRACTICAL CONSIDERATIONS

CLINICAL FEATURES

In the neonate, by the time infection is obvious clinically to the most inexperienced observer, the diagnosis has been made too late. Because of the subtlety and nuances of presentation, a high index of suspicion is required on the part of the physician. Some of the many presenting features are listed in Table 12–7. Unfortunately, there is no single set of criteria which is reliable. In our own nursery, it is the nurse who usually alerts us to the diagnosis by observing subtle changes in color, tone, activity, or ease in feeding the infant. (Unless an excellent working relationship between the nurse and physician exists, early diagnosis is impossible.) Poor temperature control may be an early indicator of infection, with hypothermia seen more commonly than elevations of temperature with infections in the newborn period. Abdominal distention, apnea, and jaundice are often quoted as early signs of infection. However, these may all be seen in normal, healthy, premature infants.

There is often little correlation between the clinical manifestations and the etiologic agent; in addition, symptomatology may occur without involvement of the system. Thus, convulsions may be seen in the absence of central nervous system involvement, or a gastrointestinal disturbance without infection in the gastrointestinal tract. On the other hand, meningitis and septicemia may present merely with lethargy, irritability, and color changes. Do not be deceived; it is not uncommon to see a seriously ill neonate apparently "look well." The clinical and some laboratory features of many serious infectious diseases overlap and tend to mimic each other in the neonate. Table 12–8 lists major diagnostic features of these diseases.

DIFFERENTIAL DIAGNOSIS

Inspection of Tables 12–7 and 12–8 with clinical data and features of neonatal septicemia reveals that many conditions can masquerade as infection. Disorders involving any organ system, ranging from hyponatremia to central nervous system malformations, may all raise the question of infection. A hemorrhage into the central nervous system, like infection, may present with lethargy, convulsion, jaundice, poor feeding, and apnea. An infant with heart failure may present with a large liver or spleen, rapid respirations, tachycardia, and poor temperature control. Because of the ease of confusion with other diseases, a positive bacteriologic diagnosis is required, and the same obviously applies to viral and protozoan infections.

LABORATORY DIAGNOSIS

In all cases where sepsis is suspected, blood, spinal fluid, ear, and urine cultures should be obtained. By definition, septicemia requires a positive *blood culture,* and when the culture is obtained, contamination

---

TABLE 12–7   CLINICAL PRESENTATION OF INFECTION*

"Not doing well"

Poor temperature control } Fever / Hypothermia

CENTRAL NERVOUS SYSTEM	SKIN
Lethargy/irritability	Rashes/erythema
Jitteriness/hyporeflexia	Purpura
Tremors/seizures	Pustules/paronychia
Coma	Omphalitis
Full fontanelle	Sclerema
Abnormal eye movements	
Hypotonia/increased tone	

RESPIRATORY SYSTEM	HEMATOPOIETIC SYSTEM
Cyanosis	Jaundice
Grunting	Bleeding
Irregular respirations	Purpura/ecchymosis
Tachypnea/apnea	Splenomegaly
Retractions	

GASTROINTESTINAL TRACT	CIRCULATORY SYSTEM
Poor feeding	Pallor/cyanosis/mottling
Vomiting (may be bile-stained)	Cold, clammy skin
Diarrhea/decreased stools	Tachycardia/arrhythmia
Abdominal distension	Hypotension
Edema/erythema abdominal wall	Edema
Hepatomegaly	

*Adapted from Gotoff and Behrman.[19]

TABLE 12-8   DIAGNOSTIC FEATURES OF SOME TRANSPLACENTALLY ACQUIRED INFECTIONS COMPARED TO ERYTHROBLASTOSIS FETALIS*

FINDING	SEPTICEMIA	CONGENITAL SYPHILIS	TOXOPLASMOSIS (GENERALIZED FORM)	CYTOMEGALIC INCLUSION DISEASE	RUBELLA SYNDROME	ERYTHROBLASTOSIS FETALIS
Jaundice	++	+++	+++	+++		+++
Anemia	++	+++	+++	++	+	+++
Thrombocytopenia	+	++	+	+++	++	+
Hepatomegaly	++	+++	+++	+++	+++	+++
Splenomegaly	+	+++	+++	+++	+++	++
Purpura	+	++	+	+++	+	+
Skin Rash	+	+	+	0	?	0
Chorioretinitis	0	+	++	+	+	0
Intracranial calcifications	0	0	+	++	?	0
Generalized edema	+	++	+	+	?	+
Small-for-dates			++	++	+++	–
Special features:	Temperature Pustules Red hands and feet with gram-negative septicemia Convulsions	Mucocutaneous lesions Periostitis Snuffles Positive serology	Convulsions Microcephaly Hydrocephaly Positive dye test Lymphadenopathy	Pneumonia Cytomegalic inclusion cells in urine Cytomegalovirus culture	Cataract Glaucoma Heart defects Deafness Microcephaly Hydrocephaly Bone lesions Rubella virus recoverable	Positive Coombs test Evidence of blood group incompatibility between mother and child Hypoglycemia

0 not described

+ present in approximately   1–25% of cases

++ present in approximately 26–50% of cases

+++ present in approximately 51–75% of cases

+++ present in approximately 76–100% of cases

*Adapted from Oski and Naiman.[28]

from the skin must be eliminated. Meticulous technique should be utilized in obtaining cultures from the cord. Merely cutting the cord and allowing the blood to drip into the bottle often results in a contaminated sample.

We have found it very helpful to use the simple technique of doubly clamping a long section of cord and thoroughly cleansing it for three to five minutes before taking the sample using a syringe.[1]

Spinal fluid should be obtained when septicemia is suspected, as one-third of infants with septicemia have meningitis. *Urinalysis* is helpful, since this may be the port of entry of the infection, or the organisms may be disseminated there by the blood stream. In uncircumcized males, the urine should be collected by suprapubic aspiration. (see Chapter 14). *Histologic examination of the cord*,[31] membranes, and placenta may aid in the diagnosis of antenatal infection, but has not been utilized in our unit. *Gastric aspiration* with smear and culture of the gastric aspirate should be carried out. If more than five polymorphonuclear leukocytes are seen per high power field, it is highly suggestive of amniotic contamination and an infected infant. The *complete blood count* may reveal important diagnostic and therapeutic data. Anemia, fragmentation of the red blood cells, reticulocytosis, and thrombopenia, together with abnormal coagulation studies, are suggestive of disseminated intravascular coagulation complicating generalized infection.

In infants suspected of infection, it is useful to make a blood smear every four to six hours, looking for the following ominous changes: (1) extreme shift to the left, (2) >50 per cent of granulocytes not segmented, (3) toxic granulocytes, (4) thrombocytes <80,000, and (5) a drop in leukocytes to <4000.

S. PROD'HOM

Direct examination of smears from any suspicious skin lesions and vesicles, together with gram stain, will help differentiate between an innocuous condition , such as erythema toxicum, characterized by the presence of eosinophils, and the potentially life-threatening pustules of staphylococcal or streptococcal infection where organisms and polymorphs may be identified.

Examination of meconium or stool with gram stain may show gram-positive pleomorphic bacilli. When these are found, there is a 95 per cent chance that listeriosis is present.

S. PROD'HOM

Intranuclear inclusion bodies or multinucleated giant-size cells may be seen with viral infections; occasionally, intracytoplasmic viral inclusion bodies may be detected. *Serologic studies* are performed according to the clinical indication. There was hope that measurement of cord blood immunoglobulins could be utilized as a generalized screening test for intrauterine infections. However, not all infants with documented intrauterine infection have elevated immunoglobulins. Those with early clinical manifestations usually have elevated IgM, but an important asymptomatic group with rubella, syphilis, or cytomegalovirus infection may go undetected in the early neonatal period if reliance is placed on this alone. Because of the high frequency of false negative results, the cord blood IgM is not an ideal screening test; however, in the presence of elevated IgM levels in the neonatal period, further evaluation should be undertaken.

The finding of an elevated IgM does not pinpoint the nature of the infecting organism. More specific direct or indirect fluorescent antibody techniques are available and required in order to do this.

1. The ultimate diagnosis depends on demonstrating the organism by gram staining or culture, or indirectly via serologic tests.

2. Blood culture, spinal fluid, complete blood count, and urinalysis should be carried out on all infants with suspected sepsis.

3. Gram staining and direct microscopic examination for all skin lesions; Papanicolaou smear where herpes infection is suspected.

4. Blood chemistry, pH, blood sugar, serum calcium, and serum bilirubin with fractionation are useful in the overall management of the patient. The direct-reacting bilirubin is frequently elevated in congenital infections, while acidosis, hypoglycemia, hypocalcemia, and hyponatremia, together with hyperkalemia and uremia, frequently complicate generalized infection.

5. A chest X-ray, even in the absence of pulmonary symptoms or signs, may reveal extensive pulmonary involvement. X-rays of the long bones may reveal the characteristic metaphysitis and periostitis of congenital syphilis or the radiolucent zone seen in the infant with congenital rubella. Cerebral calcifications evident on X-ray of the skull may be present with toxoplasmosis or cytomegalic inclusion disease. The laboratory work-up is summarized in Table 12–9.

TABLE 12–9 LABORATORY INVESTIGATIONS

Cultures: blood, spinal fluid, urine, skin lesions, and (if indicated in the mother)— blood, lochia, urine. Catheters—when removed.

Microscopy and gram stain: spinal fluid, urine, skin lesions, gastric aspirate, scraping from ear.

Complete blood count.

X-ray of chest.

Serology as indicated: immunoglobulins, specific fluorescent antibodies.

Blood chemistry: pH, sugar, calcium, coagulation studies if purpura/bleeding.

TREATMENT

Early diagnosis and vigorous treatment are essential. Otherwise, not only are the chances of survival reduced but also permanent neurologic damage may occur. Septicemia is more prominent and a greater threat to life than the undesirable effects of antimicrobial therapy. When sepsis is strongly suspected, treatment should be commenced even before the etiologic agent or its drug susceptibility is known. Treatment is initiated on the basis of the most likely pathogen, taking into account the details of the history, the age of onset, and all other available data. It is essential for the physician to be aware of the sensitivity patterns of organisms in his hospital, and to keep surveillance of the organisms in his nursery. It is, however, important to bear in mind that the metabolism of the newborn as related to absorption, breakdown, distribution, and excretion of drugs is unlike the older individual. Absorption may be impaired, and conjugation, detoxification, and excretion delayed.

The variety of antibiotics useful at present in the neonatal period, together with their dosage, some of their toxic effects, and the susceptible organisms, are summarized in Table 12–10.[21, 23] While indications for antibiotics vary, there is general agreement that "prophylactic antibiotics" are of no value and may in fact be harmful. Antibiotics are prescribed for definite infection as well as when clinical findings and history suggest probable infection or a high risk of infection. These conditions *might include:*

1. Membranes ruptured 24 hours or more prior to delivery.

2. Maternal infection at the time of delivery or shortly before it. (Such infection may be manifested by fever; malodorous, thick amniotic fluid, cystitis or pyelonephritis; cervicitis; vaginitis; gastroenteritis.)

3. Infant with respiratory distress, particularly where the etiology of the respiratory distress has not been established. (At autopsy, pneumonia is found far more frequently than suspected.[6])

4. Meconium aspiration.

5. Surgical procedures, especially involving resection of gut or manipulation of genitourinary tract.

6. Streptococcal or enteropathogenic *E. coli* outbreaks in nursery.

We treat primary septicemia (those infections occurring in the first 48 to 72 hours) with the combination of kanamycin and penicillin, although kanamycin and ampicillin are equally effective. In late septicemias, our preference is a combination of kanamycin and methicillin or oxacillin, as staphylococcus occurs more commonly. More recently, we have used Gentamycin in this situation. Antibiotic treatment should be continued for at least 7 to 10 days or until cultures have been negative for 48 hours in cases of suspected infection. Meningitis requires three weeks' antibiotic therapy. (If clinical deterioration occurs, bear in mind that it may be the drug rather than nonsensitive organisms.)

In view of the increasing reports of kanamycin-resistant Klebsiella-Aerobacter group bacteria, it might be appropriate for any individual nursery to reconsider what its initial therapy may be. In areas where the strains seem prevalent, Gentamycin may (for the moment at least) afford better protection in initial therapy before the organism has been specifically identified and its sensitivity established.

L. STERN

Although antibiotics form the mainstay of therapy for sepsis, supportive therapy is essential.

1. Maintenance of the neutral thermal environment (see Chapter 4).

2. Administration of oxygen (as indicated).

3. Careful manipulation of fluids to maintain normal electrolyte and acid-base balance.

4. Gastric dilation and increased mucus production are a feature of sepsis, so all oral feedings should be temporarily discontinued.

5. Electronic monitoring of vital signs alerts the physician to any alteration in con-

TABLE 12–10   ANTIBIOTIC THERAPY IN THE NEWBORN*

ANTIBIOTIC	INDICATIONS	TOXICITY	DOSE	COMMENT
Kanamycin	Against gram-negatives in initial therapy of neonatal infections except Pseudomonas, and in continuing therapy of gram-negatives. E. coli, Klebsiella, Proteus	Neither renal or CNS toxicity when properly used in infants. Do not use > 12 days.	15 mg./Kg./day. Divided dose I.M. 12 hourly Intrathecally 1 mg./day for 3 days	Key drug for initial therapy and for continuing therapy if etiology is non-pseudomonas gram-negative
Penicillin G	Against gram-positives; in initial therapy of neonatal infections; and in continuing therapy of hemolytic streptococcus, staphylococcus, pneumococcus	Rare cause of neuromuscular irritability in premature infants	100,000–200,000 units/Kg./day I.M. or I.V. 12 hourly	Key drug for initial therapy and for continuing therapy; do not use procaine penicillin in newborns
Semisynthetic penicillins: Ampicillin	For gram-positive organisms, except penicillin-resistant staphylococci; for gram-negative organisms, only on basis of antimicrobial susceptibility testing; usual drug of choice against Proteus, Hemophilus, Shigella, Salmonella. Streptococcus faecalis	Elevation of transaminase; rash, eosinophilia; neuromuscular irritability in excess dosage	200 mg./Kg./day. Give 6 hourly I.V. or I.M.	Useful against selected gram-negative organisms; not to be used in initial therapy instead of kanamycin but may be used with kanamycin instead of penicillin G
Methicillin Oxacillin Nafcillin	Against penicillin-resistant staphylococci only	Nephrotoxic; watch for hematuria, rising BUN, SGOT	100–200 mg./Kg./day. 6 hourly I.M./I.V.	Excessive dosage must be avoided; use on proper indication only. Used with kanamycin as drug of choice in sepsis after 72 hours
Carbenicillin	Pseudomonas, Proteus	SGOT elevation	200–400 mg./Kg./day I.V. only. Divided dosage 2–4 hourly	Limited experience in newborn. Use for Pseudomonas only
Polymyxins	Against Pseudomonas infections; kanamycin-resistant E. coli	Nephrotoxic; may cause reversible neurotoxicity	2–2.5 mg./Kg./day. 4 divided doses 6 hourly deep I.M. Colistin 4–8 mg./Kg./day I.M. Give 6 hourly	Most effective agent against Pseudomonas
Tetracycline hydrochloride	Listeria monocytogenes	Teeth-enamel defect, bone-growth retardation, intracranial hypertension	10 mg./Kg./day 12 hourly I.M./I.V. 25 mg./Kg./day 6 hourly orally	Rarely indicated in newborn

Do not use I.V. or intrathecally

*Adapted from Eichenwald.[12]

(Table continued on opposite page.)

TABLE 12–10 ANTIBIOTIC THERAPY IN THE NEWBORN* (*Continued*)

ANTIBIOTIC	INDICATIONS	TOXICITY	DOSE	COMMENT
Gentamycin	Gram-negative bacilli, *E. coli*, Klebsiella, Pseudomonas, Proteus; also most *Staphylococcus aureus*	As for kanamycin renal and CNS (ototoxic) but little information in new-born period	3–7.5 mg./Kg./day. Give 12 hourly I.M. for prematures, 8 hourly full-terms	Effective against more resistant species of gram-negative bacilli encountered clinically; also Staphylococcus
Neomycin	Against susceptible entero-pathic *E. coli* only	Renal damage is sig-nificant risk if used parenterally	50–100 mg./Kg./day, P.O. only. Divided doses 4–6 hourly	For enteropathogenic *E. coli* outbreaks in nursery
Cephalothin	Gram-positive bacteria. Gram-negative bacteria: *E. coli*, Klebsiella, Proteus	Nephrotoxic	50–100 mg./Kg./day. 4–6 hours I.M.	Experience in newborn is insufficient to evaluate. Brown/black urine to Clinitest. False positive Coombs
Streptomycin	In TB; against gram-negatives	Nephrotoxic; CNS toxicity, cardio-vascular collapse in excessive dosage; must be used with care in presence of renal insufficiency	20 mg./Kg./12 hours I.M.	Limited by rapid development of re-sistance; 10-day maximum. Use with extreme caution because of toxicity
Bacitracin	For penicillin-resistant staphylococci only	Renal; rare in infants	Full-term: 1000 units/day, every 8–12 hours. I.M. Prematures: 900 units/day, every 8–12 hours I.M.	Do not use more than 10–12 days. Rarely used systemically; ointment effective locally
Chloromycetin	Gram-negative and some gram-positive organisms *Salmonella typhi* and *H. influenzae*, Klebsiella	Gray baby syndrome, aplastic anemia	25 mg./Kg./day 4–6 hourly I.M.	Use with extreme caution following sensitivity tests where other drugs are unavailable. Do not exceed 25 mg./Kg./day in prematures.
Nystatin (Mycostatin)	Oral thrush (Candida)	None	200,000 units/day. 4 doses daily (by mouth only).	
Amphotericin B	Systemic yeast and fungus infections	GIT, kidneys	0.25–1 mg./Kg./day (slow I.V. infusion). Orally 100 mg./dose. 4 hourly	Limited experience in prematures and extremely toxic

dition. Early detection and treatment of apnea prevent permanent neurologic sequelae.

6. Blood transfusions are used to correct anemia and shock. In addition, whole blood provides specific factors enhancing the phagocytic properties of the neonate's leukocytes as well as providing small amounts of specific antibody. We therefore transfuse all neonates with septicemia; exchange transfusions are indicated for disseminated intravascular coagulation.

Since 1970, we have used repeated fresh whole citrated blood exchange transfusion in cases of severe infection, especially in the presence of severe sclerema. Three to six exchanges are given within 48 hours, and our survival rate is 14/18 in the presence of severe sclerema.

S. PROD'HOM

7. The use of pooled gamma globulin has not been demonstrated to be effective and is only indicated in specific conditions associated with agammaglobulinemia. (Hyperimmune serum is useful in neonatal vaccinia, which is very rare.[30])

8. There has been to date limited experience with specific antiviral agents, including iodo-deoxyuridine, which is effective against DNA-containing virus (e.g., herpes virus), and Amantadine, which is effective against the influenza virus.[30]

The physician dealing with an infected infant must be alert for the onset and development of shock, adrenal hemorrhage, disseminated intravascular coagulation, or metabolic derangements, including acidosis, hyponatremia, hypoglycemia, and hypocalcemia, the correction of which may produce dramatic improvement in the infant.

In assessing the results of treatment of infection in the neonatal period, it is particularly important to look at the quality of survival as well as the quantity, because the long-term sequelae of neonatal meningitis, as well as some viral illnesses, may be devastating. The increased recognition of subclinical forms of congenital and neonatal viral infection raises the intriguing question of the possible contribution of these infections to minimal degrees of neurologic dysfunction in later years. In screening programs, infants excreting cytomegalovirus have been detected who appeared normal in the neonatal period yet demonstrated neurologic deficits at a year or two.

CONTROL OF INFECTION IN THE NURSERY

Admittance to the nursery is granted only to well personnel concerned with the care of the infant, including medical and nursing personnel, clergymen, laboratory and X-ray technicians, and parents getting to know their infants.

1. Personnel and mothers with the following illnesses will be excluded from the nursery or contact with the infants:
    a. Fever of undetermined origin.
    b. Febrile respiratory infection.
    c. Gastroenteritis of bacterial or viral origin.
    d. Any communicable disease or infection, such as open draining skin lesion and herpes.

2. Infants admitted from outside nurseries must be isolated in an incubator with gown isolation until results of cultures are available. Cultures of the throat, skin, and urine are to be obtained.

3. Infants in the same room with infants with possible infection should be maintained in a forced-draft incubator.

4. Infants excluded from the nursery and to be isolated in separate rooms are those with enteropathogenic E. coli infection, herpes simplex, coxsackie myocarditis, gastroenteritis, and draining lesions.

5. Infants delivered to patients who have a communicable disease are to be excluded from the nursery.

6. Following any delivery, the infants are required to be bathed if:
    a. Amnionitis is suspected.
    b. The amniotic fluid is foul-smelling or appears infected.
    c. The membranes have ruptured 36 hours prior to delivery.
    d. The mother's temperature is 38° C or above.

Formerly, we used to recommend bathing and antiseptic skin and cord care as follows: "Begin antiseptic skin and cord care in the delivery room, as soon after birth as possible. Wash the entire skin and umbilical cord of the newborn infant thoroughly with warmed, three per cent hexachlorophene-in-detergent cleanser (pHisoHex) and rinse gently but thoroughly with sterile warm water. Wash off all vernix and all visible blood, since protein, especially blood, is an inhibitor of the antibacterial action of hexachlorophene. Be sure to wash off all the hexachlorophene."

As a result of the recently recognized problems concerning the use of hexachlorophene, particularly in low-birth-weight infants, we have discontinued the use of hexachlorophene for bathing infants and have substituted a Castile soap.* (It is not necessary to bathe all babies immediately after delivery.)

7. The incubators and cribs are washed thoroughly with antiseptic solution at least each week and after each separate occupancy. The water is changed every few days.

8. All equipment is to be sterilized before use, and respirator tubing and humidification areas are to be changed every 24 hours while infant is on the respirator.

In accordance with state regulation practices recommended by the American Academy of Pediatrics:

1. All nursing personnel shall wear short-sleeved scrub gowns in the nursery.

2. Physicians and others who enter the nursery briefly shall wear a long-sleeved gown over street clothes or a uniform.

3. All persons shall wash their hands before entering any of the nurseries. Antiseptics most useful for handwashing in the nursery are iodophor preparations and antiseptic preparations containing a three per cent concentration of hexachlorophene. The iodophors are superior because of their activity against gram-negative as well as gram-positive organisms, but may cause sensitization. Hence, both preparations should be available at the sink-side. *The containers for these preparations should be periodically sterilized.*

Antiseptic soaps should be active against gram-negative and gram-positive organisms. The introduction of pHisoHex (active against gram-positive organisms) was followed by a large outbreak of pathogenic *E. coli* diarrhea, which was cultured from the hands of nurses who had washed carefully. (No *E. coli* was found in the soap container.)

S. PROD'HOM

4. Hands should be considered contaminated unless they are washed just before and just after handling an infant, and after touching contaminated materials.

5. To examine infants in incubators, medical personnel should roll their gown

sleeves above their elbows and wash to the elbows before each handling of a baby. Gown sleeves once wet are considered contaminated.

6. If medical personnel are to hold babies in their arms or against their gowns, then they must observe individual gown technique.

7. Nurses are required to use an individual gown for each infant, washing their hands and donning a fresh gown before handling the infant. This applies whether the infant is to be held or to be cared for in an incubator. (The individual gown technique by nurses not only is an ideal method for clean handling of infants but also prevents undue irritation of the arms from the many dozens of washings the nurse does daily.)[18]

8. Proper antiseptic and cord care is observed on all infants, including daily cord cleansing with alcohol. As the cord dries and shrivels, it recedes below skin margins of the umbilicus, creating a moist skin pocket which can become an excellent culture site for staphylococci. Wash scrupulously in pocket with a cotton-tipped applicator.

9. Masks are useless for pediatricians and nurses, who know how to behave in a nursery. They are only good for surgeons. Everyone must wash his hands if he has touched his face or nose.

10. Anything wet in the nursery (e.g., emergency drain in the sink, siphon in the sink) should be thoroughly cleaned and sterilized as often as possible.

11. Any equipment that becomes wet (e.g., oxygen hoods, tubing, etc.) should be cleaned and sterilized every 24 hours.

S. PROD'HOM

Table 12–11 describes the procedures to be followed in the management of a nursery epidemic.

PRACTICAL SUGGESTIONS

1. An infant in a neonatal intensive care nursery requires close observation and easy accessibility. (Infection is not the only problem in the nursery.)

2. Rigorous handwashing and the closed incubator are our present defenses against infection.

3. Some infections in infants are highly contagious (rubella, coxsackie, etc.).

4. Infants are susceptible and easily damaged by some organisms (herpes).

5. All infants in the same room as an infant with possible infection should be housed in incubators.

*"Hexachlorophene—its usage in the nursery." Proceedings of a conference held in Stowe, Vermont, under the auspices of the University of Vermont School of Medicine, June, 1972. Pediatrics *51*: Suppl. II, 1973.

TABLE 12-11 PRINCIPLES OF MANAGEMENT DURING A MAJOR NURSERY EPIDEMIC*

1. Identify source.
2. Determine extent of outbreak (culture of contacts and nursery personnel).
3. Re-evaluate techniques (handwashing, antiseptic bathing and cord care, cleaning and sterilizing of equipment).
4. Notify local hospital infection committee and proper health authorities.
5. Follow up infants discharged from nursery previously (including cultures).
6. Continue surveillance after epidemic (culture infants, personnel, equipment, etc. May do cultures on admission and discharge).

COMMON EXAMPLES:

	E. coli	Streptococcus	Staphylococcus
Nursery	Close to new admissions. Reduce census. Culture fomites and equipment.	Do not close nursery. Culture all new admissions.	Close nursery if serious epidemic. May colonize all infants with low virulence Staphylococcus. Re-evaluate techniques.
Affected infants	Antibiotics and fluids.	Penicillin × 10 days.	Methicillin/cloxacillin.
Infant contacts	Culture stools. Antibiotics (neomycin** 50 mg./Kg./day, colistin** 10 mg./Kg./day.)	Culture cords. Oral penicillin (150,000 units/Kg. in 3 divided doses) while in nursery + 48 hours after discharge. If positive culture. treat for 10 days.	Culture cords and noses. If severe epidemic, colonize infants with low virulence Staphylococcus.
Personnel	Stool culture.	Nose and throat culture. If positive culture, move from nursery.	Culture nose. Remove personnel with Staphylococcus aureus lesions but not nasal carriers.

The six principles outlined above apply in all cases.

*Adapted from the American Academy of Pediatrics.[3]
**Give orally in four equally divided doses every six hours throughout nursery stay and for 48 hours after discharge.

6. Symptoms and signs of infection in the premature are often sudden, subtle, and rapidly progressive.

7. A high index of suspicion is required to diagnose infections. Take careful note of feeding problems, lethargy, early onset of jaundice, thermolability. Common sites of infection include umbilicus, skin, nails (paronychia), and eyes.

8. Gram-negative infections are now more common than gram-positive.

9. Investigation of an infant suspected to be suffering from sepsis includes cultures and examinations of blood, urine, stool, and cerebrospinal fluid. Serum immunoglobulin estimations may be of value in diagnosis of intrauterine-acquired infection.

10. When sepsis is strongly suspected, treatment should be commenced before etiologic agent or drug susceptibility is known.

QUESTIONS

How would you advise the parents of the following children with regard to the risk of the abnormality recurring in a subsequent pregnancy?

A. *Infant with hydrocephalus and chorioretinitis secondary to congenital toxoplasmosis.*

B. *Infant with microcephaly secondary to cytomegalic inclusion body disease.*

C. *Infant with "saddle nose" and periostitis due to congenital syphilis.*

D. *Infant with cataracts and patent ductus*

arteriosus following documented rubella during first trimester of pregnancy.

A. There is no risk of subsequent infants being affected by toxoplasmosis, as primary infection must occur during pregnancy in order to affect the baby. The mother has already been infected and they may safely attempt an addition to the family.

B. As for "A."

C. The mother requires a full course of treatment if she has not already had same; otherwise, there is a hazard of having either an abortion or stillbirth, or another infant affected by the spirochete. Following treatment, the STS will remain positive and the cord blood antibody may reflect this; however, the infant will not require treatment.

D. As for "A."

The phagocytic properties of neonatal leukocytes are reduced because of a deficient factor: (Check correct answer)
   A. *In the serum.*
   B. *In the leukocytes.*

The deficient factor is present in the serum and this is the rationale for administration of whole blood to neonates with infection.

Match the following clinical features with the most likely infectious agent:

A. *Skin pustule.*
B. *Ecthyma gangrenosum.*
C. *Swollen red eyes with purulent discharge.*
D. *Persistent lung infiltrate in premature infant with hypogammaglobulinemia.*
E. *Clinical, ECG, and radiological evidence suggesting myocarditis.*
F. *Vesicular skin lesions and keratoconjunctivitis.*
G. *Red hands and feet and septicemia.*

1. *Gram-negative septicemia*
2. *Herpes*
3. *Pneumocystis carinii*
4. *Coxsackie*
5. *Staphylococcus*
6. *Pseudomonas*
7. *Gonococcus*

A) 5, B) 6, C) 7, D) 3, E) 4, F) 2, G) 1.

You are consulted by the obstetrician who has a mother with suspected herpes progenitalis.
   A. *How can the diagnosis readily be made?*
   B. *If the diagnosis is confirmed, how should the infant be delivered?*

A. Diagnosis can be confirmed by the finding of intranuclear inclusions or multinucleated giant cells on Papanicolaou smear.

B. Cesarean section is probably indicated to protect the infant from exposure to herpes virus in the birth canal.

Examination at 8 1/2 months' gestation because of close family contact with tuberculosis revealed a positive tuberculin test with questionable parenchymal disease in a 17-year-old Negro girl. Sputum and gastric aspirate were negative. The baby at delivery appears healthy. (Check correct answer.)
   A. *The baby should be allowed to breast feed.*
   B. *The baby may room in with the mother.*
   C. *The baby requires BCG alone.*
   D. *The baby requires BCG and INH for six months.*
   E. *The baby should be separated from the mother and receive BCG.*

A and B. Because of the danger that this mother could infect the infant, he should not be allowed either to breast feed or to room in with the mother.

C. Although this infant requires BCG, this will take some six weeks before converting the tuberculin skin test, at which stage the infant is probably protected. Therefore, he also needs to be separated from the mother.

D. Although the infant requires immunization, there is no evidence that the baby is infected and requires treatment. (INH appears not to interfere with BCG conversion.)

E. Correct.

To safeguard against the spread of infection in the intensive care nursery, all visitors should wear masks, gowns, and scrub for five minutes, one minute of which should be with brushes. Comment.

Handwashing is the most important protection for the infant against spread of infection. Prolonged vigorous scrubbing with brushes results in higher bacterial counts on cultures from the hands and is contraindicated. Scrub with a brush for only one minute, but the nails should be scrupulously cleaned. No proof exists that masks are useful; no person should enter the nursery with a cold or sore throat.

If monilia is found in an infant's mouth in the intensive care nursery, he should be isolated in a separate unit and treated with mycostatin by mouth.

It is not necessary to isolate the infant in a separate area, since the incubator acts as an isolation unit. Mycostatin therapy *is* effective for oral thrush.

The recent admission of mothers to the intensive care nursery has increased the incidence of infection in infants.

There has not been an increase in infection in the intensive care nursery since the admission of mothers. Therefore the statement is false.

Because of the small drug toxicity and the high incidence of neonatal infection following 24 hours of ruptured membranes, all infants should be treated with antibiotics for seven days.

Although there is a slightly increased risk of infection following 24 hours of ruptured membranes, it is our feeling that not all infants require antibiotic therapy. Each case is assessed with regard to maternal infection, state of the amniotic fluid, clinical condition of the infant, together with laboratory data, before a decision is reached as to whether or not to treat. The infants must be cultured regardless of this decision.

Following umbilical arterial catheterization, all infants should be treated with penicillin and kanamycin for seven days.

The incidence of infection is not significantly increased following arterial catheterization. However, antibiotics may be required for the underlying disease prompting the arterial catheterization. Good data to answer this problem is not available. The statement is therefore false.

Our own experience with antibiotic coverage and umbilical catheterization, unfortunately, is at variance with this. We cover all of our arterial catheters with three days of penicillin and kanamycin. In the past, attempts to discontinue such a regimen have resulted in outbreaks of systemic infection in these

infants and we have, therefore, chosen to re-institute the regimen under these circumstances. Again, we believe that this is the kind of decision which every individual unit must make, based on its own experiences.

L. STERN

An attempt should be made to remove all umbilical venous catheters within 72 hours because of the high incidence of complications.

Every effort should be made to avoid prolonged umbilical venous catheterization because of the high incidence of sepsis and other complications. Some neonatologists recommend avoiding umbilical vein catheterization altogether. Therefore the statement is true.

Sulfonamides are not useful drugs in the management of urinary tract infections in the first week of life.

Sulfonamides are contraindicated in the first week of life, as they are bound to albumin in the serum, and will compete with bilirubin, increasing the risks of kernicterus. The statement is therefore true.

The oxygen nebulizer, the oxygen hood, and all tubing connected with the administration of oxygen should be changed every 24 hours to prevent infection.

Certain bacteria, including Pseudomonas, have a predilection for humid environments. Ideally, therefore, oxygen hoods and tubing should be changed every 24 hours. In practice, because of the quantity of equipment involved, changes are made every 48 hours.

Aspiration of meconium is frequently followed by a bacterial pneumonia; therefore, antibiotics should be given.

Meconium in vitro enhances the growth of bacteria. As it is not possible to differentiate between a chemical and bacterial pneumonia, we have elected to institute antibiotic therapy for aspiration syndromes.

A. *What steps should be taken to prevent fetal infection with gonorrhea acquired during delivery?*
B. *Is this really necessary?*

A. Instillation of a one per cent solution of silver nitrate in the conjunctival sac immediately after birth is recommended. Penicillin ointment is equally effective and less irritating.

After reviewing all the evidence, the American Academy of Pediatrics' Committee on Drugs has indicated its preference for silver nitrate over penicillin for the prophylaxis of neonatal ophthalmia. The preference is stated both because of the proven efficacy of silver nitrate in this regard and because of its lack of toxicity as opposed to the possible hazard of penicillin sensitivity initiated by its installation into the conjunctival sac. Moreover, the emergence of penicillin-resistant strains of gonococci would further support the preference for silver nitrate over penicillin in this situation.

L. STERN

B. Neonatal ophthalmia is a real hazard where prophylactic measures are not used. At Johns Hopkins Hospital, two per cent of private and almost five per cent of staff patients had gonococci in cervical cultures taken at time of admission for delivery. Therefore the answer is yes.

How should the patient with a history of rubella-like illness, or exposure to such an illness, be managed during pregnancy?

Two hemagglutination antibody titres should be measured approximately two weeks apart in order to establish the diagnosis. If the titre shows a fourfold or greater increase, the patient has had rubella and should be managed accordingly. Other viral illnesses may be clinically indistinguishable from rubella, and documented only by specific antibody tests or isolation of the virus.

CASE PROBLEMS

Case One

The mother is 24 years old, unwed, and an unemployed black woman from the inner city. Three weeks prior to delivery, she was discovered to have an E. coli urinary tract infection, which was treated with ampicillin for two weeks. The infant, a 1700-gm. female, was delivered spontaneously at 32 weeks' gestation, following 24 hours of ruptured membranes, with clear amniotic fluid. She was moderately asphyxiated; pH = 7.1, PaO_2 = 40 mm. Hg. and HCO_3 = 14 mEq. per liter. Resuscitation: sodium bicarbonate per umbilical catheter, and mask and bag ventilation. She recovered promptly. At age 2½ hours she appeared to be a normal, preterm infant.

Enumerate the factors predisposing to infection in this infant.

A. Prematurity (i.e., this is a preterm baby).

B. Premature rupture of membranes, although lethal infection does commonly occur even with intact membranes in infants born to mothers from the inner city.

c. Maternal infection. Identical organism in maternal infection and neonatal meningitis in 50 per cent of cases.

d. Asphyxia and the resuscitation requiring umbilical venous catheterization.

e. Poverty.

The following laboratory results then became available. Comment on the significance of each finding:

A. *E. coli in the throat culture.*

B. *Gastric aspirate smear showed 40 polymorphs per high power field.*

Although *E. coli* may be part of the normal throat flora in the newborn, since the mother had an *E. coli* urinary tract infection, it is a potential pathogen to the infant. Should therapy be indicated, antibiotics will be used to treat this organism.

The fact that there are more than 5 polymorphs per HPF is significant. This is associated with increased rate of infection. While presumptive diagnosis of neonatal sepsis cannot be made on the basis of polymorphs alone in the gastric fluid, a false positive test is rarely seen. (The absence of polymorphs in the gastric fluid effectively excludes the occurrence of sepsis in the first 72 hours.[33] The usefulness of the test is limited by the high incidence of false negatives—that is, normal gastric aspirate in the face of infection.

At three days of age, the infant appeared lethargic. The abdomen was distended with rare bowel sounds, and she regurgitated her feed. The rectal temperature was 36.6° C. The physical examination was unremarkable apart from diminished responses. Hematocrit = 47 per cent, Dextrostix = 60 to 90 mg. per 100 ml., calcium = 9 mg. per 100 ml., sodium = 140 mEq., potassium = 5.5, pH = 7.34, CO_2 = 19, pCO_2 = 42, chloride = 105 mEq. per liter. Chest X-ray was normal. Urinalysis = specific gravity 1.010. White blood cell = 4 per HPF; red blood cell = 2 per HPF. Cerebrospinal fluid = 20 cells, 11 polymorphs, 9 monocytes; protein = 50 mg. per 100 ml. sugar = 70 mg. Blood sugar = 85 mg. per 100 ml. Gram stain is negative. Cultures were taken of throat, skin, blood, umbilical cord, and urine, and treatment was started with penicillin (100,000 units per Kg. I.V.) and kanamycin (15 mg. per Kg. per 24 hours). Six hours later the infant was asymptomatic.

In the absence of bulging fontanel and stiff neck, was a spinal tap indicated?

Yes. The most common presenting signs and symptoms of meningitis are lethargy, abnormal temperature, poor feeding or vomiting, respiratory distress, and irritability. Bulging fontanel and stiff neck occur less frequently. In the presence of these symptoms, blood, urine, and spinal fluid should be examined and cultured.

Are the cerebrospinal fluid findings abnormal?

The chemistries are normal. However, questions may be raised regarding the presence of 11 polymorphs and 9 monocytes in the spinal fluid.

In an older child, this number of white cells would definitely be considered abnormal. In the preterm infant (as is this case), the normal range for white blood cells is sufficiently great (see Appendix 32) that cell count alone cannot be used to exclude meningitis.

Note that the incidence of meningitis, as well as the mortality, is higher in low-birth-weight infants. Predisposing factors significantly associated with meningitis are complications during labor and delivery, maternal peripartum infection, and chorioamnionitis.[29]

The history, together with the clinical condition of the infant, examination of CSF smear for organisms, and the culture of the fluid, must be used to make the diagnosis.

Were the symptoms due to infection?

Without the culture results, you are not in a position to know whether the symptoms were due to sepsis. It is possible that the symptoms were due to infection, and the subsequent improvement to a prompt response to therapy. However, in view of the rapidity of the response, this is unlikely. Therapy should be continued until all culture results are available and have been negative for 48 hours. Note that the full-blown pictures of sepsis or meningitis are late manifestations of infection in the newborn. As a result, when sepsis is strongly suspected, treatment should be commenced before the etiologic agent or drug susceptibility of the organism is known.

On the second day of therapy, the following culture results were available: Blood = two colonies of gram-negative rods per pour plate. Scanty growth of gram-negative rods on Thio and Beef Heart Infusion. CSF culture = sterile. Stool culture = non-enteropathogenic E. coli. Throat culture = E. coli. Skin and umbilical culture = hemolytic Staphylococcus coagulase negative.

What is the significance of two colonies of gram-negative rods in pour plates?

Two colonies per pour plate of gram-negative rods have been shown to be due to skin or other contaminants. True gram-negative bacteremia should have more than three colonies per pour plate (i.e., growth in both pour plates). Thus, using the Eitzman-Smith criteria,[14] this culture is insignificant.

Would you continue or discontinue therapy? Why?

Therapy should be continued. If the gram-negative rods on Thio and Beef Heart Infusion turn out to be E. coli, this infant would be regarded as having E. coli septicemia, since she has been colonized by the organism. (It might be propitious to discontinue penicillin and introduce ampicillin.)

What additional information would you ask concerning the blood cultures?

One should ask whether the colonies on the pour plate were deep or surface colonies (surface colonies = probably contaminated). One should also ask whether the correct amount (namely 1 cc.) of blood was added to the pour plate. The site from which the blood sample was drawn is also important. Blood cultures obtained from the umbilical cord or umbilical veins yield many positive results. Only a fraction of the infants with positive cord blood cultures eventually develop infection, indicating a high incidence of contamination or transient bacteremia.[1] In a study of 131 three-day-old infants, 16 per cent showed significant bacterial growth in blood cultures, which was thought to be due to contamination. All infants except one were asymptomatic. The bacteremia was transient in all except four patients.

Aerobacter aerogenes was cultured from blood culture. Is this significant? Should treatment be continued?

Although this patient's antenatal and natal history place her in the high-risk group, the evidence against sepsis is strong. There are different organisms growing from the throat *(E. coli)*, skin and umbilicus (nonpathogenic Staphylococcus), and blood *(Aerobacter aerogenes)*. Cultures of urine and spinal fluid were negative, as was stool culture. In view of the scanty growth of the Aerobacter on the pour plate and the rapid clinical response, antibiotics were discontinued. Note that high-risk infants with clinical signs and symptoms consistent with septicemia should receive therapy until the results of all cultures are available. Therapy can then be discontinued if all cultures are negative.

Case Two

At two days of age, an infant with fever (38.7° C) was transferred from an outlying hospital. The mother was a diabetic who had had antenatal care during only the last one and one-half months of pregnancy. The delivery was said to be normal. Birth weight was 3900 gm. The infant was entirely breast-fed. Admission weight was 3520 gm. Examination showed an active, pink, fat baby, with features characteristic of an infant of a diabetic mother. Peripheral hematocrit was 79 per cent. Six hours later the infant was afebrile.

Should this infant have been cultured?

Yes. All infants admitted from outside nurseries require cord, skin, and throat cultures. In addition, because this infant was febrile, blood, urine, and spinal fluid should have been cultured. These investigations would not be universally approved, especially in those parts of the world where breast feeding is widely practiced, as it would be more than a full-time job for pediatricians to do a spinal tap on every infant with a temperature.

Should this infant be treated with antibiotics?

The clinical impression was that the fever was "dehydration fever" in view of the fact that the infant had lost approximately 10 per cent from birth weight, had a high hematocrit, was breast-fed, and had received no additional fluids. Apart from the temperature elevation, there was no other indication of sepsis, and the infant was active, alert, and vigorous. Cultures were taken and I.V. fluids administered. No antibiotics were given. Within six hours, the temperature was normal.

The umbilical culture grew β-hemolytic group A streptococci. All other cultures were negative. Should this be treated?

Yes. The infant should receive penicillin therapy systematically together with with local cord therapy.

Where should the epidemiologic investigation of the infection be commenced?

Cord cultures should be taken from other infants in the nursery at the referring hospital. The mother's lochia should be cultured as well. (See Table 12–11.)

Case Three

The infant is a 1300-gm. male Negro, fed formula containing 24 calories per 30 ml., who developed diarrhea on day eight. No blood or mucus was found in the stool. This formula was discontinued and formula containing 13 calories per 30 ml. was initiated. The diarrhea promptly subsided, although an occasional stool was abnormal. The stool culture grew enteropathogenic *E. coli*. The patient continued gaining weight.

Would you treat this infant? Why?

Yes. The lull in the diarrhea is misleading, as infants may suddenly develop fulminant diarrhea with high mortality rate. Therapy with oral colistin or neomycin should be started and continued for five to seven days.

The patient was started on neomycin. Diarrhea (explosive) began on the third day of therapy and the patient became dehydrated and very lethargic. Stool pH was 5; Clinistix, 2+.

How would you proceed?

This infant needs investigation for generalized sepsis and pseudomembranous enterocolitis. Do a gram stain on the stool. If this shows gram-positive cocci, presumptive diagnosis of staphylococcal pseudomembranous enterocolitis can be made. The infant requires close monitoring of electrolytes and maintenance of hydration with I.V. fluids. Discontinue oral feedings. If gram-positive cocci are seen in stool, methicillin should be added to the therapy; otherwise, treat as for gram-negative septicemia. Reducing substances in the stool probably indicate lactose intolerance secondary to infection and antibiotics. This must be taken into account with re-introduction of oral feeding.

Case Four

A 2000-gm. male of 39 weeks' gestation (head circumference = 34 cm.) was delivered after Pitocin induction because of a falling maternal estriol level. The mother was discovered to be STS 3+ on the 12th week of gestation. She was treated with a full course of penicillin. (STS was 2+ at 28 weeks' gestation.) At birth the infant had purpura, splenomegaly, thrombocytopenia, STS ++, and IgM on cord blood 52 mg. per 100 ml.

Is this infant infected with Treponema pallidum?

This is a small-for-dates infant with features very suggestive that he is infected with *T. pallidum*, but no definitive diagnosis is possible with the available data. The placenta forms an effective barrier to the spirochete during the first trimester, when the mother received treatment. It is possible that she was re-infected during the third trimester, hence infecting the infant; however, other congenital infections may also produce a similar clinical picture (see Table 12–8). (All pregnant females require two serologic tests for syphilis during pregnancy.)

What is the significance of the elevated IgM? (For normal values, see Table 12–2.)

The elevated IgM is indicative of intrauterine infection, but not specific for syphilis. Specific treponemal fluorescent antibodies should be determined; the presence of these will clinch the diagnosis of syphilis.

Are X-rays of the skull or long bones more helpful at this stage?

X-ray of the long bones would be more helpful, metaphysitis and periosteal reaction being a feature of syphilis. The periostitis may not be present in the immediate neonatal period. "Wimbergers sign," consisting of bilateral symmetrical excavating osteomyelitis with pathologic fractures of the medial tibial metaphysis, is almost pathognomonic of syphilis but is seen later. The presence of calcification in the skull may indicate other conditions (e.g., cytomegalovirus infection).

How could diagnosis be established if mucocutaneous lesions were present?

Diagnosis of syphilis could be confirmed by detecting spirochete on dark field examination. *Note*: Rhinitis and intractable diaper rash should alert physician to the diagnosis of syphilis in the neonate. Rashes of congenital syphilis have a predilection for the buttocks and posterior thighs. (This infant did have congenital syphilis.)

REFERENCES

1. Albers, W., Tyler, C., and Boxerbaum, B.: Asymptomatic bacteremia in the newborn infant. J Pediat 69:193, 1966.
2. Altemeier, W., and Smith, R.: Immunologic aspects of resistance in early life. Pediat Clin N Amer 12:663, 1965.
3. American Academy of Pediatrics' Committee on Fetus and Newborn: *Standards and Recommendations for Hospital Care of Newborn Infants.* Evanston, American Academy of Pediatrics, 1971. 5th Edition.
4. Barnett, C., Leiderman, P., Grobstein, R., et al: Neonatal separation: the maternal side of interactional deprivation. Pediatrics 45:197, 1970.
5. Brown, G.: Recent advances in the viral etiology of congenital anomalies. Advances Tetrol 1:55, 1966.
6. Butler, N., and Alberman, E.: *Perinatal Problems.* Edinburgh, E. and S. Livingstone, 1969.
7. Cooper, L.: Rubella: a preventable cause of birth defects. National Foundation March of Dimes 4:21, 1968.
8. Davies, P.: Bacterial infection in the fetus and newborn. Arch Dis Child 46:1, 1971.
9. Desmond, M., Franklin, R., Blattner, R., et al: The relation of maternal disease to fetal and neonatal morbidity and mortality. Pediat Clin N Amer 8:421, 1961.
10. Dossett, J., Williams, R., and Quie, P.: Studies on interaction of bacteria, serum factors and polymorphonuclear leukocytes in mothers and newborns. Pediatrics 44:49, 1969.
11. Dunham, E.: Septicemia in the newborn. Amer J Dis Child 45:229, 1933.
12. Eichenwald, H.: Antibiotics and the newborn. Hosp Practice 2:51, 1967.
13. Eichenwald, H., and Shinefeld, H.: Viral infections of the fetus and of the newborn infant. Advances Pediat 12:249, 1962.
14. Eitzman, D., and Smith, R.: The significance of blood cultures in the newborn period. Amer J Dis Child 94:601, 1957.

15. Forman, M., and Stiehm, E.: Impaired opsonic activity but normal phagocytosis in low-birth-weight infants. New Eng J Med *281*:926, 1969.
16. Gluck, L., and Silverman, W.: Phagocytosis in premature infants. Pediatrics *20*:951, 1957.
17. Gluck, L., and Wood, H.: Staphylococcal colonization in newborn infants with and without antiseptic skin care. New Eng J Med *268*:1265, 1963.
18. Gluck, L., Wood, H., and Fousek, M.: Septicemia of the newborn. Pediat Clin N Amer *13*:1131, 1966.
19. Gotoff, S., and Behrman, R.: Neonatal septicemia. J Pediat *76*:142, 1970.
20. Hess, J., and Landeen, E.: *The Premature Infant: Medical and Nursing Care*. Philadelphia, J. B. Lippincott Co., 1949. 2nd Edition.
21. McCracken, G.: Gentamycin in the neonatal period. Amer J Dis Child *120*:524, 1970.
22. McCracken, G., and Shinefeld, H.: Changes in the pattern on neonatal septicemia and meningitis. Amer J Dis Child *112*:33, 1966.
23. McCracken, G., Eichenwald, H., and Nelson, J.: Antimicrobial therapy in theory and practice. II. Clinical approach to antimicrobial therapy. J Pediat *75*:923, 1969.
24. Miller, M.: Demonstration of replacement of functional defect of the fifth component in newborn serum: a major tool in the therapy of neonatal septicemia. Presented at the combined meeting of the Amer Pediat Soc/Soc Pediat Res, 1971.
25. Naeye, R., and Blanc, W.: Relation of poverty and race to antenatal infection. New Eng J Med *283*:555, 1970.
26. National Foundation March of Dimes *4*: No. 7, 1968.
27. Nyhan, W., and Fousek, M.: Septicemia of the newborn. Pediatrics *22*:268, 1958.
28. Oski, F., and Naiman, J.: *Hematologic Problems in the Newborn*. Philadelphia, W. B. Saunders Co., 1972. 2nd Edition.
29. Overall, J., Jr.: Neonatal bacterial meningitis. J Pediat *76*:449, 1970.
30. Overall, J., Jr., and Glasgow, L.: Virus infections of fetus and neonate. J Pediat *77*:315, 1970.
31. Overbach, A., Daniel, S., and Cassady, G.: The value of umbilical cord histology in the management of potential perinatal infection. J Pediat *76*:22, 1970.
32. Parmelee, A.: *Management of the Newborn*. Chicago, Year Book Medical Publishers, 1959. 2nd Edition.
33. Ramos, A., and Stern, L.: Relationship of premature rupture of membranes to gastric fluid aspirate. Amer J Obstet Gynec *105*:1247, 1969.
34. Rothberg, R.: Immunoglobulin and specific antibody synthesis during the first weeks of life of premature infants. J Pediat *75*:391, 1969.
35. Schaffer, A., and Avery, M.: *Diseases of the Newborn*. Philadelphia, W. B. Saunders Co., 1971. 3rd Edition.
36. Sever, J., and White, L.: Intrauterine viral infections. Ann Rev Med *19*:471, 1968.
37. Silverman, W., and Homan, W.: Sepsis of obscure origin in the newborn. Pediatrics *3*:157, 1949.
38. Smith, R., Platou, E., and Good, R.: Septicemia of the newborn. Pediatrics *17*:549, 1956.
39. Soothill, J., Chandra, R., and Dudgeon, J.: Some relationships between serum immunoglobulin deficiencies and infection in utero and in the early weeks of life. J Pediat *75*:1257, 1969.
40. Williams, C., and Oliver, T., Jr.: Nursery routines and staphylococcal colonization of the newborn. Pediatrics *44*:640, 1969.

Chapter 13

THE HEART

by
JEROME LIEBMAN, M.D.
and
VICTOR WHITMAN, M.D.

The most common cause of death in a pediatric referral hospital, excluding problems concerned with prematurity, is a congenital heart defect. Most of these deaths occur in the first month, especially the first two weeks.

There has been a rapid advancement in both the diagnosis and management of congenital heart disease in the neonatal period. Before surgery was available for the neonate, the majority of babies with heart disease who developed distress during the newborn period died, and the tendency was not to perform potentially dangerous investigations such as cardiac catheterization. Today, neonatal cardiology is much more sophisticated, so that all infants with suspected congenital heart disease who are in difficulty should be referred to a center with full facilities for diagnostic evaluation (including cardiac catheterization) and surgery.

In order to care for the newborn with heart disease, the physician must know which cardiac conditions are likely. Cardiac catheterization is potentially hazardous and is facilitated by having a good idea of the diagnosis before the procedure is begun. In this regard, the recent data from the New England Regional Infant Cardiac Program concerning the diagnostic distribution of critically ill infants in the first month is very helpful (Table 13–1), as are the composite autopsy data of Rowe.

Together the stress is that 70 per cent of neonates with fatal cardiac malformations will have one of the following five defects: the hypoplastic left ventricle syndrome, complicated coarctation of the aorta, transposition of the great arteries, the hypoplastic right ventricle syndrome, or severe tetralogy of Fallot.

Although we guide ourselves by what defect we expect to find, we must be prepared for the unexpected. Many infants with primary lung disease may well be confused with those having heart disease. Careful evaluation of the history, physical examination, laboratory data (including response of blood gases and arterial oxygen saturation in an enriched oxygen environment), X-ray, electrocardiogram, echogram, and sometimes cardiac catheterization, will help to define the problem.

In discussing the high-risk newborn with heart disease, one loses perspective if there is no discussion of the even more common low-risk neonate with heart disease. Therefore, this chapter is divided into two sections: the first considers the low-risk baby, including only the simple left-to-right shunt lesions; the second considers the high-risk baby, concentrating on the five major defects mentioned above. Constant reference to the pathophysiology and natural history of each lesion is recommended. Each section will be supplemented with case material and questions.

TABLE 13-1 DIAGNOSTIC
DISTRIBUTION OF CRITICALLY ILL
CARDIAC INFANTS 0 TO 30 DAYS OF
AGE. 1968-1971*

DIAGNOSIS (In Rank Order)	NUMBER	PER CENT
Transposition of the great arteries	81	14
Hypoplastic left ventricle	76	13
Coarctation of the aorta (includes simple and complicated)	51	9
Hypoplastic right ventricle (includes pulmonary atresia and tricuspid atresia group)	49	9
Tetralogy of Fallot	44	8
Ventricular septal defect	44	8
Other malpositions	31	5
Single ventricle	21	4
Patent ductus arteriosus	19	3
Atrioventricularis communis	15	3
Pure pulmonary stenosis	14	2
Myocardiopathy	12	2
Total anomalous pulmonary venous return	12	2
Truncus arteriosus	9	2
Others	108	18
Total	586	

*Adapted from Dr. D. Fyler, unpublished data.

It is important to note that these are babies who were critically ill but did not necessarily die or need surgery to live. The table is also not broken down as to day of onset of illness. Thus, a child with a ventricular septal defect who became ill at 30 days is included and is likely to survive with medical therapy.

SECTION ONE: THE LOW-RISK CARDIAC NEWBORN

Statistically, the most important defects of low-risk babies in the newborn period are the simple left-to-right shunt lesions. Consequently, the physician taking care of newborns must have an understanding of their pathophysiology and natural history. Isolated ventricular septal defect, for example, is believed to account for between 30 and 40 per cent of all congenital heart disease. Atrial septal defect and patent ductus arteriosus are less common, but important. Occasionally, difficulty occurs late in the neonatal period (three to four weeks of life) for ventricular septal defect and patent ductus arteriosus, but is unheard of in our experience for simple secundum atrial septal defect. Nonetheless, consideration of these defects by the physician is very frequent.

Three cases are illustrated in which there are no symptoms in the newborn period, but in which the physiologic events during that time are directly related to the eventual course. The pathophysiology which follows the questions not only helps to answer these questions but also should provide a basis for understanding the very complicated defects to be discussed later.

CASE PROBLEMS

Case One

At the one-month checkup, a murmur is heard for the first time in an acyanotic, well baby. The diagnosis of ventricular septal defect with left-to-right shunt is made. The family is very upset with the physician for not having heard the murmur in the newborn period.

Is the family justified? Why or why not?

Obviously the family was not justified. It is possible, though not definite, that this is a large ventricular septal defect. It is probably at least moderate sized. If the defect is moderate to large, then, by necessity, the pressure in the right ventricle and pulmonary artery will be elevated. The high pulmonary artery pressure is believed to be one of the factors in delaying maturation of the pulmonary arterioles. The delayed maturation means that pulmonary vascular resistance comes down slowly. Consequently, the left-to-right shunt begins slowly, causing the murmur to develop after the early neonatal period.

Is it at all possible that congestive heart failure will develop before the next regularly scheduled visit at two months?

The maximal left-to-right shunt is believed to develop by about one month of life, so that when congestive heart failure occurs, it is usually by two months. Occasionally, it is first recognized a little later, but in those cases referred with congestive heart failure at five to six months, it has probably been present for several months.

Is pulmonary hypertension likely to be present at this time?

The larger the defect, the higher the right ventricular pressure. Thus, with large defects and no pulmonary stenosis, high pulmonary artery pressure *must* be present no matter what the shunt. With a moderate defect, the pressure is moderately elevated. Therefore the answer is yes.

Case Two

On the first day of life, the physical examination of a full-term baby is normal, but at 48 hours, a murmur is heard by the house officer. The child is acyanotic, and the murmur is typical of a ventricular septal defect with left-to-right shunt.

Is a ventricular septal defect possible? Why?

The left ventricular pressure is now transmitted to the right side through the small restrictive ventricular septal defect. This allows the pulmonary vascular resistance to drop normally. As the pulmonary vascular resistance decreases, the RV pressure drops as it would normally. Therefore, there is a large early gradient, and an early left-to-right shunt is possible. The early murmur obviously is due to the early left-to-right shunt. The answer is yes.

Is whatever defect present likely to be small or large?

The shunt never becomes large because of the high resistance to flow through the small defect. The major key to suspecting that the defect is small is the early onset of the murmur.

Is eventual congestive heart failure likely?

Heart failure is not likely when the left-to-right shunts are small.

Is pulmonary hypertension likely?

When septal defects are small, there is great resistance to flow from one ventricle to the other; thus, there is no transmission of the high LV pressure on the pulmonary arterioles. Consequently, the pulmonary arterioles are not affected by the ventricular septal defect and mature normally. Pulmonary hypertension is thus unlikely.

Case Three

A murmur is recognized for the first time at six months of age. The child has done well and an insignificant pulmonary ejection murmur is diagnosed. At the pre-school checkup at age five years, the child is recognized as being thin, though she is asymptomatic. Because of the persistent murmur, a cardiac evaluation is obtained. The chest X-ray shows cardiomegaly with a prominent pulmonary artery and increased pulmonary vascularity. The electrocardiogram shows right ventricular hypertrophy. The diagnosis of large atrial septal defect is made.

Has harm possibly been done by missing the diagnosis?

In the presence of a large atrial septal defect with equalization of right and left atrial pressures, the shunting is determined by the difference in resistance to the two outlets from the atria. In the newborn period, because the right ventricle is thicker than the left, its compliance is less. Blood flows less easily into the right ventricle, so that there is usually no left-to-right shunt in the newborn period. As systemic vascular resistance gradually increases, the left ventricle thickens. Consequently, during infancy the left-to-right shunt gradually increases. Meanwhile, at birth the pulmonary arterioles *are not affected* by the left-to-right shunt or high pressure and they mature normally. By the time the left-to-right shunt is large, the pulmonary arterioles are mature, thin-walled, and able to dilate maximally; therefore, the pulmonary artery pressure is not elevated. Since the left-to-right shunt has increased so gradually over a long period of time, the ventricular muscle is conditioned. Thus, no harm has been done by missing the diagnosis.

Is it likely that the child has ever been in congestive heart failure?

Congestive heart failure in the presence of an ASD is very uncommon in infancy and childhood.

Is pulmonary hypertension likely?

Significant pulmonary hypertension in simple secundum type atrial septal defects is virtually unknown in childhood.

PATHOPHYSIOLOGY

It is useful to look at the hemodynamic data in the heart and great vessels of children with heart defects, using a box diagram.

The normal pressures in the heart and great vessels for the older child are noted in Figure 13–1.

The oxygen saturation in the right side of the heart is approximately 70 to 75 per cent, while that in the left side of the heart is 95 to

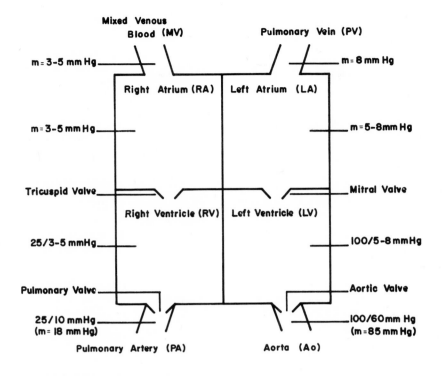

Figure 13–1   Normal pressures in the heart and great vessels of the older child. (m = mean)

98 per cent. When an end-hole catheter is passed as far into the periphery of the lung bed as possible, forward flow is eventually obstructed. The pressure measured in this position is a reflection of that in the pulmonary veins. This is the so-called pulmonary artery wedge pressure. The oxygen saturation of the blood obtained in this position should be greater than 95 per cent, irrespective of the patient's systemic arterial saturation, and is used only to judge whether the catheter position is proper. The oxygen saturations may be used to determine the direction of shunting within the heart or great arteries. For example, an increased saturation in the right atrium indicates a left-to-right shunt at atrial level. In pulmonary disease, some of the pulmonary venous blood has not been exposed to oxygen in the alveoli, effectively resulting in a right-to-left shunt within the lung. The pulmonary vein saturation will therefore be low.

It is imperative always to relate the cardiac outputs and pressures in each side of the heart to each other. Thus, an elevated pressure of 60 mm. systolic in the pulmonary artery is indicative of a greater degree of pul-

monary hypertension when the aortic pressure is *90 mm.* than when it is 120 mm. In the former case, we speak of pulmonary hypertension at two-thirds' systemic level; in the latter, it is at one-half systemic level. When the pressure in the pulmonary artery is equal to that in the aorta, we speak of "systemic level" pulmonary hypertension.

Vascular resistance (systemic or pulmonary) results from the obstruction to flow across the so-called resistance vessels, which are mainly small muscular arteries and arterioles. Thus, we must know the pressures on each side of these vessels. On the systemic side, the ΔP (the pressure drop) is systemic artery pressure minus mixed venous pressure. On the pulmonary side, the ΔP is pulmonary artery pressure minus pulmonary venous pressure. The calculation is made from a modification of Poiseuille's equation. Thus:

Pulmonary Vascular Resistance (PVR)
$$PVR = \frac{\text{pulmonary artery pressure} - \text{pulmonary venous pressure}}{\text{pulmonary flow}}$$

Systemic Vascular Resistance (SVR)
$$SVR = \frac{\text{systemic artery pressure} - \text{mixed venous pressure}}{\text{systemic flow}}$$

Obviously, the narrower the "resistance" vessels are, the greater the resistance; the wider the vessels, the less the resistance. But as we cannot measure this exactly, all we can do is to relate the flow through the entire cross-sectional area of the vascular bed to the pressure drop across the bed. Thus, this is the *calculated* pulmonary or systemic vascular resistance. If the pressure drop is measured in mm. Hg and the flow in liters per minute per meter², then the calculated resistance has been considered to be in "units." The top normal PVR is 3, while the high normal SVR is 15 to 20 units. (It is unnecessary to calculate the resistance measurement in dynes, etc., for one is merely multiplying the units by 80.)

Pulmonary Hypertension

Pulmonary hypertension is defined very specifically. It is the state of *a high pressure in the pulmonary arteries*. It does not necessarily indicate pulmonary vascular disease, nor a high pulmonary vascular resistance. According to Poiseuille's Law, *resistance,* or better yet, calculated pulmonary vascular resistance, is proportional to the reciprocal of the radius of the vessel to the fourth power (i.e., resistance is equivalent to $\frac{1}{r^4}$.) In the original experiments, Poiseuille used a rigid glass tube, but in humans, the resistance vessels are not a fixed size. If the tubes were rigid, the use of the formula $\Delta Pressure = Flow \times Resistance$ would indicate that, if the flow were doubled, the pressure would double.

It is well known that the "adult" type of pulmonary arteriole is a very thin-walled vessel which has a tremendous capacity to dilate. *In fact, the pulmonary flow can increase up to four times that of normal without an increase in pressure.* Thus $\Delta P = 4F \times R$ would indicate in the above situation that the pulmonary vascular resistance is now one-fourth normal. This adult-type vessel, present usually by one month of life, has very little capacity to vasoconstrict. On the other hand, the full-term newborn's pulmonary arterioles are thick walled and very muscular ("fetal" vessels) and have less capacity to dilate with increased flow. These vessels have a remarkable ability to vasoconstrict. Diseased vessels have intimal fibrosis with little or no capacity to either dilate or vasoconstrict. In their most diseased form, they can be considered rigid tubes with a small radius.

Other Types of Resistance

Pulmonary resistance is not the only type of resistance to flow. For example, a narrowed valve provides more resistance to blood flow than a wide-open valve; a small ventricular septal defect provides more resistance to blood flow than a large ventricular septal defect; and a thick, noncompliant ventricular chamber provides more resistance to blood flow than a thinner, more compliant ventricular chamber. Thus, we have four types of resistance quite important to us in understanding the hemodynamics of congenital heart disease. This brings up a statement which, in its simplicity, appears absurdly obvious. It is a key to understanding the various defects and their natural history: *Blood flow goes where resistance is least.*

Fetal and Neonatal Circulation

Blood enters the inferior vena cava (IVC) from the umbilical veins (UV) via the ductus venosus (DV) and enters the right atrium (Figure 13–2). Because of the anatomic relationship of the IVC to the foramen ovale, most of this blood passes from the IVC through the foramen ovale and into the left atrium. There it mixes with the small amount of blood returning from the lungs via the pulmonary veins (PV) and the mixture is propelled into the left ventricle and ascending aorta. The superior vena caval blood enters the right atrium and traverses the tricuspid valve (TV) into the right ventricle (RV). When this blood enters the main pulmonary artery, it is divided. A small amount goes through the pulmonary arteries into the lungs and the greater part enters the descending aorta via the ductus arteriosus. The elevated fetal pulmonary vascular resistance is responsible for this "right-to-left" shunt through the ductus (see Figure 13–2). In utero, the right ventricle and pulmonary arteries have systemic systolic pressure. Significantly, this enables the blood with the highest oxygen saturation to supply the cerebral circulation. Aspects of the circulation prior to birth are important in determining what happens after birth, not only for the normal but also for many congenital cardiac defects. At about 28 to 30 weeks' gestation, the left and right ventricles are about the same thickness with, on the average, perhaps the left a bit more muscular. However, there is gradual change until 37 to 40 weeks, when the right ventricle is at least as thick as the left. It might be up to one-third thicker. Part of the

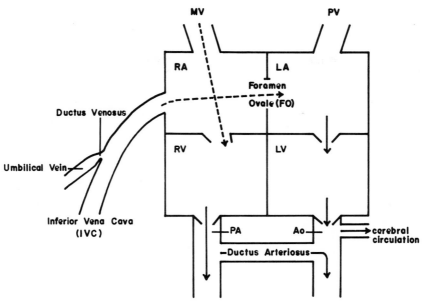

Figure 13–2 Fetal circulation.

explanation for this comes from the data of Naeye, who measured the cross-sectional area of the pulmonary and pancreatic arterioles (the resistance vessels) and found that, while they were similar at 28 to 30 weeks, the pulmonary arterioles were considerably more muscular at 37 to 40 weeks. Since the placenta provides a remarkably low resistance and permits a large flow despite the wide-open ductus arteriosus, the fetal right ventricle should be more muscular than the left.

In the fetus, no more than 10 per cent of the combined right and left ventricular output flows into the lungs. This is not secondary to coiling and kinking of vessels in the collapsed lungs, but is a result of the marked vasoconstriction of the muscular pulmonary arterioles. In classic experiments on the fetal lamb, inflation of the fetal lung with 100 per cent nitrogen does not markedly alter pulmonary blood flow; however, pulmonary flow markedly increases with oxygen inflation. Infusion of histamine or acetylcholine into the pulmonary artery will also increase the flow, even if the lung is *not* expanded.

Some of the sudden changes which occur with the first breath can therefore be explained. Oxygen enters the lungs, suddenly lowering the pulmonary vascular resistance and causing an increase in the pulmonary blood flow. Meanwhile, the clamping of the umbilical cord removes the placenta from the

circuit. Prior to birth, the placenta received more than half of the combined ventricular output; thus, after birth, functional systemic resistance increases and the transfer of gas exchange from the placenta to the pulmonary circulation is facilitated.

In the immediate neonatal period, the pulmonary vascular resistance and systemic vascular resistance are nearly equal, with the former often being a bit lower. Thus, a small left-to-right shunt through the ductus arteriosus may be present. Normally this is not large, for with oxygenation the ductus arteriosus begins to constrict. Sometime during the first 24 hours, the constriction is complete. (It is important to remember, however, that at this time and for a few days thereafter, the normal ductus has the capacity to reopen if a low PaO_2 develops for any reason.)

In this first day after birth, there is a considerable and rapid decrease in pulmonary vascular resistance (about one-half by 24 hours). This is too rapid to be due to anatomic change, but is the result of the continued release of vasoconstriction. However, anatomic change from the "fetal" type, heavily muscular resistance vessels to the "adult" type, thin-walled resistance vessels is much more rapid than was traditionally taught for many years. Although there is considerable species and intraspecies difference, the pulmonary artery pressure in the normal human infant is at or near adult level by one week and often in the first few days. *This potential for very rapid "maturation" from the high resistance fetal vessels to the low resistance adult type vessels is a most important factor in the consideration of congenital heart defects with left-to-right shunts.*

But what prevents the fetal pulmonary arteriole from "maturing?" There are *many possible* factors. Included are:

1. Elevation of pulmonary venous pressure.

2. Transmission of systemic pressure onto the pulmonary circulation.

3. High pulmonary blood flow from birth (including obligatory left-to-right shunts).

4. Low arterial oxygen tension (such as in babies born at high altitudes).

5. Idiosyncrasy — particularly of the female > male.

6. A paradoxical factor (high pulmonary artery pO_2) could be a factor causing early vascular disease.

One more step sideways is necessary before discussing some specific heart defects. We return to the above-mentioned concept that blood flow goes where resistance is least.

In a large barrel filled with fluid (Figure 13–3*A*), with a spigot on each side of the bottom, the pressure of the fluid on each side will be equal.

If the spigots are opened equally (resistance to flow equal), the amount of fluid flowing through each spigot will be the same. If one narrows the spigot on the right (increasing its resistance), most of the flow will be through the left spigot (right-to-left shunt), but the pressure of the fluid will still be equal on each side. If, on the other hand, the spigot is narrowed on the left side with the right one wide open, the flow of the fluid will be mainly through the right one (left-to-right shunt). Again the pressure of the fluid is equal on each side. If one puts a board down the middle of the barrel with a wide opening in the board so that there is still no resistance to flow from one side of the barrel to the next (Figure 13–3*B*), the pressures and flows will be identical to that described in Figure 13–3*A* when no intervening board is present. Obviously, the above can be likened to a large congenital defect, such as a large ventricular septal defect, where *the most important factor in determining whether or not the right ventricular pressure is at systemic level is the size of the defect. In an infant, a child, or an adult with a large, nonrestrictive ventricular septal defect (and in the absence of pulmonic stenosis)*, the relationship of the pulmonary to systemic resistance decides whether the shunt is (1) right-to-left, (2) nonexistent, or bidirectional, or (3) left-to-right. But in each case, there may be the same amount of pulmonary hypertension. *Pulmonary hypertension must not be equated with pulmonary vascular disease or high pulmonary vascular resistance.*

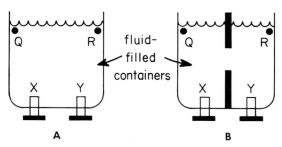

Figure 13–3 A model illustrating the effect of varying resistances. *A*. Pressures at points Q and R are equal. Pressures at spigots X and Y are also equal, provided that the resistance of the two spigots is equal. If, however, the resistance is greater in spigot X than spigot Y, a greater volume of fluid will be obtained from Y (right-to-left shunt). If the resistance is greater in spigot Y, a greater volume of fluid will be obtained from spigot X (left-to-right shunt). *B*. This is the same fluid-filled container as in *A*, except that a board with an opening has been introduced. Pressures at points Q and R are still equal, as are the pressures at spigots X and Y (provided that the resistances are equal). The requirements for right-to-left and left-to-right shunts apply as in *A*.

Atrial Septal Defect (ASD)

For our purposes here, only the very large, nonrestrictive ASD will be discussed. Occasionally, the pressure will be similar in the right and left atria. Where the blood will flow depends partially on streaming effects from the superior vena cava, inferior vena cava, and pulmonary veins, but mainly on where resistance to flow is least. Since, in the newborn period, the right ventricle is at least as thick as and up to one-third thicker than the left ventricle, resistance to flow into the right ventricle is as much as or greater than resistance to flow into the left ventricle. The thick ventricle is less compliant. Thus, not only is there no left-to-right shunt but also there could even be a small right-to-left shunt. *The pulmonary arterioles are not affected by a large atrial septal defect; therefore, normal matura-tion occurs.* The pulmonary vascular resist-ance rapidly decreases, but the thick right ventricle cannot disappear overnight. In fact, it does not disappear at all. Very slowly, the left ventricle increases its thickness, becoming about twice that of the right ventricle by six months of age. Therefore, the left-to-right shunt develops very slowly and by the time there is a large shunt, the vessels have matured nor-mally. Such thin-walled vessels, as you recall, can accept an increase in flow up to four times that of normal without an increase in pressure. Thus, *pulmonary hypertension is extremely uncommon in children with atrial septal de-fects.* Only after 20, 30, or 40 years or so of huge pulmonary flow does pulmonary vascular disease (a high pulmonary vascular resistance and pulmonary hypertension) often develop. It is of interest also that because the develop-ment of the left to right shunt is so slow, the right ventricle has plenty of time to adjust. Therefore, *congestive heart failure in infants and children with atrial septal defects is al-most as uncommon as is pulmonary hyperten-sion.* (The fool who plays four hours of tennis after not having played in many years is most likely not to arise from his bed the next day, his muscles having failed. Had he gradually conditioned himself, however, muscle failure would not have occurred.)

(In order to stress further pathophysiol-ogy, an aside must be made to mention briefly the much less common atrial septal defect of the ostium primum type, where mitral re-gurgitation is usually present. If the mitral regurgitation is severe, congestive heart fail-ure is obvious. Of greater interest is pulmonary hypertension, which may or may not be pres-ent. If there is a large atrial opening along with the mitral regurgitation, pulmonary artery pressures are usually *not* significantly ele-vated. On the other hand, if the atrial opening is small along with the mitral regurgitation, pulmonary venous pressure will be high. In addition, the concept of obligatory left-to-right shunt must be brought up, because, if there is considerable mitral regurgitation, early left-to-right shunt is inevitable no matter what the size of the atrial opening. In summary, ostium secundum atrial septal defects are not associ-ated with early left-to-right shunt nor elevated pulmonary venous pressures. Ostium primum atrial septal defects are often associated with early left-to-right shunts and/or elevated pul-monary venous pressures. Elevated pulmo-nary artery pressures may therefore occur.)

Ventricular Septal Defects (VSD)

In ventricular septal defect, the physiol-ogy is much different. In the large, *nonrestric-tive* VSD, the pressure in the right ventricle and pulmonary artery *will always be* at sys-temic level. If the thick-walled fetal pulmo-nary vessels matured normally, the vascular resistance would decrease so rapidly that there would be a tremendous left-to-right shunt, left ventricular failure, pulmonary edema, and death. Such a series of events is almost unheard of. In fact, in cases with such large VSDs, a heart murmur is not even usu-ally heard in the newborn period. The left-to-right shunt does not develop because the pul-monary resistance vessels remain heavily muscular. In the next few weeks, the vessels slowly mature but do not reach the adult-type vessel. There is considerable variation from one child to the next. Some decrease their re-sistance so that there is a 4:1 pulmonary to systemic flow ratio or greater; some decrease their resistance less so that there is a 3:1 or 2:1 flow ratio, and a rare infant ends up with a persistently high resistance and little or no left-to-right shunt. When there is a large shunt, it is usually maximal by a month of age, early enough so that congestive heart failure is com-mon, and is usually present by six weeks of age. Very infrequently, failure may occur late in the newborn period. An increasing pulmo-nary vascular resistance in childhood is very uncommon, but in the presence of a large non-restrictive ventricular septal defect, it is to be expected by adulthood.

Even in children with the largest defects and the most severe congestive heart failure, the ventricular muscle usually adjusts so that digitalis is no longer needed by the second year of life; heart failure is no longer a prob-lem. Furthermore, the defect tends to become smaller as the child ages. In childhood, large numbers of small defects close spontaneously. A smaller number of large defects close. It is not known how many defects close in adult-hood.

The majority of ventricular septal defects are very small and quite restrictive. In these children, the great resistance to flow between the left and right ventricles allows the pulmo-nary vessels to mature normally into adult-type vessels. Therefore, a left-to-right shunt can develop quickly, so that, with small de-fects, the murmur is often present even in the newborn period. Despite the low pulmonary vascular resistance, the great resistance to flow at the ventricular septal defect prevents much left-to-right shunt; therefore, congestive heart failure does not occur. Pulmonary hypertension is not present because the defect is very small and whatever shunt there is goes easily through the thin-walled, dilatable vessels. A large percentage of these small defects close spontaneously, but pulmonary hypertension does not develop even in those that remain the same size throughout life.

There are many children with moderate-sized openings as well who may have three-fourths, two-thirds, one-half, or one-third systemic pressure pulmonary hypertension, depending on the size of the defect. The amount of left-to-right shunt depends on the defect size and how much maturation occurs. Once the maximal left-to-right shunt develops, most of these children remain stable throughout childhood, or the defect becomes smaller.

Patent Ductus Arteriosus (PDA)

The principles presented for ventricular septal defect hold true for the patent ductus arteriosus, although because there is length to the ductus as well as caliber, resistance to flow is greater. Therefore, systemic level pulmonary hypertension is less common. (When it occurs, the risk of eventually increasing pulmonary vascular resistance may be greater than in ventricular septal defect.) Congestive heart failure, when it occurs, usually has its onset in the second month. Only very rarely does the failure occur late in the newborn period.

The immature infant may be born with a lower pulmonary vascular resistance than the full-term baby; therefore, if he has a ventricular septal defect or patent ductus arteriosus, the left-to-right shunt may develop quickly and congestive heart failure develop earlier than the full-term infant.

In severe respiratory distress syndrome, when oxygenation is poor and PaO_2 is low, the ductus arteriosus may remain patent. At this time, pulmonary vascular resistance is elevated and blood tends to flow right to left through the ductus. If the patient survives and the pulmonary vascular resistance falls, the ductus may still remain patent, with a left-to-right shunt. Occasionally, such infants develop such severe symptoms from the large left-to-right shunt that it is necessary to close the ductus surgically early in infancy. Why the ductus remains open even after the PaO_2 has become normal is not clear. Sometimes the ductus stays open even when the premature baby's respiratory distress syndrome is mild. In most cases, no surgery is required. Surprisingly, in many babies the ductus will close when the number of weeks of gestation plus "outside life" reaches 40 weeks. The physical findings, even in the babies where the ductus will eventually close, are typical of any significant patent ductus with left-to-right shunt. The murmur is very uneven (like water going down the Colorado rapids), frequently going into diastole, and is associated with a wide pulse pressure.

SECTION TWO: THE HIGH-RISK INFANT

SIGNS AND SYMPTOMS

The signs and symptoms of the infant presenting with severe cardiac problems in the newborn period fall into *four major categories*: (1) cyanosis, (2) respiratory distress, (3) systemic venous congestion, and (4) diminished cardiac output. A heart murmur is not usually the presenting sign and in the sickest children, murmurs are usually soft.

Generalized Cyanosis

This condition indicates a low arterial saturation and is either caused by intracardiac or intrapulmonary right-to-left shunt. In intracardiac right-to-left shunting, some venous blood bypasses the lungs and is shunted to the left side of the heart and into the systemic circulation. (A special type of central "shunting" occurs in transposition of the great arteries, where large volumes of fully oxygenated blood do not reach the systemic circulation, which continually is fed mainly unsaturated blood returning from the body.) *Cyanosis is less readily appreciated in newborns than in the older child. By the time congenital heart disease is suspected and the child is clearly blue, the PaO_2 is usually very low.* The reasons for this are not completely clear, particularly since a high hematocrit would make cyanosis more obvious. The newborn's edema may be one factor. Probably more important is the fetal hemoglobin which has a higher oxygen saturation at lower PaO_2's than does adult hemoglobin. Anxiety suggests profound hypoxemia.

Respiratory Distress

In newborns with congenital heart disease, respiratory distress may be related to pulmonary venous hypertension and pulmonary congestion. Mild to moderate degrees of hypoxemia or diminished cardiac output usually do not cause respiratory symptoms, but tachypnea may be present when hypoxemia is severe or there is attendant acidosis.

Systemic Venous Congestion

Systemic venous congestion in the neonate is usually manifested by hepatosplenomegaly and not by peripheral edema. It may be a manifestation of either right or left ventricular myocardial failure. In addition, infants with anatomical obstruction to inflow into the right ventricle may exhibit systemic venous congestion. Included here are those infants with tricuspid atresia and hypoplastic right ventricle with small tricuspid valve. In these individuals and in those with pure right ventricular failure, the degree of systemic venous congestion is governed not only by the basic problem but also by the size of the interatrial communication. Thus, an individual with tricuspid atresia and a large interatrial opening will have little systemic venous congestion, whereas with a small interatrial opening, the systemic venous congestion will be prominent.

Diminished Cardiac Output

A profound decrease in cardiac output is manifested by very poor pulses and mottling of the skin. The child with low cardiac output may also present with marked hypotonia and slight cyanosis.

There does not exist an adequately comprehensive and yet simple classification with which to approach the diagnosis of serious heart disease in the newborn. Our classification of neonates with serious congenital heart disease is based on the outstanding clinical presentation. Like any system or classification, it has its exceptions and overlaps and is obviously not complete. We have, however, found it most useful clinically.

The distressed newborn with heart disease may be placed into one of three major groups, based on the four cardinal signs and symptoms: (1) cyanosis is the outstanding feature, (2) cyanosis is outstanding with moderate respiratory distress, and (3) decreased cardiac output is outstanding with significant respiratory distress and usually no more than moderate cyanosis.

In Table 13–2 the three major groups are delineated. In Table 13–3 the three groups are described in terms of their major characteristics.

Group I: Cyanosis the Outstanding Feature

In the early days of life, a ductus may remain open, providing good pulmonary blood flow into a low-resistance pulmonary vascular bed, but unfortunately the ductus commonly persists only in patients with maximal tetralogy of Fallot with pulmonary atresia. The amount of blood going into the lungs determines the arterial saturation, and the heart murmurs result from the blood flowing into that bed. Therefore, *the more severe the disease, the softer the murmur.*

Hypoplastic Right Ventricle with Tricuspid Atresia. The right ventricle is usually very small and there is complete aplasia of the tricuspid valve (Figure 13–4A). All venous

TABLE 13–2   APPROACH TO SERIOUS HEART DISEASE IN THE NEONATE

GROUP I. CYANOSIS THE OUTSTANDING FEATURE
    A. The hypoplastic right ventricle syndrome.
        1. With tricuspid atresia.
        2. With pulmonary atresia.
    B. Severe tetralogy of Fallot.
        1. With very severe pulmonary stenosis.
        2. With pulmonary atresia.
GROUP II. CYANOSIS THE OUTSTANDING FEATURE, WITH MODERATE RESPIRATORY DISTRESS
    A. Transposition of the great arteries with intact ventricular septum.
GROUP III. EVIDENCE OF LOW CARDIAC OUTPUT OUTSTANDING, WITH RESPIRATORY DISTRESS AND MODERATE CYANOSIS
    A. Hypoplastic left ventricle syndrome.
    B. Complicated coarctation of the aorta.

TABLE 13–3 CHARACTERISTICS OF THE THREE MAJOR GROUPS

GROUP I. CYANOSIS THE OUTSTANDING FEATURE
The hearts are small and quiet, with diminished pulmonary blood flow. Evidence of low cardiac output does not occur, and there is no respiratory distress unless there is severe hypoxemia and acidosis.
GROUP II. CYANOSIS THE OUTSTANDING FEATURE, WITH MODERATE RESPIRATORY DISTRESS
The hearts are small or minimally enlarged, but hyperdynamic with increased pulmonary blood flow. Evidence of low cardiac output does not occur, and systemic venous congestion is no more than moderate.
GROUP III. EVIDENCE OF LOW CARDIAC OUTPUT OUTSTANDING, WITH RESPIRATORY DISTRESS AND MODERATE CYANOSIS
The hearts are large and hyperdynamic (unless the cardiac output is very low) with increased pulmonary blood flow. There is systemic venous congestion, and cyanosis is no more than mild to moderate.

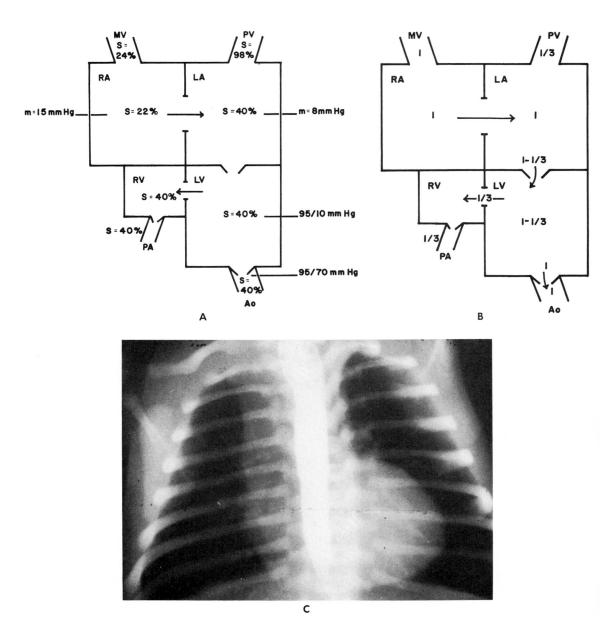

Figure 13–4 Hypoplastic right ventricle with tricuspid atresia. *A*. Pressures in mm. Hg and saturations (S) in percentages. *B*. Flows in units of cardiac output. *C*. Radiogram of chest.

blood must therefore go through an atrial opening into the left atrium. Almost invariably, blood then returns to the right ventricle by way of a ventricular septal defect and through a small right ventricular outflow tract to normally placed pulmonary arteries. Thus, there are three areas where flow can be obstructed: the atrial septum, the ventricular septum, and the right ventricular outflow tract. The left ventricle accepts the normal cardiac output plus whatever pulmonary blood flow comes back from the pulmonary veins. If pulmonary blood flow is one-third of normal, then the left ventricle will have one and one-third of the normal cardiac output (Figure 13–4*B*). The right ventricle has one-third the normal cardiac output. This extra workload on the left ventricle is not enough to cause left ventricular failure prior to surgery (Figure 13–4*C*).

The physical findings reveal a small quiet heart with a "right ventricular" impulse and a murmur of a ventricular septal defect with a left-to-right shunt. In very blue babies, this murmur may be very soft and short, but it usually obscures the first sound. There may also be a soft pulmonary ejection murmur. The electrocardiogram shows left ventricular hypertrophy, partly because of the increased left ventricular volume work but mainly because of the hypoplastic right ventricle. There is also usually an abnormally superior vector believed to be due to a conduction defect secondary to an endocardial cushion-type ventricular septal defect. The majority of the babies have no trouble in the newborn period but have difficulty later on as the ventricular septal defect gets smaller.

Hypoplastic Right Ventricle with Pulmonary Atresia. Although the embryology is similar to that of the hypoplastic right ventricle with tricuspid atresia, there are many differences in physiology (Figure 13–5). Because blood enters the right ventricle and is then obstructed, the right ventricular pressure may become very high (only a very insufficient tricuspid valve prevents this). The amount of blood entering the right ventricle is very small; essentially all right atrial blood enters the left atrium. There is no ventricular septal defect, so that pulmonary blood flow depends entirely on the ductus arteriosus. Consequently, these babies, on the average, are in grave trouble at an earlier age than are babies with tricuspid atresia and a ventricular septal defect. Such infants may even be ill before 24 hours of age. As in the babies with tricuspid atresia, the left ventricle handles a normal cardiac output plus whatever pulmonary blood flow is returning via the pulmonary veins. However, the abnormally superior vector of tricuspid atresia is *not* present, presumably because a ventricular septal defect is not present.

The physical findings may sometimes be confusing when there is a murmur at the lower left sternal border suggesting a ventricular septal defect. This murmur, however, can

Figure 13–5 Hypoplastic right ventricle with pulmonary atresia. Pressures in mm. Hg and saturations (S) in percentages.

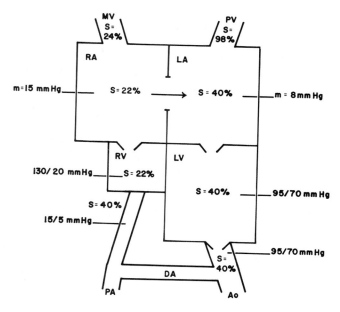

usually be noted to increase in intensity with inspiration, indicating tricuspid regurgitation.

Although the risk of surgery is very high for many reasons, all cardiologists now agree that when such babies are in trouble in early infancy, a root of aorta to right pulmonary artery anastomosis must be performed. We believe it highly desirable to have previously created a good atrial opening with a balloon catheter prior to surgery, and for the surgeon also to do a pulmonary valvotomy.

Severe Tetralogy of Fallot. The physiology of tetralogy is best understood if the condition is considered as being a large, nonrestrictive ventricular septal defect with pulmonic stenosis severe enough so that resistance to flow into the pulmonary artery is higher than resistance to flow out of the aorta. The result is right-to-left shunt. (Figure 13–6A). The right ventricle has been working at systemic pressure in utero and it is estimated that it can do so at that level without congestive heart failure well into adulthood (estimate 40 years). The more severe the pulmonic stenosis, the less volume work the heart does (Figure 13–6B). Thus, if there is only one-third normal pulmonary blood flow because of two-thirds of the right ventricular flow going right to left, the combined right and left ventricular volume work is only one and

one-third units of output compared to two units.

The murmur associated with tetralogy is that of blood flow through the pulmonary valve. There is no murmur of blood going right to left. Thus, the more severe the tetralogy, the less blood is ejected through the pulmonary valve, and the softer and shorter is the ejection murmur. Also, the more severe the tetralogy, the larger is the aorta and the more likely will there be an aortic ejection click. In the severest cases, therefore, with virtual or actual pulmonic atresia, there is an aortic ejection click after the first sound, but no murmur. The electrocardiogram demonstrates right ventricular hypertrophy.

It is very infrequent for children with tetralogy to have difficulty in the first weeks, although there is an increasing frequency of difficulty later in the neonatal period. The majority of children with tetralogy have no significant difficulty in infancy.

Differential Diagnosis. In addition to the lesions already discussed, there are two other important conditions causing severe illness to the newborn which present with cyanosis and a quiet heart. However, the hearts will be larger and there may be severe right heart failure with systemic venous congestion. Their recognition is important because (1)

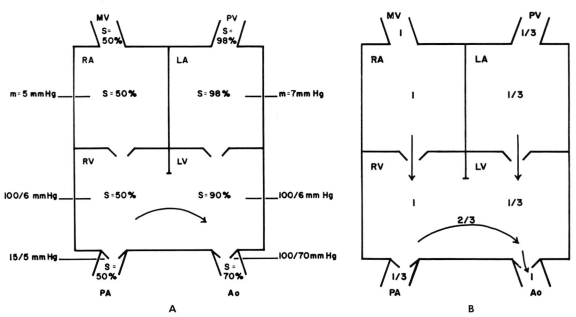

Figure 13–6 Tetralogy of Fallot. *A.* Pressures in mm. Hg and saturations (S) in percentages. *B.* Flows in units of cardiac output.

Ebstein's anomaly causes severe distress yet is best treated medically; and (2) pulmonary stenosis or atresia with intact ventricular septum must be treated surgically.

In Ebstein's anomaly, the tricuspid valve is displaced into the right ventricle and is remarkably distorted (Figure 13–7). Because of ineffective ventricular contraction against the newborn's high pulmonary vascular resistance, there is both heart failure with marked systemic venous congestion and a right-to-left shunt at the atrial level. In most cases, almost miraculously, as the pulmonary vascular resistance decreases, the heart failure lessens and there is less right-to-left shunt.

Ebstein's anomaly presenting with symptoms in the neonatal period must be extremely rare indeed. Although a number of these children are known to the Department of Cardiology in our hospital, their presentation has always been with symptoms in the somewhat older age group. Moreover, it would seem to us that the diagnosis would be heavily dependent upon the highly abnormal P waves seen on the electrocardiogram, and under normal circumstances we would not place this malformation very high on the list of possibilities to be considered for a newborn infant in trouble from congenital heart disease.

L. STERN

Severe pulmonary stenosis with intact ventricular septum (Figure 13–8) is a "curable" lesion. On the very rare occasions when difficulty occurs in the newborn period (manifested also by severe right heart failure and right-to-left shunt at the atrial level), surgery is necessary as an extreme emergency procedure. Once again we have a case in which the soft murmur is associated with severe cyanotic heart disease. Characteristically in the older child, the more severe the stenosis, the louder and longer the murmur. However, in these extremely ill neonates, there may be so little blood entering the poorly contracting right ventricle that paradoxically the murmur may be short and soft.

Group II: Cyanosis the Outstanding Feature, with Respiratory Distress

Transposition of the Great Arteries with Intact Ventricular Septum. The respiratory distress is caused mainly by an elevated pulmonary venous pressure, but severe hypoxemia with attendant acidosis may provide additional cause. The severity of the condition depends on the amount of mixing between the two sides of the circulation. The babies may be well for a day or a few days until the ductus arteriosus closes and pulmonary vascular resistance decreases. At this point, the child's survival depends upon how much blood flows through the atrial opening in both directions. In the majority, only a foramen ovale is present (Figure 13–9A and B). We stress additionally that the only murmur is due to increased flow into the pulmonary artery and is therefore soft.

Cardiac catheterization is usually done as an emergency procedure (preferably after an

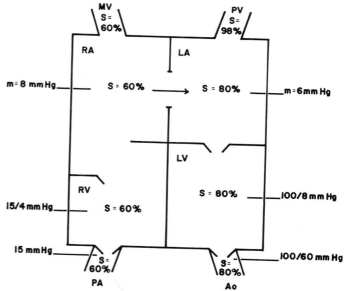

Figure 13–7 Ebstein's anomaly. Pressures in mm. Hg and saturations (S) in percentages.

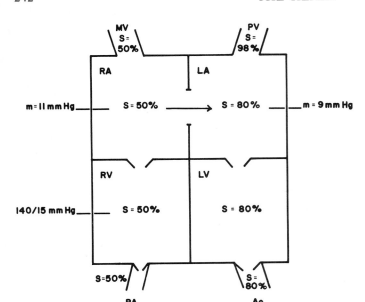

Figure 13–8 Severe pulmonary stenosis with intact ventricular septum. Pressures in mm. Hg and saturations (S) in percentages.

umbilical artery catheter is placed, as all efforts are being made to raise the pH). A balloon septostomy is performed to tear the atrial septum at the foramen ovale. The baby may improve considerably even if the foramen is only dilated. In the next days, if the arterial saturation stays above 60 to 65 per cent, no further therapy is given.

If a ventricular septal defect is also present, the pathophysiology will depend upon the size of the defect. The smaller the ventricular septal defect, the more likely will the baby act as though no defect were present; the larger the ventricular septal defect, the more likely that the problem will *not* be hypoxemia. The child may then present with congestive heart failure late in the first month, or even in the second month.

Differential Diagnosis. Included in the differential diagnosis are many conditions which are difficult to categorize. Most should not be considered if we think of the pathophysiology and understand the natural history, but the presentations in some are very perplexing.

PRIMARY LUNG DISEASE. On some occasions, it is difficult to differentiate severe cardiac anomalies from primary pulmonary disease. The characteristic grunting breathing of lung disease is frequently helpful, as is the usually clearly split second sound. However, babies with pulmonary venous obstruction may grunt and babies with lung disease and a high pulmonary vascular resistance may have a narrowly split or single second sound. Frequent measurements of arterial PaO₂ while breathing 100 per cent oxygen are also usually helpful in making the separation. On the average, babies with lung disease significantly increase their arterial PaO₂ more than do babies with heart disease. However, the more pulmonary venous obstruction and congestion the baby with heart disease has, the less clear may be the separation.

TOTAL ANOMALOUS PULMONARY VENOUS DRAINAGE. Newborns with total anomalous pulmonary venous drainage are in distress if there is marked pulmonary venous obstruction. When drainage is below the diaphragm, the pulmonary veins are invariably obstructed (Figure 13–10) and the baby will expire unless the condition is recognized early and surgery can be accomplished. Although there are cases with drainage above the diaphragm in which there is moderate or even marked pulmonary venous obstruction, most are not obstructed. The nonobstructed group is not expected to have difficulty until at least after one month of age. The babies without pulmonary venous obstruction present with marked right ventricular hypertrophy, a large, hyperdynamic heart, evidence of tremendous pulmonary blood flow with moderate pulmonary hypertension, and a low pulmonary vascular resistance. The babies with marked pulmonary venous obstruction are very different and may present in difficulty as early as the first days of life. *Many are*

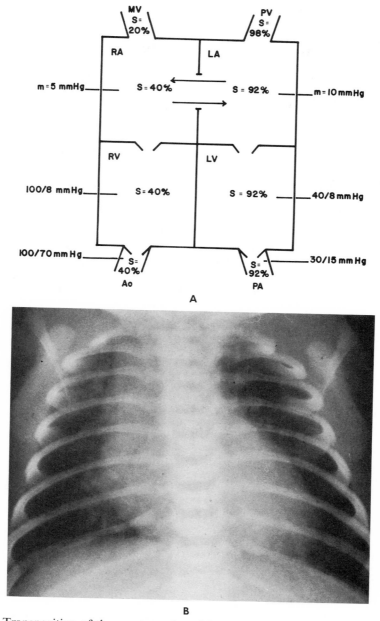

Figure 13–9 Transposition of the great arteries with intact ventricular septum. *A*. Pressures in mm. Hg and saturations (S) in percentages. *B*. Radiogram of chest.

diagnosed as having primary lung disease. They present with cyanosis, respiratory distress, and a small, quiet heart. The chest X-ray classically shows the small heart with an intense pulmonary congestion. It may be described as "ground glass," so that confusion with hyaline membrane disease is well known. The obstructed babies may have no murmur.

CEREBRAL ARTERIOVENOUS FISTULA. This condition may also be difficult to separate from an infant with lung disease. When in difficulty in the first days, the cyanosis is due to left heart failure with pulmonary venous congestion, and is mild to moderate. Despite very little murmur, the obvious clues in separation from lung disease are a very large

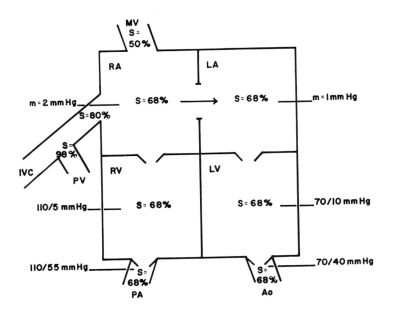

Figure 13–10 Total anomalous pulmonary venous return below the diaphragm. Pressures in mm. Hg and saturations (S) in percentages.

heart and the characteristic cranial bruit. (Diagnosis requires auscultation of the head). The prognosis is poor when the babies are symptomatic from the beginning, but attempts at tying off arterial feeders are occasionally helpful.

In the newborn infant, cerebral arteriovenous fistula almost invariably presents only as congestive heart failure and usually without any neurologic signs accompanying it. This is quite different than its presentation in the older child, in which convulsions or a subarachnoid hemorrhage may be the first diagnostic clues to its presence. Nevertheless, in the cases seen and reported by us as well as those reported in the literature, a small proportion do have additional neurologic findings which, when added to the congestive failure, strongly raise the suspicion of the diagnosis. It should be mandatory that any child with heart failure in the newborn period have his head very carefully listened to for a bruit. In its absence, the diagnosis may be suspected from an angiogram, in which dilated carotid and upper vessels can sometimes be seen. Depending upon the localization of the malformation, surgical treatment (if the diagnosis is made early enough) does afford a chance for cure provided the diagnosis is thought of and action taken early enough before intractable and severe cardiac failure has reduced the possibility for success on the operating table.

L. STERN

TRANSPOSITION OF THE GREAT ARTERIES WITH LARGE VENTRICULAR SEPTAL DEFECT; DOUBLE OUTLET RIGHT VENTRICLE WITH LARGE VENTRICULAR SEPTAL DEFECT; AND TRUE TRUNCUS ARTERIOSUS. All

three of these lesions act similarly. Usually they cause no difficulty in the first month and, if there is any, it is congestive heart failure late in the month. Occasionally the baby with true truncus is in difficulty in the first days of life, especially in association with a deformed truncus valve.

Group III: Poor Cardiac Output with Respiratory Distress

The most common time for onset of symptoms is the first week for the hypoplastic left ventricle syndrome and the second week for complicated coarctation of the aorta. Symptoms in either group may develop in the first days. In general, difficulty from the hypoplastic left ventricle syndrome develops earlier. The respiratory distress is related to the marked pulmonary venous congestion that usually develops.

The Hypoplastic Left Ventricle Syndrome. The hypoplastic left heart syndrome covers a wide spectrum, including mitral and/or aortic atresia (Figure 13–11A and B), a diminutive left ventricular cavity, and marked hypoplasia of the ascending aorta. The important concept is that, though the variation in anatomy is considerable, the hypoplastic left ventricle causes the problem. Since there is no output from the left ventricle, the pulmonary venous blood returning to the left atrium must pass through the atrial septum to the right atrium. The smaller the atrial opening, the

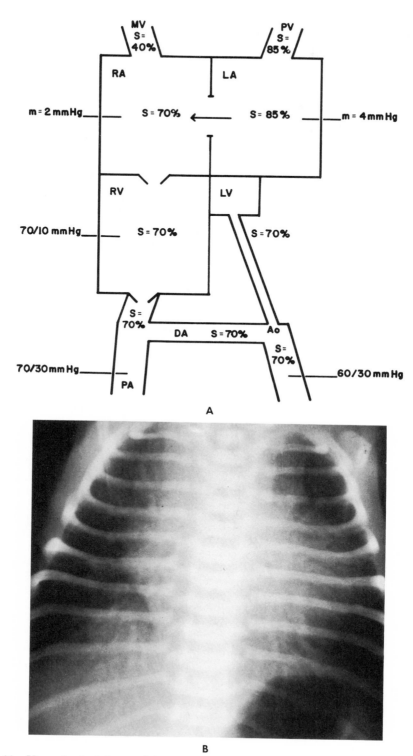

Figure 13–11 Hypoplastic left ventricle with mitral and aortic stenosis. *A.* Pressures in mm. Hg and saturations (S) in percentages. *B.* Radiogram of chest.

greater the pulmonary venous hypertension and the earlier the symptoms. The entire systemic output is supplied via right-to-left flow through the patent ductus. As the ductus narrows postnatally, there is severe impairment of systemic output. If the atrial opening permits, there may be a considerable pulmonary blood flow, and marked cyanosis is usually not present. (Early in the course, cyanosis may not even be recognized.)

At the very beginning, pulses may be within normal limits. Strikingly, they may also be intermittently very poor, as the variably low pH and PaO_2 affect the contraction of the ductus. The average age of death is usually before one week. Occasionally the babies live for many weeks if there is a wide-open ductus and a good-sized atrial septal defect. The diagnosis is not difficult. Furthermore, we, as others, have found that the echocardiogram is so characteristic that there is no need for cardiac catheterization.

Complicated Coarctation of the Aorta. The term "complicated" indicates that in addition to a significant coarctation of the aorta there is another congenital heart defect, such as patent ductus arteriosus, ventricular septal defect, or aortic stenosis. Combinations of any may be present, compounding the issue. In addition, the aortic arch may show some hypoplasia.

Mild or moderate cyanosis may be present secondary to pulmonary venous desaturation. It is not often appreciated, but if there is an associated large ventricular septal defect, there may be little or no gradient in pressure from upper to lower extremity. (The resistance to flow through the large ventricular septal defect may be so much lower than into the aorta that not enough ejectile force can be created.) Also, the congestive heart failure on admission may be so severe that a pressure gradient is difficult to demonstrate.

These babies may be very ill in the first days of life and almost always by the second week. Once ill there is very little time available. Decongestive measures and diagnostic procedures should be done rapidly, followed as soon as considered justified by surgery—at least by 48 hours.

Right ventricular hypertrophy on the electrocardiogram is to be expected no matter where the coarctation and no matter what the additional lesion, for the right ventricle has been ejecting blood through the coarctation in utero.

Differential Diagnosis. Two major le-sions are considered: simple coarctation of the aorta and valvular aortic stenosis.

SIMPLE COARCTATION OF THE AORTA. The congestive heart failure is usually not present until late in the first month of life. The diagnosis is usually readily made by the absence of markedly reduced femoral pulses with strong brachial pulses. With severe heart failure, however, there may be little pressure gradient before decongestive measures. The characteristic murmur may also not be evident until treatment has been instituted. The electrocardiogram shows pure right ventricular hypertrophy just as when the coarctation is complicated by other defects.

These children do very well medically, unless there is the complication of a considerably hypoplastic transverse arch. Therefore, surgery is not recommended in infancy. If the babies are sick early in the newborn period, they will not survive without surgery; however, if the onset of congestive failure is late in the month or after the newborn period, medical management is usually recommended. An alternative approach is that, if the coarctation of the aorta is complicated by another significant lesion, surgery is necessary; however, if the coarctation is isolated, medical management should be successful.

AORTIC STENOSIS. Patients with aortic stenosis are rarely symptomatic in the neonatal period. However, when symptoms are present, the situation is serious. These infants present much the same as do those with hypoplastic left ventricle, except later in life—generally after one month of age. The characteristic systolic ejection murmur of aortic stenosis may be absent, as these infants are in such severe heart failure that only a small quantity of blood is ejected from the left ventricle. With the use of digitalis and diuretics as the failure improves, the murmur will become audible. The electrocardiogram usually shows left ventricular hypertrophy with ST-segment and T-wave abnormality. After medical therapy and proper diagnostic procedures, surgery is imperative, since without rapid surgical intervention the mortality is high.

PRACTICAL HINTS

1. When there is little or no murmur in a symptomatic newborn with heart disease, the situation is usually grave.

2. When a heart murmur is the present-

ing problem, without symptoms, the situation is usually benign.

3. Heart sounds in most patients with congenital heart disease of a serious nature are usually abnormal. A single second sound after the first 12 hours often indicates heart disease. A well-split second sound suggests pulmonary disease rather than heart disease, although it may sometimes be present in transposition of the great arteries with an intact ventricular septum. The presence of a pulmonary systolic ejection click may be normal in the first hours, but after that a systolic ejection click of any sort is abnormal, indicating a large pulmonary artery, a large aorta, or a true truncus arteriosus.

4. Visible central cyanosis in the early newborn period usually indicates a very low arterial oxygen tension.

5. Peripheral cyanosis (acrocyanosis) is normal, and must be differentiated from central cyanosis.

6. Arterial blood gases may be helpful in differentiating pulmonary from cardiac cyanosis. A PaO_2 >100 mm. Hg in an enriched oxygen environment effectively eliminates severe heart disease with anatomic right-to-left shunt. In questionable cases, hypoxemia without significant hypercapnia (CO_2 retention) tends to suggest primary cardiac disease, although patients with severe RDS can have similar blood gases. (However, pulmonary venous congestion, as in the hypoplastic left ventricle syndrome, may result in considerable CO_2 retention.)

7. Tachypnea is a sign of cardiorespiratory difficulty. When there is little respiratory effort, congenital heart disease is suggested. Marked respiratory effort, especially with "grunting," suggests lung disease, but there may be considerable overlap.

8. Life-threatening congenital heart disease will sooner or later be associated with respiratory distress or frank cyanosis or both.

9. The presence of a large liver usually indicates systemic venous congestion, which may not necessarily indicate congestive heart failure. Many conditions in the neonatal period can produce large livers.

10. Femoral pulses must be carefully palpated in all newborn infants.

11. All infants with cardiorespiratory difficulty must have a chest X-ray. An electrocardiogram should also be strongly considered.

12. A high index of suspicion is required to diagnose congenital heart disease early.

Careful history, physical examination, and simple laboratory measurements, including chest X-ray, electrocardiogram, and blood gas studies with and without an enriched oxygen environment, will often help establish the diagnosis.

13. *When a baby with a congenital heart defect is symptomatic early in the newborn period, death is likely unless a surgical procedure or balloon septostomy can be performed.*

14. When there is difficulty in the first week, lesions not to be missed are:

Group I — The hypoplastic right ventricle syndrome with pulmonary atresia (common — needs surgery).

Group I (in differential) — Ebstein's anomaly (uncommon, usually improves without surgery); *pulmonic stenosis with intact ventricular septum* (uncommon, but needs surgery, and is important, because eventually curable).

Group II — Transposition of great arteries with intact ventricular septum (common, needs surgery, eventually curable).

Group II (in differential) — Total anomalous pulmonary venous drainage below the diaphragm (uncommon, needs surgery which is difficult); *cerebral arteriovenous fistula* (rare).

Group III — The hypoplastic left ventricle syndrome (common); *complicated coarctation of aorta* (somewhat less common, surgery necessary, eventually curable).

Group III (in differential) — Aortic stenosis (uncommon, surgery necessary).

It should be stressed that any of the defects mentioned above may cause symptoms later in the first month, while some other important lesions may occasionally cause difficulty in the first week. The latter include severe tetralogy of Fallot, the hypoplastic right ventricle with tricuspid atresia, and true truncus arteriosus.

CASE PROBLEMS

It is important to note that cyanosis due to right-to-left intracardiac shunting is difficult to recognize in the first days of life. *The degree of desaturation is usually underestimated.* It is also important to recognize two major forms of cyanotic congenital heart disease: (1) that associated with insufficient pulmonary blood flow, and (2) that in which there is increased pulmonary blood flow but in which the flow is not effective because the oxygenated blood from pulmonary vein blood does not reach the systemic circulation. (In the following cases, cyanosis is present in the newborn period.) Use of box diagrams will facilitate the solving of these case problems.

Case Four

A baby girl is considered normal at birth, but on the second day cyanosis is noted. The heart is quiet. No murmur is heard and there is no respiratory distress. On the third day, cyanosis is more obvious and the respiratory rate is increased. The child's chest X-ray shows a small heart with decreased pulmonary vascularity. The electrocardiogram shows left ventricular hypertrophy.

Can a diagnosis be suggested?

When the heart is quiet and the child is blue, insufficient pulmonary blood flow is suggested. The X-ray is consistent. These findings and the electrocardiogram indicate that perhaps the right ventricle is hypoplastic.

A cardiac catheterization is performed. The right ventricle is entered with great difficulty.

	PRESSURE (mm. Hg)	PER CENT SATURATION
SVC and RA	$m = 10$	20
RV	160/10	20
LA	$m = 5$	50
PV	$m = 5$	95
LV	80/5	50
Femoral Artery	80/50	50

Cineangiograms were done from the right atrium, right ventricle, and left ventricle.

Are the physiologic data consistent with the clinical diagnosis?

At catheterization, there is no left-to-right shunt as far as the ventricle, while the saturation of 50 per cent in LA indicates a large right-to-left shunt at the atrial level. The very high RV pressure indicates severe obstruction to outflow, while the large difference in pressure between the RV and LV reveals that there must be little or no ventricular communication. Although there is a large right-to-left shunt at the atrial level, the marked difference in pressure between RA and LA indicates that there is a small communication. Thus, the clinical diagnosis fits with the cath-

eterization diagnosis of pulmonary atresia with a hypoplastic right ventricle and an intact ventricular septum.

How does blood reach the pulmonary circulation?

Most or all of the cardiac output flows through the atrial septum into the left atrium, and then through the left ventricle and the aorta. Almost invariably there is a patent ductus arteriosus connected to normal pulmonary arteries. A normal main pulmonary artery extends to the atretic pulmonary valve.

Is there some treatment that can be done before completing the catheterization?

The atrial septum can be enlarged with the use of balloon septostomy to improve blood flow from the right atrium to the left atrium.

Should the surgeon be called?

Yes, as soon as possible.

Can the surgeon help?

Yes, by making an anastomosis between the root of the aorta and the right pulmonary artery.

What is the prognosis?

The prognosis is not known. Much depends on whether the hypoplastic right ventricle will grow. We need many more years to assess various approaches. It is also only recently that we have learned how common this condition is, and how to help these babies.

Case Five

A baby girl is considered normal at birth, but on the second day cyanosis is noted. The heart is quiet. A Grade IV full-length systolic ejection murmur at the lower left sternal border is heard. There is no respiratory distress.

At this point, in comparison to Case Four, is there any suggestion as to a different prognosis?

As in Case Four, the heart is quiet, suggesting that cyanosis is associated with decreased pulmonary blood flow. The X-ray reveals a small heart and decreased pulmonary vascularity. The most important difference is the long, loud murmur. In general, cyanotic newborns with heart disease have a better prognosis when there is a loud murmur.

On the third day, cyanosis remains minimal. The chest X-ray still shows a small heart with questionably decreased pulmonary vascularity. The electrocardiogram shows right ventricular hypertrophy.

Can a diagnosis be suggested?

The most likely diagnosis from the above information is a large ventricular septal defect with pulmonic stenosis and right-to-left shunt (tetralogy of Fallot).

Should a cardiac catheterization be performed?

Many groups catheterize virtually all cyanotic children when heart disease is suspected. It has not been our policy to do so, particularly when we are confident of the diagnosis of tetralogy of Fallot. Cardiac catheterization in infants with tetralogy of Fallot is not without risks. (Severe anoxic spells can occur.) Nothing is done when things are mild, while surgery (creation of an anastomosis of aorta to right pulmonary artery) is indicated when the infant is severely ill or having anoxic spells. We would send this child home to be followed closely.

Case Six

A baby is considered normal at birth, but on the second day cyanosis is noted. The heart is hyperdynamic. A Grade II systolic ejection murmur is heard at the upper left sternal border and there is no respiratory distress. On the third day, the cyanosis is more obvious and the respiratory rate is increased. The chest X-ray shows a normal-sized heart; however, there is a suggestion of increased pulmonary vascularity, despite which the pulmonary artery cannot be recognized. The electrocardiogram shows the normal right ventricular dominance of a newborn.

Can a diagnosis be suggested?

The most striking difference between this and Cases Four and Five is that the heart is hyperdynamic. In addition, pulmonary vascularity is shown to be increased by X-ray. Thus, the cyanosis is not likely to be due to decreased pulmonary blood flow but rather to inadequate mixing. The oxygenated pulmonary venous blood is not getting to the systemic circulation.

This, together with the fact that the pulmonary artery cannot be recognized despite increased pulmonary vascularity, suggests an abnormality of the great arteries.

A cardiac catheterization is performed.

	PRESSURE (mm. Hg)	PER CENT SATURATION
SVC	m = 5	20
RA	m = 5	40
RV	80/5	40
LA	m = 10	95
PV	m = 10	95
OV	40/10	95
Femoral Artery	80/50	40

What is the likely pulmonary artery saturation?

With a femoral artery saturation of 40 per cent, it is likely that the aorta arose from the right ventricle. The fact that the two ventricles have such different pressures indicates that there is little or no communication. Thus, double outlet right ventricle is not possible. The pulmonary artery arises from the left ventricle and its oxygen saturation will be 95 per cent (though it may be slightly less depending on how much, if any, aorta to pulmonary shunt there is through a patent ductus arteriosus).

What is the likely pulmonary artery pressure?

The pressure in the pulmonary artery can be no more than 40 mm. Hg systolic, and may be less if there is some mild pulmonic stenosis. (Pulmonary artery is fed here from left ventricle.)

Is there something therapeutic that can be done before completing the procedure?

Clearly, more mixing is needed between the two sides. The safest way to accomplish this is to create an atrial septal defect using a balloon catheter. The catheter is placed into the left atrium, blown up, and pulled back hard. The surgeon can do a better job, but obviously at great comparative risk.

Is complete repair ever possible?

Because the pulmonary artery pressure is low, pulmonary vascular disease does not as readily develop as when there is a large ventricular septal defect. Thus, the baby is an ideal candidate for eventual complete repair (age two to two and one-half years, though many surgeons are beginning to operate even earlier).

Case Seven

A baby boy is considered normal at birth, but on the second day cyanosis is noted. The heart is hyperdynamic, the pulses are good, and a Grade III systolic ejection murmur is present at the upper left sternal border. There is no respiratory distress. On the third day, the cyanosis remains mild, but the pulses (especially the femoral) are poor, there is respiratory distress, and the liver is enlarged. The X-ray shows a large heart with increased pulmonary vascularity, and there is marked right ventricular hypertrophy.

Can you explain the poor pulses, especially with the knowledge that six hours later the femoral pulses became good again?

In the newborn period, the ductus can be kept open by a low PaO_2 and low pH, which also increase pulmonary vascular resistance and depress myocardial function. No one knows the exact answer, but if the systemic circulation is dependent on flow from the pulmonary artery from a right-to-left shunt through the ductus, the peripheral pulses will become poor when the ductus constricts secondary to high pH and PaO_2. When the pH and PaO_2 drop, the ductus opens and pulses improve. Thus, systemic output must be deficient.

A cardiac catheterization was performed.

	PRESSURE (mm. Hg)	PER CENT SATURATION
SVC	$m = 8$	45
RA	$m = 8$	75
RV	100/8	75
PA	100/70	75
PV	$m = 14$	85
LA	$m = 14$	85
Descending Aorta	100/70	75

How was the aorta entered?

The aorta was entered by way of the patent ductus. The anatomy is such that usually the descending aorta is entered even if there is an ascending aorta.

What is the diagnosis?

There is a large left-to-right shunt at the atrial level, despite there being only a small opening between the two atria (RA mean pressure is 8, while LA mean pressure is 14). This high LA pressure should indicate that the left ventricle is functioning poorly or that there is marked obstruction to flow into the left ventricle. The pulmonary venous desaturation also indicates left-sided failure. Finally, the 75 per cent saturation in the descending aorta suggests that the aortic flow is coming from the pulmonary artery. The diagnosis is that of the hypoplastic left ventricle syndrome (see Figure 13–11). This condition was the cause of more deaths at Rainbow Babies' and Children's Hospital last year than any other single disease outside of those associated with prematurity.

The child may do better if a balloon septostomy or, better yet, a Blalock-Hanlon (creation of ASD by surgeon) is performed. Would you recommend this?

Although a balloon septostomy will open the atrial septum and allow the obligatory left-to-right atrial shunt to be less impeded, death is still inevitable in a short time. Consequently, probably no surgery or balloon septostomy is indicated.

The next cases involve infants who are very ill and may be pink or blue.

Case Eight

A full-term baby boy was considered to be well at birth, although at the examination there was a question of decrease in femoral pulses. The baby was discharged from the hospital at five days, eating nicely. The femoral pulses were still poor, but this was discounted as being common at this age, especially in chubby babies. At three weeks of age, the child was admitted to the hospital with respiratory difficulty. He was breathing very rapidly, was sweating profusely, and was moderately cyanotic. The liver was large. Femoral pulses were absent and brachials were not strong. Flush pressures were 70 in each arm and 60 in the legs. A Grade II short systolic ejection murmur was slightly louder in the back than the midleft sternal border. The X-ray showed a large heart with pulmonary venous congestion. The electrocardiogram showed right ventricular hypertrophy.

Can a diagnosis be suggested?

There are strong clues to the diagnosis of coarctation of the aorta, despite the lack of blood pressure gradient. The most important clues are that the femoral pulses are absent and that the murmur is maximal in the back. (Femoral pulses can appear in the presence of coarctation of the aorta, but they are usually weaker and delayed in relation to the brachials, and the murmur may be louder anteriorly than posteriorly.)

Can you explain the lack of blood pressure gradient with no femoral pulses?

In coarctation, there must be an adequate blood pressure in the lower part of the body to perfuse the kidneys. If the coarctation is very severe, the blood pressure will essentially come from collaterals. However, the pulse pressure will be *very* narrow; in order to feel a pulse, a good pulse pressure must be present. Above the coarctation, meanwhile, if there is severe congestive heart failure, the cardiac output may be very low and there may be insufficient ejectile force to create a high blood pressure. Thus, there may be little or no systolic gradient across a severe coarctation of the aorta in the presence of marked congestive heart failure.

Can you explain the cyanosis?

The cyanosis is probably due to pulmonary venous congestion as part of left heart failure.

Can the cyanosis be treated medically?

The response to medical treatment of the congestive heart failure is excellent if the coarctation is isolated (i.e., without associated left-to-right shunt). The patient will become acyanotic because the pulmonary venous saturation will normalize.

After 12 hours of acute digitalization, the pulses were strong in each brachial with flush pressures of 120 mm. Hg, while the femorals remained absent with flush pressure of 60 mm. Hg. The murmur in the back was louder (Grade III) and cyanosis was no longer seen. The heart was not hyperdynamic. Is cardiac catheterization necessary?

The diagnosis is now quite evident for simple coarctation of the aorta. There is much difference of opinion. The fact that the baby went into heart failure after the first week, responded so readily, and had such classic findings, suggests that the coarctation is likely to be isolated. However, there are some cardiologists who, knowing the poor prognosis when there is an additional lesion, insist on a cardiac catheterization to be absolutely certain. Had the onset of cardiac failure been within the first two weeks, we too would have performed the procedure.

What is the prognosis with medical therapy?

If an isolated coarctation is present, the prognosis with medical therapy is excellent. At our institution, we have never had a medical death.

Why does the patient have pure right ventricular hypertrophy?

In utero, if the coarctation is post-ductal, the right ventricle sends blood through the patent ductus, then through the coarctation to the descending aorta. Thus, the right ventricle in utero must have an additional work load.

Case Nine

A four-day-old, full-term baby boy is transferred to the hospital from the nursery because of poor feeding for two days and recent respiratory difficulties. The child is dusky, sweating profusely, and has very poor pulses. The liver is very large. The X-ray shows a large heart with pulmonary venous congestion. The electrocardiogram demonstrates no P waves and a ventricular rate of 300 beats per minute (Figure 13–12). The diagnosis of supraventricular tachycardia was made.

Should a cardiology consultant be called in immediately?

The knowledge necessary to diagnose and treat the so-called paroxysmal atrial tachycardia (PAT) of infancy cannot be left only to the cardiac consultant. There is not likely to be time for such luxury. When a child is admitted in congestive heart failure, it usually indicates that the supraventricular tachycardia has been constant for at least 48 hours. Death may be imminent.

Blood tests were drawn. Which tests would you perform and why?

The blood tests were drawn from the same vein to be used for intravenous digoxin. Whenever treating congestive heart failure, it is important to know the serum Na, K, and Cl concentrations. Of greater acute importance, however, are the pH, $PaCO_2$ and HCO_3. The child may be quite acidotic. Furthermore,

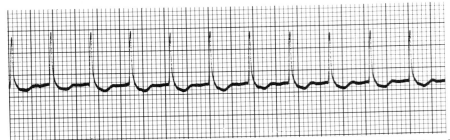

Figure 13-12 Electrocardiogram illustrating paroxysmal atrial tachycardia. Lead II Standard electrocardiogram at speed 50. Heart rate = 300 beats per minute. No P waves seen.

if the pO_2 is low secondary to pulmonary venous congestion, the low PaO_2 and pH may significantly impede successful therapy. (Particularly in the newborn period, they cause an increase in the pulmonary vascular resistance and depress myocardial function.) Despite the congestive heart failure, it is good to give sodium bicarbonate as well as oxygen.

The intern wished to start intramuscular digoxin immediately. Do you approve of this? If not, what would you do?

There is dispute in this area. However, intramuscular digoxin may be dangerous in this baby. Perfusion is poor, so that many hours after the dose digoxin may still be entering the bloodstream. Thus, it may be difficult to judge how much medication to give in succeeding doses. With intravenous digoxin, there is exact control as well as reliably fast action. Action begins in ten minutes (only five minutes later than with Cedilanid). Maximal action is in one hour. Usually one-half the calculated digitalizing dose is given immediately, with the next one-quarter dose one hour later. If the rhythm has still not converted, the final one-quarter dose may be given in another hour. Thus, digitalization can be given safely within two hours if necessary. Intravenous digoxin has another pharmacologic action that is not usually appreciated; it acutely increases systemic arteriolar resistance. Thus, there will be a *moderator* reflex and parasympathetic stimulation of the heart. The latter aids in converting the supraventricular tachycardia.

Digoxin by mouth is not reliable in babies. It does not matter if a little of the maintenance dose dribbles out of the mouth occasionally, but it does matter if much of the digitalizing dose to the sick infant does not get to the stomach. Furthermore, it takes six hours for maximal action even in the healthy child. Intramuscular digoxin may take almost as long as the per os route for maximal action.

It is difficult to give the exact dosage of digoxin because the data are being re-evaluated. The recommended digitalizing dose is at the per os level of 0.08 mg. per Kg. at one month of age, which gradually decreases to 0.04 mg. per Kg. at two years of age. Any parenteral dosage should be one-fourth less, because by mouth only 75 per cent is absorbed. In the newborn period, because some children may be very sensitive, we round off the digitalizing dose at a per os level of 0.05 mg. per Kg., gradually increasing the dose to 0.08 mg. per Kg. at one month. The maintenance dosage is then rounded off at one-quarter to one-third of the digitalizing dose. From then on it is a titration.

Are there other pharmacologic and/or manipulative avenues?

There are other avenues, but carotid pressure and/or eye-ball massage are not included. They do not work and are cruel. A better method of obtaining vagal action is to give Prostigmine after the patient has been fully digitalized. In the newborn, 0.05 mg. subcutaneously is recommended.

If the baby is hypotensive, a sympathomimetic agent should be used. Isoproterenol, epinephrine and levarterenol are contraindicated because of the high risk of ventricular fibrillation. *Methoxamine* (which causes no cardiac stimulation) is preferable; phenylephrine and metaraminol (which have very little cardiac action) are also useful if methoxamine is not available. However, the former drugs are riskier because of their cardiac action. Even if the patient is not hypotensive, and digitalization has been completed without success, methoxamine has been almost always successful in converting the babies to sinus rhythm, Methoxamine is made up as 35 mg. in 250 ml. of five per cent glucose, phenylephrine as 10 mg. in 100 ml., and metaraminol as 35 mg. in 100 ml. Each is dripped in constantly as a titration.

The use of other drugs, such as quinidine, Pronestyl, and/or propranolol, is rarely necessary during the acute period. However, occasionally a baby will go in and out of the arrhythmia for many months. In such cases, another maintenance medication, especially quinidine, has been found to be useful in control.

Is there an alternative treatment besides rapid digitalization?

The alternative treatment is that of direct current countershock (cardioversion). There are some who prefer to use this method as the one of choice, digitalizing the patient only after conversion. We prefer digitalization plus the other adjuncts as described because they are usually effective, but we cannot quarrel with those who utilize countershock. If the latter is used, however, the patient should not be acidotic nor have had too much digitalis. Furthermore, it is imperative not to use a defibrillator that cannot be synchronized to shock on the QRS, for there is a risk of ventricular fibrillation if not used properly.

What chance is there that there is something structurally wrong with the heart?

The vast majority of the children with supraventricular tachycardia or PAT have nothing structurally wrong with the heart. One rule of thumb is to predict that when the baby is a boy, there will almost invariably be nothing wrong with the heart; however, when the baby is a girl, there is a greater chance of a structural abnormality.

Is the patient likely to be prone to supraventricular arrhythmias in the future?

In the few weeks after the first episode of paroxysmal atrial tachycardia (PAT), the rhythm may intermittently revert to the abnormal in many children. In the majority of children on digoxin throughout the first year, another episode never occurs. After one year of age, when digoxin is discontinued, repeat episodes of PAT are rare. It is of great interest that an occasional boy or girl will be seen to have the Wolff-Parkinson-White syndrome. We have usually expected that the prognosis here was not as good, but have been pleased to find that the W-P-W syndrome, more often than not, also disappears.

REFERENCES

I. General Newborn Physiology and Pathophysiology

1. Adams, F., and Lind, J.: Physiologic studies on the cardiovascular status of normal newborn infants: With special reference to the ductus arteriosus. Pediatrics 19:431, 1957.
2. Blount, S., Jr., and Vogel, J.: Altitude and the pulmonary circulation. In Dock, W., and Snapper, I., Eds.: Advances in Internal Medicine. Chicago, Yearbook Medical Publishers, 1967, Vol. 13.
3. Cook, C., Drinker, P., Jacobson, H., et al.: Control of pulmonary blood flow in the fetal and newly born lamb. J Physiol 169:10, 1963.
4. Dawes, G.: Physiological changes in the circulation after birth. In Fishman, A., and Richards, D., Eds.: Circulation of the Blood: Men and Ideas. New York, Oxford University Press, 1964.
5. Dawes, G., Mott, J., Widdicombe, J., et al.: Changes in lungs of newborn lamb. J Physiol 121:141, 1953.
6. Emmanouilides, G., Moss, A., Duffie, E., Jr., et al.: Pulmonary arterial pressure changes in human newborn infants from birth to 3 days of age. J Pediat 65:327, 1964.
7. Hoffman, J., and Rudolph, A.: Natural history of ventricular septal defects in infancy. Amer J Cardiol 16:634, 1965.
8. Penaloza, D., Sime, F., Banchero, N., et al.: Pulmonary hypertension in healthy man born and living at high altitudes. Med Thoracic 19:449, 1962.
9. Rowe, R., and James, L.: Normal pulmonary arterial pressure during the first year of life. J Pediat 51:1, 1957.
10. Rudolph, A.: The changes in the circulation after birth: The importance in congenital heart disease. Circulation 41:343, 1970.
11. Rudolph, A., and Auld, P.: Physical factors affecting normal and serotonin-constructed pulmonary vessels. Amer J Physiol 198:846, 1960.
12. Rudolph, A., and Nadas, A.: Pulmonary circulation and congenital heart disease: Considerations of the role of the pulmonary circulation in certain systemic-pulmonary communications. New Eng J Med 267:968, 1962.
13. Rudolph, A., Auld, P., Golinka, R., et al.: Pulmonary vascular adjustments in the neonatal period. Pediatrics 28:28, 1961.
14. Wagenvoort, C., Newfeld, H., and Edwards, J.: Structure of the pulmonary arterial tree in fetal and early postnatal life. Lab Invest 10:751, 1961.

II. General-Disease States in the Newborn

1. Goodman, N., Scarpelli, E., and Rudolph, A.: Metabolic acidosis in children with severe cyanotic congenital heart disease. Circulation 31:251, 1963.

2. Lambert, E., Canent, R., and Hohn, A.: Congenital cardiac defects in the newborn: A review of conditions causing death or severe distress in the first month of life. Pediatrics 37:343, 1966.
3. Lambert, E., Tinglestad, J., and Hohn, A.: Diagnosis and management of congenital heart disease in the first week of life. Pediat Clin N Amer 13:943, 1966.
4. Liebman, J., and Nadas, A.: Heart disease in the newborn. Pediat Clin N Amer 5:1087, 1958.
5. Lindesmith, G., Galleher, M., Durnin, R., et al.: Cardiac surgery in the first month of life. Amer Thor Surg 2:250, 1966.
6. Rashkind, W.: Atrial septostomy in congenital heart disease. In Schulman, I., Ed.: Advances in Pediatrics. Chicago, Yearbook Medical Publishers, 1958, Vol. 10.
7. Rowe, R.: Severe congenital heart disease in the newborn infant: Diagnosis and management. Pediat Clin N Amer 17:967, 1970.
8. Rowe, R., and Mehrizi, A.: The Neonate with Congenital Heart Disease. Major Problems in Clinical Pediatrics. Philadelphia, W. B. Saunders Co., 1968, Vol. 5.
9. Talner, N., and Ordway, N.: Acid-base balance in the newborn infant with congestive heart failure. Pediat Clin N Amer 13:983, 1966.

III. Atrial Septal Defect

1. Wagenvoort, C., Newfeld, H., Dushane, J., et al.: The pulmonary arterial tree in atrial septal defect: A quantitative study of anatomic features in fetuses, infants, and children. Circulation 23:733, 1961.
2. Weidman, W., Swan, H., Dushane, J., et al.: A hemodynamic study of atrial septal defect and associated anomalies involving the atrial septum. J Lab Clin Med 50:165, 1957.

IV. Ventricular Septal Defect

1. Hoffman, J., and Rudolph, A.: Natural history of ventricular septal defects in infancy. Amer J Cardiol 16:634, 1965.
2. Wagenvoort, C., Newfeld, H., Dushane, J., et al.: The pulmonary arterial tree in ventricular septal defect: A quantitative study of anatomic features in fetuses, infants and children. Circulation 23:740, 1961.

V. Patent Ductus Arteriosus

1. Burnard, E.: A murmur from the ductus arteriosus in the newborn baby. Brit Med J 1:806, 1958.
2. Danilowicz, D., Rudolph, A., and Hoffman, J.: Delayed closure of the ductus arteriosus in premature infants. Pediatrics 37:74, 1966.
3. Neill, C., and Mounsey, P.: Auscultation in patent ductus: With a description of two fistulae simulating patent ductus. Brit Heart J 20:61, 1958.
4. Siassi, B., Emmanouilides, G., Cleveland, R., et al.: Patent ductus arteriosus complicating prolonged assisted ventilation in respiratory distress syndrome. J Pediat 74:11, 1969.

VI. Hypoplastic Left Ventricle Syndrome

1. Noonan, J., and Nadas, A.: The hypoplastic left ventricle syndrome: An analysis of 101 cases. Pediat Clin N Amer 5:1029, 1958.
2. Schiebler, G. L., Adams, P., Jr., Anderson, R. C., et al.: Clinical study of twenty-three cases of Ebstein's anomaly of the tricuspid valve. Circulation 19:165, 1959.
3. Strong, W., Liebman, J., and Perrin, E.: Hypoplastic left ventricle syndrome: Electrocardiographic evidence of left ventricular hypertrophy. Amer J Dis Child 120:511, 1970.

VII. Coarctation of the Aorta

1. Lang, H., Jr., and Nadas, A.: Coarctation of the aorta with congestive heart failure in infancy. Pediatrics 17:45, 1956.
2. Sinha, S., Kardatzka, M., Cole, R., et al.: Coarctation of the aorta in infancy. Circulation 40:385, 1969.

VIII. Aortic Stenosis

1. Hastreiter, A., Oshima, M., Miller, R., et al.: Congenital aortic stenosis syndrome in infancy. Circulation 28:1084, 1963.
2. Moller, J., Nakib, A., Eliot, R., et al.: Symptomatic congenital aortic stenosis in the first year of life. J Pediat 69:728, 1968.

IX. Hypoplastic Right Ventricle Syndrome

1. Cole, R., Muster, A., Lev, M., et al.: Pulmonary atresia with intact ventricular septum. Amer J Cardiol 21:23, 1968.
2. Luckstead, E., Mattioli, L., Crosby, I., et al.: Two-stage palliative surgical approach for pulmonary atresia with intact ventricular septum (type I). Amer J Cardiol 29:490, 1972.
3. Subramanian, S., Carr, I., Waterston, D., et al.: Palliative surgery in tricuspid atresia: Forty-two cases. Circulation 32:977, 1965.

X. Transposition of the Great Arteries

1. Liebman, J., Cullum, L., and Belloc, N.: The natural history of transposition of the great arteries. Circulation 40:237, 1969.
2. Noonan, J., Nadas, A., Rudolph, A., et al.: Transposition of the great arteries: A correlation of clinical, physiologic and autopsy data. New Eng J Med 263:592, 1960.
3. Rashkind, W., and Miller, W.: Creation of an atrial septal defect without thoracotomy: A palliative approach to complete transposition of the great arteries. JAMA 196:991, 1966.

XI. Total Anomalous Pulmonary Venous Return

1. Gathman, G., and Nadas, A.: Total anomalous pulmonary venous connection: Clinical and physiologic observations of 75 pediatric patients. Circulation 42:143, 1970.
2. Gersony, W., Bowman, F., Jr., Steeg, C., et al.: Man-

agement of total anomalous pulmonary venous drainage in early infancy. Circulation *43*: Suppl I 19, 1971.

XII. Ebstein's Anomaly

1. Kumar, A., Fyler, D., Miettinen, O., et al.: Ebstein's anomaly: Clinical profile and natural history. Amer J Cardiol *28*:84, 1971.
2. Newfeld, E., Cole, R., and Paul, M.: Ebstein's malformation of the tricuspid valve in the neonate: Functional and anatomic pulmonary outflow tract obstruction. Amer J Cardiol *19*:727, 1967.

XIII. Pulmonary Stenosis

1. Luke, M.: Valvular pulmonic stenosis in infancy. J Pediat *68*:90, 1966.

XIV. Truncus Arteriosus

1. Lee, M., Bellon, E., Liebman, J., et al.: Truncal valve stenosis. Amer Heart J *85*:397, 1973.
2. Taussig, H.: Clinical and pathologic findings in cases of truncus arteriosus in infancy. Amer J Med *2*:26, 1947.

Chapter 14

THE KIDNEY

by
WARREN E. GRUPE, M.D.

"The kidneys are commonly described as excretory organs, but the assignment of such a limited role scarcely does them justice."

R. F. PITTS, *Physiology of the Kidney and Body Fluids.* (Preface to the First Edition.)

Whether or not the fetal kidney contributes any useful function prior to delivery is undetermined. Although fetal urine contributes to the formation of amniotic fluid, and renal disease existing prenatally may influence development, the fetus with complete renal agenesis is metabolically not markedly altered, probably because the placenta assumes the regulatory functions in utero. All of this changes drastically postnatally and the rapid onset of renal function, even in the premature, shows the functional potential of the immature kidney. The immature kidney, although capable of adjusting to normal variations, is especially vulnerable to the stresses imposed by disease, injudicious management, unrealistic expectations, or unreasonable demands. This chapter will attempt to review those areas of physiology and pathology of particular interest to those caring for the neonate.

BASIC CONSIDERATIONS

DEVELOPMENTAL ANATOMY[5, 7, 8, 13, 17]

Developmental anomalies of the genitourinary tract account for 3.5 to 10 per cent of hospital admissions. The explanation for many lies in anomalies of embryonic development, for which the reader is referred to standard texts.

Defects during the time nephrons are forming have direct expression as developmental anomalies. For example, agenesis can result from any one of several developmental arrests. Absence of ureteric bud development leads to an absence of both kidney and ureter. If the ureteric duct fails to make contact with the metanephric blastema, a short, blind ureter with a normal bladder insertion results. If the ureteric bud enters the mesonephric tissue but there is a failure of induction and/or differentiation, the result is a nubbin of "aplastic," nonfunctioning tissue at the end of an otherwise normal ureter.

DEVELOPMENTAL PHYSIOLOGY[1, 6, 18]

Renal blood flow, glomerular filtration rate, and tubular function do exist, but at inadequately low levels in the fetus. Urine is produced from about the 12th gestational week through functioning but immature and developing nephrons. The loop of Henle functions by the 14th week, leading to a decrease in urine production despite a progressive increase in glomerular filtration rate. Separation

256

from the placenta, however, suddenly places increased demands on these essentially untried kidneys. A marked improvement occurs in these functions within a few days, followed by a slower, progressive rise to essentially adult levels by the end of the first year. Although several factors seem to play a role, a change in renal vascular resistance seems to be the effective mediator of this improvement. This change appears to take place at the level of the afferent arteriole, where the obstructing cells of the fetal juxtaglomerular apparatus disappear after birth. Also, in renal vessels, as in pulmonary vessels, there is a gradual change in the wall-to-lumen ratio in favor of progressive "dilatation," reducing resistance. Since cardiac output and blood pressure increase concomitantly with the decrease in vascular resistance, the hydrostatic pressure available for filtration increases approximately 100 per cent.

Even with this prompt response to the demands of independent existence, *glomerular filtration rate* in the newborn infant is still well below that of adults when corrected for body weight, body surface area, or kidney weight. The explanations for this are insufficient to account for the rates observed.

Even though the glomerulus is not functioning at a mature level, there is both anatomic and functional data demonstrating a glomerular-tubular imbalance with glomerular predominance; the *tubule* is more functionally immature than its size would indicate, and the persistently low glomerular filtration rate per nephron is still excessive relative to the tubular functional capacity. Functionally, evidence of tubular immaturity is indicated by the lower renal threshold for bicarbonate in the premature and full-term infant, the low maximal rate of reabsorption of glucose, the limited response to a saline load, and the decreased rate of sodium transport. It has also been shown that infants excrete a higher percentage of their filtered amino acids than do adults, and that the rate of tubular reabsorption of phosphate is low. These findings make the neonatal kidney very similar to the older, failing, diseased kidney, where an increased osmolar load requires a high filtration rate per nephron resulting in a glomerular tubular imbalance with glomerular preponderance.

The relative immaturity of the neonatal nephron quantitatively limits its response to changing loads which is amplified by the limited ability of the tubule to handle even the somewhat reduced load presented to it by the glomerulus. An example is the infant's limited capacity to tolerate abrupt changes in *sodium*. Although the infant is limited in his response to either an increase or decrease in sodium intake, his ability to handle excess is particularly limited. This quantitative response, though limited, appears operative over a reasonably broad range; infants ordinarily muster enough to excrete the sodium in proprietory formulas that approaches three times the load of human milk. Challenged by the present-day practices of early feeding of solids, they can defend against a load ten times that of human milk. However, balance is achieved only after significant expansion of extracellular fluid volume, which is 45 per cent of body weight as compared to only 20 per cent in the adult. This suggests that the immature control system responds only to large changes in volume. The neonate has a reduced operating reserve with which to meet stresses in excess of normal, and the "safety zone" is further reduced by both acute and chronic changes in exogenous sodium load.

Once stimulated, the direction and rate of the qualitative response is normal. It is the reduced quantitative response that renders the infant more vulnerable to a sodium load, much like that seen in older patients with renal insufficiency.

Conversely, the immature nephron also has limits producing urine low in sodium when faced with sodium deprivation.

Functional limits also render the immature infant less capable of excreting water loads, or of concentrating the urine to conserve *water*. As with sodium, there appears to be incomplete development of the control mechanism, since a young animal ceases to excrete a water load before it has all been eliminated. The immaturity of control as well as the altered absolute rate of water excretion renders the infant more vulnerable to water overload. Faced with water deprivation, the maximum urine osmolality reached by the newborn is around 700 mOsm. per liter. The major limitation here seems to reside in the smaller number of osmoles (particularly urea) excreted in the urine, reflecting the powerful anabolic state that the demands of growth create. Altering the rate of urea excretion by feeding urea or high-protein diets to newborns increases their ability to concentrate the urine. This is not without some risk, since high-protein diets are in some way irritating to the immature kidney, producing cylindruria.

The influence of renal immaturity on the

reabsorption of bicarbonate or the excretion of hydrogen ion has also been noted. Infants in general maintain a normal blood pH, a lower concentration of plasma bicarbonate, and have reduced capacity to excrete a strongly acidic urine. Although several factors play a role, the lower renal threshold for bicarbonate that has been demonstrated in young infants appears important: the bicarbonate reabsorptive tubular maximum is set at a lower threshold than in the older child and adult. Another factor involved is the smaller amount of phosphate in the urine, limiting the receptor buffer available for the manufacture of titratable acid. When they are given additional phosphate, the excretion of titratable acid increases. During the first weeks of life, infants also excrete less ammonium in their urine in response to an ammonium chloride load than do older children. When corrected for glomerular filtration rate, however, these differences become less apparent. Under usual circumstances, the lower blood bicarbonate and pH are not as much dependent on the limitations of hydrogen ion excretion as on the limited ability to reabsorb bicarbonate. There is some question again of the infantile control mechanisms, since a larger stimulus appears to be required by the neonate in order to promote hydrogen ion excretion in any form. Although the qualitative response is prompt and in the proper direction, the quantitative ability to excrete acid is limited. Whereas older infants can double or triple hydrogen ion excretion during acidosis, the neonate is normally functioning at or near his maximum, and only a modest response can be expected.

In summary, the immature kidney has the capability to alter appropriately under stress. The control mechanisms for these homeostatic operations do exist and respond qualitatively, but are sluggish and require greater stimuli to initiate a response that is quantitatively limited with incomplete end-points. A decreased glomerular filtration rate quantitatively limits the neonate's ability to respond to changes in load of a variety of substances. Glomerular-tubular imbalance with a glomerular preponderance, confirmed both anatomically and functionally, defines a tubular function at an even more reduced level. This further limits the ability of the immature kidney to handle even the reduced load presented by the glomerulus. This makes it more difficult for the infant to conserve glucose, phosphates, bicarbonate, and amino acids, and makes the infant less able to quantitatively handle hydrogen ion.

In other ways, tubular development limits the immature kidney's ability to excrete certain substances with ease. The ability to completely excrete a salt or water load is quantitatively limited not only by the decreased glomerular filtration rate but also by the function of the more mature and more developed juxtamedullary nephrons, which are designed to withstand salt and water deprivation and hinder excretion of a load.

The process of growth, with its strong anabolic drive, assists the kidney by reducing the excretory load of sodium, water, phosphorus, hydrogen, and nitrogen. By the same token, however, the limited ability of the same kidney to concentrate urine is in part due to the small amount of urea available for excretion. It is worthwhile remembering that the anabolic state reverses promptly when growth is altered by acute illness, thereby increasing the demands to excrete at a time when the kidney is possibly less able to quantitatively respond. The neonatal kidneys, often functioning at or near maximum capacity, are barely adequate for health, with very limited reserve to handle the increased demands of stress.

> This depends on your point of view, for the so-called immature kidney is much better adapted to promote growth.
>
> G. ODELL

Renal immaturity also limits the newborn's ability to excrete drugs. For example, the renal clearance of penicillin in the newborn is about one-fifth that of the adult. Barbiturates which are eliminated by the kidney, such as phenobarbital, must be used judiciously.

PRACTICAL CONSIDERATIONS[2, 3, 4, 9-12, 14-16]

THE PHYSICAL EXAMINATION

Inspection and palpation of the abdomen of the newborn is more easily accomplished during the first 24 hours of life, since muscle tone is minimal. Normally, the lower pole of both kidneys can be palpated. The bladder is also normally percussed or palpated a few centimeters above the symphysis. It is often difficult to identify the newborn bladder because of its very thin wall, unless percussion is used. Persistent distention of the bladder may be due to congenital urinary tract obstructions. *The vast majority of all palpable abdominal masses in the newborn are renal in origin.*

Congenital absence of the abdominal musculature (prune-belly syndrome) can be diagnosed at birth. The characteristic appearance is a wrinkling and atonicity of the abdominal wall (hence the name prune-belly), with the abdomen usually bulged and the flanks flaccid and limp. This may be associated with a variety of underlying genitourinary defects, including hydroureter, hydronephrosis, megacystis, polycystic kidneys, and cystic urachus, and may be associated with imperforate anus and arthrogryposis.

Although the appearance of the umbilical cord at birth is often deceiving, remnants of the urachus in the cord should be determined. Any discharge from an otherwise normal-appearing cord should be suspect of a patent urachus, particularly a moist cord that does not appear to be separating. The fluid discharge from such a cord may be present at birth, appear within the first few days, or be delayed several weeks. Examination of the fluid shows all the characteristics of urine, particularly an elevated specific gravity. Radiopaque dye injected into an urachus will outline the urachal tract and enter the bladder. Occasionally, a cystogram will demonstrate the tract along the anterior abdominal wall. Surgical excision provides the most successful therapy.

Ascites in the newborn is associated with urinary tract obstruction in a high percentage of cases. Obstruction is usually confined to the lower urinary tract and is often a posterior urethral obstruction. The ascites is usually due to rupture in the collecting system. Hydrometrocolpos and megacystis can be easily confused with ascites in the neonatal period. The differential diagnosis of ascites in the neonatal period includes hemolytic disease of the newborn, peritonitis, severe congestive heart failure, thoracic duct obstruction, hepatoportal venous obstruction, and anomalies of the urinary tract. Infants with ascites may present with severe abdominal distention, producing respiratory distress which can be an immediate threat to life. Severe abdominal distention that may mime ascites includes: meconium peritonitis, intestinal obstruction, intra-abdominal tumors, and ileus. Edema of the abdominal wall is often present with fluid in the peritoneal cavity. Ascites may also appear within a few

days of birth in congenital nephrotic syndrome. Detailed investigation is important in the presence of ascites, including complete evaluation of the urinary tract.

The evaluation of neonatal ascites includes aspiration and immediate measurement for urea, protein, and cell analysis, as well as appropriate blood chemistry. A high protein would indicate chylous ascites. If the infant has not been fed, one would not expect lipemia. Peritonitis would include pleocytosis of the fluid. If it were urine from an obstructed urinary tract, it would have a high urea content, and the infant would show evidences of azotemia and acidosis. If blood were contained in the fluid, the hemoglobin would be immediately apparent.

G. ODELL

The major concern is the detection of congenital anomalies, particularly those which may obstruct urine outflow. In the male, identifying the urethral meatus is of importance, as meatal stenosis may be associated with hydronephrosis and hydroureter. If the meatus can be visualized, phimosis does not exist. An opening on the ventral surface of the penis denotes hypospadias, while an opening on the dorsal surface is epispadias. Both can be associated with abnormalities of the upper urinary tract. It should be determined whether the testes are at the external inguinal ring or in the scrotum. Hypospadias and cryptorchidism, either alone or together, may be an expression of intersexuality as well as indicative of other major genitourinary malformations. An infant with cryptorchidism, ambiguous genitalia, or hypospadias should be investigated with chromosome karotype, buccal smear, intravenous pyelogram, and estimations of urinary 17-ketosteroids and 17-hydroxycorticosteroids. Intersexuality tends to occur in those infants with the more severe degrees of hypospadias. First degree hypospadias, where the meatus is at the base of the glans, is much less likely to have associated abnormalities. In hypospadias, the remnant hood of foreskin should not be removed, since it can be useful in later surgical procedures.

Abnormalities of the female external genitalia should also be sought. Hydrometrocolpos, detected as a bulge of the perineum through which a bluish discoloration can be seen, occurs in the absence of the usual small openings in the hymen. This can be associated with a lower abdominal cystic mass, the distended uterus, which can easily be confused with a distended bladder. The presence of a urogenital sinus should raise questions of

intersexuality. X-ray visualization with radiopaque dye in the sinus, as well as urethros-
copy, may help distinguish the origins of a
single perineal opening and the nature of the
internal organs.

A composite of clinical characteristics
that have come to be associated with a variety
of severe, irreversible abnormalities of the
kidney were recognized by Potter in association with bilateral renal agenesis. These
anomalies which include dysplasia, hypoplasia, and aplasia, are incompatible with
life. Recognition of these characteristics at
birth discourages the multitude of surgical
and investigative procedures that may ensue.
The appearance, usually in a male, is of widely
spaced eyes flanking a depressed nasal bridge
and the troussé nose with a very prominent
fold arising from the epicanthus and progressing interiorly then laterally beneath the
eyes. The chin is receded and the face is prematurely senile in appearance. The ears are
posteriorly rotated, asymmetrical, floppy,
and low-set. Oligohydramnios is often present by history and the placenta is abnormal.
Associated abnormalities include imperforate anus, hydrocephalus, meningomyelocele,
skeletal anomalies, abnormalities of the lower
extremities, and hypoplasia of the lungs. The
infants fail to pass urine. Not all die in uremia,
as might be expected; many die with cyanosis
and dyspnea or pneumothorax resulting from
the lung abnormality before uremia can inter-
cede.

URINALYSIS

Evaluation of the urine must be considered part of the physical examination of a
child who is suspected of urinary tract abnormality. It is also a useful tool in the evaluation of the general status of the infant. A newborn will usually urinate soon after birth,
which is often missed in the delivery room.
However, a delay in urination for as long as 48
hours should not be a cause for immediate
concern in the absence of palpable bladder,
and manipulative or radiographic procedures
are not necessary. Under normal circumstances, little urine is produced during the first
few days of life, with as little as 30 to 60 cc.
during the first 48 hours considered normal.
Urine output, however, may be diminished in
infants with severe disease, such as cardiac
failure, dehydration, respiratory distress syndrome, or asphyxia, and might be expected to
increase coincident with clinical improvement. The normal newborn urine is usually

quite pale in color, almost clear. However,
clouds of urates may be present. Increasing
amounts of conjugated bilirubin can produce a
yellow-brown to deep olive-green color.
Porphyrins, drugs, such as Pyridium, and
urate crystals may stain the diaper pink and
be confused with bleeding. A benzidine test
on the diaper can distinguish between hemoglobin and other red hues. Urine which contains old blood, hemosiderin, or myoglobin
is characteristically brown.

Specific gravity of neonatal urine is often
persistently low (less than 1.004), but may be
factitiously elevated by high molecular weight
solutes, such as radiographic dye, sugars, or
protein. Osmolarity is a more representative
measure of the kidney's concentrating abili-
ties. In the absence of extraneous solute, however, there is ordinarily a good correlation
between specific gravity and osmolarity. Specific gravity can be measured on as little as
two drops of urine, using the small clinical
refractometers now available. Maximum concentrating ability of the premature is approximately 750 mOsm. (specific gravity 1.018).
Occasionally a full-term infant may reach as
high as 1000 mOsm. (specific gravity 1.025).
The inability of the infant to concentrate the
urine any farther is because the newborn normally excretes such a small osmolar load. This
relatively limited concentrating capacity influences the infant's ability to tolerate restricted intake or excessive insensible fluid
losses. Under these circumstances, urinary
volume then becomes a more useful parameter
of hydration than specific gravity. In older
children, the specific gravity increases markedly with water deprivation, while in young
infants it may not.

Persistent proteinuria must be considered
pathologic until proven otherwise. Proteinuria
may be seen with asphyxia, cardiac failure,
massive doses of penicillin, dehydration, fever,
or in the presence of X-ray contrast media.
Massive proteinuria usually indicates a glomerular injury. The so-called physiologic proteinuria of the newborn does not exist. Highly
alkaline urine may cause a false positive test
for protein when the albustix are used, and a
false negative for protein with sulfosalicylic
acid or heat and acetic acid. Persistent massive proteinuria in a newborn should alert one
to consider congenital nephrotic syndrome.

Urinary Sediment

Cells. Cells in the urine can come from
anywhere in the genitourinary tract; their
origin may be difficult to determine. Specimens

collected in the usual adhesive bag, particularly from females, often have white cell contamination from the perineum or vagina. Very often, when female infants void while supine, the urine contains vaginal washings.

Hematuria. Hematuria (greater than 2 to 3 red cells per centrifuged HPF) may be seen with blood dyscrasia, infections, neoplasia, stones, trauma, congenital malformations, or disseminated intravascular coagulation. The presence of red blood cell casts indicates a glomerular irritation. Hematuria is not frequently seen in the newborn, and its occurrence calls for urgent investigation. Renal vein thrombosis must be considered after traumatic delivery, and is more common in infants of diabetic mothers and in those infants with cyanotic congenital heart disease or marked dehydration.

Editors' Comment: In our nursery, hematuria is most commonly observed in infants who have had neonatal asphyxia.

We have seen occasional microscopic hematuria following the use of kanamycin in newborns. This is often associated with cylindruria. While it has given us some concern, the red cells do tend to disappear despite continuation of the kanamycin therapy, and where indicated we have, therefore, chosen not to discontinue the drug.

L. STERN

Pyuria. Pyuria (greater than 3 to 5 white cells per centrifuged HPF) is most commonly associated with urinary tract infection, but can come from anywhere in the genitourinary tract as a manifestation of irritation. Pyuria can be seen in glomerular injury, tubular acidosis, interstitial nephritis, dehydration, or following instrumentation. White blood cell casts are always an indication of renal irritation.

Casts. Casts are the only definitive evidence of upper renal involvement. Red blood cell casts are most commonly seen in glomerular injury. White blood cell casts, however, may be seen with infection, interstitial injury, or renal inflammation. Epithelial cell casts are seen with tubular or interstitial injury. Broad casts are seen with tubular ectasia and destruction. Granular casts are usually partially decomposed cellular casts. They can be seen, however, in dehydration, interstitial injury, or tubular injury.

Urine Collection

Collection of an adequate, uncontaminated urine specimen is extremely difficult in the neonate. The so-called clean voided specimen obtained by cleaning the perineum and applying a sterile adhesive plastic bag may give erroneous results. The reliability of a catheterized specimen, particularly in a neonate, is no greater than a clean voided specimen, particularly for bacteriologic evaluation. In these circumstances, a suprapubic bladder aspiration may resolve many problems and avoid unnecessary instrumentation and study. It is a rapid procedure, subjects the infant to no more distress than a venipuncture, and greatly reduces the chance of contamination of the urine specimen or of the bladder. It is indicated in any infant who is suspected of having a urinary tract infection, particularly when the results of several clean voided specimens are confusing or conflicting. It may also be considered as the initial means of collecting urine for culture in seriously ill infants, or in infants where delay in the start of antibiotics is considered hazardous because of suspected septicemia. Suprapubic aspiration is also useful as a means of following the success of therapy in infants with urinary tract infection. When the child is on antibiotics, it is hard to determine whether minimal growth in the urine is due to urethral contamination or represents a persistent low grade infection; sterile urine by suprapubic aspiration would indicate successful therapy, while any growth must be interpreted as persistent infection and so treated. Suprapubic bladder aspiration is also useful in the diagnosis or exclusion of infection in the urinary tract in the presence of vulvovaginitis, urethritis, or balanoposthitis, particularly since catheterization from below is contraindicated because of the increased risk of contamination of the bladder. Suprapubic bladder aspiration is the method of choice whenever contamination appears to be unavoidable, as it often is in the newborn, or when standard techniques have given confusing results.

Suprapubic Bladder Aspiration

The procedure we use is as follows: In neonates, the bladder is already an abdominal organ easily palpated or percussed. The infant is placed supine and held in a frog-leg position (see Figure 14–1). We make no attempt to resist outflow by compressing the penis in the male or the urethra via a rectal digit in the female. The lower abdomen is prepared with alcohol sponge or other suitable antiseptic as for a venipuncture. The symphysis pubis is located with the index finger of the free hand.

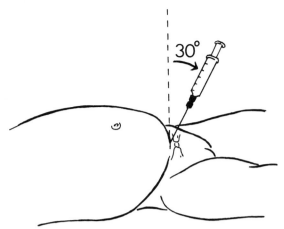

Figure 14–1   Suprapubic bladder aspiration.

We use a 5 to 10 cc. syringe with a #22, 1-inch disposable needle to puncture the abdomen in the mid-line, about 1½ to 2 cm. above the symphysis. In many newborns, a transverse lower abdominal skin crease just above the symphysis provides an excellent landmark. The needle is angled about 30° from the perpendicular, toward the fundus, and advanced into the bladder. Minimal negative pressure will aspirate the required volume of urine and the needle is withdrawn. Pressure until skin bleeding stops is all the dressing required.

X-RAY TESTS

Radiologic evaluation of the genitourinary tract in the newborn can be more difficult than in the older child, but is clearly of value. Given the poor ability of a newborn to concentrate the urine, as well as the generally low glomerular filtration rate, visualization is not always adequate when standard intravenous pyelography is performed. However, pyelography can be successful in any infant who can attain a creatinine urine/plasma ratio in excess of 15. Poor visualization can often be overcome by using 3 cc. per Kg. of 25 per cent hypaque as a single injection or by utilizing the infusion pyelography technique with 6 cc. per Kg. of hypaque. An intravenous urogram and a voiding cystourethrogram is indicated in any infant, boy or girl, with the first documented urinary tract infection. Complete radiologic investigation of the urinary tract is clearly indicated in neonates with abdominal masses, hematuria, absent abdominal musculature, single umbilical artery, and other congenital malformations known to be associated with renal malformations, such as severe hypospadias and epispadias.

EVALUATION OF RENAL FUNCTION

The accurate estimation of the glomerular filtration rate by standard creatinine clearance in neonates and infants is difficult and often virtually impossible, owing largely to incomplete or inaccurate urine collections. When properly done, however, the results are reliable. Recent investigations have shown that a clearance can be calculated from the plasma disappearance curve of a substance handled such as inulin, if the data are calculated according to a multicompartmental analysis. Such a method has been developed, using sodium iothalamate, which correlates well with inulin and creatinine clearances. This method should be considered when inconsistent results are obtained with standard creatinine clearances. Any collection for creatinine clearance in which the infant excretes creatinine at a rate less than 15 mg. per Kg. per 24 hours should be considered erroneous. Clinical methods of evaluation of the various renal functions in infants are listed in order of decreasing accuracy in Table 14–1. Table 14–2 lists normal values for various renal functions in prematures, full-term infants, and infants under two months of age.

CASE PROBLEMS

Case One

G.R., a 3600-gm. male, is transferred to your service at 18 hours of age because of a mass in the left flank. He was born at the termination of a 38-week, normal pregnancy and 12-hour spontaneous labor by a nondifficult breech extraction to a 26-year-old gravida 2 mother. Although there was a small amount of meconium in the amniotic fluid, the child had a prompt, good cry and appeared quite well. Initial examination by the nurse in the delivery room was reported as normal, and the child was transferred to the newborn nursery in good condition. An examination at 12 hours of age by the pediatrician disclosed a large left flank mass, but was otherwise within normal limits.

TABLE 14–1 RENAL FUNCTION TESTS

FUNCTION	USEFUL CLINICAL TESTS
Glomerular filtration rate	Sodium-iothalamate clearance
	Creatinine clearance
	Urea clearance
	Blood creatinine
	Blood urea
Renal plasma flow	Phenolsulfonphthalein excretion
Proximal tubular transport	
Reabsorption	Tubular maxima glucose
Excretion	Tubular maxima para-aminohippurate
	Phenolsulfonphthalein excretion
	Glycosuria
	Aminoaciduria
Distal tubular transport	Concentration and dilution (urine osmolarity)
	Maximal and minimal urine specific gravity

Your examination concurs: the infant has a large, firm, superficial, somewhat lobulated mass filling the left flank, extending from the costal margin almost to the iliac crest. He is pale with a poor suck. Temperature is 37°C, hemoglobin is 16.5 mg. per 100 ml., hematocrit is 43 per cent, WBC is 8500 per mm.³, platelets are normal, and red cell morphology is normal on peripheral blood smear.

What are your diagnostic considerations at this point?

Seventy per cent of all abdominal masses in the newborn are renal in origin; about 50 per cent of all abdominal tumors are renal. Thus, the percentages, as well as the location and feel of the mass, strongly suggest it is kidney. The superficiality of the mass might suggest splenic enlargement, but its extension deep into the flank is more supportive of a renal lesion. The breech delivery, although not difficult, coupled with the mass being easily felt anteriorly, might suggest a retrorenal hematoma, but other causes of renal enlargement (such as hydronephrosis, multiple kidneys, horseshoe kidney, ectopic kidney, renal cyst, renal vein thrombosis, cortical necrosis, or adrenal hemorrhage) should be considered.

TABLE 14–2 AVERAGE RENAL FUNCTION

	TERM		
	Premature	Neonate	Two months
Glomerular filtration rate			
Urea clearance	25	36	32
(cc./min./1.73M²)	(11–45)	(11–52)	(23–44)
Creatinine clearance	28	38	70
(cc./min./1.73M²)	(13–58)	(15–60)	(63–80)
cc./min.	3.5	5	10
(absolute)	(1.2–5.3)	(5–6.5)	(9–12)
Inulin clearance	45	40	70
(cc./min./1.73M²)			
Renal plasma flow			
PAH clearance	150	200	300
(cc./min./1.73M²)			
Tubular reabsorption			
Tm (Glucose)		60	170
(mg./min./1.73M²)			
Tubular excretion		16	50
(mg./min./1.73M²)			
Concentrating capacity			
(mOsm./Kg.)	400–700	600–1100	700–1200
Urine volume			
(cc./day)	15–40	15–60	250–450

Likewise, neoplasia, such as Wilms' neuroblastoma, or adrenal tumors cannot be excluded.

Transillumination should always be performed on large abdominal masses to determine whether they are solid or cystic. Also, a sonogram is most helpful, for it can delineate cysts versus solid masses.

G. ODELL

What is your next move?

With the above in mind, it would be appropriate to evaluate the infant's renal function by BUN, creatinine, electrolytes, and blood gases. Intravenous pyelography might define anatomically the status of both kidneys. Of prime importance, however, would be a careful examination of the urine.

At 22 hours of age, the infant passes the first recorded urine. It is grossly bloody with 1+ protein, no clots, and no casts. The infant has become less active, less responsive, with shallow, rapid respiration, refuses to suck, and has vomited a small amount of yellowish fluid once. Temperature is 35.4°C, electrolytes are normal, BUN 45 mg. per 100 ml., pH is 7.24, and bicarbonate is 15 mEq. per liter.

Does this change your thinking? What course should be followed now?

The infant is now clearly ill and has gross hematuria. The initial nurse's examination now assumes historical importance; the mass not palpable at birth but so easily palpable now would suggest sudden enlargement of one kidney. In general, only renal vein thrombosis or acute adrenal hemorrhage would produce such rapid change and such a degree of clinical illness. The gross hematuria and the size of the mass would suggest renal vein thrombosis as the more likely of the two, as does the azotemia and hypothermia. A coagulation disorder, such as disseminated intravascular coagulation syndrome, might be considered. (Intravenous pyelography and coagulation studies are indicated.)

An IVP shows a normal nephrogram on the right with calyces faintly visualized but normal. The bladder fills with radiopaque dye. Although the mass can be seen, there is no excretion of dye detectible on the left. Coagulation studies were normal.

An IVP in this situation may not even reveal a nephrogram. If renal vein thrombosis is considered, then an inferior vena cavagram should be performed to look for lack of a filling defect in the column at the level of the left renal vein.

G. ODELL

Should surgery be contemplated, or are further studies indicated?

The diagnosis appears quite clear now. The sudden enlargement of one kidney, marked clinical illness, azotemia, gross hematuria, and nonvisualization of the kidney on the involved side are quite characteristic of renal vein thrombosis. The etiology in this case is not really clear; noncomplicated breech delivery has not been implicated in this disorder, although traumatic deliveries have been suspect. Factors associated with renal vein thrombosis have included dehydration, gastroenteritis, maternal diabetes, and septicemia. Although thrombocytopenia has been reported, this has been thought to be the result of the thrombosis rather than part of a disseminated intravascular coagulation syndrome. Normal platelets, normal red cell morphology, normal coagulation studies, and the absence of systemic bleeding would eliminate this consideration in the present case.

Therapy has come under question recently. Formerly it was standard to perform a unilateral nephrectomy as a life-saving surgical maneuver. Some nephrologists have questioned the need of this, since some infants managed medically with anticoagulants have survived and done well. In this infant, left nephrectomy was performed, removing a large, tense, purple kidney. The renal vein was thrombosed.

Case Two

H.Y., a 2680-gm. female, was born to a 29-year-old gravida 7, STS negative, A+ mother, after a 38-week normal pregnancy and a two and one-half hour spontaneous labor with vaginal delivery under spinal anesthesia. She did well until three days of age, when grunting respirations with intermittent cyanosis was noted. The chest is clear on examination; abdominal palpation discloses no organ enlargement. Chest films show no abnormality of the heart or lungs. The morning of the fifth day, periorbital edema is noted, which becomes less marked as the day progresses. A urinalysis shows 3+ protein, 5 to 10 RBC per HPF, 4 to 8 WBC per HPF, and occasional granular casts. Serum electrolytes are normal, pH is 7.38, bicarbonate is 25.6 mEq. per liter, and pCO_2 is 44 mm. Hg.

Are the symptoms and signs compatible with cardiac failure? With respiratory distress syndrome? With renal disease?

The clinical picture is not that of cardiac failure or respiratory distress. There is no cardiomegaly, pulmonary vascular changes by X-ray, murmur, hepatomegaly, or tachypnea. Edema is a late finding in infants with cardiac failure, is characteristically not facial, and is usually worse late in the day. Although grunting and cyanosis could be from respiratory difficulty, the course does not fit respiratory distress syndrome, since it took three days to appear. Cyanosis in RDS accompanies severe dyspnea, retractions, and tachypnea. Edema may accompany RDS or anoxia, but again is not limited to the face or the morning. Other causes of edema in the first few days of life, such as erythroblastosis, maternal toxemia, or excessive exogenous sodium and water loading, do not appear to be operating here either.

Periorbital edema, worse in the morning and less as the day progresses, is characteristic of hypoproteinemia or renal disease. In this instance, proteinuria and cylindruria with this characteristic pattern of edema is quite compatible with a renal lesion, probably glomerular.

How would you proceed at this point?

Investigation of renal function and anatomic status would be in order. Because of the edema, components of the nephrotic syndrome (proteinuria, hypoproteinemia, and hyperlipemia) should be investigated.

The following laboratory results are obtained: BUN = 11.5 mg. per 100 ml., creatinine = 0.6 mg. per 100 ml., and total serum protein = 2.4 gm. per 100 ml. with albumin 27.5 per cent, alpha 2 globulin 39.0 per cent, and gamma globulin 5.5 per cent; cholesterol = 273 mg. per 100 ml., and total lipids = 709 mg. per 100 ml.; Kline is nonreactive; urinary protein = 0.576 gm. per 100 ml. with 0.288 gm. excreted in 24 hours; creatinine clearance is 23 cc. per minute per 1.73 M^2; intravenous pyelogram shows normal anatomic structures; and clean voided urine culture shows 10^3 col. per cc. E. coli and 10^2 col. per cc. diphtheroids.

What are the diagnostic possibilities? What is your diagnosis?

The laboratory data is consistent with some form of nephritis. Acute pyelonephritis is probably unlikely, since the proteinuria is too high, the IVP normal, and the urine culture not definitive. However, 10^3 col. per cc. E. coli on a single culture could be significant in the dilute urine of a newborn, so either a repeat clean voided culture or a suprapubic bladder aspiration would be useful. Acute tubular injury or renal cortical necrosis is not supported by the clinical course or the laboratory findings. A nephrotic syndrome is present. There is hypoalbuminemia with an elevation of alpha 2 globulin; cholesterol and total lipids are elevated for a newborn; and the proteinuria of 0.576 gm. per 100 ml. is likewise quite massive for a newborn. The diagnosis would be congenital nephrosis.

Should a renal biopsy be performed on such a young infant? Would it help, if it could be done?

Congenital nephrotic syndrome is a heterogenous group of diseases from which microcystic disease, membranous glomerulonephritis, and interstitial nephritis have been separated as histologic entities. The syndrome has been reported in association with congenital syphilis, renal vein thrombosis, Nail-Patella syndrome, and cytomegalic inclusion disease. That the spectrum of histologic alterations cannot be defined clinically suggests that renal biopsy can be useful in the diagnosis and management of these children. It can be performed on such young infants either by open surgical biopsy or by percutaneous needle biopsy under fluoroscopic guidance. In this child, needle biopsy showed the changes of microcystic disease, a form of congenital nephrosis that does not respond to any known type of therapy.

Infants with congenital nephrotic syndrome are often born prematurely, with a large, edematous placenta. They will soon develop edema and ascites. They show the usual serum alterations of the nephrotic syndrome, including low albumin and an elevation of alpha 2 globulin. The level of hypercholesterolemia and hyperlipidemia is less than that seen in the older child, but is persistently above normal for newborns. In general, these children fail to do well and do not respond to corticosteroid therapy. The outcome is usually fatal in the first year of life. However, when due to congenital syphilis, congenital nephrotic syndrome can be successfully treated with penicillin.

Case Three

F.D., a 3800-gm. newborn male, has a routine urine obtained at four days of age prior to circumcision. This urine shows 1+ protein, 25 to 30 WBC per HPF, no casts, but many motile bacteria in the spun sediment. Pregnancy, labor, and delivery were uncomplicated. Physical examination is normal. He is vigorous, with a good cry, and is afebrile. Feeding has been no problem, and his weight is only 250 gm. below birth weight.

Does this child have a urinary tract infection?

Certainly pyuria must raise the suspicion of a urinary tract infection, as does the presence of bacteria on smear. Several questions need to be answered first, however. It is not clear how this urine was obtained. Was the prepuce cleaned in any way? Was the foreskin retracted in the cleaning? The problem does not exist here, as it does in a female, of determining if the cells came from vaginal secretions washed out by vaginal reflux in the process of micturition, and one would hope that balanoposthitis has been excluded by examination as a source of "pyuria."

The presence of bacteria in the spun sediment is of little value in determining the presence of bacteria—for this, one must examine the uncentrifuged urine; moreover, it is not of value if the urine has been in the bag at room temperature for any length of time. At best, one can only suspect a urinary tract infection. Other studies are necessary before a diagnosis can be made.

What other studies should be performed?

In this child, the diagnosis has not yet been established. The next study would seem to be a re-examination of the urine with culture included. The outlook for a male infant with a urinary tract infection must be viewed with caution. The chance of developing renal insufficiency in the male is four times that of the female, and obstructive uropathy is three times more common than in the female. In the newborn, hematogenous spread of bacteria is a more common route of colonization of renal parenchyma, suggesting septicemia. Therefore, blood cultures and radiologic evaluation of the urinary tract are important when an infant, particularly a male, has a urinary tract infection.

A second urine is obtained the same day by cleaning the prepuce with pHisoHex and applying a sterile adhesive plastic bag. The specimen is removed from the bag as soon as possible. This urine shows no protein, 2 to 5 WBC per HPF, and no casts. A stained smear of uncentrifuged urine shows no organisms, but the culture shows 10^5 col. per cc. E. coli.

Can we now document the presence of a urinary tract infection?

No. A single culture, even though a pure growth of more than 10^5 col. per cc. of a single organism, is insufficient evidence for urinary tract infection in the newborn. As many as 60 per cent of normal newborns will have greater than 10^5 col. per cc. in a standard clean voided urine, about one-quarter of which will yield a pure growth of one type of organism. In the uncircumcised male, as many as 35 per cent will show "significant growth," even with very careful cleansing. Thus, in the newborn, the usual criteria for infection must be even more stringent than in the older child.

A third urine is obtained the next day by the same clean voided technique. The urinalysis is unchanged, and the culture shows 10^4 col. per cc. E. coli, 10^3 col. per cc. paracolon, and 10^3 col. per cc. Proteus. The infant's clinical state has not changed.

Are you ready to treat this child with antibiotics? What would you use?

Without a reliable diagnosis, it would not seem wise to start therapy. Since the prognosis must be guarded and the urologic evaluation more extensive in a young male, undue concern and unnecessary study might follow definitive therapy for what may prove to be an erroneous diagnosis. If a urinary tract infection were firmly established, the choice of antibiotics should be determined by the sensitivity of the organism. (In a four-day-old, without hyperbilirubinemia or evidence of hemolytic disease of the newborn, even the usual concern over sulfonamides need not apply.)

What do you do now?

The third urine and the second culture are of little help. It is now 48 hours since concern was raised. It is probable that this child does not have a urinary tract infection, but we need to know with certainty. It is in exactly this sort of confusing situation that the suprapubic bladder aspiration of urine has proved so helpful. When performed in this child, a sterile urine was obtained.

In reports now numbering in the thousands, suprapubic bladder aspiration has proved a safe, easy procedure with less complications than catheterization. One can anticipate success in over 90 per cent of attempts, with practice. There are only two contraindications to the procedure: (1) an empty bladder, as evidenced by a wet diaper or a reliable history of having voided within thirty minutes; and (2) dilated loops of bowel, from either obstruction, ileus, or inflammation. The reliability is excellent; any growth can be considered positive. Growth directly from the bladder cannot be confused with urethral or perineal contamination. The technical problems of bladder catheterization in the neonate are real, and the reliability is probably no greater than in the clean voided specimen. Therefore, we prefer the suprapubic aspiration.

The suprapubic circumvents the problem of perineal contamination or the need for repeated, confirmatory cultures and the days of delay that can accrue therefrom. It is especially important in the infant, where suspicion of sepsis is so great that a delay in antibiotic therapy until a "good" or "reliable" culture result is available would be hazardous. Here, a single suprapubic aspirate provides rapid, reliable results before starting therapy. There are very few complications. Transient gross hematuria lasting less than 24 hours (often present on only one void) occurs in about 0.5 per cent. We have had none require transfusion or surgical intervention.

Should urine cultures be part of the nursery routine?

Routine nursery cultures by the usual clean voided technique often create more difficulties than they solve. The incidence of urinary tract infection in the newborn nursery varies between 0.5 and 3 per cent. This certainly needs to be diagnosed, but the difficulty is evident. It is clear that the diagnosis of infection without a suprapubic aspirate is virtually impossible in the usual nursery situation; yet, one cannot justify a suprapubic on 60 per cent of newborns for only a one per cent yield. Therefore, we do not recommend a routine urine culture. When the clinical situation suggests infection in the child, we recommend a single clean voided urine. In any child with greater than 10^3 col. per cc. organism in that specimen, a suprapubic bladder aspiration for culture should be obtained. We do recommend a urine for analysis be routine, particularly in the high-risk nursery.

QUESTIONS

A newborn is noted to have a single umbilical artery at the time the cord is clamped and cut. How serious is this anatomic curiosity? Should further investigation be attempted?

This anomaly occurs in 0.76 per cent of deliveries (collaborative study), of whom 17 per cent had major malformations. Only about half of these will have externally evident malformations. There seems to be a high incidence of associated genitourinary developmental defects, of which 60 per cent will be lower urinary tract and 40 per cent will be associated with renal hypoplasia or agenesis. Thus, an infant with a single umbilical artery and no other external manifestations has a high risk of having a severe internal malformation, especially of the urinary tract. It would seem reasonable, then, to evaluate the genitourinary tract radiologically for structural abnormalities.

At our institution, urine examination is followed weekly, and when the infant is close to a month of age, if no other symptomatology has occurred, radiologic examination is performed by some physicians, while others wait until there are signs of renal disease.

G. ODELL

Developmental anomalies of the genitourinary system are present in about 3 to 10 per cent of hospital admissions. It is interesting how often they are seen in association with other congenital anomalies. These include: (1) absence of abdominal musculature; (2) congenital heart lesions, especially ventricular septal defect; (3) Turner's syndrome; (4) gastrointestinal abnormalities, especially anorectal anomalies; (5) severe hypospadias; and (6) hydrometrocolpos. From these associations, it would appear that the fetus is most susceptible to developing anomalies of the genitourinary tract at about 33 days' gestation.

It would seem appropriate here to include a discussion of renal agenesis (and/or hypoplasia) presenting in the newborn period. Although as originally described by Potter, at least 70 per cent of these infants have pulmonary hypoplasia, it is not generally recognized that the presenting symptomatology for these infants at birth is in fact usually severe respiratory distress due to pneumothoraces which are often bilateral and which have no other explanation. Such an occurrence, together with the characteristic physical appearance of the infant (low-set ears, spade-like hands, and usually underweight for gestational age) should raise a high index of suspicion. In our department, virtually all of the infants who present with *bilateral* pneumothoraces *immediately* at birth have suffered from some variety of severe renal hypoplasia or total agenesis. Moreover, in reviewing our autopsy material on serious renal malformations in the newborn, we have an incidence of approximately one-third in which there has been an associated pneumothorax either suspected clinically or discovered at autopsy. Since not all of these cases are associated with oligohydramnios, the explanation that the pulmonary hypoplasia is due to a lack of amniotic fluid in utero seems to us to be incorrect. A more reasonable suggestion would be the fact that the gene loci for renal and pulmonary malformations may lie sufficiently close together as to be dually involved in many such instances.

L. STERN

How might a BUN of 17 mg. per 100 ml. be compatible with severe renal disease? How might a BUN of 43 mg. per 100 ml. be compatible with normal renal function?

The level of blood urea is the difference between production and excretion. Production is influenced by nitrogen intake, tissue nitrogen catabolized, and the nitrogen incorporated into new tissues (anabolism). Excretion is a function of glomerular filtration rate and tubular reabsorption.

Without any change in renal function, the level may rise with excessive catabolism. It may also rise during periods of decreased renal plasma flow, such as is seen in dehydration, often accompanied by decreased urine flow which allows increased tubular reabsorption of urea (so-called prerenal azotemia). If protein intake is allowed to continue unchanged during these periods, the level of urea will rise still higher.

A markedly decreased protein intake, however, may allow the BUN to be 17 mg. per 100 ml. in face of severe renal disease, merely because the nitrogen load presented to the kidneys does not exceed their limited capacity to excrete, particularly if sufficient calories are available from carbohydrates and fats so that tissue catabolism is reduced to a minimum. With a normal protein intake, the BUN does not rise above normal until the glomerular filtration rate is below 40 per cent of normal. By reducing the protein intake, the BUN may not rise until the glomerular filtration rate is below 20 per cent of normal.

It is for these reasons that most nephrologists have come to rely more on the serum creatinine level as a more sensitive general screening test for general renal function. The serum creatinine concentration can be expected to double for each 50 per cent fall in glomerular filtration rate.

A 2200-gm. male infant was delivered after a 36-week normal pregnancy. The labor was normal until 30 minutes prior to delivery, when fetal heart rate was noted to be 80. At delivery, the cord was tight about the neck. Apgar at one minute = 2; at five minutes = 8. Resuscitation included intermittent positive pressure breathing plus intravenous sodium bicarbonate. Blood gases at 15 minutes: pH = 7.11, PaO_2 = 93 mm. Hg, and $PaCO_2$ = 54 mm. Hg. Examination of the first urine passed, at age 36 hours, shows 1+ protein, positive benzidine, and many granular casts. Is this acute tubular necrosis or glomerulonephritis?

Not necessarily either. Oliguria is quite common in respiratory distress syndrome and perinatal asphyxia. Proteinuria, hematuria, and cylindruria are merely the renal manifestations of the asphyxia. Prerenal azotemia may also be present. In most instances, vigorous attention to ventilation and judicious limitation of salt and water intake is the treatment of choice (follow electrolytes and weight closely). Rarely do these children require peritoneal dialysis or die of renal failure. When anoxia is corrected, urine output increases dramatically and the urine albumin clears rapidly. In some who have been severely asphyxiated, gross hematuria may be present and renal vein thrombosis must be ruled out. An occasional infant with severe anoxia may also demonstrate disseminated intravascular coagulation with renal involvement.

It is important to know where bicarbonate is given. If it is given by arterial injection, this characteristically can produce hyperviscosity and medullary necrosis of the kidney with a resultant hematuria. This is not an infrequent observation in centers where arterial catheters are used.

G. ODELL

We have had the opportunity to see a number of infants (usually following birth asphyxia) who demonstrate the syndrome of inappropriate ADH (antidiuretic hormone) response with a confusing renal picture until the syndrome is suspected and recognized. In these instances, there is very low serum osmolality, and electrolyte concentrations may fall to very low levels. We have seen situations with a serum sodium as low as 103 mEq. per liter, and potassium of less than 2. In addition, the fall in serum calcium has often provoked seizures. The child thus appears to be water-intoxicated; yet, despite this, the urine remains concentrated with a high specific gravity. It is likely that the low electrolyte levels (especially that of the potassium) may further result in renal impairment. Many of these infants are unable to feed by themselves and have been given intravenous fluids which only make matters worse, particularly if the fluids are calcium-free. In such instances, we have had to resort to initial administration of electrolytes, with hypertonic saline as well as calcium, to effect at least partial improvement in the situation. The hallmark of therapy, however, lies in fluid restriction, as the condition is generally self-limited and will improve with a return to normal serum osmolality and appropriate urinary concentrations when the cerebral insult either resolves or (as in the case of meningitis) the underlying cause is treated.

L. STERN

REFERENCES

1. Barnett, H., and Vesterdal, J.: The physiologic and clinical significance of immaturity of kidney function in young infants. J Pediat 42:99, 1953.
2. Belman, A., Susmand, D., Burden, J., et al: Nonoperative treatment of unilateral renal vein thrombosis in the newborn. JAMA 211:1165, 1970.
3. Bergstrom, T., Larson, H., Lincoln, K., et al: Studies on urinary tract infections in infancy and childhood. J Pediat 80:858, 1972.
4. Burke, E., Shin, M., and Kelalis, P.: Prune-belly syndrome: Clinical findings and survival. Amer J Dis Child 117:668, 1969.
5. Crocker, J., Brown, D., and Vernier, R.: Developmental defects of the kidney. Pediat Clin N Amer 18:355, 1971.
6. Edelman, C., and Spitzer, A.: The maturing kidney. J Pediat 75:509, 1969.
7. Fetterman, G., Shuplock, N., Phillipp, F., et al: The growth and maturation of human glomeruli and proximal convolution from term to adulthood: studies of microdissection. Pediatrics 35:601, 1965.
8. Froehlich, L., and Fujikura, T.: Significance of a single umbilical artery: Report from the collaborative study of cerebral palsy. Amer J Obstet 94:274, 1966.
9. Garrett, R., and Franken, E.: Neonatal ascites: Perirenal urinary extravasation with bladder outlet obstruction. J Urol 102:627, 1969.
10. Lincoln, K., and Winberg, J.: Studies of urinary tract infections in infancy and childhood. Acta Paediat Scand 53:307, 1964.
11. Nelson, J., and Peters, P.: Suprapubic aspiration of urine in premature and term infants. Pediatrics 36:132, 1965.
12. Newman, C., O'Neill, P., and Parker, A.: Pyuria in infancy, and the role of suprapubic aspiration of urine in diagnosis of infection of urinary tract. Brit Med J 2:277, 1967.
13. Osathanodh, V., and Potter, E.: Development of human kidney as shown by microdissection. Arch Path 76:271, 1963.
14. Potter, E.: Bilateral renal agenesis. J Pediat 29:68, 1946.
15. Sakai, T., Leumann, E., and Holliday, M.: Single injection clearance in children. Pediatrics 44:905, 1969.
16. Thompson, I., and Baker, J.: Hazards of hypospadias. Missouri Med 65:301, 1968.
17. Vernier, R., and Birch-Andersen, A.: Studies of the human fetal kidney. I. Development of the glomerulus. J Pediat 60:754, 1962.
18. Weil, W.: The evaluation of renal function in infancy and childhood. Amer J Med Sci 229:678, 1955.

Chapter 15

HEMATOLOGIC PROBLEMS

by

SAMUEL GROSS, M.D.

and

DAVID K. MELHORN, M.D.

"The great questions of the day are not decided by speeches and majority votes but by blood and iron."

BISMARCK, September 30, 1862.

This chapter, describing the nature and management of hematologic problems common to the neonate (with the exception of erythroblastosis, which is discussed in Chapter 11), is organized in a different fashion. Case problems will serve as a basis upon which discussion will be developed, and the sections on Basic Considerations, Clinical Management, and Practical Hints are incorporated into the cases. For quick reference, the following cases will be discussed in this chapter: (1) accidental blood loss, (2) vitamin K deficiency, (3) low platelets, (4) consumption coagulopathy, (5) iron deficiency, (6) vitamin E deficiency, and (7) a complicated case.

This chapter is not intended to serve as an introduction to basic hematology, for which the reader is referred to Mauer,[16] Oski and Naiman,[24] and Ratnoff.[25]

DISORDERS IN HEMOSTASIS

BLOOD VOLUME AND ACCIDENTAL BLOOD LOSS

Case One

Male infant A was the second child born to a healthy, blood type O, Rh positive mother, whose medications during pregnancy consisted solely of calcium, iron, and vitamins. Labor began spontaneously, but was then precipitously hastened following manual rupture of the membranes. The infant's birth weight (2.6 Kg.) was consistent with the estimated gestational age of 39 weeks. Examination of the placenta revealed a small 1 cm. tear at the base of the cord adjacent to its insertion. No bleeding was noted from this site. Although the baby breathed and cried spontaneously, he appeared to be moderately lethargic, and accordingly was placed in the observation nursery where he received vitamin K_1 (0.5 mg. I.M.). One hour later, lethargy was more pronounced and accompanied by pallor, tachypnea, and tachycardia (respiratory rate 70 per minute; pulse rate 165 per minute). Apart from these changes, there were no other abnormal physical findings, nor was there evidence of active bleeding. Rectal temperature at that time was 34.7°C. The umbilical vessels were catheterized and the following studies, including type and cross-match, were obtained:

Hemoglobin	10.2 gm. per 100 ml.
Hematocrit	29.5 per cent
Arterial pressure	20 mm. Hg
Arterial pH	7.15
$PaCO_2$	50 mm. Hg
Blood type	O, Rh positive
Coombs test (direct)	negative
Platelets	230,000 per mm^3
Prothrombin time	16 seconds

270

Partial thromboplastin
    time   80 seconds
Fibrinogen   200 mg. per 100 ml.
Erythrocyte mor-   normochromic,
    phology   normocytic; 12
                                     nucleated RBCs
                                     per 100 WBC.

As shown, the major abnormalities included low hemoglobin and hematocrit values, and low arterial pressure and oxygen saturation. The presumptive diagnosis was accidental blood loss with impending shock, presumed to be the result of a tear in the cord at the time of delivery. Twenty minutes later, the infant received 50 ml. (20 ml. per Kg.) of whole blood, cross-matched against both mother and infant. There followed an immediate, albeit modest, clinical improvement (arterial blood pressure rose to 28 mm. Hg, and the hematocrit rose to 32 per cent). Two hours later, an additional 50 ml. of whole blood was transfused, following which the hematocrit rose to 41 per cent, and the arterial pressure stabilized at 43 mm. Hg.

Commentary

The presence of a tear in the umbilical cord and the clinical findings of pallor, tachycardia, and tachypnea, with failure to identify either hemolytic or coagulation abnormalities, are strong presumptive evidence of accidental hemorrhage. This was further supported by the lack of any evidence for active internal bleeding (e.g., abdominal distention, shifting dullness, periumbilical ecchymoses) or hemorrhage into the central nervous system (e.g., apnea or convulsions). The association of tachypnea and tachycardia with arterial hypotension further distinguishes blood loss with impending shock from the symptoms of primary pulmonary dysfunction.

Once a hemorrhagic event is identified as a life-threatening process, the hallmarks of which are shock and hypotension, efforts to ameliorate this disorder must be carried out with deliberate haste. Ideally in such situations the measurement of choice is a blood volume determination by radioactive assay. However, in the absence of this technique, dependable estimations can be made based upon the studies of Usher et al,[30] who showed that term infants, after immediate cord clamping, had a mean blood volume of 78 ml. per Kg. (red cell volume 52 ml. per Kg.), as compared to 101 ml. per Kg. (red cell volume 51 ml. per Kg.) following a five-minute delay in clamping. In premature infants,[29] following immediate clamping only, the mean blood volume was 89 ml. per Kg. (red cell volume 51 ml. per Kg.). Insofar as identifying volume losses, reliable estimations may be applied from studies on term infants by Walgren et al,[31] who showed that a 25 per cent reduction in circulating volume halved the initial pulmonary and systemic arterial pressures, and that conversely, a corresponding increase in volume doubled the pressures. Thus, in the absence of specific information, one may estimate volume as 90 ml. per Kg. and losses in accord with arterial pressures (i.e., 50 per cent decline in arterial pressure approximates at least a 25 per cent reduction in volume).

Equally important is the knowledge of the blood-processing measures characteristic of each institution. For example, in this center, 450 ml. of donor blood is collected into a plastic bag containing 67.5 ml. of anticoagulant (acid citrate-dextrose), resulting thereby in an average hemoglobin content of 64 gm., or 12.4 gm. per 100 ml. When "routinely packed" cells are requested (i.e., a single centrifugation followed by removal of 90 per cent of the plasma volume), the resultant hemoglobin range is 19 gm. per 100 ml. to 22 gm. per 100 ml. A double centrifugation of saline-washed cells, followed by removal of both supernatant and the upper five per cent cell mass, will increase the hemoglobin range to 27 to 31 gm. per 100 ml.

Another significant factor is the basis upon which cell measurements are made. Capillary blood should not be used for such determinations.[19] During the first five days of life in term infants, and for as many as 14 days in small premature infants, peripheral stasis may result in a differential of as many as 20 percentage points between central and peripheral determinations. (The peripheral determinations are higher than the central measurements.) In addition, cord blood obtained at the time of delivery is also unsuitable for estimation of red cell mass because of difficulties in collection. Blood from the umbilical or other free-flowing veins is preferred.

Application of this information in the treatment of baby A, in whom blood loss was acute and treatment not completed until slightly over three and one-half hours had elapsed, would have provided a logical basis of therapy and a more efficacious response. The following is our approach to treatment in such cases.

1. Assume an intermediate value for blood volume (i.e., 90 ml. per Kg.). In the case of baby A, 2.6 Kg. × 90 ml. = 234 ml.

2. In slightly more than 90 per cent of term infants, the normal range in hemoglobin

and hematocrit values is 16 to 20 gm. per 100 ml. and 48 to 60 per cent, respectively. (Appendices 25 to 27). In this infant, who was symptomatic by one hour of life, these values were 10.2 gm. per 100 ml. and 29 per cent, respectively, which would indicate an estimated volume loss between 35 and 45 per cent.

3. A judgment must then be made as to the type of volume replacement. The clinical picture was one of acute blood loss and hypotension (hypovolemia). The pressing goal of therapy in such circumstances is the repair of the "effective" circulating volume. In any situation of profound hemorrhage and vascular collapse, the rapid infusion of 20 ml. per Kg. of saline containing five per cent dextrose (or 10 per cent albumin if available) will provide a temporary restoration of volume. Plasma or other fluid expanders may also be used at this stage. However, without restoration of red cell mass, the alleviation of hypoxia will be marginal at best, especially in the infant compromised by hemoglobin that contains low levels of 2,3-DPG. The treatment of choice is whole blood, cross-matched against both mother and infant. Since this procedure may not be practical in emergency situations, the initial transfusion may follow a "partial"* match or be provided from a "walking" donor of known blood type.

One effective measure is to always keep fresh frozen plasma from AB donors, which would be the ideal plasma volume expander for an acute emergency.

G. ODELL

During this period, appropriate cross-matching must be carried out prior to completing the total calculated transfusion. This should return the hemoglobin level to at least 80 per cent of the estimated loss. This case clearly underlines the need to anticipate therapy. Had a single "routinely packed" cell transfusion (hematocrit 55 to 65 per cent) been used, a 75 ml. infusion (equal in volume and cell mass to the estimated loss) would have corrected the deficit in a relatively brief period of time.

4. The arterial pressure must be monitored in all situations of neonatal hypovolemia. It is the most sensitive early index of volume repair, since the return to a normotensive state precedes restoration of normal hematocrit values. Examination of baby A's therapy demonstrates this point. The initial infusion of whole blood, although it provided transient clinical benefit, did not result in a normotensive state, nor did it correct the loss of red cell volume. The modest rise in arterial pressure indicated that further replacement therapy was necessary. Monitoring of arterial blood pressure also prevents overly vigorous attempts at volume repair with the attendant risks of overexpansion of the intravascular space.

5. Supportive efforts must include the maintenance of an unobstructed airway, adequate oxygenation, and appropriate correction of acid-base balance. In situations in which lengthy laboratory studies are needed to identify possible coagulation abnormalities or internal hemorrhage secondary to trauma, the transfusion procedures must be maintained as long as evidence for continued bleeding persists, especially if surgical intervention is anticipated. Every possible attempt should be made to ensure proper temperature control during manipulation and transfusion procedures.

6. Examination of the placenta and umbilical cord must also be included as an integral part of the initial evaluation. In this instance, identification of the tear in the umbilical cord should have immediately alerted the physician to the possibility of blood loss.

In cases of suspected fetal-maternal hemorrhage or twin-to-twin bleeding of similar clinical severity, the same procedures must be employed. In the former instance, the acid elution technique may confirm the presence of fetal cells in the maternal circulation.[32] If differences in maternal and infant blood typing exist, differential agglutination studies will also be helpful. Although fetal-maternal hemorrhage usually occurs during labor, one may, on occasion, observe pallor after delivery without signs and symptoms of acute blood loss (presumably the result of bleeding into the maternal circulation before labor). It is reasonable to treat such infants solely with iron (see section on the red cell, pp. 278–281). On occasion, blood is identified in the vomitus or stool of the infants suspected of a bleeding disorder. In such situations, the use of the hemoglobin identification test of Abt and Downey[2] will help to distinguish adult from fetal hemoglobin.

It must be remembered that the theory upon which the test is based is that fetal hemoglobin *resists* alkali denaturation. However, given sufficient time, it too will result in the same color response as adult hemoglobin (i.e., a change from cherry pink to yellow).

L. STERN

---

*In this sense, "partial" indicates a rapid cross-match.

Polycythemia

Neonatal polycythemia, by definition, is an hematocrit value in excess of 70 per cent. It occurs most commonly as a result of maternal-to-fetal transfusions, but also may occur with twin-to-twin transfusions, infants of diabetic mothers, congenital adrenal hyperplasia, infants born to thyrotoxic mothers, and infants who are small-for-gestational-age. The occurrence of neonatal polycythemia requires appropriate diagnostic studies, including the maternal history, examination of the placenta, fetal and adult hemoglobin levels, IgA levels, differential erythrocyte agglutination, and, if indicated, glucose, cortisol, and thyroxin levels. In dizygotic twins, a hemoglobin differential greater than 4.0 gm. per 100 ml. should suggest twin-to-twin transfusion.

The risks of neonatal polycythemia include arterial and venous thromboses, pulmonary hemorrhage, and hyperbilirubinemia. These risks are intensified in small premature infants who had delayed clamping of the cord. When polycythemia with hypertension is identified, removal of 10-ml. increments of whole blood, carried out in conjunction with arterial pressure monitoring, is usually sufficient to lower the hematocrit to a 60 to 70 per cent range and restore a normotensive state. In the absence of precise volume measurements, it may not be possible to distinguish between an absolute or relative volume increase. In such instances, it is safer to perform a partial exchange transfusion with whole blood (hematocrit 36 per cent) rather than risk the development of a hypovolemic state.

Although diagnostic and management procedures employed in the care of the anemic or polycythemic infant usually require catheterization of the umbilical vessels, it should be emphasized that these manipulations are not without risks, (i.e., infection, perforation, thrombosis).

VITAMIN K DEFICIENCY

Case Two

While driving home from the market, Mrs. Y, a 33-year-old gravida 6 mother of five healthy children, entered spontaneous labor and within a few minutes, in the midst of heavy downtown traffic, delivered a male infant. Further assistance was provided by the rescue squad, who subsequently transported both mother and infant to a nearby hospital. Physical examination in the nursery revealed a normal, term male (weight 3.0 Kg.). Because of the circumstances of the delivery, the baby received prophylactic penicillin and kanamycin. On the second hospital day, breast feeding was begun. On the third day, excessive oozing from a heel site following routine capillary puncture was observed. No further studies were obtained at that time. On the fourth hospital day, the infant was circumcized, and within a short time the surgical dressing and diaper were thoroughly saturated with blood. Venous blood was then obtained for screening hematologic and clotting studies.

Hematocrit	46 per cent
Platelets	205,000 per mm³
Partial thromboplastin time	68 seconds
Prothrombin time	28 seconds
Fibrinogen	255 mg. per 100 ml.

On questioning the nursery personnel, it was revealed that the infant did not receive vitamin K, an apparent result of the confusing and unusual circumstances of his birth. At this point, the presumptive diagnosis of hemorrhagic disease secondary to vitamin K deficiency was made.

Commentary

In the absence of vitamin K, the liver is unable to synthesize factors II (prothrombin), VII (proconvertin), IX (plasma thromboplastin component), and X (Stuart-Prower). In the small premature infant, hepatic synthesis of these factors is often minimal, even in the presence of large amounts of vitamin K. Furthermore, the only factors that remain within the range of normal adult values in the immediate newborn period, irrespective of gestational maturity, are factors I, V, VIII, and with rare exception, platelets (Appendix 22).

A reliable index of vitamin K deficiency is the one-stage prothrombin time determination, which, however, does not measure solely prothrombin levels. It measures the activity of factors II, V, VII, and X, but in situations of vitamin K deficiency, the prothrombin time becomes prolonged because of the progressive deficiencies of factors II, VII, and X. Factor IX is not identified in the prothrombin time determination, and factor V is not vitamin K dependent. (Figure 15–1).

The ability of the newborn infant to synthesize and utilize vitamin K is a function of both gestational and chronologic age. In term infants, prothrombin time is most prolonged at three to four days and remains increased for an additional two to three days. In the small premature infant, the prolonged time may persist for 10 to 14 days.

The initial diet of the newborn also plays a significant role in the production of vitamin K deficiency.[7] For example, cow's milk

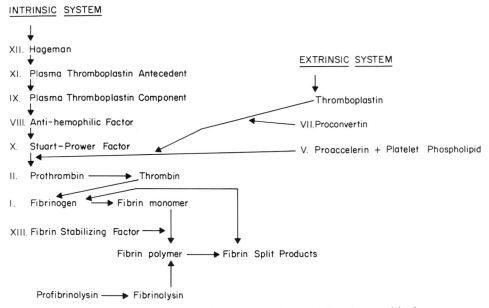

INTRINSIC SYSTEM

↓

XII. Hageman

XI. Plasma Thromboplastin Antecedent

IX. Plasma Thromboplastin Component ——— Thromboplastin

EXTRINSIC SYSTEM

VIII. Anti-hemophilic Factor ——— VII. Proconvertin

X. Stuart–Prower Factor ——— V. Proaccelerin + Platelet Phospholipid

II. Prothrombin ——→ Thrombin

I. Fibrinogen ⟷ Fibrin monomer

XIII. Fibrin Stabilizing Factor ——→

Fibrin polymer ——→ Fibrin Split Products

Profibrinolysin ——→ Fibrinolysin

Figure 15–1   The system of clot promotion, stabilization, and lysis.

contains approximately 6 μg. per 100 ml. of vitamin K, or four times the amount present in human milk. Furthermore, the frequency of a marked prolongation of prothrombin time in infants fed cow's milk preparations before 12 hours of age is approximately half that of infants whose feedings are delayed during this period.

The prolonged administration of antibiotics, which eliminate intestinal bacterial flora, may contribute to vitamin K deficiency. The combination of antibiotic therapy and formulas low in vitamin K has been related to the occurrence of serious hemorrhagic problems in infants well beyond the newborn period.

In the case of baby Y, failure to administer vitamin K was compounded by the subsequent administration of a diet low in vitamin K (breast milk). It is a moot point, however, as to whether the antibiotics administered during the first three days of life added to this problem.

Although as little as 25 μg. per 100 ml. of vitamin K_1 is sufficient to protect against the prolongation of prothrombin time in term infants, the recommended dose is 0.5 to 1.0 mg. I.M., administered immediately after birth. There is no advantage gained by the administration of vitamin K to the mother immediately prior to delivery. In cases of obvious bleeding, it is advisable to use the intravenous route in

order to avoid the occurrence of hematoma formation. In the small premature infant, as much as 2 to 3 mg. may be necessary to effect a favorable response in prothrombin time. However, prolonged bleeding may still persist in such infants, and although administration of fresh plasma may help in replacing some of the deficient factors and aid in shortening the prothrombin time, in no instance should synthetic vitamin K analogues be used. Such agents are not only slow in effecting a response; in large doses they have the attendant risk of producing hyperbilirubinemia and kernicterus when administered to premature infants. The data relative to a similar response in full-term infants is not clearly established.

Certain of the milk substitute formulas contain less than 25 μg. of vitamin K per liter. Infants receiving such preparations should have additional vitamin K in the dietary regimen in order to raise the daily intake to the levels of around 100 μg. per liter. The same holds true for infants with malabsorption disorders, such as cystic fibrosis, biliary atresia, or infants requiring prolonged parenteral nutritional supplementation. The water-soluble preparation is to be preferred and need not be administered parenterally unless there is unequivocal evidence that vitamin K absorption is impaired.

It should be noted that a prolongation of prothrombin time may reflect primary abnormalities in liver function rather than lack of dietary vitamin K. Table 15–2 contains a summation of the screening tests useful in characterizing the clotting abnormalities in vitamin K deficiency, liver disease, primary clotting factor deficiencies, and consumptive coagulopathies.

PLATELETS

Case Three

Baby boy Z was born at term to a healthy, gravida 2, blood type AB, Rh positive mother, whose pregnancy was uncomplicated and who received no drugs other than vitamins. A previous sibling, born at another hospital, had a history of chronic umbilical bleeding during the first three days of life, which allegedly did not respond to the administration of vitamin K. However, no clotting studies were performed on that infant, and only after a transfusion of fresh whole blood did the bleeding apparently cease. Immediately following delivery of baby Z, scattered petechiae were visible over the entire body, and during the ensuing three hours the subcutaneous bleeding increased and became confluent. Blood was obtained from an antecubital vein for hematologic studies. With the exception of the petechiae and ecchymoses, there were no physical abnormalities noted.

Hemoglobin	16.0 gm. per 100 ml.
Hematocrit	49.0 per cent
Blood type	A, Rh positive
Coombs test (direct)	negative
Platelets	18,000 per mm^3
Partial thromboplastin time	70 seconds
Prothrombin time	15 seconds
Fibrinogen	205 mg. per 100 ml.
IgG	650 mg. per 100 ml.
IgA	10 mg. per 100 ml.
IgM	10 mg. per 100 ml.

These studies revealed that the only identifiable abnormality was the marked reduction in platelets (18,000 per mm^3). X-rays of the skull and long bones were normal, and bacterial and viral cultures were negative. A bone marrow examination and stain for morphology revealed a slight increase in erythroid precursors, with normal myeloid activity and a modest decrease in the number of megakaryocytes, some of which were immature. The platelet count on the mother was 253,000 per mm^3. The presumptive diagnosis was iso-immune thrombocytopenia, and treatment with prednisone (1 mg. per Kg. daily) was initiated.

Therapy was discontinued after four weeks because the platelet count failed to improve. However, no further bleeding problems were noted. Eight weeks later, the platelet count was 75,000 per mm^3, and by three months of age, the count had stabilized in a range of 170,000 to 225,000 per mm^3.

Commentary

The absence of any blood group incompatibilities, coupled with normal bone marrow and X-ray examinations in an infant whose sole clinical abnormality was purpura, effectively excluded the possibilities of erythroblastosis, infection, or tumor (including congenital leukemia). The negative maternal history of drug ingestion (specifically thiazides), as well as her normal platelet count, made unlikely the possibility of an auto-immune, drug-induced thrombocytopenia. With the suggestion of a similar disorder in the previous sibling, the presumptive diagnosis of iso-immune thrombocytopenia was considered likely. Although the diagnosis was made solely by exclusion, the course of the disease was consistent with iso-immune thrombocytopenia. It should be noted that serologic tests for platelet antibodies are both difficult to perform and frequently inconclusive.[27]

The differences between iso-immune and auto-immune thrombocytopenia are usually quite distinct. Iso-immune purpura should be suspected in any otherwise healthy thrombocytopenic infant whose mother has a normal platelet count and a negative history of drug therapy. In this disorder, as in erythroblastosis fetalis, the antibody will attack both infant's and father's platelets, and successive pregnancies usually result in thrombocytopenic infants. In both disorders, it is not unusual to observe an amegakaryocytic marrow, presumably the result of a direct antibody attack on the antigenic sites of the megakaryocytes.

Corticosteroid therapy rarely is effective in the treatment of the auto-immune type, but for unknown reasons such therapy may occasionally have an ameliorating effect on the iso-immune variety. Exchange transfusion with fresh, platelet-rich whole blood may also be beneficial, possibly by providing extra sites for antibody absorption. It is possible that whenever iso-immune thrombocytopenia is anticipated, benefit might accrue from the administration of prednisone (1 mg. per Kg.) to the mother four to six hours prior to delivery.

If iso-immune thrombocytopenia is expected or suspected, treatment with washed platelet packs from the mother is the most appropriate therapy, since her platelets would not be agglutinated by the antibody, whereas most donor platelet units contain the common antigens to which the mother's antibody would be active, and very little benefit would accrue from administering such platelet packs.

G. ODELL

Other causes for neonatal thrombocytopenia include erythroblastosis fetalis (although thrombocytopenia may develop following repeated and prolonged exchange transfusions) and congenital absence of megakaryocytes as an isolated phenomenon or in association with phocomelia; it may appear as part of a pancytopenia syndrome (which may on rare occasions respond to the administration of corticosteroids and/or testosterone). Thrombocytopenia may be present in a wide variety of infectious diseases, including bacterial septicemia, herpes simplex, toxoplasmosis, cytomegalic inclusion disease, congenital syphilis, and the rubella syndrome. It is usually a feature of congenital leukemia, Down's syndrome, Wiskott-Aldrich syndrome, Letterer-Siwe's disease, and disseminated intravascular coagulation. Although rare before two months of life, it may be associated with giant hemangiomata as a result of platelet trapping.

The clinical expression of thrombocytopenia in the immediate newborn period is usually quite dramatic. Unlike the occasional scattered petechiae on the head and shoulders of an otherwise normal infant, subcutaneous bleeding sites are usually profuse and scattered over the entire body. Fortunately, bleeding is rarely of sufficient degree to impair vital function. In such instances, immediate exchange transfusion with fresh whole blood or platelet packs should be administered and followed by splenectomy (but only if megakaryocytes are clearly identified in the marrow).

Platelet counts vary in accordance with both the method of determination and, to a lesser extent, the degree of gestational maturity. In general, platelet levels, enumerated by phase microscopy, are 25,000 to 50,000 per mm³ lower than those performed under direct microscopy. In small premature infants, occasional platelet values as low as 25,000 to 50,000 per mm³ have been noted in the absence of any clinical disorder. However, this information is not intended to deter the physician from seeking an etiologic agent.

THE CONSUMPTION OF CLOTTING FACTORS

Case Four

Baby girl W was born at term (birth weight 3.9 Kg.), following an uncomplicated pregnancy and delivery. On the first postpartum day it was noted that the mother had a streptococcal breast abscess and, as a consequence, breast feeding was not allowed, although rooming-in was permitted. Capillary blood studies, obtained on the third day of life because of the presence of icterus, revealed the following: hematocrit 43 per cent; blood type O, Rh positive; direct Coombs test negative; bilirubin D/T 0.7/9.4 mg. per 100 ml. The infant appeared to be sluggish during the blood-drawing process. Twelve hours later, she suddenly became pale and voided a small quantity of burgundy-colored urine. The umbilical artery was catheterized and revealed a pressure of 25 mm. Hg. Additional blood studies performed at this point included a hematocrit of 31 per cent and a peripheral blood film which contained polychromatophilic and fragmented erythrocytes, increased numbers of normoblasts, and a marked reduction in platelets. Detailed studies are included below.

Hemoglobin	11.1 gm. per 100 ml.
Hematocrit	31.0 per cent
Reticulocyte count	17.1 per cent
Normoblasts	15/100 WBC
Peripheral smear	fragmented erythrocytes, decreased platelets
Coombs test (direct)	negative
Platelet count	35,000 per mm³
Partial thromboplastin time	> 160 seconds
Prothrombin time	> 120 seconds
Thrombin time	> 60 seconds
Fibrinogen	10 mg. per 100 ml.
Urinalysis	free hemoglobin, red cells, protein
Fibrin split products	60 mg. per 100 ml.*
Factor VIII	10 per cent*
Factor V	10 per cent*

The infant's clinical status rapidly deteriorated. She immediately received an infusion of 30 ml. of normal saline containing five per cent glucose and 10 per cent albumin, which was followed in rapid sequence by an exchange trans-

---

*These results were obtained seven hours later on pre-exchange plasma stored at −20°C.

fusion of 24-hour-old, type-specific, citrated whole blood. Bleeding from the umbilical vessels, which had been profuse prior to the exchange transfusion, ceased midway through the procedure and the arterial pressure rose to a normal level. Following the exchange transfusion, the infant was markedly improved and had normal clotting studies, which remained normal throughout the hospital stay. Blood cultures obtained from the umbilical vein prior to the exchange grew β-hemolytic streptococcus, Group A, for which the infant accordingly received 10 days of penicillin (initiated 24 hours after completion of the exchange transfusion). On the 18th hospital day, the infant was sent home in good health with a discharge diagnosis of consumptive coagulopathy (disseminated intravascular coagulation) secondary to β-hemolytic streptococcal septicemia presumably contracted from the mother.

Commentary

In 1961, Abelli and DeLamerans applied the term "secondary hemorrhagic disease" to a group of immature newborn infants with alterations in capillary permeability and abnormally low clotting factors, including fibrinogen (I), factor V, and platelets. In most of these infants, hypoxia and/or sepsis was a major clinical finding and the response to vitamin K was generally poor, although the administration of fresh whole blood occasionally effected transient improvement. In retrospect, it appears likely that many of these patients did indeed have disseminated intravascular coagulation. It is now well established that a variety of factors can either initiate or worsen disseminated intravascular coagulation. Table 15–1 lists known triggering events.

The diagnosis of disseminated intravascular coagulation (DIC) must be strongly suspected in any newborn infant (particularly the susceptible infant of a high-risk pregnancy) with a bleeding disorder secondary to a deficiency of all factors (including factors I, V,

VIII, and platelets) in association with increased levels of fibrin-split products and a peripheral smear characterized by fragmented erythrocytes. The erythrocyte abnormality is presumed to be the result of a shearing effect on the membrane following flow through an angiopathic or semioccluded blood vessel. Such cells rapidly undergo lysis within the vascular space, and because of the newborn's limited capacity to synthesize haptoglobin, free hemoglobin is usually released into the renal collecting system, with the attendant risks of tubular damage. The elevation of fibrin-split products reflects the response of the fibrinolytic system to the initial increase in clot formation. However, in cases of overwhelming disease, such elevations may not be present or even found on postmortem examination. Furthermore, the clotting abnormalities may not always occur in temporal association. As a consequence, fluctuations in these laboratory determinations are commonly seen during the course of the illness.

The present case illustrates the rapidity with which clinical manifestations of DIC may appear, and underlines the urgency in providing rapid diagnostic studies and appropriate therapy. Several procedures which are readily accomplished within minutes include: (1) estimation of platelet numbers and erythrocyte morphology by examination of routine blood films, and (2) estimation of fibrinogen content by observing the degree of flocculation of plasma heated at 56°C (no precipitate or only a fine flocculus is strong presumptive evidence of decreased fibrinogen levels). Reliable determinations of partial thromboplastin and prothrombin times, as well as fibrinogen content, can be made within five minutes on as little as 3 cc. whole blood. However, because assays for factors V, VIII, and fibrin-split products are time consuming, such determinations may be held in abeyance

TABLE 15–1 ETIOLOGIC FACTORS IN DISSEMINATED INTRAVASCULAR COAGULATION IN THE NEWBORN

Septicemia: bacterial, viral, parasitic, rickettsial, mycotic
Tissue Release:
    Antigen-antibody complexes
    Abruptio placentae
    Intravascular hemolysis
    Malignancy
    Idiopathic respiratory distress syndrome (asphyxia, hypoxia)
    Burns
Giant hemangioma (platelet trapping)
Purpura fulminans (? septicemia)
Hepatitis and cirrhosis (? tissue release)

until time permits by storage of citrated plasma in plastic tubes at $-20°C$.

Therapy should be directed against both the inciting cause, if identifiable, and the hemorrhagic event. Although heparin in a dose of 100 units per Kg., administered every four to six hours and continued until sustained improvement has been obtained, has been recommended as the treatment of choice, it is our experience that heparinization is less efficacious in the neonate than in the older child or adult. One possible explanation in this regard may relate to an estrogenic effect. For example, in the rabbit, DIC as part of the generalized Schwartzman reaction may be aborted by pretreatment with heparin, but not by heparin pretreatment in the pregnant rabbit.[11] It is conceivable that the newborn infant, with a long-term exposure to estrogen in utero, may behave in a similar fashion. The use of heparin poses the additional problem of providing a means of neutralizing its effect in order to perform follow-up clotting studies. Protamine has been used in this regard, but it too has test tube anticoagulant characteristics. The best results in our series have been obtained with the use of citrated, whole blood exchange transfusion, repeated if necessary until a favorable response is obtained.[9] For the term infant, blood less than 72 hours old has been satisfactory; for the premature infant, fresh blood is preferred. Platelet pack transfusions may also provide additional support.

The possible relationship of hypoxia and DIC in infants with the idiopathic respiratory distress syndrome (RDS) remains the subject of considerable controversy.[5, 12-14] Several investigators have identified a marked increase in fibrinogen turnover and fibrinolytic activity in such infants. It has further been postulated that failure to effect optimal perfusion of the pulmonary vasculature in premature infants, as a result of either perinatal hemorrhage or sequestered placental blood, may potentiate or actually initiate the RDS,[6] which may in turn trigger a local bleeding diathesis and the consumption of coagulation factors. However, in the absence of adequate confirmatory findings, one should at least be aware of the potential risks in such patients and obtain appropriate studies in anticipation of such events as intracerebral (or intraventricular) hemorrhage, pulmonary hemorrhage, or severe gastrointestinal bleeding—all of which may be life-threatening.

Other causes of hemorrhagic disease in the newborn may be related to iatrogenic effects, namely, overzealous flushing of an indwelling umbilical catheter with heparin, or thrombus formation secondary to an inappropriately positioned catheter.

The initial presentation of hemorrhagic disease secondary to inherited coagulation abnormalities may, on occasion, occur in the newborn period. As in all clotting disorders, appropriate studies should be obtained and treatment directed toward replacement of deficient factors. A variety of differential laboratory examinations relative to various clotting disorders are presented in Table 15-2.[25]

THE ERYTHROCYTE

IRON

Case Five

Baby girl S was born at term (birth weight 2.9 Kg.) to a healthy, blood type B, Rh positive

TABLE 15-2 CLOTTING DISORDERS AND RELATED SCREENING STUDIES IN THE NEWBORN

DEFICIENCIES OF:	PTT	PT	TT	FIBRINOGEN	FSP	PLATELETS	UREA CLOT LYSIS
Vitamin K	↑	↑	N	N	N	N	N
Factors VIII, IX or XI	↑	N	N	N	N	N	N
Factor X	↑	↑	N	N	N	N	N
Factor V,° or VII	N	↑	N	N	N	N	N
Factor XIII°	N	N	N	N	N	N	↑
Platelets	N	N	N	N	N	↓	N
Disseminated Intravascular Coagulation	↑	↑	↑	↓	N or ↑	↓	N
Liver Disease	↑	↑	↑	N	N or ↑	N or ↑	N

↑ = Increased   ↓ = Decreased   N = Normal   TT = Thrombin Time
° = Decreased in DIC   PT = Prothrombin Time   PTT = Partial Thromboplastin Time
FSP = Fibrin-Split Products

primigravida mother following an uneventful pregnancy. However, labor was complicated by vaginal bleeding which was apparently the result of marginal sinus rupture of the placenta. For this reason, delivery was accomplished by cesarean section. Initial physical examination revealed a vigorous, active infant in no distress. The placenta was not examined. Laboratory data obtained on blood from the umbilical vein included:

Hemoglobin	13.9 gm. per 100 ml.
Hematocrit	40 per cent
Peripheral smear	normocytic erythrocytes with 5 nucleated RBC/WBC
Reticulocyte count	8.7 per cent
Platelet count	425,000 per mm³

A stain of maternal peripheral blood revealed 3.5 per cent fetal cells. The infant's blood type was B, Rh positive and differential agglutination was therefore not attempted. After an uneventful four-day hospital course, the infant was discharged without further therapy. The mother was instructed to use an evaporated milk formula which was not iron supplemented, and the infant was scheduled for a follow-up return visit one month after discharge. However, the infant did not return for six months, at which time examination revealed an irritable, pale infant whose only other pertinent physical finding was a spleen tip palpable 1 cm. below the left costal margin. Laboratory data at this time included:

Hemoglobin	7.0 gm. per 100 ml.
Hematocrit	24 per cent
Peripheral smear	Marked hypochromia
Reticulocyte count	3.2 per cent
Platelet count	450,000 per mm³
Bound serum iron	35 mg. per 100 ml.
Total iron binding capacity	490 mg. per 100 ml.

On further questioning of the parents, it was learned that the sole dietary intake during the first six months of life was an evaporated milk preparation, which averaged approximately 36 ounces per 24 hours. Later during this examination the infant passed a stool which was normal in color and consistency, but which was found to be 2+ for guaiac.

Commentary

The clinical and laboratory findings were consistent with a diagnosis of iron deficiency anemia. In most normal full-term infants the most common etiologic factor in the production of iron deficiency is inadequate iron intake. This was obviously the situation in this baby. Infrequently, iron deficiency may occur as a result of chronic occult blood loss secondary to the ingestion of large amounts of unmodified cow's milk preparations. In such infants, a reduction in the total milk intake reduces the red cell losses. Bleeding as a result of vascular abnormalities of the gut will also lead to iron deficiency. Tissue desquamation losses (i.e., nails, hair, gut, etc.) account for somewhere between 0.1 and 0.3 mg. of elemental iron per day, but this loss is not sufficient to explain iron deficiency per se. Most cases of nutritional iron deficiency in term infants are rarely apparent before six months of age; in fact, they usually do not present until sometime late in the first year of life. On the other hand, premature infants not supplied with medicinal or dietary iron will present with signs of iron deficiency before six months of age because of the excessive demands secondary to rapid weight increases. Thus, in the case of Baby S, dietary deprivation was only one factor in the causation of the iron deficiency anemia, which was present at least by six months of age. The following facets of her newborn course are relevant:

1. A history of blood loss from the placenta before delivery.

2. An initial hematocrit of 40 per cent, which is abnormally low for a full-term infant.

3. Delivery by cesarean section. The manipulation of the infant during this type of extraction often results in "trapping" of a significant amount of the infant's blood volume in the placenta prior to clamping of the cord.

Unlike infants who are symptomatic as a result of profound, acute blood loss in the neonatal period, Baby S appeared deceptively normal in the newborn period, presumably because she was able to maintain adequate vascular perfusion. However, it is reasonable to implicate blood loss in the neonatal period as the major reason for part of the clinical and laboratory expression of severe iron deficiency six months following delivery.

Certain of the clinical and laboratory data noted on this infant at six months of age are worthy of comment. The finding of splenomegaly, moderate thrombocytosis, and positive stool guaiacs are not unusual phenomena in iron-deficient infants. Approximately one-fourth to one-third of all such infants have readily palpable spleens (the etiology of which is obscure) which recede to normal following appropriate therapy. The increase in platelets probably represents the overall increase in marrow response early in the course of iron deficiency. In fact, thrombocytopenia may occur later on, related solely to the deficiency of iron, or on occasion, as part of a concomitant folate deficiency. The presence of occult blood in the stool occurs as a result of profound changes within the mucosal structures caused by deficiencies in tissue iron enzymes which thereby result in loss of cellular integrity and increased exfoliation.

Had the hematologic data on Baby S been viewed with greater scrutiny in the immediate newborn period, appropriate preventive measures could have been initiated. The administration of a low-protein, iron-enriched (8 to 10 mg. of elemental iron per liter) formula offered at the time of discharge from the hospital, with the addition of iron-rich foodstuffs beginning at three to four months of age, would have in part supplied the iron necessary to allow for restoration of losses as well as maintain the needs imposed by growth. For example, the average daily intake of such a formula during the first six months of life is approximately 400 to 500 cc. (4 to 5 mg. of elemental iron) per day. With approximately 10 per cent absorption of the iron, during this interval a total iron intake of somewhere between 75 and 100 mg. would have resulted. Examination of the iron balance sheet in Table 15–3 (a retrospective study of Baby S and her hypothetical normal term counterpart) suggests that an iron-fortified, low-protein formula per se is not sufficient in such an instance. For example, the hemoglobin in the normal baby was 17.5 gm. per 100 ml. with an estimated total body iron of 200 to 220 mg. at birth. At six months of age (a time when birth weight is doubled), the ideal hemoglobin is 12 gm. per 100 ml., with a total body hemoglobin iron of around 200 mg. (representing two-thirds to three-fourths of the total body iron, or approximately 270 to 300 mg. per 100 ml.). For Baby S, the total body hemoglobin iron measured approximately 130 mg., and probably no

more than 150 mg.; the amount of available iron even in an iron-rich formula would not have been entirely sufficient to provide both maintenance and correction.

Effective treatment would consist of the administration of oral medicinal iron in a dosage of 10 mg. of elemental iron per Kg. of body weight per day for two to three months. Deleterious side effects are essentially nonexistent — only on rare occasions do oral iron preparations produce either diarrhea or constipation. It is also advisable to avoid the use of unmodified cow's milk preparations because of their greater iron binding effects than the low-protein preparations, as well as the rare chance, as noted, of initiating gastrointestinal occult red cell losses.

Under circumstances in which medical follow-up of such patients as Baby S is uncertain, more rapid replacement of iron losses is desirable. Total replacement of the iron deficit in the immediate neonatal period is easily accomplished with the use of parenteral iron preparations, calculating the deficit as outlined in Table 15–3. The usual parenteral (iron dextran) preparation contains 50 mg. of elemental iron per ml. Although it is advised to administer no more than 1 ml. per day, 2 to 3 ml. per day have been administered without untoward effect (namely, febrile response). On rare occasion, an anaphylaxis-like response is known to occur, which readily responds to treatment with oxygen and epinephrine.

Once therapy of the iron deficient state is completed, there is no further need for the use of iron supplements, provided such infants are maintained on a well-balanced dietary regimen. The authors are aware of the recent recommendations for supplemental iron during the entire first year of life for all infants (Committee on Nutrition, American Academy of

TABLE 15–3   IRON BALANCE

	NORMAL TERM INFANT	BABY S
Birth weight	2.9 Kg.	2.9 Kg.
Mean hemoglobin (gm. per 100 ml.)	17.5	13.9
Blood volume (90 ml./Kg.)	261 ml.	261 ml.
Total body hemoglobin (gm. per 100 ml.)	$17.5 \times 2.61 = 45.7$	$2.61 \times 13.9 = 36.3$
Total body hemoglobin iron (mg.)	$45.7 \times 3.4* = 155$	$3.4 \times 36.3 = 129$
Storage iron (8 mg./Kg.)**	$8 \times 2.9 = 23$	$2.9 \times ? = ?$
Tissue iron (12 mg./Kg.)**	$12 \times 2.9 = 35$	$2.9 \times ? = ?$
Total body iron (mg.)	213	129 plus
Total iron deficit at least: $213 - 129$		

*Approximately 3.4 mg. of iron per gram of hemoglobin.
**Depleted in iron deficiency anemia when total body iron stores are not maintained.

Pediatrics).[28] However, while this is appropriate for premature infants (whose requirements for hemoglobin synthesis may exceed iron intake during the rapid growth period of the first year), the normal, term infant provided with appropriate medical care and dietary instructions (which include the use of a low-protein formula) does not benefit from additional iron supplementation. In a recent carefully controlled study of formula and solid feeding practices, only those term infants fed cow's milk with the higher protein content had lower hemoglobin values. Iron supplementation for the lower protein formula-fed infants was not necessary. This is illustrated in Table 15–4.

In the United States, nutritional iron deficiency is most often a reflection of broader dietary inadequacies and the lack of optimal medical care among educationally and socioeconomically deprived families.

VITAMIN E

Case Six

Baby boy E was born prematurely to a healthy, 20-year-old mother whose pregnancy history, apart from the premature birth, was normal. Birth weight was 1.45 Kg. and the physical characteristics of the infant were consistent with an estimated gestational age of 32 weeks. A central hematocrit obtained shortly after birth was 48 per cent. At three days of age, icterus was noted (bilirubin D/T 0.5/9.0 mg. per 100 ml.). The hematocrit remained stable and there was no evidence of blood group incompatibility. Peripheral

blood film obtained shortly after birth revealed normal erythrocyte morphology. Treatment consisted of phototherapy, which was discontinued four days later following a bilirubin decline to 0.5/3.1 mg. per 100 ml. At four weeks of age, the hematocrit and reticulocyte counts were 36 per cent and 7.8 per cent, respectively. Three weeks later, the hematocrit had fallen to 24 per cent, and the reticulocyte count had risen to 14.2 per cent. The platelet count was 425,000 per mm.^{3}, and a peripheral blood smear revealed approximately 10 per cent pyknotic red cells. Venous blood was obtained for evaluation of red cell enzymes, serum vitamin E, iron, and folic acid. Laboratory results were:

Hemoglobin	8.4 gm. per 100 ml.
Hematocrit	25 per cent
Reticulocytes	14.2 per cent
WBC	8000 per mm.^{3}, with normal differential count for age
Platelets	425,000 per mm.^{3}
Serum folic acid	3.8 mμg. per ml.
Serum vitamin E	0.23 mg. per 100 ml.
Serum iron	80 μg. per 100 ml.
Glucose 6 phosphate dehydrogenase (G-6-PD)	normal
Pyruvate kinase	normal

As noted, the infant was markedly deficient in both vitamin E and folic acid (see Appendices 30, 31). However, it was concluded that neither reticulocytosis nor thrombocytosis was consistent with folate deficiency, and accordingly the infant was treated solely with a daily oral dose of 25 units per Kg. of alpha tocopherol. Repeat blood counts obtained one week later failed to reveal a change in hematocrit, reticulocytes, or serum vita-

TABLE 15–4   MEAN HEMOGLOBIN (AND PER CENT OF TERM INFANTS) WITH HEMOGLOBIN LEVELS BELOW 10 gm.* per 100 ml. IN RELATIONSHIP TO PROTEIN AND IRON CONTENT OF FORMULAS**

MONTHS	LP-I	LP	HP	HP-I
2	11.4 (1)	11.8 (1)	11.6 (1)	11.5 (2)
3	11.5 (0)	11.7 (2)	11.9 (1)	11.6 (2)
4	12.4 (0)	12.2 (0)	11.7 (1)	12.5 (0)
5	12.4 (0)	12.6 (0)	11.8 (1)	12.5 (0)
6	12.6 (0)	12.5 (0)	11.8 (1)	12.2 (1)
8	12.5 (0)	12.2 (0)	11.9 (2)	12.4 (0)
10	12.8 (0)	12.4 (0)	12.1 (1)	12.8 (0)
12	12.7 (0)	12.6 (0)	12.1 (0)	12.6 (0)

*Lowest hemoglobin was 9.0 gm. per 100 ml.
LP-I : Protein, 1.5 gm. per 100 ml.; elemental iron, 0.8 mg. per 100 ml.
LP   : Protein, 1.5 gm. per 100 ml.; trace iron
HP   : Protein, 2.4 gm. per 100 ml.; trace iron
HP-I : Protein, 2.4 gm. per 100 ml.; elemental iron, 0.85 mg. per 100 ml.
**Adapted from data of Gross.[8]

min E levels. Therapy was continued for an additional seven days, at the end of which time the hematocrit had risen to 28 per cent in association with a decline in reticulocyte count to 4.5 per cent and a rise in the level of vitamin E to 0.85 mg. per 100 ml.

Commentary

The erythrocyte of the newborn infant, as with many aspects of the clotting mechanism, is not especially suited for extrauterine life. Its hemoglobin has a reduced potential for effective oxygen release owing to a lowered 2,3-DPG content,[23] and although the activity of the glycolytic enzymes (except phosphofructokinase) is increased, glutathione peroxidase and catalase activity is diminished.[24] This results in lessened antiperoxidant protection for the red cell membrane, which in less mature infants has a lipid content 1.5 times greater than that of adult red cells. The instability in the "redox" system is further intensified by lowered levels of reduced glutathione, apparently the result of an unstable TPN system. The lack of antioxidant protection afforded the red cell of the premature infant is further compounded by vitamin E deficiency[17] (due essentially to inadequate absorption of fatty compounds), which persists in varying degrees until the infant approaches gestational maturity[18] (seven weeks of age in Baby E). In the term infant, the instability of the glutathione system is rarely apparent beyond the first week of life, while in very small premature infants, low levels of glutathione peroxidase and an unstable, reduced glutathione system may persist for four to five weeks.

The combination of increased red cell lipids and decreased levels of vitamin E render the red cell particularly susceptible to the adverse effects of peroxidant activity. The administration of agents known to enhance peroxidation, such as iron and oxygen, may further increase lipid peroxidation, resulting in cell leakage and ultimately hemolysis.

In addition to the hemolytic aspects, thrombocytosis and occasional peripheral edema have been noted. The thrombocytosis probably reflects nonspecific heightened marrow response to hemolysis, but the significance of the latter finding is not clear, and furthermore is least responsive to vitamin E therapy.

Baby E exhibited the essential characteristics of a vitamin E dependent, hemolytic anemia which responded to appropriate therapy only after he reached gestational maturity of sufficient degree to absorb the fat-soluble preparation of the vitamin (at approximately 36 to 38 weeks' gestational age). It is tempting to speculate that the consequences of vitamin E deficiency in such infants might be modified or eliminated by the routine and early administration and absorption of a biologically active water-soluble preparation.

Although the serum folic acid level was low in this infant, a finding common in many premature infants,[26] folate deficiency does not play a role in the development of the early anemia of prematurity. Evidence indicates that the administration of folic acid to such infants, even in the absence of vitamin E deficiency, does nothing more than raise the level of circulating folic acid.

The administration of iron during this early period of life, on the other hand, has a significant relationship to vitamin E. Not only does it interfere with the intestinal absorption of tocopherol[18] but also, when given in large amounts, it intensifies the hemolytic process, presumably as a result of its pro-oxidant effect in heightening peroxidation of lipid membranes. It is advisable, therefore, to defer the practice of administering large amounts of oral or parenteral iron early in the life of a small premature infant (in anticipation of a late-occurring iron deficiency) until such infants attain vitamin E sufficiency (i.e., three months of age).

Other causes of hemolytic anemia in the newborn include ABO and, to a lesser extent, Rh erythroblastosis. Less frequently occurring are the inherited disorders in the glycolytic mechanism (i.e., deficiencies of glucose-6-phosphate dehydrogenase, pyruvate kinase, etc.) or defects in structure (i.e., hereditary spherocytosis, elliptocytosis, and congenital pyknocytosis), all of which may produce significant anemia and hyperbilirubinemia (the latter of sufficient degree to require treatment with exchange transfusion). The disorders of hemoglobin synthesis, with the exception of Bart's, rarely are apparent before the middle of the first year of life.

Among the aregenerative or megaloblastic anemias, juvenile pernicious anemia usually is not apparent before three months of age. In addition, only rare cases of folic acid deficiency anemias are identified during the same interval. Equally uncommon during this period of time are any of the varieties of pancytopenia or erythroid hypoplasia.

A Complicated Case

The history and clinical course of the next newborn infant provided the physicians who cared for her with almost the entire gamut of the currently reviewed acute hematologic problems as well as many related difficulties which are considered in other sections of this book. Since diagnostic efforts and the clinical management did not necessarily represent optimal care, questions are also provided for the reader's consideration.

Baby girl H, who was transferred from another hospital two hours after birth because of suspected Rh incompatibilty, was a term product of an uncomplicated pregnancy. One previous pregnancy resulted in a full-term, living child who had no difficulties in the newborn period, although the mother stated that labor was long and painful. The mother was type O, Rh negative, and antibody titers on two occasions early in pregnancy were reported as 1:64 and 1:128, respectively.

Under these circumstances, what further maternal history should be sought, and what further investigation would have been appropriate during the pregnancy?

Detailed knowledge of the first pregnancy and delivery, including maternal antibody titers.

Once an anti-D titer (anti-Rh) is identified, amniocenteses should be carried out in order to obtain chromogen levels, which are far more reliable than anti-D titers in estimating the degree of anemia in utero.

Actually, chromogen levels were obtained during this pregnancy and were reported as being in the low zone.

How should the physician interpret the results of the amniocenteses, and how might this information have affected the course of the pregnancy?

Chromogen levels in the low zone indicate well-compensated hemolysis, or more likely, minimal hemolysis. For this reason, the decision to allow the pregnancy to go to full-term was proper. High-zone chromogen levels obtained at 34 weeks' gestation usually indicate the need for intrauterine transfusion of Rh negative cells. If mid- or high-zone levels occur after 34 weeks, consideration regarding induction of labor or early delivery should be made.

Labor was said to be long and difficult, and the obstetrician reported that considerable effort was necessary to deliver the infant vaginally. Initial physical examination revealed an infant who was pale, cold, and cyanotic. Deep gasping respirations were noted, although auscultation indicated satisfactory pulmonary air exchange. Additional physical findings included a partial left brachial palsy and a slightly distended abdomen. The liver and spleen were not palpable. The laboratory values included a cord bilirubin D/T of 0.5/5.2 mg. per 100 ml.; central venous hematocrit 30 per cent; blood type O, Rh positive; and direct Coombs test 4+.

Given the historical, clinical, and laboratory findings at this point, how would one evaluate the infant's condition?

The difficulties in labor and delivery should cause suspicion that the infant's poor clinical condition immediately after birth was in some way related to these events. In retrospect, the partial brachial palsy was indicative of the vigorous extraction efforts. The condition of the infant at birth suggested that a catastrophic event had occurred in the immediate perinatal period. Although the blood type and positive direct Coombs test in association with a moderate elevation in cord bilirubin confirmed the presence of Rh incompatibility, the shock-like clinical condition in the absence of hydrops fetalis and the lack of demonstrable hepatosplenomegaly are more consistent with either acute hemorrhage or hemolysis rather than a chronic hemolytic process. Furthermore, the low-zone chromogen studies are in keeping with this impression.

What other laboratory information should be obtained as soon as possible?

The critical nature of her condition required the following essential information:
a. Arterial blood gases, pH, and blood pressure determinations.
b. Radiologic examination of both chest and abdomen in search of internal hemorrhage (and also to provide identification of the site of catheter placement).
c. Initiation of cross-matching procedures against fresh donor blood (less than three days old).

The arterial blood pressure was 24 mm. Hg; pH was 7.2; PaO_2 was 28 mm. Hg; $PaCO_2$ was 40 mm. Hg; and HCO_3 was 18 mEq. per liter. A stained film of peripheral blood showed increased numbers of immature red cells and adequate numbers of platelets. Following catheterization and blood drawing, several bandage changes were necessary in a short period of time to control oozing.

What is the significance of these blood gas and pressure values?

The patient had a metabolic acidosis without CO_2 retention. The low arterial blood pressure is indicative of hypovolemia, or at least peripheral pooling.

This baby also had respiratory insufficiency. A pH of 7.2 with a $PaCO_2$ of 40 mm. Hg is never normal. Newborn infants without respiratory insufficiency in response to an acidosis can ventilate sufficiently to bring the $PaCO_2$ to as low as 20. Similarly, the normal bicarbonate in infants is only 18 to 20 mEq. per liter. Consequently, it would be inappropriate to include bicarbonate infusion, since it does nothing to correct hypoxia per se, whereas plasma volume expanders are most appropriate. Likewise, this circumstance could have been avoided if some of the packed cells that were available at the time of the baby's delivery had been given with appropriate monitoring of central venous pressure. This would have permitted a subsequent exchange transfusion to be done under much more physiologic circumstances after the baby makes a normal circulatory adjustment to extrauterine life.

G. ODELL

What therapeutic approach should be carried out at this point?

Prompt treatment should be directed toward the maintenance of optimal body temperature, correction of the metabolic acidosis, improvement of the arterial PaO_2, and correction of the presumed hypovolemia (hypotension). In the last instance, this may be provided by an infusion of normal saline, plasma, or plasma expanders.

What is the next course of action?

The transfusion of appropriately cross-matched O, Rh negative, "routinely packed" cells, if time permits. Otherwise, use the freshest available whole blood.

This infant received 20 ml. per Kg. of O, Rh negative whole blood, following which the arterial pressure rose to 38 mm. Hg in association with moderate improvement in the respiratory status. Laboratory values for clotting studies performed prior to the transfusion became available and revealed markedly prolonged prothrombin and partial thromboplastin times, as well as decreased levels of fibrinogen and platelets. At this point, an exchange transfusion was carried out, following which the infant's clinical condition further improved with coincident repair of blood gases and pH. However, at five hours of age, the abdomen was noted to be distended and firm, and respirations became labored.

What was the role of the exchange transfusion?

Exchange transfusion is an effective way to treat DIC. In this infant it was performed on the assumption that the fundamental problem was anemia secondary to Rh incompatibility. It is therefore probable that this procedure fortuitously helped in the treatment of two separate disorders. Although citrated whole blood exchange transfusion for the treatment of DIC is known to be effective, in DIC with vascular collapse, exchange transfusions with heparinized (200 units per 50 ml.) whole blood has been recommended.

Given the change in the infant's course, what further studies should be done?

X-ray examination of the abdomen, repeat clotting studies, and needle aspiration of the lower abdominal quadrants.

X-ray examination showed a diffuse haziness throughout the abdomen, clotting studies were normal, and a peritoneal aspiration of the left lower quadrant returned fresh blood which clotted immediately. The hematocrit had fallen from a 37 per cent post-exchange level to 29 per cent. The history of a traumatic delivery and the evidence of blood in the abdominal cavity and corrected or normal clotting studies lent strong support to the presumptive diagnosis of an additional cause of the anemia (i.e., post-traumatic bleeding).

What are the two most frequent causes of internal bleeding in a neonate, and what guide can one use in distinguishing between them?

Capsular tears in the liver or spleen. Blood loss from hepatic capsular tears is usually self-limited and hence requires no direct surgical intervention. However, splenic rupture is a life-threatening event which can be corrected only by splenectomy. If the latter procedure is contemplated, arrangements must be made to obtain adequate supplies of fresh whole blood.

Over the next twelve hours, abdominal girth and distention steadily decreased, and the hematocrit and arterial blood pressure remained stable. At 24 hours of age, the infant developed seizure activity consisting of frequent, short episodes of tonic-clonic movements of the extremities. However, the seizures did not interfere with feeding or vital functions.

What studies should be undertaken to identify the etiology of the seizure activity?

Seizure activity under these circumstances falls into one of three categories:

a. Central nervous system bleeding, possibly related to anoxic damage or trauma.

b. Metabolic disturbances incurred in the early course of therapy (possibilities include hypoglycemia, hypocalcemia, hypomagnesemia, or hyponatremia—none of which was present in this infant).

c. CNS damage secondary to a wide variety of infectious agents.

Bacterial cultures were negative, a lumbar tap revealed xanthochromic fluid with no other abnormalities, and a serum bilirubin was D/T 0.6/12.4 mg. per 100 ml.

Should the bilirubin level at this point be of concern?

The reader should refer to the section on hyperbilirubinemia for a more complete exposition of this dilemma. Briefly, however, although the infant was full term, the period of anoxia and acidosis early in life could significantly alter bilirubin metabolism and therefore increase the risk of kernicterus.

The infant's seizure activity gradually ceased during the next seven days, and she began to gain weight on oral formula feedings. The infant was discharged at 16 days of life, at which time the hematocrit was 32 per cent.

What type of follow-up should be ensured?

In addition to a careful evaluation of this infant's physical and neurologic development, the hematocrit should be closely followed in the first few months of life. Increased red cell destruction due to Rh incompatibility may continue without the production of jaundice and result in a marked anemia. In such instances, it may be necessary to transfuse with packed cells (15 to 20 ml. per Kg.) should the hematocrit fall below 20 per cent.

Are vitamin E, iron, or folic acid indicated as adjunct therapy?

Neither vitamin E nor folate levels are abnormally low in the term infant, although it is possible that the demand for folic acid could rise in response to the increase in marrow activity. The possibility of iron deficiency, in view of the past history of some external blood loss and frequent blood specimens for laboratory determinations, would indicate the need for supplemental iron, administered in accordance with the suggestions in the section of this chapter devoted to iron metabolism.

REFERENCES

1. Abelli, A., and DeLamerans, S.: Coagulation changes in the neonatal period and in early infancy. Pediat Clin N Amer 9:785, 1962.
2. Abt, L., and Downey, W., Jr.: Melena neonatorum: the swallowed blood syndrome. J Pediat 47:6, 1955.
3. Ambrus, C., Ambrus, J., Niswander, K., et al: Changes in fibrin stabilizing factor levels in relation to maternal hemorrhage and neonatal disease. Pediat Res 4:82, 1970.
4. Cade, J., Hirsh, J., and Martin, M.: Placental barriers to coagulation factors. Its relevance to the coagulation defect at birth and to hemorrhage in the newborn. Brit Med J 2:281, 1969.
5. Ekelund, H., and Fumstrom, O.: Fibrinolysis in preterm infants and in infants small for gestational age. Acta Paediat 61:185, 1972.
6. Flod, N., and Ackerman, B.: Perinatal asphyxia and residual placental blood volume. Acta Paediat 60:1, 1971.
7. Gellis, S., and Lyon, R.: The influence of diet of the newborn infant on the prothrombin index. J Pediat 19:495, 1941.
8. Gross, S.: The relationship between milk protein and iron content on hematologic values in infancy. J Pediat 73:521, 1968.
9. Gross, S., and Melhorn, D.: Exchange transfusion with citrated whole blood for disseminated intravascular coagulation. J Pediat 78:415, 1971.
10. Gross, S., and Melhorn, D.: Vitamin E, red cell lipids and red cell stability in prematurity. Ann NY Acad Sci 203:141, 1972.
11. Hjort, P., and Rappaport, S.: The Schwartzman reaction: pathogenic mechanism and clinical manifestation. Ann Rev Med 16:135, 1965.
12. Karitzky, D., Leine, N., Pringsheim, W., et al: Fibrinogen turnover in the premature infant with and without idiopathic respiratory distress syndrome. Acta Paediat 60:465, 1971.
13. Kartizky, D., Pringsheim, W., and Kumzen, W.: Fibrinogen and fibrinolysis in the respiratory distress syndrome: observations during the first day of life. Acta Paediat 59:281, 1970.
14. Markarian, M., Githens, J., Jackson, J., et al: Fibrinolytic activity in premature infants: relationship of the enzyme system to the respiratory distress syndrome. Amer J Dis Child 113:312, 1967.
15. Markarian, M., Lindley, A., Jackson, J., et al: Coagulation factors in premature infants with and without the respiratory distress syndrome. Throm Diath Haemorrh 17:587, 1967.
16. Mauer, A.: Pediatric Hematology. New York, Blakiston, 1969.

17. Melhorn, D., and Gross, S.: Vitamin E dependent anemia in the premature infant. I. Relationships between iron and vitamin E. J Pediat *79*:569, 1971.

18. Melhorn, D., and Gross, S.: Vitamin E dependent anemia in the premature infant. II. Relationships between gestational age and absorption of vitamin E. J Pediat *79*:581, 1971.

19. Newman, A., and Gross, S.: Capillary and venous hematocrits in the newborn. Clin Pediat *6*:6, 1967.

20. Nielsen, C.: Coagulation and fibrinolysis in normal women immediately post partum and in newborn infants. Acta Obstet Gynec Scand *48*:371, 1969.

21. Nielsen, C.: Coagulation and fibrinolysis in prematurely delivered mothers and their premature infants. Acta Obstet Gynec Scand *48*:505, 1969.

22. Nossel, H., Lanzkowski, P., Levy, S., et al: A comparison of coagulation factor levels in women during labor and in their newborn infants. Throm Diath Haemorrh *16*:185, 1966.

23. Oski, F., and Delevoria-Papadopoulos, M.: The red cell, 2,3-diphosphoglycerate and tissue oxygen release. J Pediat *77*:941, 1970.

24. Oski, F., and Naiman, J.: *Hematologic Problems in the Newborn*. Philadelphia, W. B. Saunders Company, 1972. 2nd Edition.

25. Ratnoff, O.: The blood clotting mechanism and its disorders. DM, pp. 1–49, 1965.

26. Shojania, A., and Gross, S.: Folic acid deficiency and prematurity. J Pediat *64*:323, 1964.

27. Shulman, N., Aster, R., Pearson, H., et al: Immunoreactions involving platelets. V. Immunoreactions of maternal isoantibodies responsible for neonatal purpura. Differentiation of a second platelet antigen system. J Clin Invest *41*:1059, 1962.

28. Statement of the Committee on Nutrition, American Academy of Pediatrics: Iron fortified formulas. Newsletter, Vol. 21. (See also Pediatrics *48*:152, 158, 1971.)

29. Usher, R., and Lind, J.: Blood volume of newborn premature infant. Acta Paediat *54*:419, 1965.

30. Usher, R., Shepard, M., and Lind, J.: The blood volume of the newborn infant and placental transfusion. Acta Paediat *52*:497, 1963.

31. Walgren, G., Barr, W., and Rudhe, U.: Haemodynamic studies of induced acute hypo- and hypervolemia in the newborn infant. Acta Paediat *53*:1, 1964.

32. Zipursky, A., Hull, A., White, F., et al: Foetal erythrocytes in the maternal circulation. Lancet *1*:451, 1959.

Chapter 16

NEUROLOGIC PROBLEMS

by

SAMUEL J. HORWITZ, M.D.

"As for intelligence, there is a little friend of mine who three days after birth weighed only 950 grams. She is seven years old and speaks French and German. I think that the allegations regarding the permanent bodily and mental debility of weaklings . . . are entirely without foundation."

PIERRE BUDIN, *The Nursling*

The integrity and function of the nervous system are of utmost concern to the physician, nurse, and parents of the high-risk newborn infant. The aim is for intact survival. Primary disorders of the brain, spinal cord, muscle, and nerve account for a relatively small proportion of the neurologic problems of the infant. More frequently, the nervous system disorder is secondary to metabolic, physical, infectious, or environmental conditions, which may leave permanent sequelae. Conversely, the recognition and careful management of systemic disorders can and does minimize or entirely prevent permanent neurologic deficits.

The past decade has seen a remarkable change in the care of the high-risk infant. Previously, the physician caring for children with retardation and "cerebral palsy" regarded the high-risk neonatal unit as a continuing source of referral.[2, 3, 7, 11, 16] Today, this is no longer true[21, 22] and our own experience in the neurologic clinics suggests that the flow of patients being referred from the newborn nurseries has been reduced to a trickle.

Disease involving the brain of the infant is a source of major anxiety for the parents. The physician must maintain a considerate attitude and avoid gloomy prognostication unless he is absolutely certain that the prognosis is poor (e.g., in major congenital abnormalities).

There are many disorders that affect the nervous system of the neonate, but it is not possible to discuss all of these in this chapter. Instead, emphasis will be placed on remediable conditions, and the major thrust will be directed to the recognition and management of seizures, hypotonia, and the effects of hypoxia on the brain.

PATHOPHYSIOLOGIC CONSIDERATIONS

The nervous system of the newborn infant is extremely immature anatomically, chemically, and physiologically. The cerebral hemispheres show poor differentiation of gray and white matter; the majority of neuronal cells are present at birth but are immature in appearance and function. In the premature infant there is little myelination, and polysynaptic connections are only just beginning to form. The neurologic function is largely at brain stem and spinal cord level. The primitive infantile reflexes such as Moro, grasping, stepping, and placing reactions represent primitive released neuronal function largely uninhibited by higher cerebral control. Alterations of these primitive responses are usually nonspecific in terms of localizing the lesion, and may occur with either cortical or lower brain dysfunction. However, they may be of clinical value, particularly if asymmetrical reflexes or changes in the reflexes are noted.

Cortical function is difficult to evaluate. However, determination of visual perception has been a useful clinical index of cortical function in our experience.

The neonatal cortex is capable of producing abnormal neuronal discharges in the form of seizures which may manifest clinically in a variety of ways.

A large variety of primary structural nervous system abnormalities, as well as many causes of brain dysfunction secondary to systemic disorders, are described in the literature. An abbreviated list of some of these conditions is seen in Table 16–1.

The role of drugs as causes of nervous system malfunction secondary to systemic disorders should not be underestimated in terms of drugs administered either to the mother or postnatally to the infant himself. It must be remembered that when any drug is given to the mother, the fetus becomes an unwanted recipient of such an agent. Although commonly associated with depression (morphine, Demerol, etc.), intoxication with local anesthetic agents, either by direct puncture or from absorption through injudiciously administered paracervical block, can cause serious, and if not recognized early enough, fatal seizures. Depression and hyperexcitability can result from these agents.

Hyponatremia can occur both as a result of the inappropriate ADH response syndrome (see Chapter 14) and following the use of diuretic agents in the mother just prior to birth. In addition, hypernatremia has been implicated in the production of CNS hemorrhage and is capable of producing CNS damage in the experimental animal.

Finally, in addition to hypomagnesemia, which can result in seizures, hypermagnesemia secondary to the use of magnesium sulphate in the treatment of pre-eclamptic and eclamptic women has resulted in serious depression of the newborn. Recognition of this possibility is crucial, since it can be effectively treated by exchange transfusion with citrated blood (the citrate will bind magnesium, which is a divalent cation, thereby inactivating it in addition to simply reducing the total level, which the exchange transfusion with either citrated or heparinized blood would do).

L. STERN

Because of the lack of structural and functional maturity of neuronal tissue, there is a limited and stereotyped clinical response to a variety of pathologic conditions (see Table 16–2). Thus, the newborn infant with neurologic disorders (primary or secondary) may present a clinical picture in which the cause of

TABLE 16–1 CAUSES OF NERVOUS SYSTEM MALFUNCTION IN THE NEONATAL PERIOD

Primary in Central Nervous System

Prenatal:	*Congenital malformations:* microcephaly, hydrocephalus, hydranencephaly, encephalocele, meningomyelocele, polymicrogyria, megalencephaly, porencephalic cysts, chromosomal abnormalities, including trisomy 13–15, trisomy 18, trisomy 21, cri-du-chat syndrome
	Infections: cytomegalic inclusion disease, rubella, toxoplasmosis, congenital syphilis
	Neurocutaneous syndromes: neurofibromatosis, tuberous sclerosis
Birth:	*Mechanical birth injury:* tearing of dural sinuses and bridging veins, subdural, subarachnoid, intraventricular hemorrhage, depressed skull fracture, spinal cord injury (breech delivery), brachial plexus injuries

Secondary to Systemic Disorders

Prenatal and Birth:	*Infections:* Maternal sepsis Disseminated herpes simplex
	Drugs: Narcotics (heroin, Demerol) Barbiturates General anesthetic agents Local anesthetics
Postnatal:	*Hypoxia*
	Infections: bacterial meningitis, viral encephalitis
	Metabolic endocrine: Hypoxia; acidosis, hypoglycemia; hypocalcemia; hyponatremia; hypernatremia; hyperbilirubinemia; pyridoxine dependency; hypomagnesemia; aminoacidurias—phenylketonuria, maple syrup urine disease, hyperlysinemia; galactosemia; hyperammonemia; hypothyroidism
	Hemorrhage: Secondary to bleeding disorder including thrombocytopenia, disseminated intravascular coagulation
	Physical: Hypothermia, hyperthermia

Peripheral Nervous System and Muscle Disorders
Spinal muscular atrophy (Werdnig-Hoffman)
Neonatal myasthenia gravis
Myopathies—myotonic dystrophy

the problem is difficult to determine from the neurologic examination alone.

It is neither necessary nor desirable for the physician to memorize a handbook of differential diagnosis in order to solve the neurologic problem of a high-risk infant. More important is to realize that permanent struc-

TABLE 16–2 CLINICAL FEATURES OF NERVOUS SYSTEM DYSFUNCTION IN THE NEONATE

DECREASE IN NEURAL FUNCTION
Crying—absent, weak
Sucking—diminished, weak, incoordination of suck/swallow
Swallowing—absent, weak, with choking
Respiration—apnea, irregular
Limb movements—infrequent, asymmetrical
Tone—hypotonic
Primitive reflexes—diminished, absent, asymmetrical
Deep tendon reflexes—depressed
Visual perception—diminished

RELEASE OF ABNORMAL NEURAL FUNCTION
Cry—high-pitched, screaming
Tone—spasticity, rigidity, opisthotonus convulsions
"Jitteriness"—stimulus-sensitive myoclonus
Abnormal postures
Deep tendon reflexes—hyperactivity, sustained clonus

tural changes can and do occur in the brain if systemic disorders are not recognized and corrected promptly. Therefore, the causes of reversible, treatable abnormalities of function *must* be considered first in clinical management.

HYPOXIA

Experimental hypoxia in animals has produced a variety of lesions, often affecting brain-stem nuclei, but these are not generally consistent with the pathologic lesions noted in asphyxiated human infants. Term monkey fetuses subjected to episodes of partial asphyxia exhibit injury to structures in the hemispheres. This damage, when severe, may consist of a total bilateral hemispherical necrosis. With less severe injury, the necrosis may be restricted to the paracentral region and/or the basal ganglia. *After prolonged survival,* areas of necrosis are transformed into areas of nodular cortical atrophy, white matter sclerosis, and status marmoratus of the basal ganglia. These eventual long-term static lesions closely compare to the lesions of the human perinatal injury or cerebral palsy. The acute lesions in full-term infants most commonly found at our institution are degeneration of nuclear chromatin of neuronal cells in the hippocampus and pons. Only in extremely severe and rare instances are necrotic changes seen in cells of the remainder of the cerebral cortex.[23] In contrast, prematures most commonly develop subependymal hemorrhages which may rupture into the ventricles. Small

hemorrhages in the cerebellum and subarachnoid space are fairly frequent findings. Periventricular leukomalacia was demonstrated by Banker and Larroche[1] to be a highly typical lesion in prematures, but this has not been a frequent finding at this hospital. The lesions in midbrain and basal ganglia, often described in experimental hypoxia, are not found in human infants.[23] The reader is referred to the extensive work of Myers,[17–19] Towbin,[28–30] Banker,[1] Windle,[31] and Ross[25] for further details of the pathology of human and experimental neonatal hypoxia.

The clinical effects and non-neurologic sequelae of asphyxia are considered in Chapter 1. Perinatal asphyxia is associated with myocardial injury and heart failure. A vicious cycle is established, with asphyxia leading to diminished ventricular contractility and cardiac output. The consequent arterial hypotension contributes to the development of brain damage because of diminished cerebral perfusion. At the same time, impaired circulation to the heart increases the probability of myocardial injury. The development of myocardial injury in turn further impairs circulation. The neurologic picture of infants who have been asphyxiated is extremely variable. While some appear completely normal initially, others are severely depressed or comatose. Close observation of these infants in the early phases may reveal a paucity of spontaneous movements, absent or diminished crying, poor suck with incoordination of swallowing and depressed gag reflex, depression of primitive reflexes, and alterations of tone. Jitteriness may be seen for many days, as well as a wide range of abnormal movements, including all types of seizures.

A high-pitched cry, excessive irritability, hyperactivity, and exaggerated primitive reflex responses may also be observed. Respiration should be closely monitored, as periods of apnea may develop. These infants require intensive clinical observation with careful recording of neurologic status.

HEMORRHAGE

Mechanical tearing of the dural sinuses may occur following traumatic delivery in term infants, usually in the region of tentorium and falx, resulting in a massive hemorrhage which is usually fatal.

Focal intracerebral hemorrhage is often suspected but very rarely substantiated clinically or pathologically.

Subdural hemorrhage, with a thin layer of blood overlying the cerebral hemisphere, is common in cases of bleeding associated with tears of the sinuses or bridging veins. Development of secondary membranes, liquefaction of blood clots, and further fluid accumulation take place over a period of days or weeks. Thus, isolated, localized, space-occupying collections of subdural fluid are very rare in the immediate neonatal period. Review of the literature reveals very few cases of isolated subdural hematoma in the first week of life,[12, 26, 32] and our own experience corroborates this.

Intraventricular hemorrhage in immature infants may result from hypoxia with periventricular hemorrhagic infarction and rupture of the poorly supported deep veins into the ventricles.

Subarachnoid hemorrhage represents a very common site of bleeding in immature infants. It is associated not only with birth trauma but also with hyaline membrane disease. (The majority of infants dying with hyaline membrane disease who have received some form of assisted ventilation will have evidence of cerebral bleeding!) The bleeding usually occurs in the subarachnoid and/or intraventricular space, but its cause is as yet not fully established. The clinical picture in infants with hyaline membrane disease is characterized by catastrophic collapse developing over 15 minutes, usually occurring on the second or third day following a prolonged anoxic episode. The picture is that of shock, with pallor, cyanosis of mucous membranes, mottled skin, and poor pulses. Neurologic signs including squinting, sun-setting appearance, nystagmus, and jerking movements of the limbs may be observed.

We usually find persistent apnea followed by poor tone with minimal movements.

G. ODELL

Temperature often falls. There is a sudden onset of severe metabolic acidosis together with a fall in arterial oxygen tension and a drop in hematocrit. All infants developing these symptoms die within a few hours of their occurrence despite continued intermittent positive pressure respiration, administration of bicarbonate, and increasing environmental oxygen.[10]

The intraventricular hemorrhage seen in small infants who die of the respiratory distress syndrome is, we believe, a terminal anoxic phenomenon. Studies using radioactive iron have demonstrated that it is in fact so time-related in the course of the disease. It is, therefore, in our view, not at all related to the use of the respirators; its finding in infants who die following respirator therapy is a reflection only of the severity of the disease which necessitated the use of the respirator in the first place. It is also, in our experience, relatively rare in larger infants with hyaline membrane disease, suggesting that it is the smaller, more immature baby whose vessels (usually the anterior terminal vein) are more susceptible to hypoxic injury with resultant hemorrhage occurring.

L. STERN

Spinal tap may be of value in diagnosing subarachnoid and intraventricular hemorrhage (the CSF must be persistently heavily blood-stained to substantiate this diagnosis). Normal spinal fluid findings may be found in Appendices 34 to 36.

Cytologic examination of the spinal fluid in cases of cerebral hemorrhage shows a large number of macrophages containing erythrocytes or hemoglobin (erythrophagic). This finding may help in diagnosing small central nervous system hemorrhages. (Work is in progress.)

S. PROD'HOM

The presence of large quantities of blood may interfere with absorption of cerebrospinal fluid through the arachnoid granulations and may result in transient or permanent communicating hydrocephalus.[14] Serial head circumference measurements are imperative in order to recognize this late complication of subarachnoid hemorrhage.

ALTERATIONS IN TONE

The evaluation of tone in the newborn infant requires considerable experience, practice, and patience on the part of the physician. A detailed description of the assessment of tone in the newborn is included in Chapter 3, to which the reader is referred. Although much has been written about the hypotonic or floppy infant, establishing the cause of hypotonia is difficult and fraught with many pitfalls. The reader is referred to the excellent monograph by Dubowitz[6] (see also Appendix 37) for detailed study of this important group of disorders, the diagnostic features of which are summarized in Table 16–3. When a physician is confronted with a hypotonic infant, the history should be carefully reviewed and a detailed physical examination completed prior to the "taken for granted" meticulous neurologic examination. Electrodiagnostic study and muscle biopsy are indicated only if the clinical

TABLE 16–3 APPROACH TO THE DIAGNOSIS OF HYPOTONIA

ANATOMIC SITE		CEREBRAL	SPINAL CORD	ANTERIOR HORN CELL	NEUROMUSCULAR JUNCTION	MUSCLE
Pathogenesis		Malformation Hemorrhage Anoxia Metabolic Infection Drugs	Injury	Spinal muscular atrophy (Werdnig-Hoffman)	Neonatal myasthenia gravis	Congenital myopathy Myotonic dystrophy Glycogen storage
Clinical features	Alertness	Poor	Good	Good	Good	Good
	Cry	Poor	Normal	Normal/weak	Weak	Good
	Eye movements	Occasionally abnormal	Normal	Normal	Abnormal	Normal
	Tongue fasciculation	No	No	Yes	No	No
	Deep tendon reflexes	Normal or increased	Decreased or increased	Absent	Normal	Decreased or normal
Laboratory aids	Muscle bulk	Normal	Normal	Decreased	Normal	Decreased
	Electromyography	Normal	Normal	Neurogenic pattern	± Normal	Myopathic pattern
	Muscle biopsy	Normal	Normal	Neurogenic group atrophy	Normal	Myopathic change
	Muscle enzyme (CPK)*	Normal	Normal	Normal	Normal	Normal or elevated
	Prostigmin test	Negative	Negative	Negative	Positive	Negative

*CPK = Creatine phosphokinase.
CPK is grossly elevated in Duchenne dystrophy, which does not usually manifest as hypotonia in neonates.

features point clearly to a structural neuro-muscular disorder.

Neonatal myasthenia gravis is a life-threatening disorder which requires prompt diagnosis. A history of maternal myasthenia gravis is the diagnostic giveaway. The clinical picture of hypotonia with respiratory weakness should always raise the possibility of this entity. The infants frequently have difficulty in eye closure, the jaw hangs open, and there is weak sucking and swallowing. The diagnosis is confirmed by intramuscular Prostigmin (0.1 to 0.2 mg.), which will produce dramatic clinical improvement within 30 minutes. The condition is transient and will usually subside within six weeks. During this time, administration of Prostigmin (0.2 mg. every six hours) will be necessary.

SEIZURES

The physiologically and morphologically immature neonatal cerebrum is capable of producing seizure discharges, but the clinical appearance of the seizures is considerably different from that manifested by the mature brain.[8, 9, 20, 22, 24, 27] Classical *grand mal convulsions* with tonic followed by clonic phase are not usually seen in the neonate. Similarly, the typical Jacksonian march of motor seizures and petit mal spells are most uncommon. On the other hand, the relatively advanced maturation of the subcortical structures, such as the hippocampal formation and its descending connections, results in considerable spread of discharges to adjacent neurons. This manifests in the production of primitive subcortical seizure movements, including respiratory arrest, chewing movements, ocular deviation, episodes of rigidity or acute flaccidity, and vasomotor changes. In place of the mature grand mal tonic and clonic seizure, the neonate demonstrates either migratory clonic jerking or sometimes alternating hemiconvulsions.[9]

Sustained, irregular focal jerking is fairly common and may affect different parts of the body in succeeding seizures. *Focal or generalized myoclonic jerking* may be seen either singly or repeated in clusters (infantile spasms, infantile myoclonic seizures). The generalized myoclonic seizure resembles the Moro reflex fairly closely. It should be clearly understood that the Moro reflex is induced by a sudden extension of the head on the trunk, and a startle reflex can be evoked by jolting the in-cubator. In contrast, myoclonic seizures are generally spontaneous and unprovoked. In "jittery" infants, the Moro reflex may be followed by several very rapid clonic jerks of the extremities, especially of the arms. These clonic movements should not be regarded as seizures. Rapid clonic jerking follows spontaneous movements of the arms and legs in these infants. Only a period of prolonged observation establishing relationship of the "jittery" movements to spontaneous movements of the limbs or startle reflex can differentiate them from seizures. "Jitteriness" is frequently noted in hypoglycemia and following hypoxia; often no cause is found, and this phenomenon may be transient without any permanent residua.

Status Epilepticus. Status epilepticus may be defined as frequently recurring seizures without full recovery of consciousness between seizures. Single seizures lasting beyond twenty minutes may also be regarded as constituting status epilepticus. Drug therapy in this situation should always be by intravenous route (See Table 16–6).

Epilepsia partialis continua. This condition is manifested by continuous jerking of one part of the body (e.g., a hand, or the mouth). This form of seizure is not harmful to the infant per se, but its presence usually indicates a significant structural lesion, such as infarction, cortical venous thrombosis, or serious infection. These seizures are extraordinarily difficult to stop with medication, and the physician is cautioned against over-vigorous therapy. Intravenous therapy should be avoided. Maintenance therapy with phenobarbital and diphenylhydantoin should be instituted.

Apnea. Apnea as the single manifestation of a seizure is extremely difficult to evaluate. Immaturity, metabolic derangements (e.g., hypoglycemia), sepsis, and respiratory distress, among others, are much more frequent causes of apnea than are seizures. The diagnosis of seizure in cases with apnea alone can only be made definite by use of electroencephalographic monitoring.[5]

CLINICAL APPLICATIONS

In the high-risk neonate, diagnosis of neural dysfunction requires the physician to answer the following questions:

1. Are the clinical features those of neurologic dysfunction?

2. Is the cause primarily in the nervous system or secondary to systemic disorder?

3. What diagnostic information is available from thorough history-taking and clinical examination?

4. Which pertinent laboratory tests should be ordered?

These questions must be asked in the framework of a critical concept. *Remediable disease must not be missed—protect the brain from damage!*

Prior to commencing the physical examination, it is of the utmost importance to observe the infant for a few minutes—observing respiration, cry, tone, limb movements, abnormal movements, or postures. (See Table 16-2.)

Asymmetrical movements of one side of the body usually indicates some structural lesion of the opposite cerebral cortex or of the brain stem. These are best documented by watching the spontaneous movements of the infant.

Deep tendon reflexes are normally symmetrical; the patellar, biceps, and triceps reflexes are generally the most easily elicited. The plantar responses are either extensor or show forced grasping.

It is especially important that the infant's head be maintained in the midline position during evaluation of reflexes, tone, and spontaneous movements; otherwise, asymmetry may occur from invoking the tonic neck reflex, and a faulty interpretation may be made as a result of this physiologic reflex.

As part of the routine neurologic examination, head circumference should be measured, eyegrounds examined in detail, and the skull transilluminated.

Head Circumference Measurement. Normal values are well established (see Appendix 16). Daily measurements are essential. Excessively rapid growth is always to be regarded with suspicion, hydrocephalus or subdural fluid collection being most likely causes.

Funduscopic Examination. This is a routine clinical examination and elicitation of the "red reflex" only is insufficient. The eye must be examined carefully and all quadrants of the retina evaluated. (Dilatation of the pupil with 10 per cent Neo-synephrine eye drops is essential for adequate visualization.) Congenital abnormalities, chorioretinitis, and hemorrhages are the most common lesions that may be found. Small retinal hemorrhages are not infrequently seen in otherwise well infants and are not pathologic per se. Large, subhyaloid hemorrhages usually denote intracranial

bleeding, especially in the subarachnoid and subdural spaces.

Transillumination of the Head. The infant must be taken into a completely dark room. The examiner must wait a few minutes for dark adaptation to occur. A flashlight is used with two "D" cells and a tight-fitting rubber cone over the front of the flashlight. The head is transilluminated systematically. If the halo of transillumination from the edge of the rubber cone exceeds *two centimeters* in the frontal regions and one centimeter in the occipital region, it is abnormal and the conditions listed in Table 16-4 should be considered.

Excessive transillumination is sometimes seen in premature infants because of the thin, poorly calcified calvarium. Subdural blood clots may not transilluminate until a few days have elapsed and liquefaction with fluid accumulation occurs. Therefore, repeat the test if the diagnosis of subdural hematoma is suspected.

Excessive transillumination should be further studied by echogram.

G. ODELL

PRACTICAL HINTS

1. In the neonate, the stereotyped clinical response of a variety of pathologic conditions makes differentiation of the underlying cause extremely difficult on the basis of clinical examination alone.

2. The neonate in his early hours of independent life may still have functional abnormalities due to carry-over or dependence on the maternal health (e.g., drugs, myasthenia gravis).

3. In assessing neurologic status, especially tone, note time of examination in relationship to feeding schedule and state of wakefulness of the infant. The ideal time to evaluate

TABLE 16-4 ABNORMAL
TRANSILLUMINATION OF HEAD

Scalp	Caput succedaneum
	Infiltration of I.V. infusion
Subgaleal	Cephalhematoma, encephalocele
Skull	Bony defects, thin calvarium
Meninges	Subdural hematoma or hygroma
	Arachnoid cysts
Brain	Hydrocephalus, hydranencephaly, porencephalic cyst, atrophy

neurologic function is just prior to a feed, when the baby is wide awake. Immediately after a seizure, the neurologic examination is not an accurate tool for assessment of the underlying cause or prognosis of the nervous system. In evaluating the symmetry of movements and tone, the head must be maintained in the midline to avoid changes due to the physiologic tonic neck reflex. The fundi cannot be said to have been examined adequately unless the pupils have been dilated.

4. Be reluctant to diagnose congenital cerebral defects in the absence of significant abnormalities of the head, facies, extremities, or internal organs.

5. Permanent structural changes can occur in the brain if systemic disorders are not recognized and corrected promptly (e.g., hypoglycemia). (See Table 16–5). Children with asphyxial convulsions are often damaged by failure to attend to supportive measures, such as treatment of hyponatremia and cerebral edema.

In the specific treatment of seizures secondary to intoxication with local anesthetic agents, a more important maneuver than the simple attempt at suppression of the seizures with anticonvulsants is exchange transfusion to remove or lower the concentrations of the agent in the infant's plasma and tissue compartments. Cases of such intoxication both from direct needle puncture accidentally during caudal anesthesia and from systemic absorption from paracervical block too close to the placental areas, unless recognized, have terminated fatally, with repetitive uncontrollable seizures. We have identified such an infant in whom, after paracervical block, measurable concentrations of mepiva-

TABLE 16–5 NEONATAL SEIZURES

Those Requiring Specific Treatment:
   Hypoglycemia
   Hypocalcemia
   Hypomagnesemia
   Hyponatremia and hypernatremia
   Pyridoxine dependency
   Drug withdrawal (heroin)
   Local anesthesia
   Septicemia, meningitis
   Aminoaciduria—phenylketonuria, maple syrup urine
      disease

Supportive and Symptomatic Treatment Necessary for Seizures due to:
   Developmental anomalies
   Cerebral birth trauma
   Cerebral hemorrhage (intracerebral, intraventricular, subarachnoid, subdural), cerebral thrombosis
   Anoxic encephalopathy
   Infection—Bacterial meningitis, encephalitis, toxoplasmosis, cytomegalic inclusion disease, herpes simplex

caine (Carbocaine) have been isolated from blood, urine, and CSF. These infants present with intractable seizures immediately upon birth, accompanied by bradycardia. Recognition of the syndrome with immediate exchange transfusion has been reported as life saving.

L. STERN

6. One-third of perfectly normal premature infants under 12 to 15 days of age and weighing below 2 Kg. have apnea. This does not signify central nervous damage.

7. The clinical features of sepsis are so similar to anoxia that only the history and confirmation by bacteriologic study can differentiate this from central nervous dysfunction due to hypoxia.

8. I have often been at the bedside and observed a seizure which has not been recognized by inexperienced staff. Chewing and swallowing movements, often with nystagmoid deviation of the eyes and vasomotor changes, such as pallor or flushing, are not uncommon types of neonatal seizures. Full-blown grand mal seizures with tonic followed by clonic phases as seen in older children are uncommon in newborn infants.[22]

9. The most critical therapy is that of any underlying metabolic cause producing seizures. Convulsions due to asphyxia or epilepsia partialis continua cannot be stopped readily without the use of large doses of anticonvulsants, which may be extremely dangerous and depress respiration.

10. The electroencephalogram (EEG) may be of value in identifying neonatal seizures; however, therapy should not be postponed where EEG facilities are not available. Interpretation of EEG in the neonate is fraught with diagnostic pitfalls.[4, 5]

11. In the treatment of status epilepticus, diazepam (0.5 to 2.0 mg., given very slowly intravenously) is the drug of choice[15] and in our experience has been most effective and safe. (No significant complication with the use of this drug has occurred in neonates treated in the past three years.)

Diazepam does not directly cause hyperbilirubinemia. However, the contained sodium benzoate will cause displacement of protein-bound bilirubin and should not be used in jaundiced infants.

G. ODELL

Administration should be discontinued immediately if seizures stop or respiratory depression is noted. The latter is a constant threat with anticonvulsants given via the intravenous route, and the physician must always have facilities available to administer respiratory assistance. Diazepam may be repeated as necessary. Maintenance therapy of phenobarbital and/or diphenylhydantoin intramuscularly may be given immediately. In refractory cases, paraldehyde (four per cent solution) intravenously is a useful adjunct (Table 16–6).

12. Phenobarbital (3 to 7 mg. per Kg. per day I.M.) may be given as maintenance therapy to prevent further seizures. If this dose does not effect full control, diphenylhydantoin (Dilantin, 5 to 8 mg. per Kg. per day) may be added. Subsequent maintenance doses may be administered orally every eight hours. Duration of therapy will be dependent on cause and course of seizures and should be judged individually.

13. Constant attention to nutrition, temperature regulation, respiratory status, and metabolic balance is essential, no matter how severe the central nervous system disorder may appear.[15] There should be no gloomy prognosis given to the parents unless you are 100 per cent sure that permanent damage to the central nervous system has taken place.

Specific therapy for hypomagnesemia is worthy of mention not only because its therapy requires the administration of magnesium but also because its presentation is often confused with that of hypocalcemia,

TABLE 16–6 TREATMENT OF SEIZURES

General Measures
  Maintain airway.
  Oxygen if required.
Specific Therapy
  Hypoglycemia—I.V. glucose.
  Hypocalcemia—I.V. calcium gluconate.
  Pyridoxine dependency—I.V. pyridoxine.
Anticonvulsant Drugs
  Maintenance therapy (I.M. or P.O.)
    Phenobarbital (3–7 mg./Kg./day). If seizures continue, add diphenylhydantoin (5–8 mg./Kg./day).
  Status epilepticus (be prepared to intubate)
    Diazepam (Valium, 0.5–2.0 mg) *intravenously*, slowly (0.5 mg./minute).
    Repeat diazepam as required.
    Discontinue any single dose as soon as seizures stop or respiratory depression ensues.
  If Valium does not control seizures:
    Paraldehyde (4% solution*) intravenously over 10–15 minutes. (2.5–4.0 ml./Kg. of 4% solution)
    Repeat as required. Discontinue any single dose as soon as seizures stop or respiratory depression ensues.
    Start maintenance therapy as listed above.

  *10 ml. paraldehyde in 250 ml. of 2½% D/W in ½ normal saline or similar solution. Shake often.

which may, in fact, serve as an adequate screening test for hypomagnesemia itself. Thus, the hypocalcemia and hypomagnesemia usually occur together; however, in the presence of hypomagnesemia, the hypocalcemia is unresponsive to the administration of even massive amounts of calcium. The relationship between the two is not well understood, but it has been proposed that under conditions of hypomagnesemia there is interference with the release of calcium from bone and thus prevention of the normal turnover of calcium, which enables a normal serum calcium level to be maintained. Under such circumstances, both the low magnesium and low calcium levels will respond to the administration of magnesium (given as intramuscular magnesium sulphate) *alone*. The diagnosis, of course, should be suspected when magnesium levels indicate a low value (less than 1 mEq. per liter); however, magnesium determinations are not routine in most institutions and therefore the diagnosis may be missed. A good clinical guideline, therefore, as to when the magnesium determination should be done in order to ascertain a possible cause for convulsions is the failure of a hypocalcemic infant to respond to adequate calcium administration with persistence both of hypocalcemia and symptoms. In such instances, magnesium determination will often reveal the true nature of both the hypocalcemia and the resultant symptomatology, and appropriate steps can then be taken to correct them.

L. STERN

QUESTIONS

True or False

Intravenous phenobarbital cannot terminate seizures due to hypoglycemia.

Phenobarbital is a powerful anticonvulsant and may control seizures, irrespective of the underlying cause. Therefore, response to anticonvulsant drugs cannot be used as a therapeutic test. Therefore the statement is false.

In addition to acting as an anticonvulsant and thereby controlling the seizures of hypoglycemia, there is evidence that phenobarbital may have an additional specific effect on terminating hypoglycemic seizures. Experimental evidence suggests that animals made hypoglycemic with insulin, who have been pretreated with phenobarbital, have a greater partition between central nervous system and blood glucose; that is, there is more glucose in the brain for the equivalent amount in plasma. This suggests that the phenobarbital may have enhanced the enzyme system responsible for transport of glucose in the brain, and, since the hypoglycemic convulsions are dependent not on the amount of glucose in the blood but on that available for metabolism in the brain tissue, the advantage afforded by such a mechanism is obvious. It adds an additional reason as to why hypoglycemic convulsing infants should be treated not only with glucose but also with phenobarbital simultaneously. We cannot, however, agree that all seizures will respond to anticonvulsant drugs to the same extent, irrespective of their cause. In our experience, hypocalcemic seizures do not do well with phenobarbital, and hypomagnesemic convulsions are totally unresponsive to either anticonvulsants or calcium. Finally, the seizures due to metabolic inborn errors (i.e., pyridoxine deficiency or dependency) have, in our experience, been totally unaffected by such medication; indeed, the failure to elicit an even minimal response should alert the physician to the fact that the seizures may be of such underlying hereditary metabolic origin.

L. STERN

Continuous convulsive twitching of the mouth should be terminated with prolonged infusion of diazepam.

This continuous twitching (epilepsia partialis continua) may respond transiently to anticonvulsants; however, the seizures almost inevitably recur, and the continued use of large doses of drugs can and does lead to undesirable effects, especially respiratory depression. Therefore the statement is false.

Hemiparesis is most often due to a single large intracerebral hematoma which requires urgent diagnosis and surgical evacuation.

Isolated intracerebral hematoma in the newborn infant is extremely rare. Furthermore, surgical evacuation has no proven therapeutic benefit compared with conservative medical management. The statement is therefore false.

Jitteriness in the neonate may be an isolated and benign finding.

Careful physical examination is essential to look for an underlying cause, and laboratory tests are necessary in order to exclude hypoglycemia, hypocalcemia, or electrolyte disturbance. The statement, however, is true.

Cephalohematomas that transilluminate should be drained by needle aspiration.

These hematomas absorb spontaneously; therefore, needle aspiration is unnecessary and could initiate infection in the hematoma. Therefore the statement is false.

A cerebrospinal fluid protein level of 120 mg. per 100 ml. is normal in a 2000-gm. premature at age 16 days.

Protein levels may be very high in prematures (see Appendix 36). Therefore the statement is true.

Papilledema is an important sign in the diagnosis of hydrocephalus or cerebral edema in the neonate.

Papilledema is very rarely seen in small infants, because splitting of the cranial sutures and the open fontanel act as "safety valves" and pressure buildup in the optic nerve is thus prevented to a large extent. The statement is therefore false.

Cerebral edema secondary to hypoxia is not clinically evident in the neonate.

Bulging of the fontanel in the absence of acute intracranial hemorrhage is strong presumptive clinical evidence of cerebral edema. Furthermore, in fatal cases, the brain often shows the pathologic features of edema. Therefore the statement is false.

A bulging fontanel at age 24 hours is an absolute indication for subdural taps.

The fullness of the fontanel could be due to cerebral edema, subarachnoid or intraventricular hemorrhage, meningitis, or hypercapnia. If these causes were ruled out by appropriate diagnostic measures, subdural taps may be indicated. Therefore the statement is false.

Amyotonia congenita cannot be diagnosed in a floppy newborn infant.

Amyotonia congenita is a meaningless term, denoting no pathologically defined entity. There is no justification to continue the use of this term in pediatric diagnosis. Therefore the statement is true.

If a newborn infant has had asphyxial convulsions but at the time of discharge from hospital the neurologic examination is normal, this child has an 80 to 90 per cent possibility of normal brain function.

Provided that there are no residual neurologic signs, prognosis for infants with seizures in the neonatal period is excellent. Therefore the statement is true.

A repeatedly isoelectric EEG in a full-term infant denotes brain death, but this is not true in premature infants.

An isoelectric EEG on at least two occasions is evidence of cortical necrosis in term infants but not immature infants. Therefore the statement is true.

The EEG may be of predictive value for the neurologic outcome of neonates with seizures.

Rose[24] found that neonates with seizures and a normal EEG had an 86 per cent chance of normal development at age four years, regardless of other clinical data. In contrast, neonates with either a "flat," "periodic," or "multifocal" EEG had only a seven per cent chance of normal development. Unifocal EEG abnormalities do not show this correlation. Therefore the statement is true.

CASE PROBLEMS

Case One

T. G., a 2680-gm. male infant, was born at term to a 26-year-old mother, a known epileptic treated throughout pregnancy with phenobarbital (120 mg.) and diphenylhydantoin (300 mg. daily). The baby appeared normal until 30 hours of age, when he was noted to be lethargic, jaundiced, crying weakly, hypotonic, and Moro-depressed. The deep tendon reflexes were normal, and the tongue did not fasciculate. Fontanel was full but not tense, and the neck was supple. Head circumference was 33.5 cm. Transillumination was negative, and funduscopic examination was normal. Temperature was 35.3° C.

What could be the possible relationship between the anticonvulsant drugs taken by the mother and the hypotonia in the infant?

There is no significant cerebral depression of the infant whose mother is taking usual, therapeutic doses of anticonvulsants. However, anticonvulsants taken during pregnancy can cause coagulation defects in the neonate; thus, cerebral hemorrhage may occur more frequently. (The bleeding disorder associated with maternal anticonvulsant therapy responds to vitamin K and fresh frozen plasma.) In this infant, all coagulation studies were normal. It is unlikely that drugs taken by the mother will cause depression and hypotonia only at age 30 hours. Drugs affecting the fetus will usually cause problems at birth or soon thereafter.

What diagnostic steps are indicated?

Inspection of Table 16–3 reveals that an infant with hypotonia, lethargy, a poor cry, with normal deep tendon reflexes, is most likely to have central "cerebral" as opposed to peripheral nervous system disease. The fact that the baby, a normal size for gestational age, term infant, was perfectly well for the first 30 hours of his life, together with the rapid onset of symptomatology, is strong evidence against anoxic encephalopathy, cerebral birth trauma, or congenital malformation. (Infection or a metabolic derangement causing cerebral depression and hypotonia are more likely.) With realization of this information, this infant requires: CBC; spinal tap; cultures of blood, urine, skin, and throat; blood sugar, calcium, sodium, potassium, and pH determinations; X-ray of chest; and urinalysis. (With this clinical picture, I do not believe that muscle enzymes, EMG, or biopsy of muscle should even be considered.) Results of investigation: Hematocrit was 52; WBC was 12,200 with 60 per cent segmented polymorphs; urinalysis was normal; blood sugar was 42 mg. per 100 ml.; Ca was 8.0 mg. per 100 ml.; Na was 134; K was 4.6 mEq. per liter; pH was 7.37; pCO_2 was 32; and chest X-ray was negative. Spinal fluid was xanthochromic, 96 WBC with 60 polymorphs; sugar was 10 mg. per 100 ml.; protein was 279 mg. per 100 ml.; gram-stain of the spinal fluid was negative for organisms. (Refer to Appendices 34 to 36 for normal values.) There is thus an increase of white cells in the CSF, with low sugar and elevated protein.

In view of the negative gram stain of CSF, should this baby be treated immediately as a presumptive case of septicemia and meningitis?

Most definitely. The clinical picture together with the CSF abnormalities is highly suggestive of bacterial meningitis. Absence of a stiff neck and the fact that the fontanel was flat should not deceive the physician, as it is extremely rare to see neck stiffness in the early phase of bacterial meningitis in the newborn period.

[Culture of blood and CSF grew out of *E. coli* after 48 hours. The mother subsequently manifested a urinary tract infection with *E. coli,* and it would appear as if this were the source of the infection (see Chapter 12). One-third of cases of neonatal septicemia will be complicated by meningitis.]

Case Two

E. R., a 2700-gm. male infant, was born to a 26-year-old primigravida. The five-minute Apgar score was 9. Physical examination was normal.

Head circumference was 34.0 cm. Fundi were normal. At seven hours of age, the infant began having frequent brief hemiconvulsions, mainly left-sided, sometimes followed by transient weakness of the left leg. The baby was "jittery" between seizures, but no other physical abnormalities were detected on complete physical examination.

What laboratory tests should be done immediately?

Because hemiconvulsions can occur with metabolic disorders which are usually correctable, blood sugar, blood gases, electrolytes, calcium, and magnesium estimations should be performed, followed by a spinal tap. In this instance, the results were all normal.

What is the main purpose of the spinal tap?

The major purpose is to diagnose hemorrhage or infection, especially bacterial meningitis. A full spinal fluid analysis is essential in all cases; otherwise, useful data may be lost (e.g., low sugar levels).

What should the physician do next? Should he obtain neurosurgical consultation because of the predominance of left-sided seizures and transient hemiparesis?

It is time to treat the seizures. The immediately correctable disorders appear to have been ruled out. Pyridoxine (50 mg. I.V.) was given as a diagnostic test for the rare condition of pyridoxine dependency, but recurrences of seizures within 20 minutes negated this diagnosis. Treatment was started with I.M. phenobarbital (3 mg. per Kg.) stat. Seizures gradually became less frequent with maintenance therapy, but jitteriness remained. Neurosurgical consult was not obtained because a surgically correctable lesion causing seizures at this age is extraordinarily rare.

At age 48 hours, the infant was having approximately one brief seizure two to three times per day. He was feeding well.

What could the parents be told now?

No cause for the seizures has been found to date. As this baby looks well, has no obvious congenital malformations, sepsis, or evidence of cerebral hemorrhage and is responding to therapy, a serious and permanent underlying disorder is unlikely. The prognosis is guardedly good.

What additional investigations should be carried out?

Rare conditions, such as toxoplasmosis, cytomegalic inclusion disease, and aminoacidurias, require the appropriate laboratory tests. Skull X-ray, EEG, and STS should be checked, and a cerebral sonogram performed.

If all these tests are negative, can this be called "idiopathic epilepsy"?

Definitely not. This diagnosis is almost impossible in the neonatal period, and seizures at this age are always to be regarded as symptomatic (secondary).

Thorough re-evaluation of the case by the resident physician included a most important interview with the mother. She admitted to chronic heroin addiction, and the diagnosis was then clear.

Addicted mothers are notoriously unreliable informants concerning their drug habits, which often extend to substances other than heroin. The infants of addicts are often undergrown in utero, and there is also a tendency to premature delivery. Congenital malformations appear more commonly. Symptoms of withdrawal usually develop within the first 24 hours of life. The initial symptoms are those of neurologic disturbance, including a characteristic shrill cry, excessive yawning, coarse flapping tremors, irritability, hyperactivity, and seizures. Hyperpyrexia and excessive sweating are seen frequently. Gastrointestinal disturbances including vomiting and diarrhea are later manifestations. Symptoms may persist for weeks, particularly if the infants do not receive therapy. This is an extremely high-risk group of infants, and mortality — if symptomatic infants are untreated — is high.[13] Tremors, a shrill cry, and irritability are the most widely used indices of withdrawal manifestations, and may be used as indications for commencing therapy. Therapy includes careful attention to the thermal environment and close monitoring of fluid and electrolyte requirements. Drug therapy with Valium (diazepam), chlorpromazine, phenobarbital, or paragoric is successful for controlling symptoms. (More recently, withdrawal symptoms have also been reported for infants whose mothers took phenobarbital during pregnancy.)

Remember that *"cerebral" hypotonia is much more frequently the result of systemic disorders acting on the brain than primary disease originating in the brain.*

Case Three

J.P., a 1900-gm. female infant, was born to a 19-year-old primigravida at 33 weeks' gestation. In the last week of pregnancy, the mother became toxemic with blood pressure 160/100, and six hours prior to spontaneous onset of labor she had a brisk antepartum hemorrhage. Labor lasted three hours, and delivery was per vaginum. The infant did not breathe spontaneously, and required resuscitation for four minutes. The Apgar scores were 3 and 5 at one and five minutes, respectively. Acidosis was corrected promptly with sodium bicarbonate. Mild respiratory distress syndrome was present, and the infant was maintained in 40 per cent oxygen. At age 14 hours, she began having occasional spontaneous myoclonic jerks, and at 16 hours had an episode of apnea with chewing movements and rolling eye movements, lasting two minutes. Thereafter she had frequent (two to three per hour) episodes of generalized or focal jerking, accompanied by pallor and respiratory arrest lasting 30 to 60 seconds. Between seizures she was lethargic, would not suck, had a weak cry, and was hypotonic with deep tendon reflexes 1+. (Although this picture following preeclampsia might suggest hypoglycemia, the blood sugar, blood gases, serum calcium, and electrolytes were normal at this time.) The Moro reflex was absent. Seizures were controlled with intravenous diazepam and I.M. phenobarbital. All seizure activity ceased at 48 hours of age. At 60 hours, the baby was still limp, had no Moro reflex, and sucked very poorly. The cry was now high pitched and shrill. The urine was scanty, contained albumin, many casts, and 40 RBC per HPF. The anterior fontanel was full and bulging slightly.

What is the most likely cause of all the problems in this infant?

Perinatal asphyxia followed by anoxic encephalopathy with secondary renal effects could explain the clinical picture very adequately.

During the acute phase, what should the parents be told?

The cause of the infant's problems could be briefly outlined, mentioning that the seizures are a manifestation of cerebral dysfunction. A description of the clinical picture is helpful, together with your plans for therapy. At this stage it is not possible to predict whether any permanent cerebral damage has occurred. The physician should avoid the use of the term "brain damage."

What is the significance of the full fontanel?

Cerebral edema secondary to anoxia is the most likely explanation. This brain swelling may result in further neuronal damage although this is difficult to prove. Treatment of cerebral edema with dexamethasone is reasonable, but the ultimate benefit of this therapeutic measure in neonates has not been clearly proved.

We are quite concerned about the occurrence of cerebral edema following anoxic birth injury, since it may not only further potentiate the damage but also, by increasing intracerebral pressure, actually be a cause of debility and death in such infants. We have found the use of mannitol (1 to 2 gm. per Kg. given over a four-hour period) to be quite effective in reducing the edema and would much prefer it to the use of dexamethasone. Moreover, some of the symptomatology encountered initially in such infants may be due not to the anoxia but to the edema itself, and considerable improvement may often be anticipated once the edema has been controlled and/or subsides by itself.

L. STERN

How may damage to the infant's brain be prevented?

Prevention of further hypoxemia and elevated bilirubin, and careful attention to metabolic status and fluid and electrolyte balance, maintenance of blood sugar, calcium, and pH at normal values, together with prompt treatment of apnea, will prevent further insults to the central nervous system.

At age three weeks, the baby was doing very well, and the neurologic examination was normal.

What prognosis could the physician now give to the family?

A perfectly normal examination at this time indicates a strong possibility that no permanent damage resulted from the hypoxia, and the physician should indicate this. Statements such as, "We will have to wait until she starts to school to see if there is brain damage," should be strenuously avoided.

How long must the anticonvulsants be continued?

There is no absolute period. If no further seizures occur after approximately three to four weeks, the drug should be tapered and discontinued over a two to three week period. A normal EEG at this time is helpful in making this decision.

What long-term precautions should be taken by the parents with this girl?

None. Treat and regard her as a normal infant.

When can routine immunizations be started?

At the usual time.

REFERENCES

1. Banker, B., and Larroche, J.: Periventricular leukomalacia of infancy. Arch Neurol 7:386, 1962.
2. Brand, M., and Bignami, A.: The effects of chronic hypoxia on the neonatal and infantile brain. Brain 92:233, 1969.
3. Dann, M., Levine, S., and New, E.: A long-term follow-up study of small premature infants. Pediatrics 34:945, 1964.
4. Dreyfus-Brisac, C.: The electroencephalography of the premature infant and full-term newborn: Normal and abnormal development of waking and sleeping patterns. In Kellaway, P., and Petersen, I., Eds.: Neurological and Electroencephalographic Correlative Studies in Infancy. New York, Grune and Stratton, 1964, pp. 186–207.
5. Dreyfus-Brisac, C., and Monod, N.: Electroclinical studies of status epilepticus and convulsions in the newborn. In Kellaway, P., and Petersen, I., Eds.: Neurological and Electroencephalographic Correlative Studies in Infancy. New York, Grune and Stratton, 1964, pp. 250–72.
6. Dubowitz, V.: The Floppy Infant. Lavenham, Spastics International Medical Publications, 1969.
7. Fisch, R., Gravem, H., and Engel, R.: Neurological status of survivors of neonatal respiratory distress syndrome. J Pediat 73:395, 1968.
8. Freeman, J.: Neonatal seizures – diagnosis and management. J Pediat 77:701, 1970.
9. Gastaut, H., Ouachi, S., and Roger, J.: Non-Jacksonian hemiconvulsive seizures. Epilepsia 3:56, 1962.
10. Harrison, V., de V. Heese, H., and Klein, M.: Intracranial hemorrhage associated with hyaline membrane disease. Arch Dis Child 43:116, 1968.
11. Heimer, C., Cutler, R., and Freedman, A.: Neurological sequelae of premature birth. Amer J Dis Child 108:122, 1964.
12. Ingraham, F., and Matson, D.: Subdural hemorrhage in infancy. J Pediat 24:1, 1944.
13. Kahn, E., Neumann, L., and Polk, G.: The course of heroin withdrawal syndrome in newborn infants treated with phenobarbital or chlorpromazine. J Pediat 75:495, 1969.
14. Kibler, R., Cauch, R., and Crompton, M.: Hydrocephalus in the adult following spontaneous subarachnoid hemorrhage. Brain 84:85, 1961.
15. Lombroso, C.: Treatment of status epilepticus with diazepam (Valium). Neurology 16:629, 1966.
16. Lubchenco, L., Horner, F., Reed, L., et al: Sequelae of premature birth. Amer J Dis Child 106:101, 1963.
17. Myers, R.: The clinical and pathological effects of asphyxiation in the fetal rhesus monkey. In Adamson, K., Ed.: Diagnosis and Treatment of Fetal Disorders. New York, Springer-Verlag, 1969, pp. 226–49.
18. Myers, R.: Two patterns of perinatal brain damage and their conditions of occurrence. Amer J Obstet Gynec 112:246, 1972.
19. Myers, R., Beard, R., and Adamsons, K., Jr.: Brain swelling in the newborn rhesus monkey following prolonged partial asphyxia. Neurology 19:1012, 1969.
20. Prichard, J.: The character and significance of epileptic seizures in infancy. In Kellaway, P., and Petersen, I., Eds.: Neurological and Electroencephalographic Correlative Studies in Infancy. New York, Grune and Stratton, 1964, p. 273.
21. Rawlings, G., Stewart, A., Reynolds, E., et al: Changing prognosis for infants of very low birth weight. Lancet 1:516, 1971.
22. Robertson, A., and Crichton, J.: Neurological sequelae in children with neonatal respiratory distress: Infants with low birth weight. Amer J Dis Child 117:271, 1969.
23. Roessman, U.: Personal communication.
24. Rose, A., and Lombroso, C.: Neonatal seizure states: A study of clinical, pathological, and electroencephalographic features in 137 full-term babies with a long-term follow-up. Pediatrics 45:404, 1970.
25. Ross, J., and Dimmette, R.: Subependymal cerebral hemorrhage in infancy. Amer J Dis Child 110:531, 1965.
26. Schipke, R., Riege, D., and Scoville, W.: Acute subdural hemorrhage at birth. Pediatrics 14:468, 1954.
27. Schwartz, J.: Neonatal convulsions. Clin Pediat 4:595, 1965.
28. Towbin, A.: Cerebral hypoxic damage in fetus and newborn: Basic patterns and their clinical significance. Arch Neurol 20:35, 1969.
29. Towbin, A.: Mental retardation due to germinal matrix infarction. Science 164:156, 1969.
30. Towbin, A.: Central nervous system damage in the human fetus and newborn infant: Mechanical and hypoxic injury incurred in the fetal-neonatal period. Amer J Dis Child 119:529, 1970.
31. Windle, W.: Brain damage at birth: functional and structural modifications with time. JAMA 206:1967, 1968.
32. Yashon, D., Jane, J., White, T., et al: Traumatic subdural hematoma of infancy: Long-term follow-up of 92 patients. Arch Neurol 18:370, 1968.

JEFFERSON DAVIS HOSPITAL   TRANSITIONAL CARE NURSERY
ADMISSION SHEET

NAME	HOSPITAL NUMBER

BIRTH DATE _____ TIME _____ a.m. / p.m.   WHITE ☐   MALE ☐   NEGRO ☐   FEMALE ☐

ADMISSION TIME _____ a.m. / p.m. | Brought to Nursery by   Doctor ☐   Nurse ☐ | Brought to Nursery   In Incubator ☐   Carried in Arms ☐

Placed in   Isolette ☐   Gordon ☐   Armstrong ☐ | Admission   Heart Rate _____   Respiratory Rate _____   Temperature _____ | Dr._____ (NAME) Notified of Admission _____ a.m. at _____ p.m.

CONDITION ON ADMISSION

ADMISSION APGAR SCORE _____ SILVERMAN SCORE _____

COLOR: Cyanosis _____ Acrocyanosis _____ Pallor _____
Flushed _____ Mottled _____ Vasomotor Instability _____
Other _____

OXYGEN: Required Stat. _____ 1 or 2 Sources _____

SKIN: Warm or Cool to Touch _____ Meconium Staining _____ Petechiae _____
Ecchymosis _____ Forcep Marks _____ Rash _____

RESPIRATION: Regular _____ Irregular _____ Labored _____
Apneic _____ Apneic Pauses _____ Seesaw _____
Gasping _____ Nasal Flaring _____ Expiratory Grunt _____
Intercostal Retraction _____ Xiphoid Retraction _____ Subcostal Retraction _____
Other _____

CORD: Normal _____ Small _____ Large _____
Meconium Stained _____ Oozing _____ Pulsating _____
Number of Vessels _____ Other _____

ABDOMEN: Normal _____ Scaphoid _____ Distended _____
Other _____

ACTIVITY: Inactive _____ Hypoactive _____ Normal _____
Hyperactive _____ Other _____

MUCUS: None _____ Moderate _____ Excessive _____

PASSED MECONIUM: _____ VOIDED: _____

ANY ABNORMALITY OR ANOMALY: _____

OTHER: _____

ROUTINE ADMISSION CARE

TIME GIVEN: _____ a.m. / p.m.   If Deferred, State Why: _____

CREDE EYE CARE _____ CORD BLOOD _____
BATH _____ SEROLOGY _____
CORD CARE _____ TYPE, RH, & COOMBS _____
BIRTH WEIGHT _____ LENGTH _____ F.O.C. _____ CHEST _____

Admission sheet to transitional care nursery. (Jefferson Davis Hospital, Houston, Texas.)

JEFFERSON DAVIS HOSPITAL
TRANSITIONAL CARE NURSERY

		AGE								ADDITIONAL NOTES
DATE		TIME								
BED	Isolette	—	—	—	—	—	—	—		
	Gordon Armstrong	—	—	—	—	—	—	—		
OXYGEN CONCENTRATION										
HUMIDITY										
FEEDING	No Feeding	—	—	—	—	—	—	—		
	P. O. Feeding	—	—	—	—	—	—	—		
	I. V. Feeding	—	—	—	—	—	—	—		
	P. O. + I. V. Feeding	—	—	—	—	—	—	—		
CYANOSIS	No cyanosis – No O_2	—	—	—	—	—	—	—		
	Cyanosis in air – pink in O_2	—	—	—	—	—	—	—		
	Cyanosis in O_2	—	—	—	—	—	—	—		
ACRO-CYANOSIS	Absent	—	—	—	—	—	—	—		
	Present	—	—	—	—	—	—	—		
COLOR VARIATIONS	Normal	—	—	—	—	—	—	—		
	Flushed	—	—	—	—	—	—	—		
	Pallor	—	—	—	—	—	—	—		
	Vasomotor instability	—	—	—	—	—	—	—		
	Other – describe in notes	—	—	—	—	—	—	—		
JAUNDICE	None	—	—	—	—	—	—	—		
	Moderate	—	—	—	—	—	—	—		
	Severe	—	—	—	—	—	—	—		
ACTIVITY	No Activity	—	—	—	—	—	—	—		
	Diminished	—	—	—	—	—	—	—		
	Normal	—	—	—	—	—	—	—		
	Increased	—	—	—	—	—	—	—		
	Tremulous or jittery	—	—	—	—	—	—	—		
	Seizures	—	—	—	—	—	—	—		
	Other – describe in notes	—	—	—	—	—	—	—		
RESPIRATION RATE										
RESPIRATORY PATTERN	Normal	—	—	—	—	—	—	—		
	Seesaw	—	—	—	—	—	—	—		
	Irregular or apneic pauses	—	—	—	—	—	—	—		
	Other – describe in notes	—	—	—	—	—	—	—		
NASAL FLARING	None	—	—	—	—	—	—	—		
	Transient or mild	—	—	—	—	—	—	—		
	Severe	—	—	—	—	—	—	—		
EXPIRATORY GRUNT	None	—	—	—	—	—	—	—		
	Transient or mild	—	—	—	—	—	—	—		
	Severe	—	—	—	—	—	—	—		
RETRACTIONS	INTERCOSTAL None	—	—	—	—	—	—	—		
	Transient or mild	—	—	—	—	—	—	—		
	Severe	—	—	—	—	—	—	—		
	XIPHOID None	—	—	—	—	—	—	—		
	Transient or mild	—	—	—	—	—	—	—		
	Severe	—	—	—	—	—	—	—		
	SUBCOSTAL None	—	—	—	—	—	—	—		
	Transient or mild	—	—	—	—	—	—	—		
	Severe	—	—	—	—	—	—	—		

JEFFERSON DAVIS HOSPITAL
TRANSITIONAL CARE NURSERY

	AGE		ADDITIONAL
DATE	TIME		NOTES

SILVERMAN SCORE

CHEST BARRELLING	Absent								
	Present at rest								
	Present with stimulation								

RALES AND RHONCHI	Absent								
	Few or scattered								
	Generalized								

HEART RATE

HEART SOUNDS	Regular — fixed								
	Regular — not fixed								
	Labile								
	Other — describe in notes								

| HEART MURMUR | Absent | | | | | | | | |
| | Present — describe in notes | | | | | | | | |

ABDOMEN	Scaphoid								
	Normal								
	Distended								

BOWEL SOUNDS	Not heard								
	Hypoactive								
	Normal								
	Hyperactive								

RESPON-SIVENESS	No response								
	Diminished								
	Normal								
	Increased								

TONE	UPPER EXTREMITIES	Hypotonic								
		Normal								
		Hypertonic								
	LOWER EXTREMITIES	Hypotonic								
		Normal								
		Hypertonic								

RESPONSE TO STIMULA-TION	No response								
	Brief								
	Normal								
	Excessive								

CRY	DURATION	No cry								
		Brief								
		Normal								
		Excessive								
	CHARACTER	No cry								
		Brief								
		Normal								
		Excessive								

EDEMA	None								
	Mild								
	Marked								

MUCUS	None								
	Moderate								
	Excessive								

| MECONIUM | No | | | | | | | | |
| | Yes | | | | | | | | |

| VOIDING | No | | | | | | | | |
| | Yes | | | | | | | | |

NAME OF OBSERVER

APPROACHES TO FETAL ASSESSMENT

OBSTETRIC HISTORY AND EXAMINATION

Date of last menstrual period
Date when fetal movement first noted—normally 16 weeks' gestation
Date when fetal heart first heard—normally about 20 weeks' gestation
Height from symphysis pubis to top of uterine fundus
Screening of patients prenatally for syphilis, gonorrhea, and evidence of past rubella infection
Screening for evidence of infection of birth canal; e.g., herpes and increased use of cesarean section to enable infant to bypass infected birth canal
Emphasis on maternal nutrition (with less limitation on total weight gain) as relating to effects of malnutrition on developing brain

MATERNAL STUDIES THAT REFLECT THE STATUS OF THE PREGNANCY AND/OR THE PLACENTA

Estriol—most widely used
Diamine oxidase
Folic acid
Serum copper
Serum alkaline phosphatase
Chorionic gonadotropin
Placental lactogen

STUDIES ON AMNIOTIC FLUID

A. Examination of Cells from Amniotic Fluid

Sexing by (a) staining cells for chromatin
        (b) culturing for karyotype, to identify male fetuses with sex-linked diseases; e.g., hemophilia, muscular dystrophy
Cell culture for karyotype, to identify chromosomal abnormalities; e.g., translocation Down's syndrome
Cell culture for enzyme assay, to identify inherited metabolic disease; e.g., G-6-PD (hemolytic anemia); galactose-1-phosphate uridyl transferase (galactosemia)

Direct biochemical analysis of amniotic fluid cells, utilized to detect metabolic diseases; e.g., Pompe's disease, Tay-Sachs disease
Cytology for fetal age (squamous and fat cells)

B. Examination of Metabolites in Amniotic Fluid

Bilirubin in hemolytic disease
Pregnanetriol in congenital adrenal hyperplasia
Phospholipids (lecithin to sphingomyelin ratio) for fetal (especially pulmonary) maturity
Creatinine for fetal age

C. Examination of Color of Amniotic Fluid by Amnioscopy

Bilirubin staining—hemolytic disease
Meconium staining—fetal distress

FETAL SCALP BLOOD SAMPLING

Acidosis—fetal distress
Anemia—hemolytic disease; feto-maternal hemorrhage
Abnormal metabolites (placental excretion usually will prevent accumulation of metabolites by the fetus)

FETAL HEART MONITORING

Electrocardiogram—heart rate; specific patterns of change in fetal heart rate

ULTRASONOGRAPHY

Localization of placenta
Measurement of fetal biparietal diameter
Diagnosis of multiple pregnancy
Diagnosis of fetal abnormalities—hydrocephalus; anencephaly

RADIOLOGIC TECHNIQUES FOR FETAL SIZE AND AGE

Fetogram (classic) to determine size of fetus
fetal age (ossification centers)
fetal position
multiple pregnancy
fetal abnormalities
Dye injection into amniotic cavity to outline fetus (subcutaneous fat)

Appendix 3

COMPLICATED TRANSITION (NEONATAL MORBIDITY)

COMPLICATION	TRANSITION	COMPLICATIONS AND CARE

Immaturity
Transition is more difficult because of structural and metabolic handicaps, such as anatomically inefficient lungs, immature liver and kidneys, large surface area, and immature central nervous system.
	Slower reaction during transition.
	Prolonged and less clear-cut period of transition
	  initial tachycardia and unresponsive interval are delayed; secondary reactivity period begins at a later age (12 to 18 hours).
	Responses to repetitive stimuli more readily fatigued
	  not infrequently flaccid and nonreactive at delivery; maintains tone briefly (therefore, alerting behavior characteristic of term infant seldom seen).
	The more mature infant of low birth weight reacts like a larger infant of comparable gestational age in regard to temperature control, first reactivity period, etc.
		Observe for:
		1. Onset of respiratory distress early in the first reactivity period.
		2. Onset of apnea with bradycardia during the second reactivity period.
		3. Onset of apneic attacks as the tachypnea associated with respiratory distress changes over to irregular breathing with apneic pauses.
		
		Neurologic hyperexcitability.
		Lowered threshold for seizure activity.

Low Apgar Score (0–6) Poor response at birth may be related to inhalation anesthesia, drug depression, asphyxia, or intrinsic disease (infection, congenital anomalies, anemia, birth injury, etc., or combinations of these factors.	Do not follow predictable course. Have poor or unsustained response to birth stimuli. May show marked delay in transition: attain same peak heart rate and respiratory rates as term infants but peak is delayed; prolonged initial fall in temperature; delay in passage of air through GI tract and appearance of meconium stool. May exhibit exaggerations of normal respiration—grunting, retraction, apneic pauses. Excessive mucus—gagging. Neural hyperexcitability—hypertonus, tremulousness, abnormal eye movements, vasomotor instability. Majority recover rapidly (within 48 hours).	Infants not doing well by 48 hours may have complications (jaundice, septicemia, anemia, concealed bleeding, seizures, residual drug depression, etc.) Three complications noted during recovery appear to be significant: 1. Seizures. 2. Apneic attacks. 3. Feeding difficulty—suck is inefficient, swallowing may be uncoordinated with sucking, gag reflex is exaggerated or diminished.
Maternal Medications Condition at birth variable. May or may not require resuscitation.	First reactivity period usually normal. When effects of stimulation of birth process recede, infant demonstrates: shallow breathing with absence of deep breaths; barrelled chest; early scaphoid abdomen with delay of passage of gas through the bowel, delayed passage of meconium, and eventual abdominal distention; diminution of spontaneous activity with brief response to stimulation; normal cry of brief duration; normal or increased tone; poor sucking response; thermal instability.	Determine: 1. Need for artificial ventilatory assistance. 2. Need for parenteral fluids—when sucking and swallowing responses are poor. 3. Evidence of hypoglycemia—may have been masked by sedative drugs. 4. Time at which drug effects are diminishing—at this point the infant begins to perceive stimuli.

(Appendix 3 continued on opposite page.)

COMPLICATION	TRANSITION	COMPLICATIONS AND CARE
Abnormal Intrauterine Environment Infant survives by adapting to abnormal intrauterine conditions: 1. Maternal diabetes. 2. Chronic metabolic disease (thyroid, parathyroid). 3. Mothers on therapeutic or self-administered drugs (pyroxidine, tranquilizers, alcohol, narcotics).	May manifest abnormal clinical behavior during first days after birth. Must not only adapt to new extrauterine environment but also must re-program or abandon abnormal intrauterine metabolism.	Depending on cause of abnormal intrauterine environment, observe for complications, e.g., hypoglycemia, hypocalcemia, drug-withdrawal effects, etc.
Intrinsic Disease Infection Anemia and blood dyscrasia. Congenital anomaly. Birth injury. Inborn errors of metabolism. Must be diagnosed against a background of changing physical findings associated with transition.	Alters the orderly pattern of transition. In turn, the physical signs related to the disease process may be modified by the physical signs of transition.	

Appendix 4

HIGH-RISK FACTORS CONTRIBUTING TO PERINATAL MORTALITY AND MORBIDITY IN INFANTS

PRECONCEPTION—An awareness of the risk factor will place the decision about further procreation squarely with the parents

Family History

Serious hereditary and familial abnormalities—cystic fibrosis, osteogenesis imperfecta, Down's syndrome
Significant congenital anomalies involving the central nervous system, heart, or skeletal system
Blood dyscrasias—sickle cell disease
Socioeconomic problems—poor nutrition, unmarried and adolescent mother, ethnic background, medical indigency

Maternal History

Metabolic disease in the mother
    Endocrine—thyroid disease
    Amino acid—phenylketonuria
    Carbohydrate—diabetes
    Mucopolysaccharidoses
History of reproductive failures
    Miscarriage
    Toxemia of pregnancy
    Prolonged period of infertility
    Size of infant—history of previous premature or "small-for-dates" births
Anemia
    Sickle cell disease
    Thrombocytopenic purpura
    Hematocrit below 32 per cent
Height and weight
    Height under 60 inches

Prepregnant weight of less than 20 per cent under or over the standards for
   weight and height
Smoking

Obstetrical Factors

Maternal age
   Elderly primipara (over 35 years)
   Age over 30 years after short interpregnancy periods
   Age under 16 years
Excessive multiparity (over 5), especially when the gravida is over 35 years
   of age
Obstetric complications, past or present
   Blood group incompatibility
   Toxemia of pregnancy
   Placental separation
   Polyhydramnios or oligohydramnios
Paternal age over 40

PRENATAL — A number of factors occurring during pregnancy will alert the
          physician to the possibility of complications in the fetus, or
          ultimately in the newborn infant

Medical Factors

Maternal infection (Table 12–6)
Maternal medications (Appendix 7)
Maternal drug addiction — narcotics, barbiturates, amphetamines, LSD
Socioeconomic problems
   Poor nutrition
   Illegitimacy
   Absence of father
   Lack of prenatal care — long-delayed or absent
Stressful events
   Severe emotional tension
   Hyperemesis gravidarum
   Operations for surgical problems during pregnancy, especially under general
      anesthesia — appendicitis, cholecystisis, intestinal obstruction, pelvic
      neoplasm
   Critical accidents
Radiation
Cardiovascular disease
   Congenital heart disease
   Hypertension
Renal disease
Diabetes
Myasthenia gravis
Intercurrent chronic disease — pyelonephritis, malignancy

Obstetrical Factors

Abnormal presentation — breech, transverse, unengaged presenting part at term
Fetus that fails to gain normally or is disparate in size from that expected

Fetus over 42 weeks' gestation
Multiple birth
Toxemia of pregnancy (eclampsia and preeclampsia)
Fetal heart aberrations
Rh sensitization
Hemorrhagic complications—abruptio placentae, placenta previa, rupture of
   marginal sinus
Uterine rupture
Indication for cesarean section
Polyhydramnios or oligohydramnios
Cord prolapse

NATAL—A high-risk situation may occur only during labor or following
           delivery; hence the importance of constant observation and
           monitoring during labor and delivery and postnatally

Maternal or Fetal Conditions During Labor

Fever, other signs of infection
Premature onset of labor
Premature rupture of membranes
Fetal distress (tachycardia, bradycardia, meconium staining of amniotic fluid)
Fetal scalp blood showing asphyxia (pH 7.2 or lower)
Prolonged labor
Precipitous delivery
Complicated delivery
Cesarean section
Tight nuchal cord
Cord prolapse
Uterine rupture
Abruptio placentae
Heavy maternal sedation and/or anesthesia

Infant at Birth

Congenital anomalies (choanal atresia, micrognathia with cleft palate,
   diaphragmatic hernia, tracheo-esophageal fistula, cardiovascular anomalies,
   imperforate anus)
Single umbilical artery
Breech or other abnormal delivery
Meconium staining
Low Apgar score, especially at five minutes
Placental abnormality (massive infarction, amnionitis, amnion nodosum)
Multiple birth
Prematurity
Disproportion between weight or length and gestational age
Depression
Birth trauma
Abnormal respiration
Sepsis
Severe blood loss
Severe hemolytic disease

POSTNATAL

Infant In The Nursery

Abnormal respiration
Apneic episodes
Tremors
Convulsions
Vomiting
Abdominal distention
Failure to pass meconium (24 hr.)
Melena
Pallor
Petechiae
Jaundice — especially in first 24 hours
Thermal instability
Lethargy
Failure to void
Failure to regain birth weight by 10 days of age

Appendix 5

```
UNIVERSITY OF COLORADO MEDICAL CENTER          Date

   Newborn and Premature Infant Center          Ward
                                                Name
      MORBIDITY MODEL                           Hosp. No.

       Encircle the scores which apply and add to get morbidity score.

   Variable                                                 Score

    1.  Birth weight          1500 grams or less             61.7
                              1501 to 2000                   55.0
                              2001 to 2500                   15.8
                              2501 to 3500                    4.3
                              3501 or more                    5.0

    2.  Gestational age       27 weeks or less               21.6
                              28 - 31                        18.4
                              32 - 33                        15.0
                              34 - 35                         9.0
                              36 - 37                         3.8
                              38 weeks or more                1.1
                              unknown                         2.7

    3.  Mother's age          Less than 15 years              7.4
                              15 - 19                         1.9
                              20 - 34                           0
                              35 years or more                3.9

    4.  Condition at birth    good   (Apgar 8-10)               0
                              fair   (Apgar 5-7)              3.1
                              poor   (Apgar 0-4)             11.0

    5.  Toxemia                                                4.5
    6.  Diabetes                                              34.7
    7.  Fetal distress                                         4.2
    8.  Saddle, Spinal, Caudal anesthesia                      2.4
    9.  Labor complications*                                   4.1
   10.  PROM (24 hours or more before delivery)                6.3
   11.  Abnormal delivery                                      5.3
   12.  Positive pressure resuscitation                        6.4
   13.  Stimulants in delivery room                           11.8
   14.  Habitual aborter (3 or more)                          10.4
   15.  If male baby                                           4.1


                             Total score equals       ┌──────────┐
                             percentage risk of        │          │
                                 morbidity             └──────────┘

 *Induction, pit stimulation, uterine inertia, prolapsed cord, contracted pelvis,
  transverse arrest, antepartum hemorrhage, other.
```

Neonatal morbidity model. (Courtesy of Dr. L. Lubchenco.)

```
UNIVERSITY OF COLORADO MEDICAL CENTER      Date

  Newborn and Premature Infant Center       Ward
                                            Name
     NEONATAL DEATH MODEL                    Hosp. No.
```

Encircle the scores which apply and add to get neonatal death score.

	Variable		Score
1.	Birth weight	500 grams or less	68.6
		501 - 1000	61.1
		1001 - 1250	36.4
		1251 - 1500	14.4
		1501 - 2000	7.5
		2001 - 2500	1.4
		2501 - 3500	.7
		3501 - 4000	0
		4001 or more	1.4
2.	Gestational age	27 weeks or less	21.7
		28 - 29	8.0
		30 - 31	4.4
		32 - 33	2.2
		34 - 35	.7
		36 - 39	.2
		40 - 41	0
		42 - 43	.5
		44 weeks or more	.7
		Unknown	.7
3.	Mother's Age	Over 40	2.3
4.	Previous Neonatal Death		17.5
5.	Fetal deaths (more than 2)		1.3
6.	Condition at birth	good (Apgar 8-10)	0
		fair (Apgar 5-7)	.6
		poor (Apgar 0-4)	9.5
7.	Toxemia		2.2
8.	Fetal distress		.9
9.	Multiple birth		-4.9
10.	Positive pressure resuscitation		1.4

Total score equals percentage
risk of infant dying

Neonatal mortality model. (Courtesy of Dr. L. Lubchenco.)

Appendix 7

POSSIBLE EFFECTS OF MATERNAL MEDICATION ON THE FETUS OR NEWBORN*

NAME OF DRUG	EFFECT ON THE FETUS OR NEWBORN
Inhalation anesthetics: (cross placenta rapidly; neonatal depression directly related to depth and duration of anesthesia)	
Ether	Depresses infant by direct narcotic effect.
Cyclopropane	
Nitrous oxide	No significant depression if oxygen concentration administered to mother is adequate (20 per cent or more).
Trichloroethylene (Trilene)	No significant depression unless mother deeply anesthetized.
Methoxyflurane (Penthrane)	
Halothane (Fluothane)	No significant depression if drug given to mother for short duration. Danger of maternal hypotension with possible fetal hypoxia.
Local anesthetics:	
Lidocaine (Xylocaine)	Indirect effect of maternal hypotension with possible fetal hypoxia.
Mepivacaine (Carbocaine)	
Procaine (Novocain)	Direct injection into fetus—intoxication.
Tetracaine (Pontocaine)	
Hypnosis	Maternal hyperventilation, excessive bearing down.
Narcotics: (dose and time interval between administration and delivery are important in neonatal depression)	
Morphine	Depression of fetal respirations, bradycardia, hypothermia. Decreased responsiveness of newborn.
Meperidine (Demerol)	
Heroin	Babies born to narcotic addicts develop withdrawal symptoms of hyperirritability, shrill cry, vomiting. Can be fatal.
Methadone (Dolophine)	
Alphaprodine (Nisentil)	
Levorphanol (Levo-Dromoran)	
Dihydrocodeine	
Narcotic antagonists:	
Nalorphine (Nalline)	May in themselves have respiratory depressant action.
Levallorphine (Lorfan)	
Sedatives:	
Barbiturates:**	
Phenobarbitol	All barbiturates and thiobarbiturates cross the placenta. In usual clinical doses they cause minimal fetal depression.
Amobarbitol (Amytal)	
Secobarbitol (Seconal)	Larger doses—apnea, depression, depressed EEG.
Pentobarbitol (Nembutal)	Neonatal bleeding.
Thiopental (Pentothal sodium)	Increased rate of fetal or neonatal drug metabolism.
Thiamylal (Surital)	Decreased responsiveness and poor sucking ability in early neonatal period.
Chloral hydrate	No evidence of effects on fetus or neonate.
Ethchlorvynol (Placidyl)	No evidence of effects on fetus or neonate.
Paraldehyde	If given in large doses to mother, may cause respiratory depression or drowsiness of infant.
Thalidomide	Congenital anomalies, especially extremity anomalies (phocomelia).
Ethyl alcohol	No neonatal depression. May decrease uterine contractions. Withdrawal symptoms of twitching, hyperirritability, sweating, fever in babies born to chronic alcoholic mothers.

*Adapted from Bowes, W., Jr., Brackbill, Y., Conway, E. et al: The effects of obstetrical medication on fetus and infant. Monogr Soc Res Child Develop, Serial No. 137, Vol. 35, No. 4, June 1970.

**Barbiturates and some tranquilizers may potentiate the effects of inhalation agents and narcotics.

(*Appendix 7 continued on opposite page.*)

NAME OF DRUG	EFFECT ON THE FETUS OR NEWBORN
Tranquilizers:**	
Chlorpromazine (Thorazine)	No appreciable depressant action on fetus or neonate.
Promethazine (Phenergan)	Alterations of postnatal clinical behavior (withdrawal syndrome) appear during the neonatal period and during early infancy, and last for a period of months.
Prochlorperazine (Compazine)	
Hydroxyzine (Atarax, Vistaril)	
Meprobamate (Equanil, Miltown)	
Benzodiazepines (Librium, Valium)	
Reserpine	Nasal congestion with respiratory distress, excessive secretions, lethargy, decreased activity, bradycardia, hypothermia.
Skeletal muscle relaxants: (neuromuscular blocking agents)	
Curare	In usual clinical doses, these drugs do not cross placenta in amounts that cause any noticeable effect on fetus.
Gallamine triethiodide (Flaxedil)	
Succinylcholine chloride (Anectine)	
Decamethonium iodide (Syncurine)	
Steroids:	
Cortisone	Possible relation to cleft palate.
Hydrocortisone	
Prednisone	
Prednisolone	
Dexamethasone (Decadron)	Placental insufficiency syndrome, fetal distress during labor. Not fully substantiated.
Progestin	Masculinization of female fetus (nonadrenal pseudohermaphroditism of the female).
Testosterone	
Diethylstilbestrol	
Thyroid compounds:	
Desiccated thyroid extract	Crosses the placenta slowly but no known untoward effect on fetus.
Tri-iodothyronine (Cytomel)	
Antithyroid drugs:	
Propylthiouracil	All antithyroid drugs cross the placenta and can result in fetal goiters and hypothyroidism.
Methimazole (Tapazole)	
Potassium Iodide	Iodine compounds in excessive amounts (for control of asthma, expectorants) cause fetal nontoxic goiter.
I^{131}	I^{131} administered to the pregnant woman, even in the first trimester of pregnancy, may be disastrous for the fetus (athyrotic cretin).
Antidiabetic drugs:	
Insulin	No proven untoward effect.
Chlorpropamide (Diabinese)	Respiratory distress and neonatal hypoglycemia. Teratogenic effects suggested but not proved.
	Treated diabetic mothers have three times the incidence of fetal death in utero as compared with diabetic gravidas on insulin and diet alone.
Tolbutamide (Orinase)	Teratogenic effects suggested but never proved.
Anticoagulants:	
Heparin	No untoward effect.
Coumarins (Warfarin and Dicumarol)	Risk of fetal hemorrhage and death in utero. Hemorrhagic manifestations in newborn.
Antihistamines and antiemetics:	
Dimenhydrinate (Dramamine)	No evidence of adverse effect in human beings.
Cyclizine (Marezine)	
Meclizine (Bonine)	
Antimicrobial agents:	
Cephalothin (Keflin)	No untoward effect demonstrated.
Chloramphenicol (Chloromycetin)	"Gray syndrome" (gastrointestinal irritability, circulatory collapse, death) in newborns treated with this drug. Never proved to occur in newborn if drug given only to mother.
Erythromycin	No untoward effects demonstrated.
Kanamycin	Ototoxicity suspected but never proved in infants born to mothers treated for prolonged periods.

**Barbiturates and some tranquilizers may potentiate the effects of inhalation agents and narcotics.

(Appendix 7 continued on following page)

NAME OF DRUG	EFFECT ON THE FETUS OR NEWBORN
Novobiocin	Increase in hyperbilirubinemia if newborn treated, but not proved to occur if drug given only to mother.
Penicillin	No untoward effect.
Ampicillin	No untoward effect.
Streptomycin	Hearing loss (very rare) in infants whose mothers have been treated for prolonged periods in early pregnancy.
Tetracycline (Achromycin) Chlortetracycline (Aureomycin) Oxytetracycline (Terramycin) Demethylchlortetracycline (Declomycin)	Staining of deciduous teeth. Inconclusive association with congenital cataracts. Potential for bone growth retardation but not proved to occur in utero.
Sulfonamides: Short-acting Sulfadiazine Sulfisoxazole (Gantrisin)	Fetal and maternal levels equilibrate in two to three hours. Competes with bilirubin for binding sites on albumin.
Long-acting Sulfamethoxypyridazine (Kynex) Sulfadimethoxine (Madribon)	Present in fetal blood in two hours. Newborn serum levels present 506 days. Sulfonamides compete with bilirubin for binding sites on albumin but no untoward effect on newborn proved if only mother received drug.
Metronidazole (Flagyl)	No untoward effect.
Griseofulvin	No untoward effect.
Isoniazid (INH)	Unconfirmed, retrospective, and circumstantial evidence of psychomotor retardation.
Quinine, quinidine	Early reports of ototoxicity and congenital malformations unsubstantiated by extensive experience of many other authors. Danger of fetal damage probably minimal. Thrombocytopenia has been reported.
Nitrofurantoin (Furadantin)	Megaloblastic anemia in fetus with glucose-6-phosphate dehydrogenase deficiency.
Cancer chemotherapeutic agents: Aminopterin Amethopterin (Methotrexate)	Fetal death and multiple malformations; congenital anomalies.
Miscellaneous: Hexamethonium Ammonium chloride Thiazides Salicylates (Aspirin)	Paralytic ileus. Acidosis. Neonatal thrombocytopenia. No untoward effect in usual amounts. Death in utero. Hemorrhagic manifestations in newborn. Congenital salicylate poisoning reported in mother who took overdose.
Vitamin K and analogues Menadione sodium bisulfite (Hykinone) Phytonadione (AquaMephyton)	Hyperbilirubinemia, kernicterus.
Vitamin D_2 (irradiated ergosterol)	Large quantities administered to pregnant mother may cause congenital cardiac malformation.
Intravenous fluids	Electrolyte imbalance, usually hyponatremia (lethargy, poor muscle tone, poor color).
Smoking	Intrauterine growth retardation.
Radiation	Fetal death in utero or congenital anomalies (microcephaly, etc.). Actual teratogenic dose of ionizing radiation in man not yet determined. 1 rad to fetus may probably be harmless; up to 10 rads may be potentially dangerous; 10 rads or more probably harmful. Numerous individuals received 25 rads and infants normal.
Heavy metals (environmental pollution) Lead Mercury	Abortion; growth retardation; congenital anomalies.
Hallucinogens Lysergic acid (LSD), Mescaline, etc.	"Fractured chromosomes," anomalies (?).

EQUIPMENT FOUND ON THE UMBILICAL CATHETERIZATION TRAY, UNIVERSITY HOSPITALS, CLEVELAND, OHIO

2 2 cc. Luer-lock syringes.
1 Small needle holder.
2 Curved mosquito hemostats.
1 Straight iris scissors.
2 Straight mosquito hemostats.
1 Straight suture scissors.
1 Smooth straight iris forceps.
2 Smooth deep-curved iris forceps.
1 Medicine glass.
2 Cord ties (10 inches long).
2 3-way stopcocks.
4 3 × 3 gauze sponges.
1 Size 5-0 silk suture set with needle (#682).
1 Eye treatment sheet.
2 Needle caps.

Appendix 9

CONVERSION OF POUNDS AND OUNCES TO GRAMS

POUNDS	OUNCES 0	1	2	3	4	5	6	7	8	9	10	11	12	13	14	OUNCES 15
0	—	28	57	85	113	142	170	198	227	255	283	312	340	369	397	425
1	454	482	510	539	567	595	624	652	680	709	737	765	794	822	850	879
2	907	936	964	992	1021	1049	1077	1106	1134	1162	1191	1219	1247	1276	1304	1332
3	1361	1389	1417	1446	1474	1503	1531	1559	1588	1616	1644	1673	1701	1729	1758	1786
4	1814	1843	1871	1899	1928	1956	1984	2013	2041	2070	2098	2126	2155	2183	2211	2240
5	2268	2296	2325	2353	2381	2410	2438	2466	2495	2523	2551	2580	2608	2637	2665	2693
6	2722	2750	2778	2807	2835	2863	2892	2920	2948	2977	3005	3033	3062	3090	3118	3147
7	3175	3203	3232	3260	3289	3317	3345	3374	3402	3430	3459	3487	3515	3544	3572	3600
8	3629	3657	3685	3714	3742	3770	3799	3827	3856	3884	3912	3941	3969	3997	4026	4054
9	4082	4111	4139	4167	4196	4224	4252	4281	4309	4337	4366	4394	4423	4451	4479	4508
10	4536	4564	4593	4621	4649	4678	4706	4734	4763	4791	4819	4848	4876	4904	4933	4961
11	4990	5018	5046	5075	5103	5131	5160	5188	5216	5245	5273	5301	5330	5358	5386	5415
12	5443	5471	5500	5528	5557	5585	5613	5642	5670	5698	5727	5755	5783	5812	5840	5868
13	5897	5925	5953	5982	6010	6038	6067	6095	6123	6152	6180	6209	6237	6265	6294	6322
14	6350	6379	6407	6435	6464	6492	6520	6549	6577	6605	6634	6662	6690	6719	6747	6776
15	6804	6832	6860	6889	6917	6945	6973	7002	7030	7059	7087	7115	7144	7172	7201	7228
16	7257	7286	7313	7342	7371	7399	7427	7456	7484	7512	7541	7569	7597	7626	7654	7682
17	7711	7739	7768	7796	7824	7853	7881	7909	7938	7966	7994	8023	8051	8079	8108	8136
18	8165	8192	8221	8249	8278	8306	8335	8363	8391	8420	8448	8476	8504	8533	8561	8590
19	8618	8646	8675	8703	8731	8760	8788	8816	8845	8873	8902	8930	8958	8987	9015	9043
20	9072	9100	9128	9157	9185	9213	9242	9270	9298	9327	9355	9383	9412	9440	9469	9497
21	9525	9554	9582	9610	9639	9667	9695	9724	9752	9780	9809	9837	9865	9894	9922	9950
22	9979	10007	10036	10064	10092	10120	10149	10177	10206	10234	10262	10291	10319	10347	10376	10404

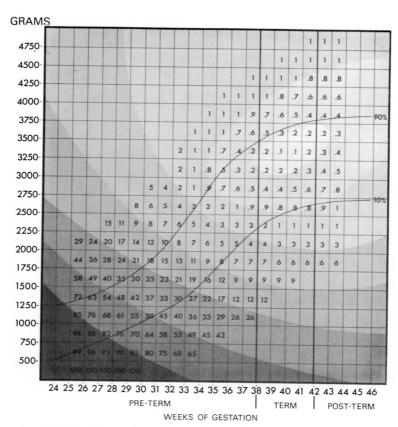

Classification of newborn infants and mortality risk. Newborn classification by birth weight and gestational age. Interpolated data are based on mathematical fit from original data from the University of Colorado Medical Center newborns, 7/1/58 to 7/1/69. Figures in each cell = per cent mortality risk. (Courtesy of Dr. L. Lubchenco.)

Appendix 11

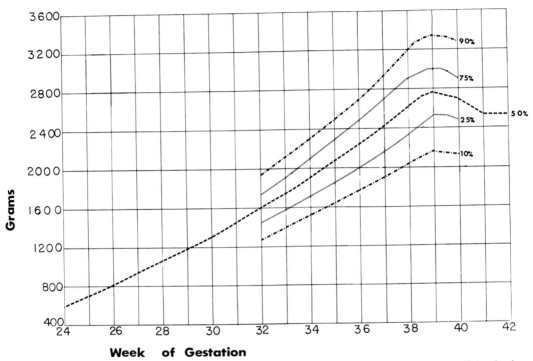

Dichorionic twins: intrauterine growth charts for both sexes. The weights of liveborn dichorionic twins at gestational ages from 24 to 42 weeks are graphed as percentages. (Naeye, R., Benirschke, K., Hagstrom, J., et al: Intrauterine growth of twins as estimated from liveborn birthweight data. Pediatrics *37*:409, 1966.)

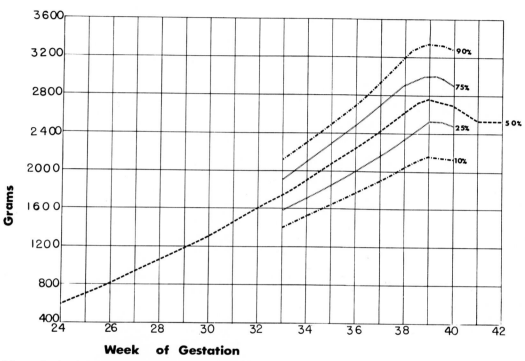

Monochorionic twins: intrauterine growth charts for both sexes. The weights of liveborn monochorionic twins at gestational ages from 24 to 42 weeks are graphed as percentages. (Naeye, R., Benirschke, K., Hagstrom, J., et al: Intrauterine growth of twins as estimated from liveborn birthweight data. Pediatrics *37*:409, 1966.)

Appendix 13

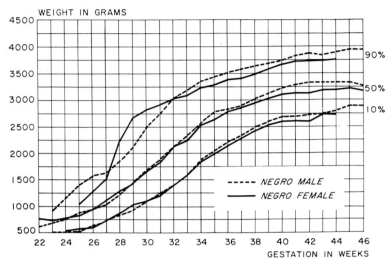

Negro infants: intrauterine growth chart. Male and female indigent Negro deliveries are graphed as percentiles. (Freedman, M., Graves, W., and Thompson, R.: Indigent Negro and Caucasian birth weight—gestational-age tables. Pediatrics *46*:9, 1970.)

	6 months 28 weeks	6½ months 30 weeks	7 months 32 weeks	7½ months 34 weeks	8 months 36 weeks	8½ months 38 weeks	9 months 40 weeks
I. POSTURE	Completely hypotonic	Beginning of flexion of thigh at hip	Stronger flexion	Frog-like attitude	Flexion of the four limbs	Hypertonic	Very hypertonic
2. HEEL TO EAR MANOEUVRE							
3. POPLITEAL ANGLE	150°		110°	100°	100°	90°	80°
4. DORSI-FLEXION ANGLE OF FOOT			40-50°		40-50°		Premature reached 40wk. 40° Full term
5. 'SCARF' SIGN	'Scarf' sign complete with no resistance		'Scarf' sign more limited		Elbow slightly passes midline		Elbow almost reaches midline
6. RETURN TO FLEXION OF FOREARM	Upper limbs very hypotonic lying in extension			Flexion of forearms begins to appear, but very weak	Strong 'return to flexion'. Flexion tone inhibited if forearm maintained 30 sec. in extension	Strong 'return to flexion' Forearm returns very promptly to flexion after being extended for 30 sec.	

Neurologic evaluation of Amiel-Tison. *A*. Active tone. *B*. Passive tone. *C*. Reflexes. (Amiel-Tison, C.: Neurologic evaluation of the maturity of newborn infants. Arch Dis Child *43*:89, 1968.)

Appendix 14B

	6 months 28 weeks	6½ months 30 weeks	7 months 32 weeks	7½ months 34 weeks	8 months 36 weeks	8½ months 38 weeks	9 months 40 weeks
1. LOWER EXTREMITY	—	Beginning of extension of lower leg on thigh upon stimulation of soles in lying position	Good support when standing up but very briefly (see illustration below)	Excellent righting reaction of leg - - -→ - - - - - - - → - - - - - - →			
2. TRUNK	—	—	—	± transitory	Good righting of trunk with infant held in vertical suspension (see illustration below)	Good righting of trunk with infant held in walking position (see illustration below)	
3. NECK EXTENSORS Baby pulled backward from sitting position	—	—	Head begins to right itself with great difficulty	Still difficult and incomplete	Good righting but cannot hold it	Begins to maintain head which doesn't fall back for few seconds	Keeps head in line with trunk for more than a few seconds
4. NECK FLEXORS Baby pulled to sitting position from supine	— Head pendulant	— Head pendulant	Contraction of muscles is visible but no movement of head	Head begins to right itself but still hanging back at end of movement	At first head is hanging back, then with sudden movement head goes forward onto chest	Head begins to follow trunk, keeps in line for few seconds in upright position	Difference between Extensors and Flexors has diminished (see illustration below)
			Straightening of legs 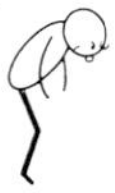		Straightening of trunk 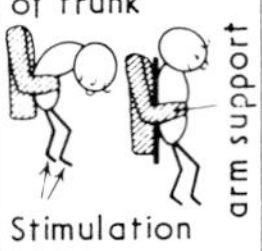 Stimulation arm support		Straightening of head and trunk together 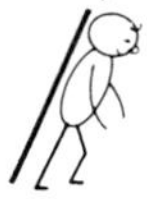

	6months 28weeks	6½months 30weeks	7months 32weeks	7½months 34weeks	8months 36weeks	8½months 38weeks	9months 40weeks
1. SUCKING REFLEX	Weak and not really synchronized with deglutition		Stronger and synchronized with deglutition	Perfect ---➤	-----------➤	----------➤	------➤
2. ROOTING REFLEX	Long latency period. Response is slow and imperfect		Complete and more rapid. Hand-to-mouth attraction established	Brisk Complete --➤ Durable	-----------➤	----------➤	------➤
3. GRASP REFLEX	Finger grasp is good and reaction spreads up whole upper limb but not strong enough to lift infant up off bed		Stronger	Stronger	The reaction of upper limb is strong enough to lift ---➤ infant up off bed	----------➤	------➤
4. MORO REFLEX	Weak, obtained just once, and not elicited every time		Complete reflex ➤ -------➤			----------➤	------➤
5. CROSSED EXTENSION	Flexion and extension in a random pattern, purposeless reaction		Extension but no adduction	Still incomplete	Good response with :- 1. Extension 2. Adduction ----➤ 3. Fanning of the toes	----------➤	
6. AUTOMATIC WALKING	—	—	Begins tip-toeing with good support on sole and a righting reaction of legs for a few seconds	Pretty good Very fast Tip-toeing		• A premature who has reached 40 weeks. Walks in a toe-heel progression or tip-toes • A full-term new born of 40 weeks. Walks in a heel-toe progression on whole sole of foot	

Appendix 15

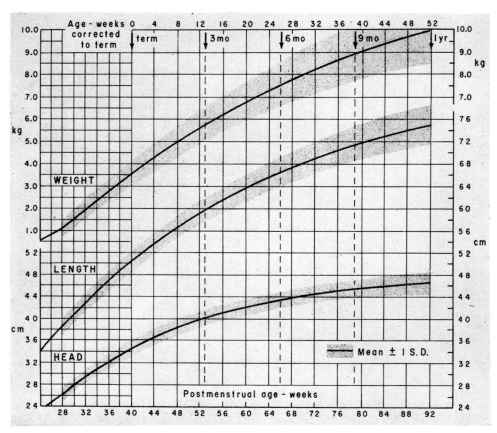

Growth record for infants in relation to gestational age and fetal and infant norms (combined sexes), University of Oregon. (Babson, S.: Growth of low-birthweight infants. J Pediat *77*:11, 1970.)

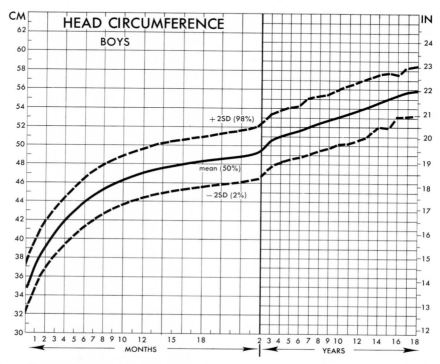

Head circumference. *A*. Boys. *B*. Girls. (Nellhaus, G.: Composite international and interracial graphs. Pediatrics *41*:106, 1968.)

Appendix 16B

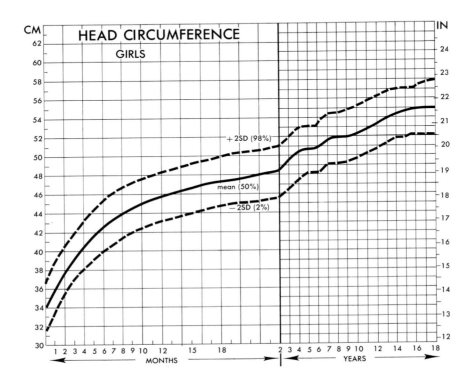

UNIVERSITY HOSPITALS OF CLEVELAND
PEDIATRIC HYPERALIMENTATION FORM

DATE _____

Physician Signiture _____

Patient's Name
Hospital Number
Date of Admission
Doctor's Name

PEDIATRIC HYPERALIMENTATION-BASE FORMULA ... EACH 1000 ml. CONTAINS

Protein Hydrolysate ....29 Gm.
Fructose ....58 Gm.
Dextrose ....195 Gm.
Sodium ....30 mEq.
Calcium ....9 mEq.
Magnesium..................9 mEq.
Potassium.................18 mEq.
Chloride ....21 mEq.
Phosphate ....25 mEq.
    Protein ....23 Gm.
    Calories 995
Phytonadione (Vit. K-1)......2 mg.
Folic Acid ....1 mg.
Vitamin B-12 ....10 mcg.

M.V.I. *Concentrate ....5 ml.

    M.V.I.*Concentrate 5cc provides:

Ascorbic Acid (C) ....500 mg.
Vitamin A.......................10,000 USP Units
Vitamin D (ergocalciferol)..........1,000 USP Units
Thiamine HCl (B_1).........................50 mg.
Riboflavin (as 5-phosphate) (B_2).............10 mg.
Pyridoxine HCl (B_5).........................15 mg.
Niacinamide ....100 mg.
Dexpanthenol ....25 mg.
Vitamin E (di-alpha tocopheryl ....5 int. Units
    acetate)

Heparin, Sodium...........................975 Units

ADDITIONAL REQUIREMENTS/1000 ml.

SODIUM (as chloride) . . . . _____ mEq/1000 ml.

CALCIUM (as gluconate) . . . . _____ mEq/1000 ml.

MAGNESIUM (as sulfate) . . . . _____ mEq/1000 ml.

POTASSIUM (as chloride) . . . . _____ mEq/1000 ml.

       (as phosphate) . . . . _____ mEq/1000 ml.

ABSOLUTE ALCOHOL. . . . . _____ ml/1000 ml.

OTHER_____

Rate of Flow_____ ml/Hr.

24-hour requirement. . . . in ml. _____ in _____ of containers
                                                 (Number)

Pediatric hyperalimentation form. (University Hospitals, Cleveland, Ohio.)

Appendix 18

RESPIRATORS AND THEIR MANUFACTURERS

Amsterdam Infant Ventilator
  G. L. Loos and Company's
  Fabrieken N.V.
  Postbus 663
  Amsterdam, Holland

Beaver Mark III
  British Oxygen Co., Ltd., Medical Dept.
  Hammersmith House
  London W6, England

Bennett
  Bennett Respiration Products, Inc.
  1639 Eleventh Street
  Santa Monica, California

Bird Mark VII and Mark VIII
  Bird Corporation
  Mark 3 Respirator Lane
  Palm Springs, California

Bourns Pediatric
  Bourns, Inc.
  6135 Magnolia Avenue
  Riverside, California

Cyclator
  British Oxygen Co., Ltd., Medical Dept.
  Hammersmith House
  London W6, England

East Radcliffe
  H. G. East and Co., Ltd.
  Sandy Lane West
  Littlemore, Oxford, England

Engstrom
  Mivab Elekro-Medicinska Apparater
  Luntmakargatan 12
  Stockholm, Sweden

Starling Pump
  C. F. Palmer (London), Ltd.,
  Myographic Works
  Effra Road
  Brixton, London SW2, England

DRUGS USED FOR CARDIAC PATIENTS IN THE FIRST MONTH OF LIFE

Digoxin	The P.O. level digitalizing dosage is 0.05 mg. per Kg. in the newborn period, rising to 0.08 mg. per Kg. at one month. The parenteral dosage is one-fourth less. *Indication* — Congestive heart failure; supraventricular tachycardia.
Quinidine	2 to 10 mg. per Kg. every 3 to 6 hours I.M. Total dosage per day — 10 to 30 mg. per Kg. (I.V. not recommended). *Indication* — Refractory supraventricular tachycardia, with digitalis; occasionally ventricular arrhythmias.
Procaineamide (Pronestyl)	10 to 100 mg. (One per cent solution, 10 mg. per cc.) — start with 1.5 to 2.0 mg. per Kg. — diluted in intravenous drip and titrated. (Can be repeated in 10 to 30 minutes; watch for hypotension). *Indication* — Refractory supraventricular tachycardia and ventricular arrhythmias.
Lidocaine (Xylocaine)	50 mg. in one per cent solution (10 mg. per cc.) — start with 1.5 to 2.0 mg. per Kg. — intravenous drip and titrated. (Can be repeated in 10 minutes). Watch for hypotension. *Indication* — Ventricular arrhythmias.
Propranolol (Inderal)	I.V. — 0.01 to 0.05 mg. per Kg. P.O. 0.5 to 1.0 mg. per Kg. per day in four doses. *Indication* — Supraventricular arrhythmia; anoxic spells as in severe tetralogy.
Edrophonium (Tensilon)	0.1 to 0.2 mg. per Kg. I.V. *Indication* — Supraventricular tachycardia.
Atropine	0.01 to 0.03 mg. per Kg. I.V. Max. 0.4 mg. per dose S.C. *Indication* — Bradycardia.
Prostigmine	0.04 mg. per Kg. I.M. *Indication* — Supraventricular tachycardia after digitalization.
Morphine	0.1 to 0.2 mg. per Kg. I.M. *Indication* — Anoxic spells as in severe tetralogy of Fallot; pulmonary edema.
Methoxamine	35 mg. in 250 cc. Titrated to bring blood pressure above normal. *Indication* — Anoxic spells as in severe tetralogy of Fallot; supraventricular tachycardia.
Epinephrine (adrenalin)	0.5 to 1.5 μg. per Kg. per min. I.V. 3 to 4 cc. (1:1000) in 250 cc. (ampules are 1:1000). *Indication* — Hypotension; severe refractory congestive heart failure.
Isoproterenol (Isuprel)	0.2 to 0.5 μg. per Kg. per minute 15 cc. (1:5000) in 250 cc. (ampules are 1:5000). *Indication* — Hypotension.
Ethacrynic Acid	1.0 to 1.5 mg. per Kg. I.V. 2 to 3 mg. per Kg. P.O. *Indication* — Diuresis.
Lasix	1.0 to 1.5 mg. per Kg. I.V. 2.0 to 3.0 mg. per Kg. P.O. *Indication* — Diuresis.
Mercuhydrin-aminophylline	Start aminophylline I.V. drip — 5 mg. per Kg. per 8-hour period; after 30 minutes give Mercuhydrin I.M. — 0.1 to 0.25 cc.

Appendix 20

NORMAL HEMATOLOGIC VALUES

VALUE	GESTATIONAL AGE (WEEKS)		FULL-TERM CORD BLOOD	DAY 1	DAY 3	DAY 7	DAY 14
	28	34					
Hb (gm./100 ml.)	14.5	15.0	16.8	18.4	17.8	17.0	16.8
Hematocrit (%)	45	47	53	58	55	54	52
Red cells (cu. mm.)	4.0	4.4	5.25	5.8	5.6	5.2	5.1
MCV (cu. micra)	120	118	107	108	99	98	96
MCH (picogm.)	40	38	34	35	33	32.5	31.5
MCHC (%)	31	32	31.7	32.5	33	33	33
Reticulocytes (%)	5–10	3–10	3–7	3–7	1–3	0–1	0–1
Platelets (1000's/cu. mm.)			290	192	213	248	252

MCV—mean corpuscular volume.
MCH—mean corpuscular hemoglobin.
MCHC—mean corpuscular hemoglobin concentration.

BLOOD CHEMISTRY VALUES IN PREMATURE INFANTS DURING THE FIRST SEVEN WEEKS OF LIFE* (BIRTH WEIGHT 1500-1750 GM.)

CONSTITUENT	AGE ONE WEEK			AGE THREE WEEKS			AGE FIVE WEEKS			AGE SEVEN WEEKS		
	Mean	*S. D.*	*Range*	*Mean*	*S. D.*	*Range*	*Mean*	*S. D.*	*Range*	*Mean*	*S. D.*	*Range*
Na (mEq./liter)	139.6	±3.2	133–146	136.3	±2.9	129–142	136.8	±2.5	133–148	137.2	±1.8	133–142
K (mEq./liter)	5.6	±0.5	4.6–6.7	5.8	±0.6	4.5–7.1	5.5	±0.6	4.5–6.6	5.7	±0.5	4.6–7.1
Cl (mEq./liter)	108.2	±3.7	100–117	108.3	±3.9	102–116	107.0	±3.5	100–115	107.0	±3.3	101–115
CO_2 (mM./liter)	20.3	±2.8	13.8–27.1	18.4	±3.5	12.4–26.2	20.4	±3.4	12.5–26.1	20.6	±3.1	13.7–26.9
Ca (mg./100 ml.)	9.2	±1.1	6.1–11.6	9.6	±0.5	8.1–11.0	9.4	±0.5	8.6–10.5	9.5	±0.7	8.6–10.8
P (mg./100 ml.)	7.6	±1.1	5.4–10.9	7.5	±0.7	6.2–8.7	7.0	±0.6	5.6–7.9	6.8	±0.8	4.2–8.2
BUN (mg./100 ml.)	9.3	±5.2	3.1–25.5	13.3	±7.8	2.1–31.4	13.3	±7.1	2.0–26.5	13.4	±6.7	2.5–30.5
Total protein (gm./100 ml.)	5.49	±0.42	4.40–6.26	5.38	±0.48	4.28–6.70	4.98	±0.50	4.14–6.90	4.93	±0.61	4.02–5.86
Albumin (gm./100 ml.)	3.85	±0.30	3.28–4.50	3.92	±0.42	3.16–5.26	3.73	±0.34	3.20–4.34	3.89	±0.53	3.40–4.60
Globulin (gm./100 ml.)	1.58	±0.33	0.88–2.20	1.44	±0.63	0.62–2.90	1.17	±0.49	0.48–1.48	1.12	±0.33	0.5–2.60
Hb. (gm./100 ml.)	17.8	±2.7	11.4–24.8	14.7	±2.1	9.0–19.4	11.5	±2.0	7.2–18.6	10.0	±1.3	7.5–13.9

*Adapted from Thomas, J., and Reichelderfer, T.: Premature infants: analysis of serum during the first seven weeks. Clin Chem *14*:272, 1968.

Appendix 22

COAGULATION FACTOR LEVELS, SCREENING STUDIES, AND FIBRINOLYSIS TIMES IN RELATION TO GESTATIONAL MATURITY

FACTORS	I	II	V	VII and X	VIII	IX	XI	XIII	PLATELETS	PTT	PT	TT	FT
	mg./100 ml.	*Per Cent of Normal*			*Mean*			*Titer*	*$\times 10^3/mm.^3$ (+S.D.)*	*Seconds*			
<1500 gm. 28–32 weeks	215	21	64	42	50	—	—	—	300 (70)	117	21	—	326
1500–2000 gm. 32–36 weeks	220	25	67	37	44	—	—	1/8	260 (60)	113	18	14	214
2000–2500 gm. 36–40 weeks	240	35	66	48	67	—	—	1/8	325 (75)	77	17	10	214
>2500 gm. Term	210	60	92	56	67	26	42	1/8	325 (70)	71	16	9	95
Mothers of premature infants	520	92	110	178	—	—	—	—	225 (45)	73	14	7	—
Mothers of term infants	500	92	110	206	196	130	69	1/16	215 (41)	75	14	8	278

PTT – Partial thromboplastin time
PT – Prothrombin time
TT – Thrombin time
FT – Fibrinolysis time
References: See Hematologic Problems, references 4, 15, 20, 21, and 22.

RESULTS OF COAGULATION TESTS ON NORMAL CORD BLOOD*

TEST	RESULT	AUTHORS
Clotting time	4 minutes (1–10 minutes)	Larrieu et al., 1952
		Fresh et al., 1956
Platelets	190,000±94,000/cu. mm.	Ablin et al., 1961
One-stage prothrombin	80%	Sanford et al., 1942
True prothrombin	53.5%	Douglas et al., 1955
	24.0%	Dyggve, 1958
Factor V	Normal	Quick et al., 1952
	100%	Fresh et al., 1956
Factor VII complex	29%	Loeliger et al., 1952
	43%	Douglas et al., 1955
Fibrinogen	231 mg./100 ml.	Taylor, 1957
	344 mg./100 ml.	Fresh et al., 1956
Factor XI	10–67%	Hilgartner and Smith, 1965

*Oski, F., and Naiman, J.: *Hematologic Problems in the Newborn*. Philadelphia, W. B. Saunders Co., 1966.

GLUTATHIONE LEVELS (MEAN) IN MG./100 ML. RBC PRE- AND POST-INCUBATION WITH ACETYLPHENYLHYDRAZINE

	PRE-INCUBATION	POST-INCUBATION
<1500 gm.	130	20
28–32 weeks		
1500–2000 gm.	120	20
32–36 weeks		
2000–2500 gm.	100	20
36–40 weeks		
>2500 gm.	70	35
Term		

HEMATOCRIT (PER CENT) –
MEAN ± [1 S.D.]

WEEKS	3 DAYS	1	2	3	4	6	8	10
<1500 gm.	54	48	42	35	30	25	25	28
28–32 weeks	[5]	[5]	[4]	[4]	[3]	[2]	[2]	[3]
1500–2000 gm.	59	51	44	39	36	28	28	29
32–36 weeks	[6]	[5]	[5]	[4]	[4]	[3]	[3]	[3]
2000–2500 gm.	59	51	45	43	37	31	31	33
36–40 weeks	[6]	[5]	[5]	[4]	[4]	[3]	[3]	[3]
>2500 gm.	59	51	46	43	37	33	34	36
Term	[6]	[5]	[5]	[4]	[4]	[3]	[3]	[3]

MEAN CORPUSCULAR HEMOGLOBIN CONCENTRATION (PER CENT)*

WEEKS	3 DAYS	1	2	3	4	6	8	10
<1500 gm.								
28–32 weeks	32	32	32	33	33	33	33	32
1500–2000 gm.								
32–36 weeks	32	32	32	33	33	33	33	32
2000–2500 gm.								
36–40 weeks	32	32	33	33	33	33	33	33
>2500 gm.								
Term	32	33	33	33	33	33	33	33

*MCV and MCH, the mean corpuscular volume and mean corpuscular hemoglobin in cu. micra and picogm. respectively, depend upon red cell counts which are not generally reliable.

HEMOGLOBIN (GM./100 ML.)
—MEAN ± [1 S.D.]

WEEKS	3 DAYS	1	2	3	4	6	8	10
<1500 gm.	17.5	15.5	13.5	11.5	10.0	8.5	8.5	9.0
28–32 weeks	[1.5]	[1.5]	[1.1]	[1.0]	[0.9]	[0.5]	[0.5]	[0.5]
1500–2000 gm.	19.0	16.5	14.5	13.0	12.0	9.5	9.5	9.5
32–36 weeks	[2.0]	[1.5]	[1.1]	[1.1]	[1.0]	[0.8]	[0.5]	[0.5]
2000–2500 gm.	19.0	16.5	15.0	14.0	12.5	10.5	10.5	11.0
36–40 weeks	[2.0]	[1.5]	[1.5]	[1.1]	[1.0]	[0.9]	[0.9]	[1.0]
>2500 gm.	19.0	17.0	15.5	14.0	12.5	11.0	11.5	12.0
Term	[2.0]	[1.5]	[1.5]	[1.1]	[1.0]	[1.0]	[1.0]	[1.0]

Appendix 28

RETICULOCYTE COUNT
(PER CENT)—MEAN ± [1 S.D.]

WEEKS	3 DAYS	1	2	4	6	8	10
<1500 gm.	8.0	3.0	3.0	6.0	11.0	8.5	7.0
28–32 weeks	[3.5]	[1.0]	[1.0]	[2.0]	[3.5]	[3.5]	[3.0]
1500–2000 gm.	6.0	3.0	2.5	3.0	6.0	5.0	4.5
32–36 weeks	[2.0]	[1.0]	[1.0]	[1.0]	[2.0]	[1.5]	[1.5]
2000–2500 gm.	4.0	3.0	2.5	2.0	3.0	3.0	3.0
36–40 weeks	[1.0]	[1.0]	[1.0]	[1.0]	[1.0]	[1.0]	[1.0]
>2500 gm.	4.0	3.0	2.0	2.0	2.0	2.0	2.0
Term	[1.5]	[1.0]	[1.0]	[1.0]	[0.5]	[0.5]	[0.5]

SERUM BOUND IRON
(μG./100 ML.) – MEAN $\pm$ [1 S.D.]

WEEKS	1	2	3	4	5	6	7	8	9	10
<1500 gm.	90	90	75	75	70	65	60	55	50	
28–32 weeks	[10]	[10]	[7]	[7]	[7]	[6]	[6]	[6]	[5]	
1500–2000 gm.	100	100	100	100	90	85	80	75	65	60
32–36 weeks	[12]	[12]	[12]	[12]	[10]	[8]	[8]	[7]	[6]	[6]
2000–2500 gm.	110	105	105	95	90	85	80	80	75	65
36–40 weeks	[12]	[12]	[12]	[10]	[10]	[8]	[8]	[8]	[7]	[6]
>2500 gm.	115	110	105	105	95	90	90	80	80	80
Term	[12]	[12]	[12]	[10]	[10]	[10]	[10]	[8]	[8]	[8]

Appendix 30

SERUM FOLIC ACID (SFA) —
MμG./ML.*

AGE	RANGE	MEAN ± S.D.
Normal premature infants		
1–4 days	7.17–52.00	29.54±0.98
2–3 wk.	4.12–15.62	8.61±0.55
1–2 mo.	2.81–11.25	5.84±0.35
2–3 mo.	3.56–11.82	6.95±0.50
3–5 mo.	3.85–16.50	8.92±0.86
5–7 mo.	6.00–12.25	9.02±0.74
Normal children		
1–6 yr.	4.12–21.25	11.37±0.82
Normal adults		
20–45 yr.	4.50–28.00	10.29±1.14

*Adapted from Shojania, A., and Gross, S.: Folic acid deficiency and prematurity. J Pediat *64*:323, 1964.

SERUM VITAMIN E (MG./100 ML.) — MEAN ± [1 S.D.]

WEEKS	1	2	3	4	5	6	7	8	9	10
<1500 gm.	0.40	0.30	0.25	0.25	0.25	0.25	0.25	0.25	0.35	0.45
28–32 weeks	[0.05]	[0.04]	[0.03]	[0.03]	[0.03]	[0.03]	[0.03]	[0.03]	[0.04]	[0.05]
1500–2000 gm.	0.45	0.40	0.40	0.45	0.45	0.45	0.50	0.50	0.60	0.70
32–36 weeks	[0.05[	[0.05]	[0.05]	[0.05]	[0.05]	[0.05]	[0.05]	[0.05]	[0.06]	[0.06]
2000–2500 gm.	0.50	0.45	0.50	0.60	0.70	0.75	0.75	0.75	0.75	0.80
36–40 weeks	[0.05]	[0.05]	[0.05]	[0.06]	[0.06]	[0.06]	[0.60]	[0.60]	[0.60]	[0.70]
>2500 gm.	0.55	0.55	0.55	0.60	0.75	0.80	0.85	0.85	0.85	0.85
Term	[0.60]	[0.60]	[0.60]	[0.60]	[0.70]	[0.70]	[0.80]	[0.80]	[0.80]	[0.80]

Appendix 32

WHITE CELL AND DIFFERENTIAL COUNTS IN PREMATURE INFANTS DURING FIRST FOUR WEEKS OF POSTPARTUM LIFE

BIRTH WEIGHT:	<1500 GM.			1500–2500 GM.		
Age in Weeks	1	2	4	1	2	4
Total Count (× 10³/mm.³)						
Mean	16.8	15.4	12.1	13.0	10.0	8.4
Range	6.1–32.8	10.4–21.3	8.7–17.2	6.7–14.7	7.0–14.1	5.8–12.4
Per Cent of Total						
Polymorphs						
Segmented	54	45	40	55	43	41
Unsegmented	7	6	5	8	8	6
Eosinophils	2	3	3	2	3	3
Basophils	1	1	1	1	1	1
Monocytes	6	10	10	5	9	11
Lymphocytes	30	35	41	9	36	38

THE WHITE BLOOD CELL COUNT AND THE DIFFERENTIAL COUNT DURING THE FIRST TWO WEEKS OF LIFE*

AGE	LEUKOCYTES	NEUTROPHILS			EOSINOPHILS	BASOPHILS	LYMPHOCYTES	MONOCYTES
		Total	Seg	Band				
BIRTH								
Mean	18,100	11,000	9400	1600	400	100	5500	1050
Range	9.0–30.0	6.0–26.0			20–850	0–640	2.0–11.0	0.4–3.1
Mean %	—	61	52	9	2.2	0.6	31	5.8
7 DAYS								
Mean	12,200	5500	4700	830	500	50	5000	1100
Range	5.0–21.0	1.5–10.0			70–1100	0–250	2.0–17.0	0.3–2.7
Mean %	—	45	39	6	4.1	0.4	41	9.1
14 DAYS								
Mean	11,400	4500	3900	630	350	50	5500	1000
Range	5.0–20.0	1.0–9.5			70–1000	0–230	2.0–17.0	0.2–2.4
Mean %	—	40	34	5.5	3.1	0.4	48	8.8

*Oski, F., and Naiman, J.: *Hematologic Problems in the Newborn*. Philadelphia. W. B. Saunders Co., 1966.

Appendix 34

CEREBROSPINAL FLUID FINDINGS IN FIRST 24 HOURS OF LIFE IN FULL-TERM INFANTS*

	RANGE	MEAN	2 S.D.
Red blood cells	0–1070	9	0–884
Polymorphs	0–70	3	0–27
Lymphocytes	0–20	2	0–24
Proteins	32–240	63	27–144
Sugar	32–78	51	35–64
Chloride	680–760	720	660–780

*Naidoo, T.: The cerebrospinal fluid in the healthy newborn infant. South Afr Med J *42*:933, 1968.

CEREBROSPINAL FLUID FINDINGS ON FIRST AND SEVENTH DAYS IN FULL-TERM INFANTS*

	DAY 1		DAY 7	
	Range	*Mean*	*Range*	*Mean*
Red blood cells	0–620	23	0–48	3
Polymorphs	0–26	7	0–5	2
Lymphocytes	0–16	5	0–4	1
Protein	40–148	73	27–65	47
Sugar	38–64	48	48–62	55
Chloride	680–760	720	720–760	720

*Naidoo, T.: The cerebrospinal fluid in the healthy newborn infant. South Afr Med J *42*:933, 1968.

Appendix 36

CEREBROSPINAL FLUID FINDINGS IN PREMATURE INFANTS

NUMBER	PER CENT XANTHROCHROMIC	PER CENT BLOODY	LEUCOCYTES PER CU. MM.	PROTEIN MG./100 ML.	REFERENCE
20	90	10	0–13 mean = 12	50–180 mean = 105	Wolf and Hoepffner*
100	97	1	7–44	1st wk. = 100 2nd wk. = 128	Otila**

*Wolf, H., and Hoepffner, L.: The cerebrospinal fluid in the newborn and premature infant. World Neurol 2:871, 1961.

**Otila, E.: Studies on the cerebrospinal fluid in premature infants. Acta Paediat Scand 35:(suppl. 8) 9, 1948.

SUGGESTED CLASSIFICATION
OF THE FLOPPY INFANT*

I. *Paralytic Conditions (weakness with incidental hypotonia)*
   1. *Proximal spinal muscular atrophies — neurogenic atrophies*
      (a) Infantile spinal muscular atrophy (Werdnig-Hoffmann's disease)
      (b) Benign variants
   2. *Congenital myopathies*
      (a) 'Structural' — Central core disease
                Nemaline myopathy
                Myotubular myopathy
                Mitochondrial abnormalities
                Miscellaneous
      (b) Metabolic — glycogenoses
   3. *Other neuromuscular disorders*
      (a) Muscular dystrophy — early onset Duchenne dystrophy
      (b) Congenital muscular dystrophy
      (c) Dystrophia myotonica
      (d) Myasthenia gravis
      (e) Periodic paralysis
      (f) Polymyositis
      (g) Peripheral neuropathies
II. *Non-Paralytic Conditions (hypotonia without significant weakness)*
   1. *Disorders of the central nervous system*
      (a) Nonspecific mental deficiency
      (b) Hypotonic cerebral palsy, athetosis, ataxia
      (c) Metabolic disorders: abnormalities of amino acid metabolism,
                abnormalities of mucopolysaccharide metabolism, lipidoses
      (d) Mongolism
      (e) Birth trauma, intracranial hemorrhage, anoxia
   2. *Hypotonia-obesity syndrome (Prader-Willi)*
   3. *Connective tissue disorders*
            Congenital laxity of the ligaments; Marfan's syndrome;
            Ehlers-Danlos syndrome; osteogenesis imperfecta; arachnodactyly
   4. *Metabolic, nutritional, endocrine*
            Hypercalcemia, renal tubular acidosis, rickets, celiac disease, hypothyroidism
   5. *Acute illness*
            Infection, dehydration
   6. *Miscellaneous*
            Congenital heart disease
   7. *Benign congenital hypotonia; "essential hypotonia."*

*Dubowitz, V.: *The Floppy Infant.* Lavenham, Spastics International Medical Publishers, 1969.

INDEX

Note: Page numbers in *italic* indicate illustrations.
Page numbers followed by t indicate tables.

Abdomen, masses in, transillumination of, 264
  scaphoid, in neonate, 33
Acidosis, in newborn, diagnosis of, 17
AGA (appropriate for gestational age) infant(s), 37, *37*
Adaptation, chemical, problems in, 168–182
Addict(s), and high-risk pregnancy, 6t
Addiction, maternal, effect of, on neonate, 298
Admission sheet, for transitional care nursery, *301*
Adoption, and behavior problems, 105
Alkali infusion, effects of, 19
Alkali therapy, in hyaline membrane disease, 140
Amiel-Tison, neurologic evaluation of, *323, 324, 325*
Aminopterin, effects of, on fetus, 24
Amnioscopy, in fetal assessment, 8, 26
Amniotic fluid, in fetal assessment, 26, 33
  studies of, 7, 304
Amphotericin B, indications for, in neonate, 217t
Ampicillin, in primary septicemia, 215
  indications for, in neonate, 216t
Analeptic(s), effect of, during secondary apnea, 18
Anemia, and high-risk pregnancy, 6t
  cesarean section and, 20
  hemolytic, in full-term infant, 200
Anesthetic(s), effects of, on fetus, 314t
Anomaly, Ebstein's, 241, *241*
Antibiotic(s), and vitamin K deficiency, 274
  in neonatal infection, 216t, 222
Antibody(ies), acquired by fetus, 207t
Anticoagulant(s), effects of, on fetus, 315t
Aorta, coarctation of, 246
Aortic pressure, measurement of, *126, 127*
Apgar score in newborn, 10, 11t, 12
Apnea, after feeding, 147
  and brain damage, 147
  as manifestation of seizure, 292
  effect of CPAP on, 154
  in immature infant, 144, *145*
  monitoring in, 146
  primary, 2, 11, 18
  secondary, 2, 12, 18
Argyle Umbilical Artery Catheter, 16
Arteriosus, true truncus, in neonate, 244
Artificial respiration, selecting infants for, 133t. See
  also *Ventilation, assisted.*
Ascites, in neonate, 259
Aspiration, suprapubic bladder, 261, *262*
  in pyuria, 267
Asphyxia, ability of newborn to survive, 4
  and brain damage, 3, 14
  and cerebral dysfunction, 299
  and convulsions, 19
  and lactic acid levels, 14

Asphyxia *(Continued)*
  and stillbirths, 7
  biochemical changes during, 4
  cesarean section and, 19
  circulatory changes during, 3
  duration of, 18
  effect of temperature on, 69
  in rhesus monkey, 2, *2*
  maternal diabetes and, 19
  pathophysiology of, 2
  renal manifestations of, 268
  sequelae to, 19
  treatment of, in utero, 8
Atresia, pulmonary, with hypoplastic right ventricle,
  239, *239*
  trucuspid, with hypoplastic right ventricle, 237, *238*
Atrial septal defect, in six-month-old infant, 230
  ostium primum type, 235
  physiology of, 234

Baby. See *Neonate.*
Bacitracin, indications for, in neonate, 217t
Balloon septostomy, 247, 248, 250
Barbiturates, effects of, on fetus, 24, 314t
  on neonate, 32
Barrelling of chest, in neonate, 33
Battered child syndrome, 106
Beckwith syndrome, in association with hypoglycemia,
  173
Behavior, of mother, during pregnancy, 99, 100, 100t
  toward neonate, 98–118
Bicarbonate, reabsorption of, by neonate, 258
Bilirubin, and exchange transfusion, *202*
  elevation of, in infant of diabetic mother, 201
  formation of, 183, *184*
Bilirubin-albumin binding, 190, 191
Bilirubin reduction light(s), and eye damage, 198
  color change in infant under, 200
  use of, 199
Birth weight, in relation to gestational age, 37, *37*
Bladder, suprapubic aspiration of, 261, *262*
Bleeding, cerebral, hyaline membrane disease and, 290
  internal, causes of, 284
Blood chemistry values, in prematures during first
  seven weeks of life, 333t
Blood circulation, fetal, 232, *233*
  neonatal, 234
Blood gas(es), changes in, during mechanical
  ventilation, 161, 165, 166
  during first days of life, *124*

Blood gas(es) *(Continued)*
  measurement of, 126, 127
  record sheet for, *148*
Blood loss, accidental, 270, 271
Blood pressure, vs. resistance, 233, *234*
Blood urea, and renal function, 268
Blood volume, in neonate, 271
Blood volume replacement, approach to, 272
Bloxom positive pressure oxygen-air lock, as
  resuscitative technique, 1
Body rocking, as resuscitative technique, 1
Brain damage, apnea and, 147
  following asphyxia, 14
Bronchopulmonary dysplasia, in neonate, 137, 139
  oxygen toxicity and, 147
  vs. pulmonary dysmaturity, 137t
Brown fat, function of, 60
Budin, Pierre, theories of, 98

Calcium, in fetus, 173
  in intravenous fluids, 84
  in neonate, 173, *174*
Caloric requirements, in neonate, 79, 79t
Cancer, and high-risk pregnancy, 6t
Carbenicillin, indications for, in neonate, 216t
Carbohydrate store(s), in SGA infant, 52
Cardiac. See also *Heart.*
Cardiac massage, external, as resuscitative
  technique, 10
Cardioversion, in supraventricular tachycardia, 253
Care, of mother, following stillbirth, 109
  with diabetes, 113
Cast(s), in neonate, 261
Catheter(s), radiopaque, 15
Catheterization, and neonatal infection, 222
  as cause of infection, 209
  complications of, 15
  in heart disease, 249, 251
  of umbilical vessel, 15
Cell growth, nutrition and, 81
Cell measurement(s), in neonate, 271
Cephalothin, indications for, in neonate, 217t
Cerebral arteriovenous fistula, vs. transposition of
  great arteries, 243
Cerebral dysfunction, following asphyxia, 299
Cerebral hemorrhage, 290
Cerebrospinal fluid findings, in prematures, 348t
  on first and seventh days of life, 347t
  on first day of life, 346t
Cesarean section, and anemia, 20
  and asphyxia, 19
  gastric aspiration following, 20
Chickenpox, effects of, on fetus, 211t
Chloromycetin, indications for, in neonate, 217t
Chvostek sign, in hypocalcemia, 175
Circulation, of newborn, changes in, during asphyxia, 3
  types of, *120*
Cleft palate, neonate with, 112
Clot formation, disorders of, in newborn, 278t
  system of, 273, *274*
CNP (continuous negative pressure), vs. oxygen, 154
Coagulation, disseminated intravascular, 277, 277t
Coagulation factor levels, in relation to gestational
  maturity, 334t
Coagulation tests, results of, on normal cord blood, 335t
Coagulopathy, consumptive, 276
Cold injury, neonatal, 67, *69*

Colon, perforation of, following umbilical vessel
  catheterization, 15
Convulsions, 292, 294, 294t, 295t
  in infant of heroin-addicted mother, 298
Cooney, Martin child hatchery of, 98, *99*
Cot nursing, advantages of, 65, *66*
Coxsackie virus, effects of, on fetus, 210t
CPAP (continuous positive airway pressure), 153, *153*
  nasal, 154, *155*
    guidelines for use of, 156t
  technique for, 153
Creatinine, in fetal assessment, 26
Creatinine level, of amniotic fluid, 7
Crigler-Najjar syndrome, 187, 190
Cryptorchidism, in neonate, 259
Cyanosis, during mechanical ventilation, 166
  heart defects and, 236, 237
  in congestive heart failure, 251
  in heart disease, 247, 248
  in hyaline membrane disease, 129
  in pneumothorax, 143
  in transient tachypnea, 141
  oxygen tensions and, 121
Cylindruria, in neonate, 257, 261
Cytology, of amniotic fluid, 7
Cytomegalic inclusion disease, vs. erythroblastosis
  fetalis, 213t
  effects of, on fetus, 210t

Death, intrapartum, 7
  neonatal, care of parents following, 117
    effect of, on mother, 109
Dehydration fever, 72, 225
Delivery, reaction of neonate to, 28
Dextrostix, in hypoglycemia, 177
  value of, 124, 126
Diabetes, care of expectant mother with, 113
  hypocalcemia in infant of mother with, 175
  hypoglycemia in infant of mother with, 170, 172, 180
  infant of mother with, prognosis for, 114
  maternal, and asphyxia, 19
    and high-risk pregnancy, 6t
    infant management in, 225
Diarrhea, in infant with *E. coli,* 225
Diazepam, in jaundiced infant, 294
Digoxin, in supraventricular tachycardia, 252
Dipalmityl lecithin, value of, 131
Drugs, analeptic, as resuscitative technique, 1
  effect of, on secondary apnea, 18
  for cardiac patients in first month of life, 331t
  maternal, effects of, on fetus, 34, 314t
    on neonate, 32
  hazards of, 24
Dubin-Johnson syndrome, 188

Ebstein's anomaly, 241, *241*
E. coli infection, in immature infant with diarrhea, 225
  maternal, infant management in, 223
Edema, pulmonary hemorrhagic, in neonate, 142
EEG, in neonate with seizure, 297
  isoelectric, 296
"En face" position, *101*
Endotracheal intubation, technique for, *13*
Endotracheal tube(s), in mechanical ventilation, 159,
  159, 160

Environment, neutral thermal, 71, 74
  of neonate, 58–76
    sensory, 70
    thermal, 58
      and body growth, 72
      disorders of, 67
      physiological considerations of, 60
      practical applications in, 63
Epidemic, in nursery, management of, 220t
Epilepsia partialis continua, 292, 296
Epinephrine, administration of, during resuscitation, 12
  in treatment of hypoglycemia, 173
Epispadias, in neonate, 259
Erythroblastosis, with hypoglycemia, 198
Erythroblastosis fetalis, 213t
Erythrocyte, in neonate, 278, 282
Estriol, function of, 26, 33
Estriol/creatine ratio, 5
Ethyliodophenylundecylate, in diagnosis of gestational
  age, 27
Examination, of neonate, neurologic, 45
  physical, 31
Exchange transfusion. See Transfusion, exchange.
Eye, examination of, 293

Fallot, tetralogy of, 240, 240
Feeding, apnea following, 147
  in hypoglycemic infant, 172
  intravenous, of full-term infant, 88
  of low-birth-weight infant, 77–89
    caloric requirements in, 79, 79t
    first, 83
    gavage, 83
    hints for, 85
    physiologic considerations in, 77
    practical considerations in, 83
    principles of, 82
    protein requirement in, 80
    suggested schedule for, 84
    vitamin requirements in, 80, 80t
    water requirements in, 79
  proper position for, 102
  oral value of, 79
Fetal assessment, approaches to, 304
Fetal growth, cell size and, 38
  drug addiction and, 41
  genetic factors and, 40
  hypertension and, 42
  infection and, 40
  malnutrition and, 38
  multiple births and, 41
  smoking and, 41
  toxemia and, 42
  X-ray and, 41
Fetal weight, vs. maternal weight, 39, 39
Feto-maternal unit, definition of, 25
Feto-placental unit, evaluation of, 5
Fetus, assessment of, 26, 304
  behavior of mother toward, 100
  effects of drugs on, 24
Flip-flop phenomenon, 150
  in hyaline membrane disease, 135
Floppy infant, 290, 291t
  suggested classification of, 349t
Fluid losses, in neonate, 79
Folic acid, serum, in neonate, 342t
Formula, composition of, 84, 84t

Galactosemia, in neonate, 187
Gantrisin, in hyperbilirubinemia, 200
Gastrointestinal tract, function of, in neonate, 81, 82
Gastroschisis, transporting neonate with, 95
Gavage feeding, procedure for, 83
Gel-filtration, in kernicterus, 192
Gentamycin, in late septicemia, 215
  indications for, in neonate, 217t
Gestational age, assessment of, 37, 42
  by head circumference, 46, 48
  neurologic examination in, 52
  scoring in, 43t, 44, 45t, 46, 47
  diagnosis of, 27
  estimation of, 7
  in relation to birth weight, 37, 37
Gilbert's syndrome, 187
Glomerular filtration rate, estimation of, 262
  in neonate, 257
Glucagon, in treatment of hypoglycemia, 172
Glucose, in fetus, 168
  in neonate, 169, 169
Glutathione levels, pre-and post-incubation, 336t
Glycogen, hepatic, function of, 4
  in fetus, 169
Gonorrhea, prevention of infection from, 222
Gram, conversion of pounds and ounces to, 318t
Greenhouse effect, 69, 70
Grief, as syndrome, 109
Growth, in relation to gestational age and fetal and
  infant norms, 326
Growth chart, intrauterine, for dichorionic twins, 320
  for monochorionic twins, 321
    for Negro infants, 322
  for premature infant, 78

Head, transillumination of, 293, 293t
Head circumference, in boys, 327
  in girls, 328
  measurement of, 293
Heart, hyperdynamic, in neonate, 249
  normal pressures in, 231, 231
Heart defects, 228–255
  diagnostic distribution in, 229
  in high-risk neonate, 236–253
    cyanosis in, 236, 237
    diminished cardiac output in, 237
    practical hints for, 246
    symptoms of, 236
    tetralogy of Fallot, 240, 240
  in low-risk neonate, 229–236
    atrial septal defects, 234
    patent ductus arteriosus, 236
    ventricular septal defects, 235
  pathophysiology of, 230
Heart disease. See also Heart defects.
  in neonate, approach to, 237t, 238t
Heart failure, 235
  in three-week-old infant, 250
  transporting neonate with, 97
Heart rate, fetal, changes in, during uterine
  contractions, 8, 8
Heat loss, in immature infant, 72
  in neonate, 61, 63, 66t
Heat production, in neonate, 60
  in utero, 62, 63
Heat regulation, in neonate, equipment for, 64, 64, 65
Helicopter, in transporting high-risk neonate, 95

Hematocrit, normal range for, in term infants, 272
Hematocrit levels, in neonate, 337t
Hematologic values, normal, 332t
Hematology, problems of, 270–286. See also *Blood*.
   disseminated intravascular coagulation, 277
   iron deficiency anemia, 279
   low platelet count, 275
   polycythemia, 273
   thrombocytopenia, 275
   vitamin E deficiency, 281
   vitamin K deficiency, 273
Hematuria, in neonate, 261
Hemoglobin, in relation to formula content, 281t
   normal range for, in term infants, 271
Hemoglobin concentration, 339t
   mean corpuscular, 338t
Hemorrhage, accidental, 270, 271
   fetal-maternal, treatment of, 272
   in immature infant, 290
Hemostasis, disorders in, 270
Henderson-Hasselbach equation, 120
Henle, loop of, 256
Heparin, in disseminated intravascular coagulation, 278
Hepatitis, effects of, on fetus, 210t
Heroin addiction, maternal, effect of, on neonate, 298
Herpes progenitalis, diagnosis of, 221
Herpes simplex, effects of, on fetus, 210t
Hexachlorophene, use of, in nursery, 218
Homeostasis, fetal to neonatal, *28*
Homeotherm, definition of, 60
Hyaline membrane disease, alkali therapy in, 140
   alveolar function in, 130, *130*
   clinical management of, 132
   differential diagnosis of, 124, *125*
   early signs and symptoms of, 129
   effects of, on lung, 129
   effect of sensory stimulation on, 146
   etiology of, 130
   oxygen concentration in, 147
   oxygen therapy in, 135, 139, *140*
   pathologic findings in, 129
   physiologic abnormalities in, 129
   prognosis in, 128t
   recovery phase in, 135
   therapeutic tools for, 135
Hydrogen ion, excretion of, by neonate, 258
Hydrometrocolpos, in neonate, 259
Hyperalimentation, in neonate, 86
    precautions during, 87
   pediatric, form for, *329*
Hyperbilirubinemia, 183–204. See also *Jaundice*.
   causes of, 186t
   due to overproduction, 185
   due to undersecretion, 187
   exchange transfusion in, 192, 192t
   from breast milk, 188
   in immature infant on respirator, 203
   in premature infant, 188
   intrauterine infections and, 189
   neonatal sepsis and, 189
   of hypothyroidism, 187
   phototherapy as treatment for, 195
   respiratory distress syndrome and, 189
   Rhogam as treatment for, 195
   treatment of, 192, *197*
Hyperparathyroidism, maternal, hypocalcemia and, 176
Hypertension, and high-risk pregnancy, 6t
   pulmonary, 232, 234
Hyperthermia, in neonate, 62, 69

Hypnosis, effect of, on fetus, 314t
Hypocalcemia, 173
   and classical neonatal tetany, 176
   and maternal hyperparathyroidism, 176
   as result of magnesium deficiency, 178
   "first day," 175
   following exchange transfusion, 176, 178
   in convulsing infant, 179
   in infant of diabetic mother, 175
   metabolic background of, 173
   methodology in, 174, *174, 175*
   precipitating factors in, 173
   prognosis in, 177
   seasonal variation in, 177
   symptoms of, 175
   treatment of, 176
   vitamin D and, 178
   vs. hypoglycemia, 171
   with hypoproteinemia, 176
Hypoglycemia, 168
   definition of, 170
   differential diagnosis in, 171t
   following exchange transfusion, 178
   in infant of diabetic mother, 170, 171, 177, 180
   in postmature infant, 179
   in small-for-dates infant, 180
   in SGA infant, 53
   metabolic background of, 168
   methodology in, 170
   occurrence of, in neonate, 49
   prognosis in, 173
   symptoms of, 170, 170t
   syndromes of, 171, 172
   transient symptomatic neonatal, 171, 171t, 177, 178
   treatment of, 172
   vs. hypocalcemia, 171
Hypomagnesemia, 177
   and seizures, 295
Hypoplastic right ventricle, with pulmonary atresia, 239, *239*
   with tricuspid atresia, 237, *238*
Hypoplastic left ventricle syndrome, 244, *245, 250*
Hypospadias, in neonate, 259
Hypothermia, 67, 149
   as resuscitative technique, 9, 10
Hypothyroidism, in neonate, 187
Hypotonia, 297
   diagnosis of, 290, 291t
Hypovolemic shock, treatment of, 14
Hypoxemia, in 2100-gm. male, 149
Hypoxia, and neurologic disorders, 289
   effects of, 120

Icterus. See *Hyperbilirubinema* and *Jaundice*.
Immunoglobulin value(s), in neonate, 207t, 208
Incubator, and heat regulation, 64
   servo-controlled, 66, 72
Incubator temperature, and survival rate, 60t
   in relation to relative humidity, 59
Infant. See also *Neonate*.
   low-birth-weight, classification of, 36–57
   of diabetic mother, prognosis for, 114
   post-term, definition of, 37
   preterm, definition of, 37
   term, definition of, 37
Infection, intrauterine, and fetal growth, 40
   maternal, effects of, on neonate, 33, 210t

Infection *(Continued)*
  neonatal, 205–227. See also *Septicemia.*
    antibiotic therapy for, 216t
    clinical presentation of, 212, 212t
    control of, in nursery, 218
    defense mechanisms against, 206, 207t
    differential diagnosis in, 212
    due to umbilical venous catheterization, 18
    history of, 205
    in nursery, 221
    incidence of, 206, 206t
    laboratory diagnosis in, 212, 215t
    mortality in, 205
    pathogenesis of, 208, 208t
    serologic studies in, 214
    significance of, 206
    treatment of, 215, 219
Influenza, effects of, on fetus, 210t
INPV(intermittent negative pressure ventilator), 163, 167
  problems of, 164
Insulin, in fetus, 169
Intensive care nursery, mobile, 90, *91*
Intensive care unit(s), neonatal, benefits of, 90, 91t
Intersexuality, in neonate, 259
Intrauterine growth retardation, and asphyxia, 49
  hypoxemia and, 52
Intubation, of the newborn, equipment for, *11, 12, 13*
Iron, serum bound, in neonate, 341t
Iron balance, in term infant, 280
Iron deficiency anemia, in neonate, 279

Jaundice, 183. See also *Hyperbilirubinemia* and *Kernicterus.*
  in infant of diabetic mother, 188
  mucoviscidosis and, 189
  pathologic, 185
  physiologic, 184, 199

Kanamycin, in primary septicemia, 215
  indications for, in neonate, 216t
Kernicterus, clinical manifestations of, 190
  in premature infant, 190
  with low bilirubin level, 198
Kidney(s), 256–269. See also *Renal.*
  developmental physiology of, 256
  function of, 32
  irreversible abnormalities of, 260
  left flank mass in 12-hour-old infant, 262
  physical examination of, 258
  tubular functional capacity of, 257
  X-ray examination of, 262
"Kinderbrutanstalt," 98, *99*

Labor, monitoring fetus during, 7
Lactic acid levels, in relation to Apgar score, 14
Laryngoscope blade(s), 14
LGA (large for gestational age) infant(s), 37, *37*
  of diabetic mother, 54
Light, effect of, on neonate, 70
Listeriosis, effects of, on fetus, 210t
Loop of Henle, 256

Lung. See also *Pulmonary.*
  air pressure volume curves of, *129*
  effects of hyaline membrane disease on, 129
  physiology of, 119
Lupus erythematosus, and high-risk pregnancy, 6t

Malaria, effects of, on fetus, 210t
Malformation(s), congenital, intrauterine growth retardation and, 40
Malnutrition, intrauterine, effects of, 39, 51, 52
  maternal, effects of, 24, 32
  postnatal, effects of, 38
Measles, effect of, on fetus, 211t
Meconium aspiration, and pulmonary disease, 141
Medication, maternal, effects of, on fetus, 314t
Meningitis, bacterial, 297
  in immature infant, 224
Mental retardation, in relation to birth weight, 38
Metaraminol, in supraventricular tachycardia, 252
Methicillin, indications for, in neonate, 216t
Methoxamine, in supraventricular tachycardia, 252
Mikity-Wilson syndrome, 143, *144, 145*
  vs. bronchopulmonary dysplasia, 137t
Minamata Bay disease, 25
Monilia, treatment of neonate with, 222
Monitoring, in apnea, 146
  of fetus, 7
Morphine, effects of, on fetus, 24
Mother, behavior of, 98–118
  care of, 98–118
    practical considerations in, 107
  with diabetes, care of, 114
Mother-child relationship, effect of isolation on, 106, 115
Mother-infant separation, effects of, 106
  evaluation of, 102, *102,* 103t, *104*
Mourning response, 109, 113, 117
Mouth-to-mouth resuscitation, 1, 10
Mucoviscidosis, and jaundice, 189
Mumps, effects of, on fetus, 210t
Myasthenia gravis, neonatal, 292
Mycoplasma, effects of, on fetus, 210t
Mycostatin, indications for, in neonate, 217t
Myelomeningocele, transporting neonate with, 95

Nafcillin, indications for, in neonate, 216t
Nalorphine, administration of, to infant of drug-addicted mother, 14
Narcotic(s), effects of, on fetus, 314t
Neomycin, indications for, in neonate, 217t
Neonatal morbidity, model of, *312*
Neonatal mortality, model of, *313*
Neonate. See also *Infant.*
  and mortality risk, classification of, *319*
  behavior of mother toward, 98–118
    disorders in, 105, *105*
    "en face" position, *101*
  care of, 23–35
    recommendations for, 31
  effect of environment on, 58–76
  effect of smoking on, 24
  evaluation of, 27
  examination of, 30
  infection in, 205–227
  management of withdrawal in, 34

Neonate *(Continued)*
  prenatal care of, 25
  reaction of, to delivery, 28
  transition of, 27
  transportation of, 90–97
  with cleft palate, 112
Nephrotic syndrome, congenital, 265
Nervous system malfunction, in neonatal period,
      causes of, 288t
    clinical features of, 289t
    drugs and, 288
Neurologic disorders, in neonate, 287–300
    alterations in tone, 290, 291t
    hemorrhage, 289
    hypoxia, 289
    pathophysiology of, 287
    seizures, 292
Newborn. See *Neonate.*
Nursery, control of infection in, 218
    high-risk, obstetrical indications for alerting, 9t
    management of epidemic in, 220t
    prevention of infection in, 221, 222
    transitional care, admission sheet for, *301*
      equipment for, 32
Nutrition, and cell growth, 81
    in neonate, 63
Nystatin, indications for, in neonate, 217t

Overheating, effects of, on neonate, 71
Oxacillin, indications for, in neonate, 216t
Oxygen, administration of, prevention of infection
      during, 222
    effect of, on retina, 135
    hyperbaric, as resuscitative technique, 1
    intragastric, as resuscitative technique, 1
Oxygen consumption, effect of environmental
      temperature on, 59, *59*
    physiology of, 120, *121,* 122t
Oxygen dissociation curve, 121, *121*
Oxygen therapy, in hyaline membrane disease, 135
Oxygen toxicity, in neonate, 137, *138, 139*

Papilledema, in hydrocephalus, 296
Parabiosis syndrome, 40, 51
Paroxysmal tachycardia, atrial, 251, *252*
Patent ductus arteriosus, in neonate, 236
Penicillin, in primary septicemia, 215
Penicillin G, indications for, in neonate, 216t
Perforation of colon, following umbilical vessel
      catheterization, 15
Perinatal mortality, high-risk factors contributing to,
      308t
Periorbital edema, in nephritis, 265
Peristalsis, gastric, during transition period, 33
Phenobarbital, in hyperbilirubinemia, 198
    in treatment of seizures, 295
Phenothiazines, effects of, on neonate, 30
Phenylephrine, in supraventricular tachycardia, 252
pHisoHex, use of, in nursery, 218, 219
Phototherapy, as treatment for hyperbilirubinemia, 195
Plantar creases, in neonate, *44*
Platelets, reduction of, in neonate, 275
Pneumonia, aspiration, 147
Pneumothorax, 142
    absorption of, *123*

Pneumothorax *(Continued)*
    in SGA infant, 54
    mechanical ventilation and, 162, 166
    transporting neonate with, 95
Poikilotherm, definition of, 60
Poiseuille's law, 232
Poliomyelitis, effects of, on fetus, 210t
Polycythemia, 273
    in SGA infant, 49
Polyhydramnios, in infant of diabetic mother, 55
Polymyxin(s), indications for, in neonate, 216t
Portal vein thrombosis, following umbilical vessel
      catheterization, 15
Positive pressure ventilation, as resuscitative
      technique, 1
Pounds, conversion of, to grams, 318t
Pregnancy, behavioral changes of mother during, 99,
      100, 100t
    high-risk, definition of, 23
      identification of, 5, 6t
Premature. See also *Neonate.*
    care of, history of, 98, 99, *100*
    criteria for discharge of, 116
    management of mother of, 115
    nurseries for, 98, 99
Pressure(s), changes in, following delivery, 233
    pulmonary artery wedge, 231
    vs. resistance, 233, *234*
Prostigmine, in supraventricular tachycardia, 252
Protein requirements, in neonate, 80
Proteinuria, in neonate, 260
Prothrombin time, in vitamin K deficiency, 273
Prune-belly syndrome, 259
Pulmonary dysmaturity, in premature, 143, *144, 145*
    oxygen toxicity and, 147
Pulmonary hemorrhage, 142
Pulmonary hypertension, 232
Pulmonary lung disease, vs. cardiac anomalies, 242
Pulmonary stenosis, vs. tetralogy of Fallot, 241
    with intact ventricular septum, 241, *242*
Pulmonary venous drainage, anomalous, vs.
      transposition of great arteries, 242, *244*
Purpura, iso-immune, 275
Pyuria, 261
    treatment of, 266

Q-10 Effect, 61

Rauwolfia, effects of, on neonate, 30
Renal agenesis, 267
    irreversible abnormalities in association with, 260
Renal biopsy, in diagnosis of congenital nephrotic
      syndrome, 265
Renal disease, and high-risk pregnancy, 6t
Renal function, blood urea and, 268
    evaluation of, 262
    tests for, 263t
Renal immaturity, 257
    and drug excretion, 258
Renal vein thrombosis, 264
Respiration, effect of temperature on, 70
    problems of, 119–151
      apnea, 144
      diagnosis in, 124
      differential diagnosis of, *125*

Respiration *(Continued)*
  problems of, hyaline membrane disease,
      128
    meconium aspiration, 141
    pneumothorax, 142
    practical hints in, 146
    prognosis in, 127
    pulmonary dysmaturity, 143
    pulmonary hemorrhage, 142
    transient tachypnea, 141
  restoration of, in SGA, distressed infant, 17. See
      also *Resuscitation.*
Respirators, manufacturers of, 330
Respiratory distress, diagnosis in, 129
  essentials of care in, 136t
  heart defects and, 237
Respiratory distress syndrome, 128, 149, 150. See also
    Hyaline membrane disease.
  CPAP in, 153
Respiratory failure, clinical manifestations of, 153
  conditions associated with, 153t
  definition of, 152
Resuscitation, and brain damage, 14
  effect of delayed, 19t
  in SGA, distressed infant, 17
  of newborn, 1–22
  preparations for, 10, 11
  techniques for, 9
Reticulocyte count, in neonate, 340t
Retina, effect of bilirubin reduction lights on, 198
  effect of oxygen on, 135, 146
Retrolental fibroplasia, in neonate, 136, 137, 145
Rh sensitization, 200
  and high-risk pregnancy, 6t
Rickets, 81
Roentgenography. See also *X-ray.*
  in estimation of gestational age, 7
Rotor's syndrome, 188
Rubella, congenital, and fetal growth, 40
  diagnostic features of, 213t
  effects of, on fetus, 211t
  management of patient with, 223
Rubeola, effects of, on fetus, 211t

Salicylate saturation test, in kernicterus, 191
Sarah Morris Hospital, premature nurseries of, 99
Scalp sampling, of fetus, procedure for, 8
Sclerema, definition of, 67
Sedative(s), effects of, on fetus, 314t
Seizure(s), 292, 294, 294t
  in depressed neonate, 33
  transporting neonate with, 97
  treatment of, 295, 295t
Sensory stimuli, effects of, on neonate, 70
Sepsis, neonatal, and hyperbilirubinemia, 189
    catheterization and, 209
    supportive therapy for, 215
Septicemia. See also *Infection.*
  diagnostic features of, 213t
  etiology of, 209, 209t
  gram-negative, 207
  with meningitis, 214
"Setting sun" sign, in kernicterus, 190
SGA(small for gestational age) infant, 37, *37*
  appearance of, 49, 52
  causes for, 38
  hypoglycemia in, 49
  mortality rate in, 52

SGA infant *(Continued)*
  polycythemia in, 49
  practical hints for care of, 50
  thermal regulation in, 49
  twin pregnancy and, 52
  vs. immature infant, 50t
Shake test, 7
Shivering, and body temperature, 72
Shock, hypovolemic, treatment of, 14
Shunt defects, left-to-right, 229, 230
Shunt equation, 121
  graphic representation of, *122*
Siggaard-Andersen nomogram, *134*
Size, of neonate, 37
Smallpox, effects of, on fetus, 211t
Smoking, effects of, on neonate, 24
Sodium, neonatal response to changes in, 257
Sodium bicarbonate, as treatment for fetal hypoxia, 9
Sonatone, premature, 126
Sound, effect of, on neonate, 70
Spectrophotometric analysis, of amniotic fluid, 7
Status epilepticus, 292
Stenosis, pulmonary, vs. tetralogy of Fallot, 241
    with intact ventricular septum, 241, *242*
Steroids, effects of, on fetus, 315t
Stethoscope, monitoring of fetus with, 7
Stillbirth, effect of, on mother, 109
Streptomycin, indications for, in neonate, 217t
Sucking, in neonate, 81
Suctioning, following instillation of endotracheal
    tube, 159
Sulfonamides, in first week of life, 222
Surfactant, pulmonary, alteration of, in hyaline
    membrane disease, 130, 131
Swaddling, effect of, on temperature, 71
Swallowed blood syndrome, 186
Swallowing, in neonate, 81
Syndrome. See names of specific syndromes.
Syphilis, congenital, and fetal growth, 40
    diagnosis of, 213t, 226
    maternal, effects of, on fetus, 211t, 221

Tachycardia, paroxysmal atrial, 251, *252*
  supraventricular, 251
    prognosis in, 253
Tachypnea, transient, in neonate, 141
Temperature, effect of, on asphyxia, 69
  on neonatal growth, 63
  elevated, in neonate, 18
  environmental, effect of, on mortality, 72
    on oxygen consumption, 61, *62*
  in incubator. See *Incubator temperature.*
  maintenance of, during resuscitation, 20
  neutral thermal environmental, 67, 68t
  regulation of, in immature infant, 74
    in postmature infant, 75
    in respiratory distress, 73
Tetany, neonatal, hypocalcemia and, 176
Tetracycline hydrochloride, indications for, in
  neonate, 216t
Tetralogy of Fallot, in high-risk neonate, 240, *240*
Thalidomide, effects of, on fetus, 24
Tham, in hyaline membrane disease, 140
  in hyperbilirubinemia, 193
Thrombocytopenia, clinical manifestations of, 276
  iso-immune, 275
Touch, effect of, on neonate, 70

Toxemia, and high-risk pregnancy, 6t
Toxoplasmosis, diagnostic features of, 213t
    effects of, on fetus, 211t, 221
Tracheostomy, in mechanical ventilation, 159
Tranquilizers, effects of, on fetus, 315t
Transfusion, exchange, 199
    albumin administration prior to, 198
    alternatives to, 195
    and hypoglycemia, 198
    complications of, 195, 195t
    in disseminated intravascular coagulation, 284
    indications for, 192t
    mortality rate in, 199
    on hydropic infant, 194
    technique of, 194
    types of, 193t
Transillumination, on abdominal masses, 264
Transition, of neonate, 29
    complicated, 30, 306t
Transportation, of high-risk neonate, 90–97
    equipment for, 94t
    information form for, 96
    physician duties during, 92, 92t, 93
    principles of, 92
    problems in, 97
    procedure for, 92
    reassuring mother during, 94
Transposition of great arteries, shunting in, 236
    with intact ventricular septum, 241, 243
        differential diagnosis of, 242
        vs. cerebral arteriovenous fistula, 243
        vs. primary lung disease, 242
        vs. total anomalous pulmonary venous drainage,
            242, 244
Trisomy-21, and fetal growth, 40
Trousseau sign, in hypocalcemia, 175
Tuberculosis, maternal, and high-risk pregnancy, 6t
    effects of, on fetus, 211t
    infant management in, 221
Twins, and SGA infants, 52
    dichorionic, intrauterine growth chart for, 320
    monochorionic, intrauterine growth chart for, 321
Twin transfusion syndrome, 40, 51

Ultrasonagraphy, monitoring of fetus with, 7
    value of, 27
Umbilical artery, single, 267
Umbilical catheterization tray, equipment on, 317
Umbilical vessel catheter, vs. peripheral I.V., 15
Umbilical vessel catheterization, technique for, 15, 16

Urachus, patent, 259
Urinalysis, neonatal, 260
Urinary estriol excretion, serial determinations of, 5
Urine, neonatal, characteristics of, 260
Uterus, as "transport incubator," 92

Vaccinia, effects of, on fetus, 211t
Varicella, effects of, on fetus, 211t
Venous congestion, systemic, in neonate, 237
Ventilation, assisted, 152–167
    and bronchopulmonary dysplasia, 137
    background of, 152
    indications for, 157
    vs. controlled, 161
    controlled, cycling frequency of, 161
    mechanical. See also Ventilation, assisted.
        and pneumothorax, 164
        and water condensation, 164
        changes in blood gas status during, 161
        checklist for, 160
        in tetanus neonatorum, 164
        indications for, 157, 157
        maintaining infant during, 161
        principles of, 158
        weaning from, 163
Ventilator(s), care of, 163
    types of, 158
Ventricular septal defect, in first days of life, 230
    in one-month-old infant, 229
    physiology of, 235
Vitamin requirement, in neonate, 80, 80t
Vitamin E, serum, in neonate, 343t
Vitamin E deficiency, 281
Vitamin K deficiency, 273
    clotting abnormalities in, 278t

Water requirement, in neonate, 79
White cell count, during first two weeks of life, 345t
    in prematures, 344t
Wilson-Mikity syndrome, 143, 144, 145
Withdrawal syndrome, management of neonate with,
    32, 34
Wolff-Parkinson-White syndrome, 253

X-ray, in fetal assessment, 27
X-ray examination, of genitourinary tract, 262

Start _____
      Date   Time

Finish _____
      Date   Time

ACTIVITY
++ = ACTIVE
+ = ACTIVE (STIMULATED)
− = LIMP
A = IRRITABLE
B = TWITCHY

COLOR
P = PINK
W = PALE
D = DUSKY
B = BLUE
J = JAUNDICE
M = MOTTLED

Patient's Name
Hospital Number
Date of Admission
Doctor's Name

Time	Age	O₂ conc	Hood / Inc.	S / R	BP	P	R	Grunt ± or Resp. Press.	P.D. W.B.	++ + − A.B.	Type	Amt.	Total	

Column group headers: **TEMPERATURE** (Hood/Inc., S/R), **VITAL SIGNS** (BP, P, R, Grunt ± or Resp. Press.), **COLOR** (P.D. W.B.), **ACT.** (++ + − A.B.), **INTAKE** (Type, Amt., Total), **DRUGS**

CODE TO THE NEONATE INTENSIVE CARE RECORD

TEMPERATURE
Hood/Incubator
Skin/Rectal

VITAL SIGNS
Blood Pressure
Pulse
Respirations

OUTPUT
Urine
Stool
Other